Essential Revision Notes for Intercollegiate MRCS Book 1

PasTest
Dedicated to your success

Essential Revision Notes for Intercollegiate MRCS Book 1

Claire Ritchie Chalmers BA BM BCh MRCS
Clinical Research Fellow, Hepatobiliary Department,
St James's Hospital, Leeds

Sam Andrews MA MS FRCS (Gen)
Consultant General and Vascular Surgeon, Department of General and Vascular Surgery, Maidstone Hospital, Maidstone

Catherine Parchment Smith
BSc(Hons) MBChB(Hons) MRCS(Eng)
Specialist Registrar in General Surgery, Yorkshire Deanery

PasTest
Dedicated to your success

Egerton Court
Parkgate Estate
Knutsford
Cheshire
WA16 8DX

Telephone: 01565 752000

First Published 2006
Reprinted 2009

ISBN: 1 904627 36 6
978 1904627 36 4

A catalogue record for this book is available from the British Library.

Text prepared by Saxon Graphics Ltd, Derby
Printed and bound in the UK by Page Bros, Norwich

Contents

Acknowledgements

I would like to thank everyone who has worked so hard to complete this book with me – fellow editors, contributing authors and the PasTest team, Kirsten, Amy and Maria. Thanks especially to Cathy, whose excellent teaching eased my early passage through basic surgical training and whose subsequent advice, friendship and *joie de vivre* is invaluable.

I have been fortunate enough to be surrounded by fantastic friends and colleagues. There are too many to list everyone by name (you know who you are) and I appreciate all your support. Particular gratitude must go to Sarah Perry, Gill Hawcroft, Angela Graham, Giles Toogood and Steve Pollard.

I am extremely grateful to have a family whose encouragement has been life-long, my parents Jean and Ken and my sister Hayley. Last but not least, thanks to my husband Roy who is a constant and irreplaceable source of support, patience and good cheer.

Claire Ritchie Chalmers

Preface

This book has been designed to present topics in core surgical knowledge in a format suitable for revision. The title has been revised and updated and includes new chapters covering surgical research methods, critical appraisal, ethics and legal issues, and peri-operative management and critical care.

It is accompanied by a second volume (Book 2) which covers systems and specialities, and these two books together encompass the syllabus for the MRCS.

Although this book is not a substitute for detailed reading of the STEP course and other set texts, it is our hope that the structure in which each topic is presented will give you a framework on which to base both your understanding and your carefully thought out answers to those tricky exam questions!

Although the format of surgical examinations in the UK is changing, the principles of core surgical knowledge remain the same, and often a good exam answer starts with a structured summary followed by expansion of individual points.

We have, therefore, arranged each topic in this format, and we have used boxes, bullet points and diagrams to highlight important points. There is additional space around the text for you to annotate and personalise these notes from your own experience.

My dad is fond of saying that the harder you work, the luckier you get – so GOOD LUCK!

Claire Ritchie Chalmers

Contributors

Contributors to the Second Edition

Editors

Claire Ritchie Chalmers BA BM BCh MRCS
Clinical Research Fellow, Hepatobiliary Department, St James's Hospital, Leeds

Sam Andrews MA MS FRCS (Gen)
Consultant General and Vascular Surgeon, Department of General and Vascular Surgery, Maidstone Hospital, Maidstone

Catherine Parchment Smith BSc(Hons) MBChB(Hons) MRCS(Eng)
Specialist Registrar in General Surgery, Yorkshire Deanery

Contributors

Amer Aldouri MBChB MRCS
Specialist Registrar in Hepatobiliary and Transplantation Surgery, Hepatobiliary and Transplantation Surgery Unit, St James University Hospital, Leeds

David Crabbe MD FRCS
Consultant Paediatric Surgeon, Clarendon Wing, Leeds General Infirmary, Leeds

Nerys Forrester
Specialist Registrar in Clinical Radiology, Yorkshire Deanery

Sheila M Fraser MBChB MRCS
Clinical Research Fellow, Institute of Molecular Medicine, Epidemiology & Cancer Research, St. James's University Hospital, Leeds

Sunjay Jain MD FRCS (Urol)
Clinical Lecturer in Urology, University of Leicester, Leicester

Shireen N. McKenzie MB.ChB MRCS(Ed)
Specialist Registrar in General Surgery, Airdale General Hospital, Keighley, West Yorkshire

Professor Kilian Mellon MD FRCS (Urol)
Professor of Urology, University of Leicester, Leicester

Sally Nicholson BSc MBChB
Senior House Officer in Yorkshire School of Surgery, ENT Department, Leeds General Infirmary, Leeds

Susan Picton BM BS FRCPCH
Consultant Paediatric Oncologist, Leeds Teaching Hospitals Trust, Leeds

Catherine Sargent BM BCh (Oxon) MRCP
Specialist Registrar in Infectious Diseases/General Medicine, The John Radcliffe Hospital, Oxford

Contributors to the First Edition

James Brown MRCS
Specialist Registrar in Surgery, South East Thames Surgical Rotation
Neoplasia

Alistair R K Challiner FRCA FIMC.RCSEd DCH
Consultant Anaesthetist and Director Intensive Care Unit, Department of Anaesthetics, Maidstone Hospital, Maidstone, Kent
Intensive Care and Peri-operative Management 1

Nicholas D Maynard BA Hons (OXON) MS FRCS (Gen)
Consultant Upper Gastrointestinal Surgeon, Department of Upper Gastrointestinal Surgery, John Radcliffe Hospital, Headington, Oxford
Peri-operative Management 2

Gillian M Sadler MBBS MRCP FRCR
Consultant Clinical Oncologist, Kent Oncology Centre, Maidstone Hospital, Maidstone, Kent
Neoplasia

Hank Schneider FRCS (Gen. Surg)
Consultant General Surgeon, Department of Surgery, The James Paget Hospital, Great Yarmouth, Norfolk
Trauma

Introduction

This book is an attempt to help surgical trainees pass the MRCS exam by putting together the revision notes they need. It was written (in the main) and edited by trainees for trainees and while we do not claim to be authorities on the subjects by any means, we hope to save you some work by expanding our revision notes and putting them in a readable format. Medical students interested in surgery may also find it a good general introduction to the surgical specialties.

This new edition of *Essential Revision Notes for the Intercollegiate MRCS* is in two parts: Book 1 and Book 2. It builds on the tremendous popularity of the previous editions of *Essential Revision Notes* for the MRCS Core Modules and Systems Modules. We have aimed to help SHOs who are faced with the huge task of learning the information in the syllabus of the new intercollegiate MRCS exam, firstly for the Applied Basic Sciences and Clinical Problem Solving papers, and then yet again for the oral/viva exam. We've listened to what SHOs loved about those first books, and then added what we think they need for the new intercollegiate exam. This time we've used a bigger team of contributors, and have re-written everything to fit in with the revision-note style we wanted. We've used the cleverest, most clear-thinking SHOs and junior registrars that we could find to write the revision notes, and we've asked the most sensible, reliable young consultants we know to look over the chapters and write the bits we didn't know enough about.

Along with its companion volume, this book:

- Covers every major subject in the new intercollegiate MRCS syllabus
- Works systematically through every general surgical topic likely to come up in the exam in enough detail for the EMQs and MCQs
- Highlights the important principles of surgery 'in a nutshell' and then explains them in appropriate detail so you have a structure for discussion in the viva
- Emphasises and reviews the applied basic sciences such as pathology, physiology and anatomy in each relevant section to prepare you for these viva stations
- Contains standardised, easy to learn 'operation boxes' and 'procedure boxes' for all the common cases you should know for the MCQ/EMQ papers and the Operative Surgery viva
- Has expanded sections on paediatric oncology, clinical governance, audit, statistics, consent, and research (in Book 1) and on elective neurosurgery, endocrine surgery and cardiothoracics (in Book 2) in line with the new college syllabus
- Is designed to work alongside the Royal College of Surgeons of England STEP course workbooks
- Is written in the easy, informal 'revision-note' style, with the punchy bullet point format that made the original book so popular

- Highlights important lists to learn and vital points to remember
- Is clearly laid out with numerous line drawings to aid understanding

We are surgical trainees, not specialists or experts on any of these subjects. We wanted to produce a book that's relevant to other trainess and the exam. We have tried to make this book as complete, concise, easy to understand, and as painless to read as possible. We hope we have compiled a useful set of revision notes for the new Intercollegiate MRCS Exam. You read them, sit the exam, and then tell us what you think.

GOOD LUCK!

Claire Ritchie Chalmers
Catherine Parchment Smith
Sam Andrews

The Intercollegiate Membership of the Royal College of Surgeons (MRCS) Examination

This new examination was agreed by, and is common to, the Surgical Royal Colleges of Great Britain and Ireland. It replaces the MRCS Eng, MRCS Glas, AFRCS Ed, and MRCSI, which used to have different formats, papers, pass rates, and syllabi. The intercollegiate exam was introduced in October 2004 and the old examinations were phased out simultaneously. It forms part of the requirement for the Certificate of Completion of Basic Surgical Training (CCBST) which requires:

- Possession of an acceptable primary medical qualification (MBChB)
- Pass in all parts of the MRCS intercollegiate examination
- Successful completion of 24 months' training in recognised posts from defined specialities
- Completion of mandatory courses

The CCBST is the minimum requirement for applicants for a Higher Surgical Training rotation in surgery. Successful applicants are awarded a National Training Number and become specialist registrars in their chosen surgical speciality. Higher Surgical Training culminates in the Certificate of Completion of Specialist Training (CCST) which, in general surgery at least, is awarded only after passing the 'exit' or Intercollegiate Examination (ICE). This CCST enables the holder to take up a post as an independent practitioner (consultant) in their speciality.

Eligibility for the intercollegiate MRCS

- Candidates must possess an acceptable primary medical qualification (MBChB)
- Candidates may apply to sit Part 1 at any time after gaining their primary medical qualification (eg during house jobs)
- Candidates must have commenced Basic Surgical Training (BST) before entering Part 2 of the exam
- Candidates may sit Part 1 and Part 2 in any order, and with any of the British and Irish colleges candidates may sit Part 1 and Part 2 at different colleges
- Candidates may re-sit Part 1 and Part 2 as many times as they wish

Candidates have a time limit of three-and-a-half years in which to complete all parts of the examination dating from their first attempt at Part 2, even if they sit Part 2 before Part 1. Three-and-a-half years after sitting Part 2, if candidates have not passed both the clinical and the viva sections of Part 3, they will never be allowed to re-sit any part of the examination.

Structure of the intercollegiate MRCS

PART 1 Applied Basic Sciences Multiple True-False paper
Duration: 3 hours

PART 2 Clinical Problem Solving Extended Matching Questions paper
Duration: 3 hours

- Held three times a year simultaneously worldwide
- Candidates must pass both papers before proceeding to Part 3

PART 3.1 Oral component

This consists of three 20-minute vivas on:

- Applied surgical anatomy and operative surgery
- Applied physiology and critical care
- Applied surgical pathology and principles of surgery

Candidates must pass the overall oral component before proceeding to the clinical component.

PART 3.2 Clinical component

There are six bays in total: four clinical bays and two communication bays.

The four 15-minute clinical bays require candidates to examine, diagnose, elicit physical signs and show that they are familiar with the treatment of patients. These four bays are:

- Trauma and orthopaedics
- Vascular
- Breast, skin, head and neck
- Trunk, groin and scrotum

The two bays of communication test skills during a session of 30 minutes, thus:

- Taking a history to reach a diagnosis
- Giving information to patients, relatives, or other healthcare professionals

Candidates who fail the clinical component will not be required to re-take the oral component, but will have to pass the clinical component within three-and-a-half years of sitting Part 2.

The structure, timing, regulations, and requirements for these examinations are constantly changing as the exams are updated. The above outline was accurate at the time of writing, but you should not rely on this or any other printed or verbal information because it may be out of date as soon as it is reaches you. Contact your Royal College; their website is often the most up-to-date source of information.

The Royal College of Surgeons of England

35–43 Lincoln's Inn Fields
London WC2A 3PE
Tel: + 44 20 7 405 3474
http://www.rcseng.ac.uk/

The Royal College of Surgeons of Edinburgh

Information Section
Adamson Centre
3 Hill Place
Edinburgh EH8 9DS
Tel: + 44 131 668 9222
http://www.rcsed.ac.uk/

The Royal College of Physicians and Surgeons of Glasgow

232–242 Vincent Street
Glasgow G2 5RJ
Tel: + 44 141 221 6072
http://www.rcpsglasg.ac.uk/

The Royal College of Surgeons in Ireland

123 St Stephens Green
Dublin 2
Tel: +353 1 402 2223
http://www.rcsi.ie/

Chapter 1

Basic Surgical Knowledge and Skills

Claire Ritchie Chalmers

Section 1
Physiology of wound healing

1.1 SKIN ANATOMY AND PHYSIOLOGY

In a nutshell ...

A core knowledge of skin anatomy and physiology is essential to understand fully the processes involved in wound healing.

The skin is an enormously complex organ acting both as a highly efficient mechanical barrier and also as a complex immunological membrane. It is constantly regenerating with a generous nervous, vascular and lymphatic supply, and has specialist structural and functional properties in different parts of the body.

All skin has the same basic structure, although it varies in thickness, colour and the presence of hairs and glands in different regions of the body. The external surface of the skin consists of a keratinised squamous epithelium called the **epidermis**. The epidermis is supported and nourished by a thick underlying layer of dense, fibroelastic connective tissue called the **dermis** which is highly vascular and contains many sensory receptors. The dermis is attached to underlying tissues by a layer of loose connective tissue called the **hypodermis** or subcutaneous layer which contains adipose tissue. Hair follicles, sweat glands, sebaceous glands and nails are epithelial structures called epidermal appendages that extend down into the dermis and hypodermis.

The four main functions of the skin:

- **Protection:** against UV light, and mechanical, chemical and thermal insults; it also prevents excessive dehydration and acts as a physical barrier to micro-organisms
- **Sensation:** various receptors for touch, pressure, pain and temperature
- **Thermoregulation:** insulation, sweating and varying blood flow in dermis
- **Metabolism:** subcutaneous fat is a major store of energy, mainly triglycerides; vitamin D synthesis occurs in the epidermis

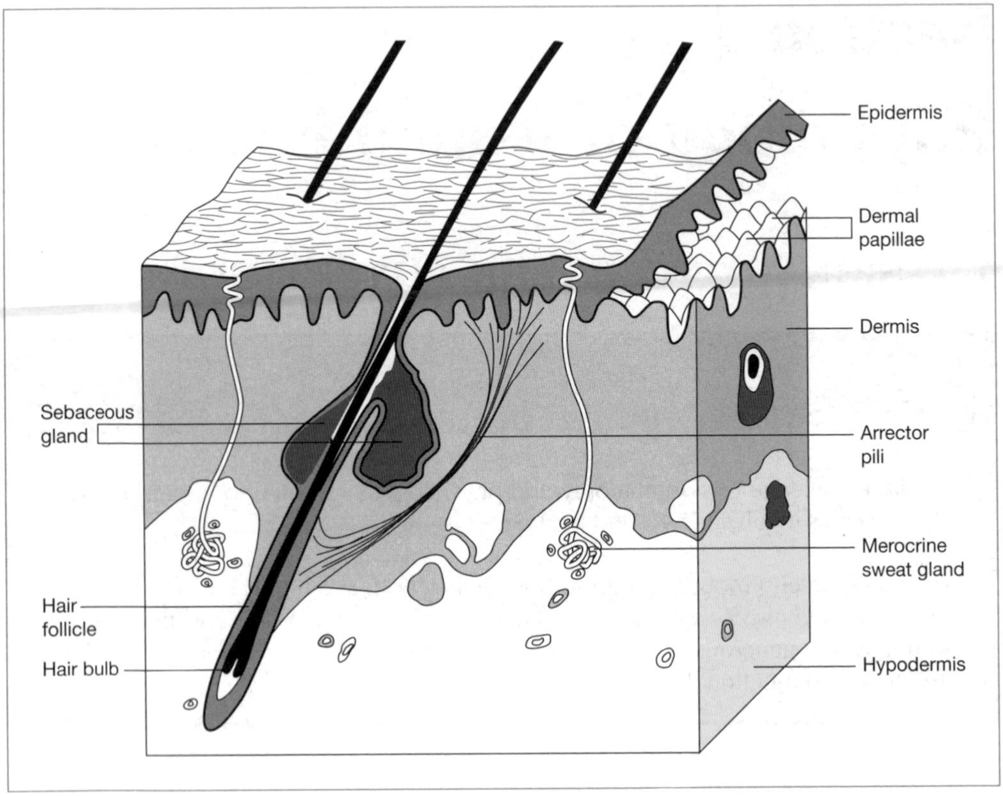

Figure 1.1a *Skin anatomy*

Skin has natural tension lines, and incisions placed along these lines tend to heal with a narrower and stronger scar, leading to a more favourable cosmetic result (see Fig. 1.1b). These natural tension lines lie at right angles to the direction of contraction of underlying muscle fibres, and parallel to the dermal collagen bundles. On the head and neck they are readily identifiable as the 'wrinkle' lines, and can easily be exaggerated by smiling, frowning and the display of other emotions. On the limbs and trunk they tend to run circumferentially, and can easily be found by manipulating the skin to find the natural skin creases. Near flexures these lines are parallel to the skin crease.

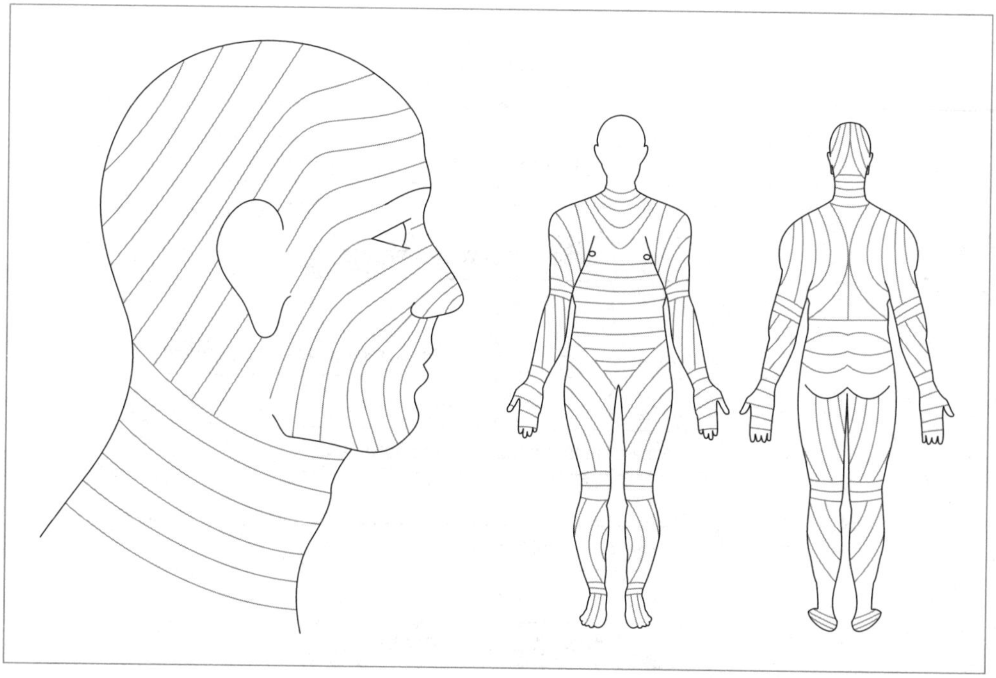

Figure 1.1b *Langer's lines. The lines correspond to relaxed skin and indicate optimal orientation of skin incisions to avoid tension across the healing wound*

1.2 PATHOPHYSIOLOGY OF WOUND HEALING

In a nutshell ...

Wound healing consists of three phases:

- **Acute inflammatory phase** (see Chapter 2 *Infection and Inflammation*)
- **Proliferative phase** (cell proliferation and deposition of extracellular matrix, ECM)
- **Maturation phase** (remodelling of the ECM)

Different tissues may undergo specialised methods of repair (eg organ parenchyma, bone and nervous tissue).

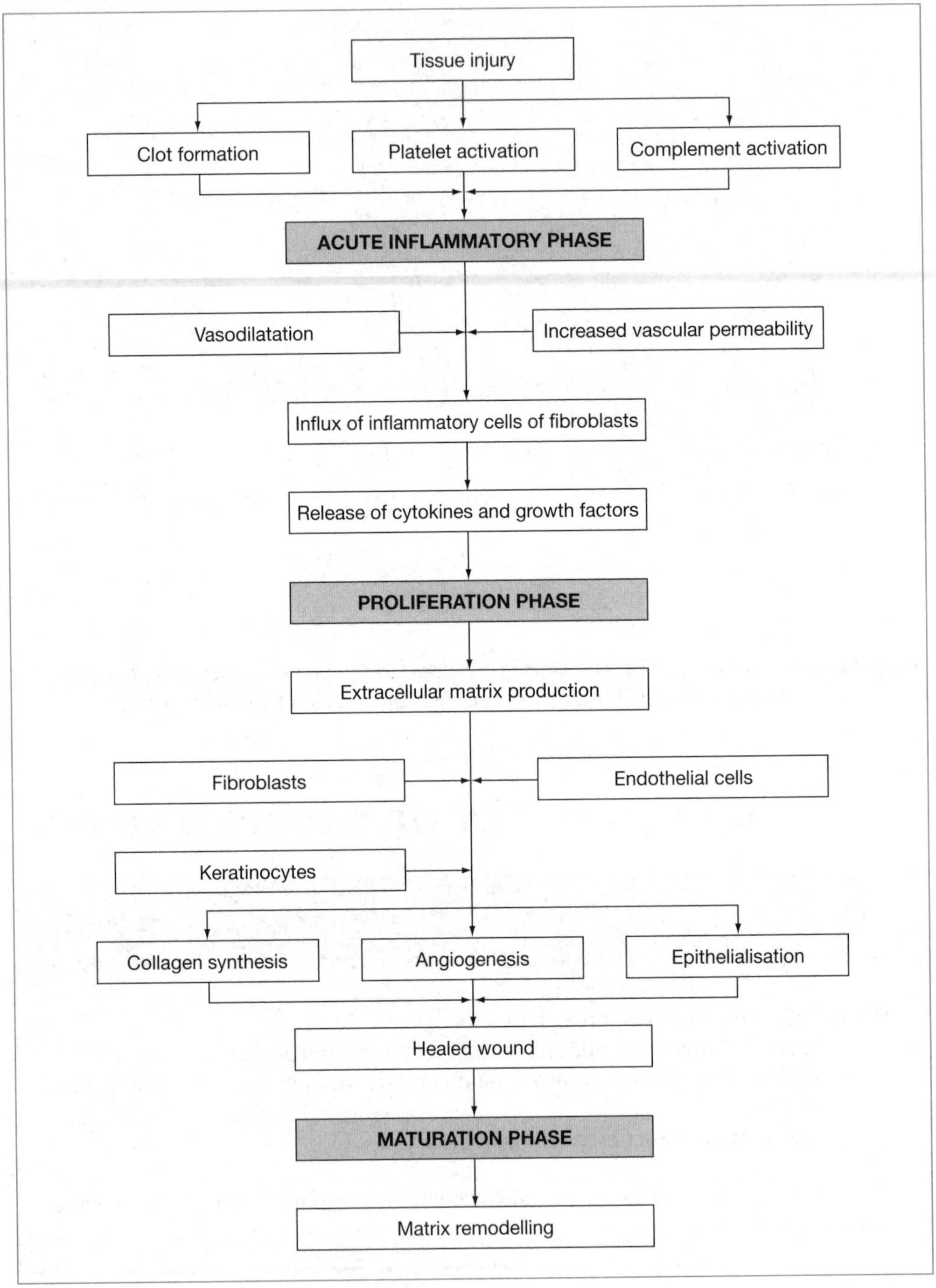

Figure 1.2a *Wound healing*

All surgeons deal with wounds and it is essential to understand fully the exact pathophysiological mechanisms involved in wound healing, how this may be optimised, and how it may be compromised, leading to wound dehiscence, delayed healing and incisional hernia formation.

The aims of wound healing are a rapid restoration of tissue continuity and a rapid return to normal function.

The inflammatory phase

Tissue damage starts a typical acute inflammatory reaction by damage to cells and blood vessels.

The inflammatory phase of wound healing involves:

- Vasodilation and increased vascular permeability
- Influx of inflammatory cells (neutrophils) and fibroblasts
- Platelet activation and initiation of the coagulation and complement cascades, leading to clot formation and haemostasis

The acute inflammatory response is generic to all forms of injury and noxious insult. It is discussed in detail in Chapter 2 *Infection and Inflammation*.

The proliferative phase

The proliferative phase is characterised by migration and proliferation of a number of cell types:

- **Epithelial cells:** within hours of injury epithelial cells at the margins of the wound begin to proliferate and migrate across the defect; epithelial closure is usually complete by 48 hours
- **Fibroblasts:** fibroblasts migrate into the wound, proliferate and synthesise extracellular matrix (ECM) components including collagen and ground substance (4–5 days)
- **Endothelial cells:** the development of new blood vessels (angiogenesis) occurs simultaneously with activation of fibroblasts – proliferation and migration of endothelial cells depend on the proteolytic activity of matrix metalloproteinases (for which zinc is an essential cofactor)

Cell types involved in wound healing and time of appearance in wound	
Platelets	Immediate
Neutrophils	0–1 day
Macrophages	1–2 days
Fibroblasts	2–4 days
Myofibroblasts	2–4 days
Endothelial cells	3–5 days

Granulation tissue is a temporary structure which forms at this stage. It consists of a rich network of capillary vessels and a heterogeneous population of cells (fibroblasts, macrophages and endothelial cells) within the stroma of the ECM. It has a characteristic pinkish, granular appearance. Additionally the wound contracts due to the action of myofibroblasts.

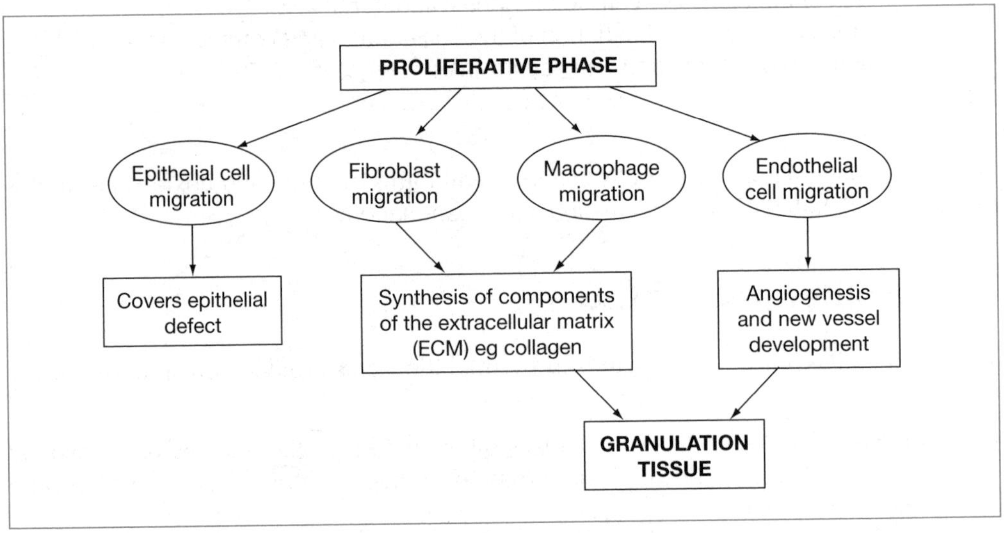

Figure 1.2b *The proliferative phase*

The maturation phase

Matrix remodelling

- This stage lasts for many months after the wound is clinically healed
- The scar becomes less vascular – hence the change in colour
- The scar tensile strength increases due to modifications made to collagen. The collagen molecule is a triple α-helix. Multiple molecules orientate to form a fibril. The cross-linkage of collagen fibrils by formation of covalent bonds (aided by the action of vitamin C) increase the tensile strength of the scar

Regaining strength in the wound

During matrix remodelling the scar regains its strength. The tissue types and thickness involved in the scar will determine the length of time to regain strength. Bowel and muscle regains virtually full strength within 1 month and skin takes up to 6 months. Strength tends to increase very quickly over the first 7–10 days although full maturation of a scar can take up to 12–18 months. Choice of wound closure materials should reflect this. Abdominal incisions through muscle layers will take many weeks to regain their strength, achieving sufficient strength at 3–4 months to no longer require suture support and about 80% of their former strength after many months. Closure is therefore performed either with loop nylon that will persist in the wound, or a strong, slowly absorbing suture material such as PDS that will support the wound. Superficial skin wounds require minimal support and so can be closed with a quickly absorbable suture material or by interrupted sutures or staples that can be removed within days.

1.3 HEALING IN SPECIALISED TISSUES

Classification of wound healing

In a nutshell ...

Wound healing can be classified into:

- First (primary) intention
- Second (secondary) intention
- Third (tertiary) intention

In addition different tissues have different healing properties. You should be aware of the healing properties of:

Skin
Bone
Nerve
Bowel
Solid organs (liver, kidney, spleen, heart)
Non-regenerative organs (eg eye)

First (primary) intention

This typically occurs in uncontaminated wounds with minimal tissue loss and when the wound edges can easily be approximated with sutures, staples or adhesive strips, without excessive tension. The wound usually heals by rapid epithelialisation and formation of minimal granulation tissue and subsequent scar tissue.

Second (secondary) intention

Usually secondary intention occurs in wounds with substantial tissue loss, when the edges cannot be apposed without excessive tension. The wound is left open and allowed to heal from the deep aspects of the wound by a combination of granulation, epithelialisation and contraction. This inevitably takes longer, and is accompanied by a much more intense inflammatory response. Scar quality and cosmetic result are poor.

Wounds which may be left to heal by secondary intention:

- Extensive loss of epithelium
- Extensive contamination
- Extensive tissue damage
- Extensive oedema leading to inability to close
- Wound reopened (eg infection, failure of knot)

Third (tertiary) intention

The wound is closed several days after its formation. This may well follow a period of healing by secondary intention, for example when infection is under control or tissue oedema is reduced.

Healing in different tissues

Different tissues heal in a remarkably similar way, albeit at different rates – the scalp and face heal very quickly, at least in part because of increased vascularity. Healing rates are quickest early in life, and decline with advancing years. Surgery performed on the fetus in utero leaves no scarring at all as it occurs by regeneration. Some tissues possess the ability to regenerate their specialised cells following injury, with the result that significant tissue loss can be replaced by regenerated specialised cells, with no – or minimal – loss of function (eg bone, intestine). Conversely, some tissues have little regenerative ability (eg cardiac tissue) and wounds heal by simple scar formation – significant tissue loss will result in significant loss of function. Nervous tissue possesses very limited regenerative capacity and partial function may be regained through slow neuronal growth in peripheral nerve injuries.

Skin

Skin consists of two layers – the keratinised stratified epidermis and the connective tissue of the dermis. Following injury to the skin, healing essentially follows the pattern outlined above. Blood lost into the wound clots into a fibrin meshwork (the scab). Inflammatory cells, fibroblasts and capillaries invade the clot to form a contractile granulation tissue that draws the wound margins together. Neutrophils release cytokines and growth factors that activate fibroblasts and keratinocytes, which alter their anchorage to the surrounding cells, ECM and basal lamina. Protease secretion by the keratinocytes allows them to migrate through the fibrin mesh of the clot and the cut epidermal edges to move forward to cover the denuded wound surface. A new stratified epidermis with underlying basal lamina is then re-established. Epidermal appendages (eg sweat glands and hair follicles) do not regenerate.

Bone and callus

Bone is unique in its ability to repair itself as it re-activates processes that normally occur during embryogenesis.

Primary bone healing

This occurs when the fracture gap is small (1–2 mm) and when there is absolute stability between the fracture fragments. Bone remodelling units cross the small gap and Haversian remodelling occurs (without callus formation); this type of bone healing is seen when there has been an anatomical reduction and stable internal fixation of the fracture (an intact blood supply is required).

Secondary bone healing

Haematoma formation

- Formed by rupture of blood vessels within medullary cavity
- Haematoma fills the fracture gap and spills out into the surrounding tissue
- Haematoma provides a fibrin mesh that seals off the fracture site and provides a framework for the influx of inflammatory cells, fibroblasts, and capillary vessels

Inflammatory phase

- Necrotic material at the fracture site releases inflammatory mediators, promoting chemotaxis of neutrophils
- Inflammatory cells release cytokines (eg TGF-β and fibroblast growth factor which activate osteoprogenitor cells)

Repair phase

- By the end of the 1st week the organised haematoma is being replaced by soft callus (it provides some anchorage but no structural rigidity)
- Soft callus gradually changes from fibrinous matrix, through a cartilaginous phase, to bony callus (resembles embryonic endochondral ossification and is similar to process occurring at the physis)
- Around the periphery, under the periosteum, osteoblasts deposit a layer of woven bone – the hard callus (process resembles embryonic intra-membranous ossification)
- So the fracture ends are bridged by a bony callus that gains strength as it mineralises (giving the fracture increasing stability, and allowing early weight-bearing)

Remodelling phase

- Remodelling occurs over the months and years following a fracture
- Callus and new bone (formed initially) is bulky and relatively disordered; it is replaced with lamellar bone through Haversian remodelling
- Internal architecture of any bone alters in response to loads placed on it (the same holds true at the fracture site); this phenomenon is known as Wolff's law

Times for healing of nerves, tendons and bone (general guide)

Tendon repair

- 3–5 weeks to protected mobilisation
- 6–12 weeks to full mobilisation
- > 12 weeks to full strength

Nerve repair

- 4–6 weeks of cast immobilisation of neighbouring joints
- > 6 weeks to free mobilisation

Fracture of upper limb

- 3–4 weeks in a cast (mobilise rest of limb)

Fracture of lower limb

- 6–8 weeks in a cast
- Protected weight-bearing from 3–4 weeks if the cast is a stable fracture
- May take 12–16 weeks for full unprotected weight-bearing

Factors that impede fracture healing

- Infection
- Diabetes mellitus
- Vascular insufficiency
- Calcium, phosphate, or vitamin D deficiency
- Displaced and comminuted fractures:
    - Large areas of periosteal stripping result in large volume of devitalised bone
    - Devitalised bone is gradually revascularised or resorbed
    - Increased volume of callus is produced and increases the process of remodelling
- Inadequate immobilisation
    - Normal constituents of callus don't form if there is constant significant movement of the fracture site
    - Callus mainly consists of fibrous tissue and cartilage, perpetuating instability, resulting in delayed union and non-union
- Drugs: steroids and possibly NSAIDs delay fracture healing

Nerve injury and repair

In a nutshell ...

In order of increasing degree of injury:

- **Neuropraxia (I):** no axonal disruption
- **Axonotmesis (II):** axonal disruption/supportive tissue framework preserved
- **Neurotmesis (III–V):** supportive tissue framework disrupted

Principles of surgical repair of nerves:

- Accurate apposition of nerve ends
- Healthy surrounding tissue
- No tension
- Minimal dissection

There are many variations of nerve injury. A common classification was described by Seddon, dividing injuries into three groups: neuropraxia, axonotmesis, and neurotmesis. Sunderland's classification expands the category of neurotmesis and refers to categories of increasing severity.

Neuropraxia (I)

This is the mildest form of nerve injury, referring to a crush, contusion or stretching injury of the nerve without disruption of its axonal continuity. There is a reduction or block in conduction of the impulse down a segment of the nerve fibre. This may be caused by local biochemical abnormalities. There is a temporary loss of function which is reversible within hours to months of the injury (average 6–8 weeks). Motor function often suffers greater impairment than sensory function, and autonomic function is often retained.

Axonotmesis (II)

This is the loss of the relative continuity of the axon and its covering of myelin with preservation of the connective tissue framework of the nerve (epineurium and perineurium). It is a more serious injury than neuropraxia. Wallerian degeneration occurs and there is a degree of retrograde proximal degeneration of the remaining axon. Recovery occurs through regeneration of the axons (which grow along the existing preserved framework of the nerve). Regeneration requires time and may take weeks or months, depending on the size of the lesion. The proximal end of the lesion grows distally (2–3 mm per day) and the distal end of the lesion grows proximally (1 mm per day).

Neurotmesis (III, IV and V)

This is the loss of continuity of both axons and nerve structural connective tissue. It ranges in severity, with the most extreme degree of neurotmesis being transection. Most neurotmetic injuries do not produce gross loss of continuity of the nerve but rather internal disruption of the architecture of the nerve sufficient to involve perineurium and endoneurium as well as the axons and their myelin sheath. There is a complete loss of motor, sensory and autonomic function. If the nerve has been completely divided, axonal regeneration causes a neuroma to form in the proximal stump.

In grade III injuries, axonal continuity is disrupted by loss of endoneurial tubes (the neurolemmal sheaths) but the perineurium is preserved. This causes intra-neural scarring and regenerating axons may re-enter the sheaths incorrectly.

In grade IV injuries, nerve fasciculi (axon, endoneurium, perineurium) are damaged, but nerve sheath continuity is preserved.

In grade V injuries, the endoneurium, perineurium, and epineurium, which make up the entire nerve trunk, are completely transected. This may be associated with perineural haematoma or displacement of the nerve ends.

Bowel

The layers of the bowel involved in the anastomosis heal at different rates. Optimal healing requires good surgical technique and apposition of the layers.

The intestinal mucosa is a sheet of epithelial cells that undergoes rapid turnover and proliferation. It may sustain injury as a result of trauma (from luminal contents or surgery), chemicals (eg bile), ischaemia or infection. Injury to the mucosa resulting in breaches of the epithelial layer is though to render patients susceptible to bacterial translocation and systemic sepsis syndromes. Minor disruption to the mucosa is thought to be repaired by a process separate to proliferation called 'restitution', instigated by cytokines and growth factors and regulated by the interaction of cellular integrins with the ECM. After uncomplicated surgery to the GI tract, mucosal integrity is thought to have occurred by 24 hours.

The other muscular layers of the bowel undergo the general phases of inflammation, proliferation and maturation as outlined above. Anastomotic healing results in the formation of collagenous scar tissue. Scarring may eventually contract resulting in stenosis.

Solid organs

Solid organs either heal by regeneration (through a process of cell proliferation) or by hypertrophy of existing cells. Some organs heal by a combination of the two processes. In organs in which the cells are terminally differentiated, healing occurs by scarring or fibrosis.

Liver

The liver has remarkable regenerative capacity. The stimulation for regeneration is reduction in the liver mass to body mass ratio (eg surgical resection) or the loss of liver functional capacity (eg hepatocyte necrosis by toxins or viruses). Regeneration is achieved by proliferation of all the components of the mature organ – hepatocytes, biliary epithelial cells, fenestrated epithelial cells and Kupffer cells. Hepatocytes, which are normally quiescent and rarely divide, start to proliferate to restore hepatic mass and function. This occurs initially in the areas surrounding the portal triads and then extends to the pericentral areas after 48 hours. After 70% hepatectomy in animal models, the remaining hepatocytes divide once or twice and then return to quiescence. About 24 hours after the hepatocytes start to proliferate, so do all the other cell types and ECM is produced, including the structural protein, laminin. Eventually the cell types re-structure into functional lobules over 7–10 days. The stimulus for hepatocyte proliferation is thought to be TNF and the IL-6 family of cytokines. Subsequently HGF and TGF-α are responsible for continued cell growth. Regeneration is terminated after about 72 hours by the action of cytokines such as TGF-β1.

Kidney

The cells of the kidney are highly specialised, reflecting their terminal state of differentiation. Healing in the kidney predominantly occurs by scarring and fibrosis.

Spleen

Splenic regeneration is controversial. Increases in size and weight of the residual splenic tissue have been recognised after partial splenectomy (eg for trauma) and, hypertrophy of missed splenunculi after splenectomy for haematological and glycogen storage diseases (eg Gaucher's) may also occur. However, there is little evidence that this increase in size of the residual splenic tissue results in functional regeneration and the increase in size may be due to infiltration of the tissue with cells characteristic of the underlying haematological or other disorder.

Heart and lung

Cardiac tissue is commonly damaged by ischaemia and occasionally by trauma. The inflammatory response is particularly important in the healing of cardiac tissue and is instigated by release of cytokines such as tumour necrosis factor-alpha (TNF-α or interleukin-6 (IL-6) from the damaged myocardium. These cytokines have been implicated in the regulation of myocyte survival or apoptosis, myocyte hypertrophy, defects in myocyte contractility, proliferation of myofibroblasts and angiogenesis/vasculogenesis and, to a limited extent, progenitor cell proliferation. The cytokine response lasts about a week and the infarcted myocardium is gradually replaced by scar tissue. Within this scar tissue there is a degree of regeneration of myocytes and blood vessels and current research is focused on facilitating this process for an improvement in myocardial function post infarct.

Non-regenerative tissues

Non-regenerative tissues, such as the cornea of the eye, heal by collagen deposition and scarring. This is obviously accompanied by complete loss of function.

1.4 DELAYED WOUND HEALING

In a nutshell ...

Wound healing is affected by:

Local factors (factors specific to the wound)
Wound classification
Surgical skill

General factors (factors specific to the patient)
Concomitant disease
Nutrition

Factors affecting wound healing

Local risk factors

- Wound infection
- Haematoma
- Excessive mobility
- Foreign body
- Dead tissue
- Dirty wound
- Surgical technique
- Ischaemia
  - Acute; damage to blood supply; sutures too tight
  - Chronic; previous irradiation
  - Diabetes
  - Atherosclerosis
  - Venous disease

General risk factors

- Elderly
- Cardiac disease
- Respiratory disease
- Anaemia
- Obesity
- Renal (uraemia) or hepatic failure (jaundice)
- Diabetes mellitus
- Malnutrition (vitamins and minerals)
- Malignancy
- Irradiation
- Steroid or cytotoxic drugs
- Other immunosuppressive disease or drugs

Nutritional factors

- Proteins are essential for ECM formation and effective immune response
- Vitamin A is required for epithelial cell proliferation and differentiation
- Vitamin B6 is required for collagen cross-linking
- Vitamin C is necessary for hydroxylation of proline and lysine residues. Without hydroxyproline, newly synthesised collagen is not transported out of fibroblasts; in the absence of hydroxylysine, collagen fibrils are not cross-linked
- Zinc is an essential trace element required for RNA and DNA synthesis and for the function of some 200 metalloenzymes
- Copper plays a role in the cross-linking of collagen and elastin

Optimising wound healing

Wound failure may be minimised by attention to the risk factors listed above. Ensure good delivery of blood and oxygen to the wound (and be aware of the importance of good hydration and respiratory function). Debride devitalised tissues and handle other tissues with care to prevent tissue necrosis. Sutures that are tied very tightly will cause tissue hypoxia. Avoid tension on the wound. Careful aseptic technique should be used. Heavily contaminated wounds or the abdominal cavity should be washed with copious amounts of warmed saline until clean. Patient nutrition is also very important and critically ill patients may require support either via NG feeding or parenteral nutrition.

On occasions the patient may be in such a poor condition (eg be elderly, have septic shock, be on steroids) and the circumstances of the operation so hostile (emergency, faecal contamination, disseminated malignancy) that the chance of good wound healing is very low. Under these circumstances, there are various surgical options:

- Bring out a stoma rather than perform a primary bowel anastomosis
- Leave the skin and subcutaneous fat open in a heavily contaminated abdomen for delayed primary closure – this wound can then be packed as required (be aware that changing dressings on large wounds may require return visits to theatre)

- Close the wound with additional deep tension sutures
- The abdominal wall itself may be left open (a laparostomy) or partially closed with an artificial mesh to reduce intra-abdominal pressure after surgery for intra-abdominal catastrophe and prevent abdominal compartment syndrome

1.5 WOUND DEHISCENCE AND INCISIONAL HERNIAS

In a nutshell ...

The same risk factors predispose to:
- Failure of wound healing
- Wound dehiscence
- Incisional herniation

- Wound dehiscence is the partial or total disruption of any or all layers of the operative wound. Risk factors for wound dehiscence are the same as those for factors affecting wound healing
- Evisceration ('burst abdomen') is rupture of all layers of the abdominal wall and extrusion of the abdominal viscera (usually preceded by the appearance of blood-stained fluid – the pink-fluid sign)
- Wound dehiscence without evisceration should be repaired by immediate elective re-closure. Dehiscence of a laparotomy wound with evisceration is a surgical emergency with a mortality rate of > 25%. Management involves resuscitation, reassurance, analgesia, protection of the organs with moist sterile towels, and immediate reoperation and closure (usually with deep tension sutures)

Incisional hernias are still common despite modern suture materials. They occur at sites of partial wound failure or dehiscence. Risk factors for incisional hernia are therefore the same as those for dehiscence. Symptoms include visible protrusion of the hernia during episodes of raised intra-abdominal pressure and discomfort. Incisional hernias usually correspond to a wide defect in the abdominal wall and so do not often incarcerate. Treatment depends on symptoms and size of defect (eg. conservative measures including a truss/corset and surgical repair). Further details on incisional hernias and methods of repair are covered in the *Abdomen* chapter of Book 2.

Section 2
Creation and care of the surgical wound

2.1 CLASSIFICATION OF WOUNDS

In a nutshell ...

Wounds can be classified in terms of:
- **Depth:** superficial vs deep
- **Mechanism:** incised, lacerated, abrasion, degloved, burn
- **Contamination or cleanliness:** clean, clean contaminated, contaminated, dirty

Depth of wound

Superficial wounds

Superficial wounds involve only the epidermis and dermis and heal without formation of granulation tissue and true scar formation. Epithelial cells (including those from any residual skin appendages such as sweat or sebaceous glands and hair follicles) proliferate and migrate across the remaining dermal collagen.

Examples:

- Superficial burn
- Graze
- Split skin graft donor site

Deep wounds

Deep wounds involve layers deep to the dermis and heal with the migration of fibroblasts from perivascular tissue and formation of granulation tissue and subsequent true scar formation. If a deep wound is not closed with good tissue approximation, it heals by a combination of contraction and epithelialisation, which may lead to problematic contractures, especially if over a joint.

Mechanism of wounding

The mechanism of wounding often results in characteristic damage to the skin and deeper tissues. Wounds are categorised as follows:

- **Incised wounds:** surgical or traumatic (knife, glass) where the epithelium is breached by a sharp object
- **Laceration:** an epithelial defect due to blunt trauma or tearing, that results from skin being stretched and leading to failure of the dermis and avulsion of the deeper tissues. It is usually associated with adjacent soft tissue damage, and vascularity of the wound may be compromised (eg pre-tibial laceration in elderly women, scalp laceration after a blow to the head)
- **Abrasion:** friction against a surface causes sloughing of superficial skin layers
- **Degloving injury:** a form of laceration when shearing forces parallel tissue planes to move against each other leading to disruption and separation. Although the skin may be intact, it is often at risk due to disruption of its underlying blood supply. This occurs when, for example, a worker's arm gets caught in an industrial machine
- **Burns**

Contamination of wounds

Wounds may be contaminated by the environment at times of injury. Surgical procedures and accidental injuries may be classified according to the risk of wound contamination.

- Clean (eg hernia repair)
- Clean contaminated (eg cholecystectomy)
- Contaminated wound (eg colonic resection)
- Dirty wound (eg laparotomy for peritonitis)

Ideal conditions for wound healing

- No foreign material
- No infection
- Accurate apposition of tissues in layers (eliminating dead space)
- No excess tension
- Good blood supply
- Good haemostasis, preventing haematoma

For a discussion of factors causing delayed wound healing see section 1.4.

2.2 INCISIONS AND CLOSURES

Fig. 2.2a shows all commonly used incisions, and the table that follows shows different routes of access to different organs.

The commonest reason for a difficult operation is inadequate access. This may be because the organ is difficult to access (gastro-oesophageal junction, gastrosplenic ligament, lower rectum), or because the body shape is unfavourable, or the wrong incision has been used. The surgeon can affect only the last of these, and it is extremely important, having considered the likely course of the operation, to plan the incision before starting. Remember when planning that you may wish to extend your incision if access proves difficult!

If it is considered that different incisions may give identical access, then that incision which leads to better healing and cosmesis should be used. As a general rule, transverse incisions heal better than vertical ones. Plan your closure at the same time as the incision – if the incision is complicated it is valuable to mark lines perpendicular to the incision in ink before you begin. These lines then show how the edges should be brought together accurately for closure.

COMMON INCISIONS

Organ	Approach
Oesophagus	Cervical
Upper thoracic	Right 4/5 postero-lateral thoracotomy
Mid thoracic	Right 5/6/7 postero-lateral thoracotomy
Lower thoracic	Right 5/6/7 postero-lateral thoracotomy Left 6/7 postero-lateral thoracotomy Left thoracoabdominal
Abdominal	Left thoracoabdominal Rooftop Upper midline
Stomach	Left thoracoabdominal Rooftop Upper midline
Liver	Right thoracoabdominal
Biliary tree	Rooftop Upper midline Right paramedian Kocher Transverse
Pancreas	Rooftop
Duodenum	Upper midline Right paramedian Kocher Transverse

Organ	Approach
Small intestine	Midline Paramedian Transverse
Colon	Right midline Right paramedian Right transverse Rutherford Morrison Gridiron
Appendix	Gridiron Lanz Left midline Left paramedian Left transverse
Rectum	Midline Left paramedian Left transverse Perineal
Uterus, ovaries	Midline Pfannenstiel
Aorta	Midline Transverse
Iliac vessels	Midline Transverse Rutherford Morrison
Bladder	Lower midline Pfannenstiel
Kidney	Midline
Adrenal glands	Kocher 12th rib incision

Abdominal incisions

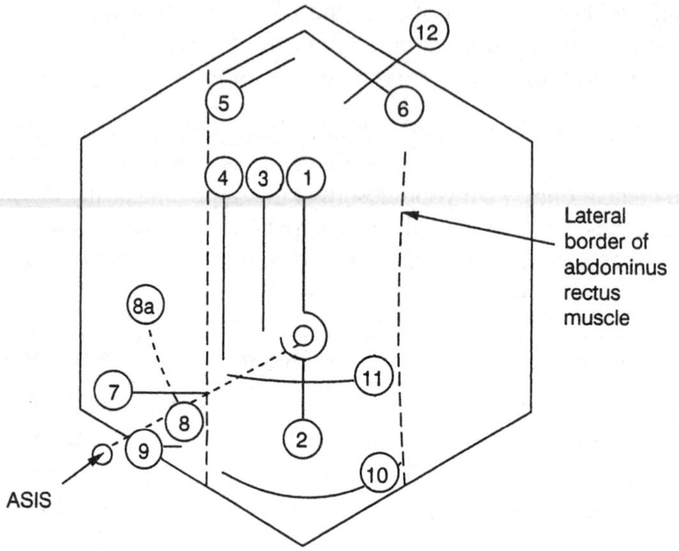

Figure 2.2a *Common abdominal incisions*

(1) **Mid-line incision through linea alba:** provides good access. Can be extended easily. Quick to make and close. Relatively avascular. More painful than transverse incisions. Incision crosses Langer's lines so it has poor cosmetic appearance. Narrow linea alba below umbilicus. Some vessels cross the mid-line. May cause bladder damage.
(2) **Sub-umbilical incision:** used for repair of para-umbilical hernias and laparoscopic port.
(3) **Para-median incision:** 1.5 cm from mid-line through rectus abdominus sheath. This was the only effective vertical incision in the days when catgut was the only available suture material. Takes longer to make than mid-line incision. Does not lend itself to closure by 'Jenkins rule' (length of suture is 4 × length of wound). Poor cosmetic result. Can lead to infection in rectus sheath. Other hazards: tendinous intersections must be dissected off; need to divide falciform ligament above umbilicus on the right; if rectus is split more than 1 cm from medial border, intercostal nerves are disrupted leading to denervation of medial rectus (avoid by retracting rectus without splitting).
(4) **Para-rectal 'Battle's' incision:** now not used because of damage to nerves entering rectus sheath and poor healing leading to post-operative incisional hernias.
(5) **Kocher's incision:** 3 cm below and parallel to costal margin from mid-line to rectus border. Good incision for cholecystectomy on the right and splenectomy on the left – but beware superior epigastric vessels. If wound is extended laterally too many intercostal nerves are severed. Cannot be extended caudally.
(6) **Double Kocher's (rooftop) incision:** good access to liver and spleen. Useful for intra-hepatic surgery. Used for radical pancreatic and gastric surgery and bilateral adrenalectomy.
(7) **Transverse muscle-cutting incision:** can be across all muscles. Beware of intercostal nerves.
(8) **McBurney's/Gridiron incision:** classic approach to appendix through junction of the outer and middle third of a line from the ASIS to the umbilicus at right angles to that line. May be modified into a skin crease horizontal cut. External oblique aponeurosis is cut in the line of the fibres. Internal

oblique and transversus abdominus are split transversely in the line of the fibres. Beware: scarring if not horizontal; ilio-hypogastric and ilio-inguinal nerves; deep circumflex artery.
(8a) **Rutherford Morrison incision:** gridiron can be extended cephalad and laterally, obliquely splitting the external oblique to afford good access to caecum, appendix and right colon.
(9) **Lanz incision:** lower incision than McBurney's and closer to the ASIS. Better cosmetic result (concealed by bikini). Tends to divide ilio-hypogastric and ilio-inguinal nerves, leading to denervation of inguinal canal mechanism (can increase risk of inguinal hernia).
(10) **Pfannenstiel incision:** most frequently used transverse incision in adults. Excellent access to female genitalia for Caesarean section and for bladder and prostate operations. Also used for bilateral hernia repair. Skin incised in a downward convex arc into supra-pubic skin crease 2 cm above the pubis. Upper flap is raised and rectus sheath incised 1 cm cephalic to the skin incision (not extending lateral to the rectus). Rectus is then divided longitudinally in the mid-line.
(11) **Transverse incision:** particularly useful in neonates and children (who do not have the sub-diaphragmatic and pelvic recesses of adults). Heals securely and cosmetically. Less pain and fewer respiratory problems than with longitudinal mid-line incision but division of red muscle involves more blood loss than longitudinal incision. Not extended easily. Takes longer to make and close. Limited access in adults to pelvic or sub-diaphragmatic structure.
(12) **Thoraco-abdominal incision:** access to lower thorax and upper abdomen. Used (rarely) for liver and biliary surgery on the right. Used (rarely) for oesophageal, gastric and aortic surgery on the left.

Thoracic incisions

A summary of the important features of these incisions is presented below. For further discussion of thoracic incisions and closures see in the *Cardiothoracics* chapter of Book 2.

Median sternotomy

This common incision is used in a number of surgical disciplines and is the most frequently used approach to the heart. The patient is placed supine with the neck extended. It is a midline incision extending from 2 cm below the sternal notch to the xiphoid. The sternum is divided using a pneumatic reciprocating saw or a jiggly saw. Gives access to:

- Heart (including aortic and mitral valves)
- Great vessels (especially ascending aorta)
- Structures in the anterior mediastinum (eg thymus, retrosternal thyroid)

Antero-lateral thoracotomy

This is the procedure of choice for emergency, resuscitation room procedures for management of cardiac or thoracic injuries, often in the context of major haemorrhage or cardiac arrest. The incision extends from the lateral edge of the sternum following the rib interspace laterally. It may be performed through the 5th interspace according to indication. Gives access to:

- Heart (control of bleeding)
- Lung hilum (control of bleeding)
- Lung parenchyma (control of bleeding)
- Descending aorta

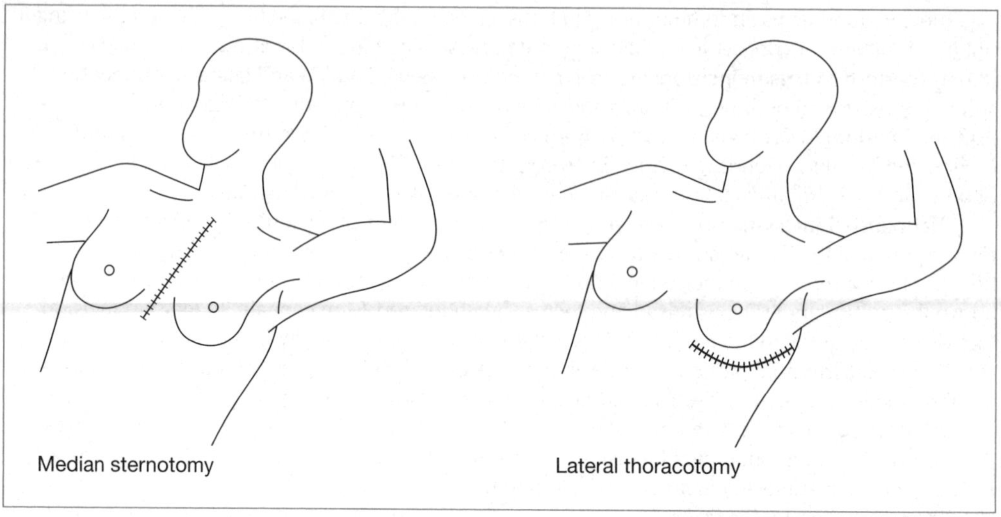

Figure 2.2b *Thoracic incisions*

Postero-lateral thoracotomy

Although there are many variants upon the thoracotomy, this is the commonest incision through which elective thoracic procedures are performed. The incision is curved and passes from the middle of the posterior border of the scapula, below the angle of the scapula to a point midway between the angle of the scapula and the nipple. This may be performed at either the 5th or 7th interspace.

- Via 5th interspace
  - Lung and hilum
  - Mid oesophagus
- Via 7th interspace
  - Lower oesophagus
  - Diaphragm
  - Heart and pericardium

Laparoscopy

Both the abdominal and thoracic cavities can be accessed by means of a laparoscope. The principles of this access are similar with insertion of a large access port to transmit a camera and a number of smaller instrument ports. Minimal access surgery is discussed in section 3.5 of this chapter. This is also discussed in detail in the *Abdomen* and *Cardiothoracics* chapters of Book 2.

Closure techniques

Good surgical technique optimises wound healing and cosmesis.

Closure techniques

Principles of wound closure include the following:

- Incise along natural tension lines
- Avoid haematoma and obliterate potential spaces
- Eliminate all dead tissue and infection
- Ensure good apposition of tissues
- Avoid excess wound tension
- Ensure good blood supply
- Handle tissues gently
- Use appropriate suture material
- Choose appropriate closure technique

Abdominal closure

At closure there is an increase in intra-abdominal pressure and some tension on the suture line is inevitable. Abdominal incisions can be closed either in layers or by a mass closure technique. The mass closure includes all layers of the abdominal wall except subcutaneous fat and skin, and has been shown to be as strong as a layered closure with no greater incidence of later wound complications such as dehiscence or incisional hernia formation. This is now the preferred closure method of most surgeons. Other abdominal incisions are closed in layers, apposing the tissues (eg rectus sheath to rectus sheath).

Procedure box: Mass closure of the abdomen

Don't ask a senior surgeon to let you close the abdomen unless you understand all the principles in this box.

- Carefully re-position abdominal contents into the abdominal cavity and cover with the omentum; abdominal contents may be temporarily protected with a large swab or plastic guard (NB bowel guards must be removed before the closure is complete)
- Use a non-absorbable (eg loop nylon 0/0) or slowly absorbable (eg PDS 0/0) continuous suture on a large curved needle (some surgeons use blunt-ended needles for safety reasons)
- Use a suture which is four times the length of the wound (in practice two or more sutures are used starting from opposite ends of the wound, meeting in the middle)

- Obey the 1-cm rule (Jenkins 1976) – each bite of the abdominal wall should be a minimum of 1 cm, and adjacent bites must be a maximum of 1 cm apart. These measurements refer to the rectus sheath only, not the fat or peritoneum or rectus muscle. To develop good technique, before you place each stitch you should identify two things: the site of the last stitch and the cut edge of the anterior rectus sheath. Only then can you apply Jenkins' rule correctly
- Generally in a mass closure you should include in each stitch all layers of the abdominal wall and peritoneum, except subcutaneous fat and skin but it is important to recognise that it is the fascia of the rectus sheath which gives the wound its strength
- Place each suture under direct vision to avoid accidental damage to the bowel
- Remember that the posterior rectus sheath is deficient in the lower abdomen

Thoracic closure

Thoracic closure is covered in the *Cardiothoracics* chapter in Book 2. The basic principles include:

- Haemostasis in the chest cavity and of the wound edges
- Closure of the bony layer (with wire for the sternum and heavy nylon ties in a figure-of-eight loop for the ribs of the lateral incisions)
- Closure of the subcutaneous layer
- Closure of the skin

Closure of the subcutaneous layers

Subcutaneous fascial layers may be apposed accurately with interrupted or continuous absorbable sutures. This aids in the elimination of dead space and helps prevent fluid collections. It also aids subsequent accurate apposition of the skin.

Thick deposits of adipose tissue heal poorly and are susceptible to collection of serous fluid from their large surface area. This predisposes the wound to risks of dehiscence and later hernia formation. Absorbable sutures placed in the deep adipose tissue itself are rarely helpful. If there is a thick layer of adipose tissue (eg bariatric surgery) a drain may be placed in the subcutaneous layer and large deep tension mattress sutures may be placed across the wound to support the adipose tissue as it heals.

Closure of the skin

There is no evidence that any different form of skin closure leads to a better cosmetic result in the long term, and the choice is usually down to cost, indication, and the surgeon's preference. A good incision made boldly at a perpendicular angle through the skin aids eventual cosmesis. Cross-hatching of scars is not a problem as long as the sutures or staples are not left in too long. Subcuticular closure is cheaper than using staples but is not suitable for heavily contaminated wounds as wound infection may require drainage of superficial collections of pus.

Skin closure options

- Staples or skin clips
- Subcuticular sutures
- Interrupted or continuous sutures
- Glue
- Self-adhesive strips
- Adequate apposition of tissues under the skin may eliminate the requirement for skin closure

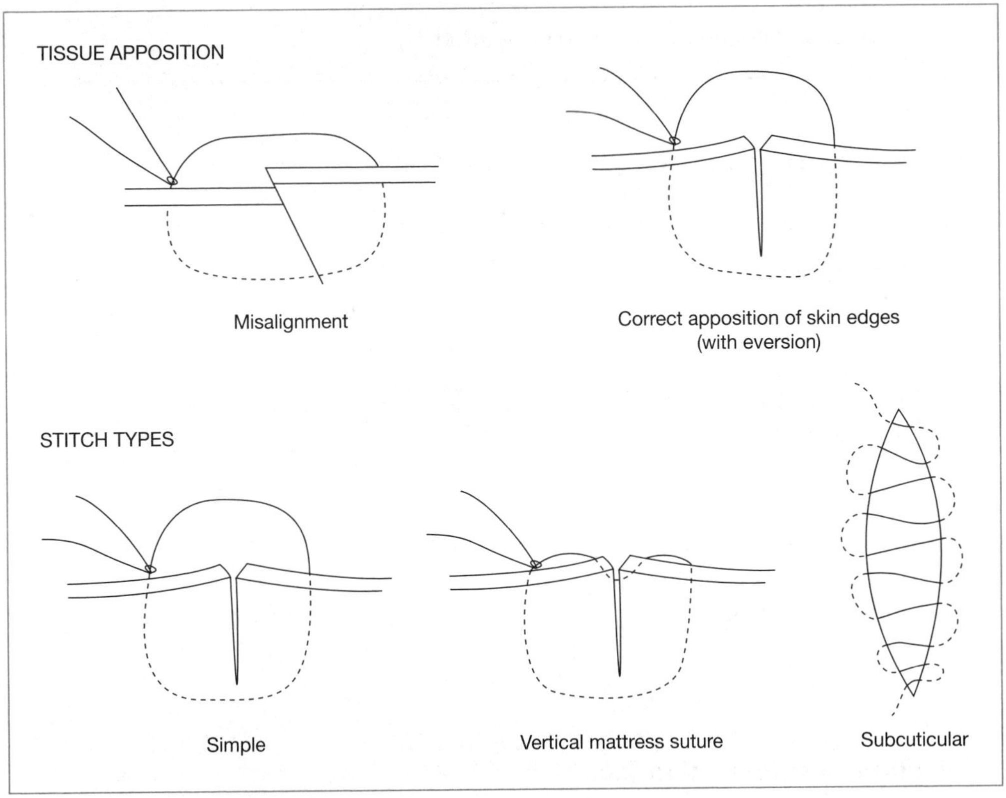

Figure 2.2c *Skin closure techniques*

2.3 NEEDLES AND SUTURES

In a nutshell ...

Choose your suture with regards to:
Size of suture (depends on strength required)
Characteristics of materials

- Structure (monofilament vs braided – depends on handling vs knotting requirements)
- Absorbancy (non-absorbable vs absorbable – depends on duration of required support)
- Needle (depends on tissue to be sutured)

Sutures and ligatures

Features of ideal suture material

- Monofilament
- Strong
- Easy handling
- Minimal tissue reaction
- Holds knots well
- Predictable absorption

Classification of sutures

- Absorbable vs non-absorbable
- Monofilament vs multifilament
- Synthetic vs natural

Types of sutures

Selection of suture materials

Absorbable sutures for tissues which heal quickly (eg bowel anastomosis).

Non-absorbable sutures for tissues which heal more slowly (eg abdominal wall closure).

Smooth (monofilament) sutures for running stitches (eg vascular surgery) as they slide easily through tissues.

Braided sutures for knotting properties (eg ligating pedicles).

Smaller sutures for fine stitching (eg 6/0 or 7/0 proline for tibial arteries).

Biological sutures (catgut, silk) cause an inflammatory reaction and fibrosis in the skin and undergo enzymatic absorption, thus persistence in the tissues and strength are unpredictable.

Non-absorbable sutures

Silk

- Biological origin from silk worm
- Braided multifilament
- Dyed or undyed
- May be coated with wax

Linen

- Biological origin from flax plant
- Twisted multifilament
- Dyed or undyed
- Uncoated

Cotton

- Biological origin from cotton seed plant
- Twisted multifilament
- Dyed or undyed
- Uncoated

Polyester

- Man-made
- Multifilament
- Dyed or undyed
- Coated or uncoated
- Trade names Ethibond™ or TiCron™, and Mersilene™ or Dacron™ (uncoated)

Polyamide

- Man-made
- Monofilament or multifilament
- Dyed or undyed
- Trade names Ethilon™ or Dermalon™ (monofilament) and Nurolon™ (braided) or Surgilon™ (braided nylon)

Polypropylene

- Man-made
- Monofilament
- Dyed or undyed
- Trade name Prolene™

PVDF

- Man-made
- Monofilament
- Dyed or undyed
- Trade name Novafil™

Steel

- Man-made
- Monofilament or multifilament

Absorbable sutures

Polyglycolic acid

- Man-made homopolymer
- Braided multifilament
- Dyed or undyed
- Coated or uncoated
- Tradename Dexon™

Polygalactin 910

- Man-made copolymer
- Coated with calcium stearate, glycolide and lactide
- Tradename Vicryl™

Polydioxanone sulfate

- Man-made copolymer
- Monofilament
- Dyed or undyed
- Referred to as PDS

Polyglyconate

- Man-made copolymer
- Monofilament
- Dyed or undyed
- Tradename Maxon™

Types of needle and their uses

Needles are categorised according to shape, thickness and type.

Shape of needle

- Straight
- Curved
- Circular (proportion of circumference)
- J-shaped

Size of needle

- Needle thickness should be appropriate to the weight of suture selected
- The choice of a larger or smaller curved needle may aid suture placement
- Large for large bites of tissue (eg abdominal closure)
- Small for accurate placement (eg vascular anastomoses)

Point and profile of needle

Blunt needle

- Rounded end helps to prevent splitting tissues
- Advocated by some surgeons for abdominal closure (safety issue)
- Usually also round bodied

Round-bodied needle

- Round profile with a pointed end
- Tend to spread rather than cut tissue (useful for placing sutures in organ parenchyma or viscera)

Cutting needle

- Triangular profile with a cutting edge on either the internal or the external curvature of the needle referred to as 'cutting' or 'reverse cutting' respectively
- Useful for tough fibrous tissue like skin

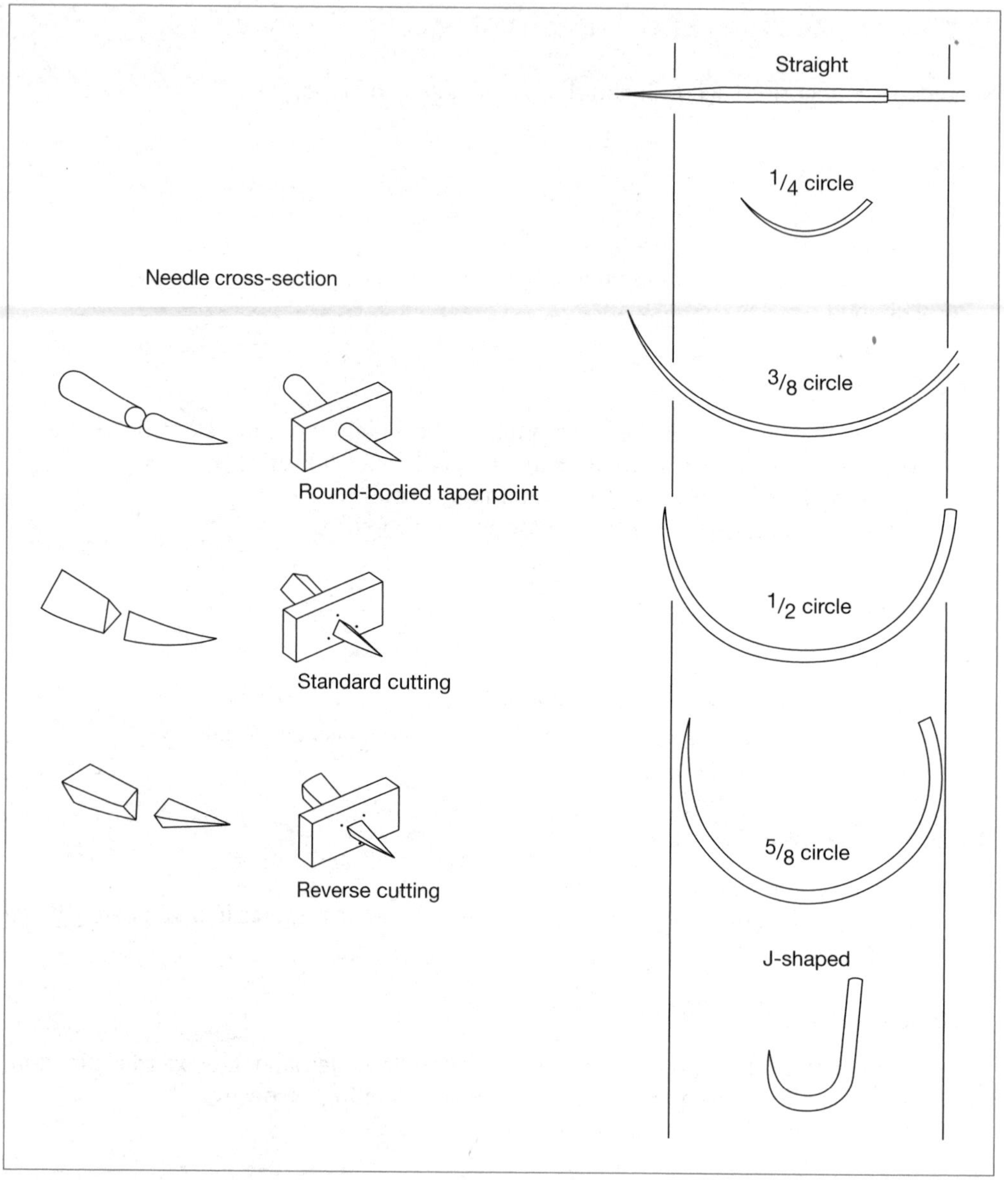

Figure 2.3a *Types of needle*

Staples

Staples can now have a variety of uses. They are more expensive than traditional methods but are often much quicker. They are made of titanium and tend to be hypoallergenic. They are removed with a device which bends the central area of the staple and releases the teeth.

Staples for skin closure

The teeth of the staples should be used to draw the dermis together and evert the wound edge (misalignment of the closure is a common complication of staple use and impedes wound healing). Alternate staples may be removed as the wound heals or to allow the escape of pus in infected areas.

Staples for bowel anastomosis

There are many stapling guns used in bowel surgery. Some are linear, some are circular, and some are combined with a cutting device which cuts between two staple lines.

Staples may be used:

- To divide the bowel without spilling contents and to reduce contamination
- To reduce the risks of anastomotic leakage
- To reduce the incidence of anastomotic stenosis – however, note that the incidence of stenosis is higher in stapled anastomosis if the diameter is small (eg high gastro-oesophageal anastomosis in the chest)
- To improve access if technically difficult (eg circular staples introduced PR in low anterior resection)
- During laparoscopic surgery
- To add strength (eg stapling of the stomach pouch in bariatric surgery)
- To reduce operative time

Disadvantages include the potential to damage or split the bowel. Failure of the stapling device often makes it extremely difficult to perform a subsequent hand-sewn anastomosis.

Staples for pedicle ligation and haemostasis

- Clips can be used instead of ties on small vessels (eg laparoscopic cholecystectomy)
- Large pedicles should be tied but some staplers are designed for haemostasis and are useful for division of smaller pedicles

Suture removal

Timing of removal of skin closure materials will vary according to the site of the wound. Good subcutaneous apposition of tissues allows the skin closure material to be removed relatively early, thus minimising scarring. Subcuticular closures with quickly absorbable sutures will not require removal. Areas that have a great deal of mobility may require longer to heal. Infection in wounds may require early removal of the staples or sutures to let pus out.

As a rough guide:

Face	4–5 days
Scalp	6–7 days
Hands and limbs	10 days
Abdominal wounds	10–20 days

2.4 SURGICAL DRAINS

In a nutshell ...

Drains are used for a variety of purposes, and overall the use of drains is reducing. Drains are used:

- **To minimise dead space** in a wound and prevent fluid collecting (eg following axillary nodal clearance, mastectomy, thyroidectomy)
- **When there is a risk of leakage** (eg pancreatic surgery, bowel anastomosis)
- **To drain actual fluid collections** (eg radiologically placed drain for subphrenic abscess)
- **To divert fluid** away from blockage or potential blockage (eg biliary T-tube, suprapubic urinary catheter, ventricular CSF drain)
- **To decompress** and allow air to escape (chest drain)

Types of surgical drains

- Drains can be **open** (into dressings) or **closed** (into container) systems
- Drains can be **suction** or **non-suction** drains (passive gravity drainage)
- Suction drains provide better drainage but may damage adjacent structures (eg bowel) and precipitate a leak
- Closed systems reduce the risk of introducing infection

Examples of surgical drains:

- Suction drains (closed) – Redivac drain, suction chest drain
- Non-suction drains (open) – Penrose drain, corrugated drain
- Non-suction drains (closed) – Robinson drain, T-tube, urinary catheter, chest drain

Complications of surgical drains

- Infection via drain track
- Lets in air (eg chest drain)
- Injury to adjacent structures by drain or during placement (eg bowel)
- Anastomotic leakage
- Retraction of the drain into the wound
- Bleeding by erosion into blood vessel
- Pain (eg chest drain irritating diaphragm)
- Herniation at the drain site

Routine drainage of a bowel anastomosis is controversial. The drains may cause more problems than they solve. They can directly damage the anastomosis, and can prevent formations of adhesions to adjacent vascular structures through which the anastomosis would expect to gain an extra blood supply. If the anastomosis is not watertight (eg biliary or urological) a drain is usually used to prevent build-up of a collection which may otherwise hinder healing.

After draining a fluid collection, removal of the drain may result in the formation of a tract of scar tissue circumferentially along the passage of the drain. A mature tract allows continued drainage from an area. Over time, this will heal in the same manner as a fistula.

2.5 DRESSINGS

In a nutshell ...

Types of dressings
- Hydrocolloids
- Hydrofibre
- Hydrogels
- Semipermeable film dressings
- Alginates
- Foam dressings
- Antimicrobial dressings
- Artificial and living skin equivalents

Dressings can make a huge contribution to the healing of a wound.

The optimum healing environment for a wound is:

- Moist
- Free of infection, with minimal slough
- Free of chemicals and foreign bodies (eg fibres from dressing)
- At the optimum temperature
- Reduce wound disruption (minimal changes of dressings)
- At the correct pH

Different dressings are appropriate for different stages of wound healing, and therefore good wound management necessitates a flexible approach to the selection and use of dressings. It is sensible to observe wounds regularly in order to assess changes in requirements.

Requirements of dressings

- Provide protection from infection and trauma
- Allow debridement, both mechanical and chemical
- Be absorbent and remove excess exudates, while keeping wound moist
- Maintain temperature and gaseous exchange
- Be comfortable and cosmetically acceptable
- Stimulate healing
- Be inexpensive and easy to change

Commonly used dressings

Traditional dressings such as gauze and 'Gamgee' have few indications for the modern treatment of wounds. Modern dressings can be classified thus:

Hydrocolloids

- Available in pastes, granules, and wafers
- Consist of a mix of carboxymethylcellulose, pectins, gelatins and elastomers
- Form a gel (on contact with wound secretions) that absorbs secretions
- Example: Granuflex™

Hydrofibres

- Consist of carboxymethylcellulose spun into a fibre
- Form a gel (on contact with wound secretions) that absorbs secretions
- Good for heavily exudating wounds
- Example: Aquacel™

Hydrogels

- Consist of insoluble polymers, water and propylene glycol
- Absorb large volumes of exudates and are effective at desloughing/debriding
- Available in sheets or gels

Semipermeable film dressings

- Clear polyurethane film coated with adhesive
- Not suitable if excessive exudate

Alginates

- Extracted from seaweed
- Absorb secretions to form gel to optimise moist wound healing
- Available in sheet form or ribbon for packing
- Examples: Kaltostat™, Sorbsan™

Foam dressings

- Consist of polyurethane or silicone foam
- Very absorbent
- Use for flat wounds and cavity wounds (two forms are available for cavity wounds: liquid foam polymer and hydrocellular cavity dressing)

Antimicrobial dressings

- Usage has declined in recent years
- Little evidence of benefit
- Examples: Inadine™, Bactigras™

Artificial and living skin equivalents

- Increasing interest in these in recent years
- Can facilitate cell proliferation, production of ECM components and increase concentrations of growth factors in the wound
- Epidermal components (eg Vivoderm™)
- Dermal components (eg Dermagraft™)
- Composite grafts (epidermal and dermal components) (eg Apligraf™)

2.6 SCARS AND CONTRACTURES

In a nutshell ...

The final appearance of a scar depends upon:

Wound factors
Site
Classification
Tissue loss

Patient factors
Risk factors for poor wound healing
Predisposition to keloid or hypertrophy

Surgical factors
Positioning of incisions
Correct alignment during closure
Correct management of traumatic wounds using the reconstructive ladder

Mechanism of scarring

As a scar forms, the strength increases rapidly within 7–10 days, and it is at this stage that sutures are normally removed. It is usually many months, however, before the scar regains full strength. As fibrous tissue is laid down, this tissue is continually digested to modify the shape of the scar, and these two competing influences are usually in balance. If too little fibrous tissue is laid down, or excessive breakdown takes place, the wound will fail to heal adequately, and this leads to wound dehiscence (early) or hernia formation (late). Conversely, if excessive scar tissue is laid down, the scar may be hypertrophic or keloid.

Minimisation of scarring

- Use lines of skin tension or hide the scar in naturally occurring lines including:
  - Langer's lines
  - Natural wrinkle lines (nasolabial fold, glabellar wrinkles, forehead wrinkles)
  - Natural junction lines that draw the eye from the scar (eg the junction between nose and face, nostril rim, vermillion border of the lip)
  - Hidden sites (eg eyebrow, hairline) where an incision parallel to the hair follicle, rather than perpendicular to the skin, avoids a hairless scar line caused by sectioning the follicles
- Appose tissues correctly (if the wound is irregular, identify landmarks on either side which fit together allowing the jigsaw to be accurately sutured back together)
- Close in layers to reduce tension (skin may be undermined to improve mobility)
- Clean tissues thoroughly of dirt to prevent infection and tattooing of the skin
- Use the smallest suitable diameter suture (to minimise foreign material in the wound and the inflammatory response, to reduce tissue compression and additional injury)
- Remove sutures as early as possible (tracks will become epithelialised and therefore visible if sutures are left)
- Recommend massage which prevents adherence to underlying structures and improves the colour of the scar (can be performed after initial healing)
- Advise patient to avoid exposure of new scars to sunshine (causes pigmentation)

Contractures

These occur as the scar shortens. They may lead to distortion of adjacent structures (eg near the eye) or limited flexibility in joints. They may also be caused by extravasation injuries. Contractures can be both prevented and treated by using a Z-plasty to break up the scar. Physiotherapy, massage, and even splintage can be used to prevent contractures when scars cross joint surfaces.

Scars

Hypertrophic scars

Most wounds become red and hard for a while but after several months spontaneous maturation leads to a pale soft scar. Occasionally this excessive scar tissue remains, but is *limited* to the site of the original wound.

- Due to fibroblast overactivity in the proliferative phase; eventually this is corrected (usually by 1 year) and a more normal scar results
- Commonly results from large areas of skin damage (eg abrasion or burns)

Keloid scars

- Excessive scar tissue which extends beyond the original wound
- Intense fibroblast activity continues into the maturation phase
- Complications include cosmesis, contractures and loss of function
- Prevention: use Langer's lines, ensure meticulous wound closure without undue tension, avoidance of infection, and judicious use of pressure garments

Risk factors for hypertrophic and keloid scars
- Young age
- Male sex
- Dark pigmented skin
- Genetic predisposition
- Site (sternum, shoulders, head and neck)
- Tension on wound
- Delayed healing

Treatment of hypertrophic and keloid scars
- Excision (usually leads to recurrence)
- Excision and radiotherapy (not always successful and cannot be repeated)
- Intra-lesional steroid injection (variable response rates)
- Pressure garments
- Silastic gel treatment
- CO_2 laser (variable response rates)

Malignant change in scars

Rarely squamous cell cancers can form in scars (so-called Marjolin ulcers). Any unusual ulceration or appearance in a scar should be biopsied.

Other scars

Other kinds of scarring may also occur. Scars may be widened and stretched if there is movement in that region which puts tension on the suture line. A scar may become tethered to underlying structures and puckered. Failure to remove dirt or surgical marker pen may result in permanent tattooing of a scar. Failure to properly align tissues and not correctly everting skin edges may result in a scar that appears 'stepped'. Scars can be revised by means of Z-plasty or by direct revision after about 18 months.

Section 3
Basic surgical techniques

3.1 ANASTOMOSIS

In a nutshell ...

An anastomosis is a join between two parts of a tubular structure with the result that the lumen becomes continuous. A surgical join occurs commonly between:

Blood vessels (eg arteries, veins, vascular grafts)
Hollow organs (eg GI tract, genito-urinary tract)
Ducts (eg the common bile duct)

Any anastomosis is at risk of infection, leak or rupture.

Vascular anastomosis

Vascular anastomosis may be between arteries, veins, prosthetic materials or combinations of these.

Autologous vein with native vein

- eg long saphenous vein graft or composite arm vein graft for femoropopliteal bypass
- eg vessels of a free flap graft for reconstruction (eg tram flap)

Donated organ vessels to native vessels

- eg anastomosis of the recipient vena cava to the donor liver vena cava in transplantation

Prosthetic graft to connect native vessels

- eg Gortex™ graft for AAA repair
- eg PTFE graft for femoro-femoral cross-over

Principles of vascular anastomoses

Non-absorbable monofilament suture with continuous stitches only (eg Proline™)
Use smallest needles and suture strong enough to hold anastomosis
Evert edges to prevent intimal disruption (reduces thrombogenicity)
Adequate graft length to eliminate tension
Place sutures drawing the needle from the inside of the vessel to the outside of the vessel
Prophylactic antibiotics (especially anti-staphylococcal cover and especially if prosthetic material implanted)
No holes or leaks (good surgical technique)

Early complications of vascular anastomosis

- Haemorrhage or leak
- Thrombosis

Late complications of vascular anastomosis

- Infection
- Stenosis (fibrosis, disease recurrence, neointimal hyperplasia)
- Pseudoaneurysm formation at the suture line
- Rupture

Hollow organs: GI and genito-urinary anastomosis

Principles of anastomosis in a hollow organ

Good blood supply
Good size approximation (avoid mis-match) and accurate apposition
No tension
No holes or leaks (good surgical technique)

Good surgical technique

- Do not perform anastomoses in areas supplied by a vascular 'watershed'
- Ensure adequate mobilisation of the ends
- Invert the edges to discourage leakage and appose mucosa

- Consider pre-op bowel preparation to prevent mechanical damage to the anastomosis by passage of faeces
- Consider the type of suture material (absorbable vs non-absorbable, continuous vs interrupted vs stapled
- Give prophylactic antibiotics: to cover bowel organisms including anaerobes
- Single layer vs double layer: the risk–benefit ratio must be considered. A single layer anastomosis may be more prone to leak but a double layer is more prone to ischaemia or luminal narrowing.

In the presence of the conditions which increase the risk of anastomotic dehiscence, if the bowel is of dubious viability, or if there is great size disparity, it may be worth considering a defunctioning colostomy proximal to the anastomosis. Some size disparity may be overcome by performing a side-to-side anastomosis or cutting the bowel of smaller diameter at an oblique angle to try to match the circumference.

Early complications of anastomosis in a hollow organ

- Anastomotic leak
- Bleeding

Late complications of anastomosis in a hollow organ

- Stenosis (fibrosis, disease recurrence eg tumour)

Duct anastomosis

Principles of anastomosis in a duct

Good blood supply
Good size approximation (avoid mismatch) and accurate apposition
No tension
No holes or leaks (good surgical technique)

Good surgical technique

- Do not perform anastomoses in areas supplied by a vascular 'watershed'
- Ensure adequate mobilisation of the ends
- Invert the edges to discourage leakage and appose mucosa
- All ducts should be sutured using monofilament absorbable sutures (eg PDS) to minimise the risk of residual suture creating a nidus for subsequent stone formation
- Many duct anastomoses may be performed over a stent that is removed at a later date (eg ureteric stent, T-tube in the CBD) to minimise subsequent stenosis

Early complications of anastomosis in a duct

- Anastomotic leak

Late complications of anastomosis in a duct

- Stenosis (fibrosis, disease recurrence eg tumour)
- Intra-ductal stone formation (stitch nidus)

Anastomotic dehiscence

Any anastomosis is at risk of leak, particularly oesophageal and rectal.

Factors responsible for anastomotic dehiscence

Poor surgical technique
Pre-morbid factors (eg malignancy, malnutrition, old age, sepsis, immunosuppression, steroids, radiotherapy)
Peri-operative factors (eg hypotension)

Predisposing factors for anastomotic leak

General factors

- Poor tissue perfusion
- Old age
- Malnutrition
- Obesity
- Steroids

Local factors

- Tension on anastomosis
- Local ischaemia
- Poor technique
- Local sepsis

Presentation of bowel anastomotic leakage

- Peritonitis
- Bowel contents in wound or drain
- Abscess
- Ileus
- Systemic signs of sepsis
- Occult (eg arrhythmia, UTI)
- Fistula

Diagnosis of bowel anastomotic leak

- Not always obvious
- Should have high index of suspicion in the post-op period
- May be made at laparotomy
- Radiological contrast study/enema/swallow are helpful to visualise leak

Treatment of bowel anastomotic leak

- Resuscitate
- Conservative (nil by mouth, IV fluids, antibiotics, intravenous nutritional support)
- May require radiological drainage
- Surgical repair (may necessitate temporary bypass eg colostomy)

Anastomosis and infection

Bowel preparation

Preparation of the bowel to remove faecal matter and reduce bacterial load has traditionally been performed prior to colorectal surgery. This minimises the flow of intestinal contents past the join in the bowel while the anastomosis heals. It is thought that this reduces rates of anastomotic leakage and infective complications. Interestingly there is no clear advantage shown in recent meta-analyses looking at bowel preparation for elective surgery. The evidence for on-table preparation in the acute situation is less clear.

Bowel preparation is achieved by:

- Emergency procedure: diversion of the stream (eg proximal defunctioning colostomy) or on-table lavage of the proximal colon
- Elective: the bowel is emptied pre-operatively by the use of laxatives and enemas

In recent years, many colorectal surgeons are moving away from routine bowel preparation, however indications vary with each procedure, patient and surgeon. It is always wise to familiarise yourself with each consultant's preference, and be aware of the commonly used bowel preparation regimens. These regimens consist of:

- Clear fluids only the day before surgery
- Repeated oral laxatives (eg two or three spaced doses) of one of the following:
  - Klean-prep™ – polyethylene glycol
  - Fleet™, sodium picosulfate
  - Picolax™ – magnesium sulfate stimulates release of cholecystokinin (CCK) (promotes intestinal motility and thus diarrhoea)
  - Citramag™
- Rectal enema (eg phosphate, Fleet™ micro-enema, Microlax™)

Arguments against bowel preparation

- Quality of bowel preparation may be variable (eg worse in those with chronic constipation)
- Unpleasant for the patient
- Dehydration due to fluid and electrolyte shifts with some agents (may be minimised by oral or IV fluid replacement)
- Contamination in modern procedures with stapled anastomoses is less likely
- The advantage of full bowel preparation in a right hemicolectomy or subtotal colectomy, for example, is not clear, as there will not be any large bowel contents proximal to the anastomosis
- Solid faeces is easier to control than liquid faeces

3.2 BIOPSY

In a nutshell ...

Biopsy is the retrieval of part or all of tissue or organ for histological evaluation to ascertain future management. Options include:

- Fine needle aspiration cytology (FNAC)
- Brush cytology
- Core biopsy
- Endoscopic biopsy
- Incisional biopsy
- Excisional biopsy

Techniques of biopsy

Biopsy is used specifically to:

- Determine tissue diagnosis where clinical diagnosis in doubt (eg Tru-cut liver biopsy for cirrhosis of unknown aetiology)
- Ascertain whether benign or malignant (eg gastric ulcer biopsy)
- Ascertain extent of spread of disease (eg sentinel node biopsy in melanoma)
- Determine different therapeutic pathways (eg lymph node biopsy in lymphoma)
- Excise whole skin lesion for histological analysis and local treatment (eg excision biopsy for rodent ulcer)

Biopsy is merely a form of special investigation and should be interpreted in the light of the clinical picture. Note that biopsy may alter the morphology of a lesion (eg by haemorrhage) and so should be performed AFTER diagnostic imaging wherever possible.

Fine-needle aspiration biopsy for cytology (FNAC)

This is performed by inserting a fine bore needle into a lesion, aspirating cells and performing a smear on a slide to allow cytological examination.

It can be performed:

- Directly into a lump (eg thyroid lump FNAC)
- Under ultrasound control (eg breast lump FNAC)
- Under CT guidance (eg liver lesion FNAC)

Advantages of FNAC

- Simple and minimally invasive
- Easily repeatable
- Cheap

Disadvantages of FNAC

- Gives cytological, but not architectural histology
- Potential for spread of malignant cells
- Sample may be insufficient, or only blood may be aspirated
- May alter morphology of lesion for subsequent imaging
- Depends on expertise of cytologist – may be operator dependent

Procedure box: Fine-needle aspiration for cytology

Use a large syringe (10-mL or 20-mL) and a green needle.

- Fix the mass to be biopsied with your left hand
- Place the needle into the lump and then aspirate creating suction within the syringe
- Retaining the needle tip in the mass make several passes maintaining suction on the syringe
- Release the suction before withdrawing the needle
- Pressure on the biopsy site

Brush cytology

Is performed by collecting exfoliated cells usually using a brush, from intra-luminal lesions and performing a smear on a slide to allow cytological examination.

It can be performed:

- Endoscopically for gastroduodenal lesions
- At ERCP for biliary or pancreatic lesions
- Bronchoscopically for pulmonary or bronchial lesions

Advantages/disadvantages are as for FNAC, except in addition false negatives may occur as the tumour may not be reached, or may not shed sufficient cells.

Core biopsy

Uses a circular cutting device to retrieve a core of tissue, either manually or with a trigger device (Tru-cut, Bioptigun). Core biopsy may be direct, ultrasound or CT controlled. Useful for breast, liver and lymph node biopsy.

Advantages of core biopsy

- Simple, easily repeatable
- Provides a core of tissue architectural and cytological evaluation

Disadvantages of core biopsy

- Insufficient sample for histological examination
- May cause bleeding
- May be painful or distressing to patient
- Potential for spread of malignant cells
- May alter morphology of lesion for subsequent imaging (always image first)

Procedure box: Core biopsy

- Infiltrate with LA
- Make a small incision through the skin (biopsy needle introduced through the incision)
- Take a core of tissue and place in formalin for formal histology
- Press on biopsy site if superficial (eg breast)
- Will require patient to remain supine and undergo at least 6 hours of observation with regular haemodynamic measurements to exclude haemorrhage if deep structure biopsied (eg liver)

Endoscopic biopsy

Used for hollow viscus or organ (eg GI tract, airways, sinuses, bladder, uterus).

Advantages of endoscopic biopsy

- Avoids open surgery

Disadvantages of endoscopic biopsy

- Operator-dependent (lesions may not always be seen or reached)
- Bleeding
- Perforation
- Small samples (malignant areas may be missed)

Incisional biopsy

This is where part of a lesion is removed to allow histological diagnosis.

- May be performed laparoscopically or open
- May be useful when other biopsy techniques have failed
- Performed when the lesion is too big or too fixed to allow complete excision

Excisional biopsy

This is performed when the whole lesion is excised to give histological diagnoses. Usually applies to skin tumours like BCC and melanoma.

Frozen section

Is where fresh tissue is sent for rapid histological assessment, during the course of an operative procedure, to allow therapeutic decisions to be made at the time of surgery. The tissue is frozen in liquid nitrogen then rapidly sectioned and examined, and the result phoned back to the theatre.

Advantages and uses

- Assessment of operability (eg to examine lymph nodes in pancreaticoduodenectomy)
- Localise tissues (eg parathyroids)
- Assessment of tumour margins
- Assessment of malignant status where pre-op diagnosis is in doubt and more radical surgery may be required

Disadvantages

- Operator- and histologist-dependent
- Occasional false positives and false negatives
- May delay surgical procedure

3.3 BASIC PLASTIC SURGERY

Management of traumatic wounds

In a nutshell ...

The principles of managing a traumatic wound are as follows:

- Identify extent and nature of tissue loss
- Debride devitalised tissue
- Identify local and distant tissue sources for reconstruction
- Replace tissue deficits with like tissue
- Follow the reconstructive ladder
- Avoid tension

Tissue loss and tissue viability

Tissue loss can occur for a number of reasons:

- Congenital absence
- Trauma (eg burns, avulsion injury, degloving injury)
- Tumours (eg invasion, ablative tumour surgery with wide margins)
- Infections (eg meningococcal septicaemia, necrotising fasciitis)

Viable tissue can be identified by colour, capillary return and bleeding from the cut edge (colour may sometimes be masked by bruising).

The function of nerves should be identified and documented before administration of LA, if possible.

Under anaesthetic the tissues should be cleaned, debrided if necessary and surviving tissue replaced to its correct anatomic position. It is then possible to assess type and extent of tissue loss.

If there is a large amount of tissue with borderline viability then wounds may be left open with careful observation, undergoing further debridement at a later stage when tissue viability has declared itself. This may require assessment to be performed as a multistep procedure but will preserve as much tissue as possible and may make a significant difference to functionality in the long term.

Principles of debridement

Debridement is the process of removing non-viable tissue from areas of tissue damage such as wounds, burns and ulceration. Non-viable tissue will undergo necrosis allowing bacterial contamination and subsequent infection and abscess formation. These processes will delay wound healing. However, not all wounds need debridement. Sometimes it is better to leave a hardened crust of dead tissue, called an eschar, than to remove it and create an open wound.

The four major debridement techniques are surgical, mechanical, chemical, and autolytic. Increasingly other techniques (eg biological) are being developed.

Surgical debridement ('sharp' debridement)

- Uses scalpel, scissors, or other instrument to cut dead tissue from a wound
- Quick and efficient
- Subjective assessment of tissue viability by the surgeon (it can be performed in stages when the viability of a tissue is in doubt)
- Risk of damage to underlying structures

Mechanical debridement

- Occurs during vigorous cleaning of a wound (eg under anaesthesia)
- May occur on removal of dressings (necrotic tissue adheres to the dressing)

Chemical debridement

- Uses certain enzymes and other compounds to dissolve necrotic tissue
- More selective than mechanical or surgical debridement

A pharmaceutical version of collagenase is available and is highly effective as a debridement agent. Any crust of dead tissue is etched in a cross-hatched pattern to allow the enzyme to penetrate. A topical antibiotic is also applied to prevent introducing infection into the bloodstream. A moist dressing is then placed over the wound.

Autolytic debridement

- Takes advantage of the body's own ability to dissolve dead tissue
- Dressings are used to keep the wound moist and trap wound fluid that contains growth factors, enzymes, and immune cells that promote wound healing
- More selective than any other debridement method, but also takes the longest to work
- It is inappropriate for wounds that have become infected

Biological debridement

- Uses biological agents (eg maggots) to clear the wound area of dead tissue, leaving a healthy base (eg ischaemic ulcers caused by PVD)

Soft tissue reconstruction

The reconstructive ladder

The reconstructive ladder is used as a guide to soft tissue reconstruction. Reconstruction should always take the simplest form (NB bear cosmesis in mind).

- **Secondary intention:** the wound is left to heal from the base upwards. Suitable for small wounds, infected wounds, ischaemic wounds. Scar contracture will close the wound but may cause distortion
- **Primary closure:** direct closure of the wound for the best cosmetic result. Suitable for small, tidy wounds without infection. Not suitable if there is tissue loss (causes tension)
- **Delayed primary closure:** allows a period of secondary intention to bring wound edges together and for any concerns about infection to be resolved. May be speeded up by the use of certain dressings or treatments (eg vac-pack (vacuum suction) or stepwise debridement)

Skin grafting

Skin grafts act as a biological dressing for a de-epithelialised wound. They also provide a cellular source to start the regeneration process by means of autotransplantation.

Skin grafts can be categorised according to the structure of the skin, ie split-skin or full-thickness grafts.

Split-skin grafts (epidermal layer + small part of the dermis only)

The recipient site may not have suffered a full thickness injury – transplantation of epithelial cells alone will be sufficient to cover the deficit. This graft is generated by using a dermatome to shave epidermis from a donor area. The donor site will regenerate its epidermis from the cell islands left behind and the epidermal layer which extends down the hair follicles and sweat glands into the dermis is transferred to the recipient site.

Advantages of split-skin grafts

- Can be processed to cover large areas such as extensive burns
- Very thin, so conform to underlying contours well
- Large number of potential donor areas
- Allow regeneration of donor areas and thus repeated use of the same site
- May take in areas of more marginal blood supply

Disadvantages of split-skin grafts

- Poor cosmetic outcome
- Grafts tend to contract as they heal
- Meshing may be visible in the finished scar
- Poor matching of colour and texture

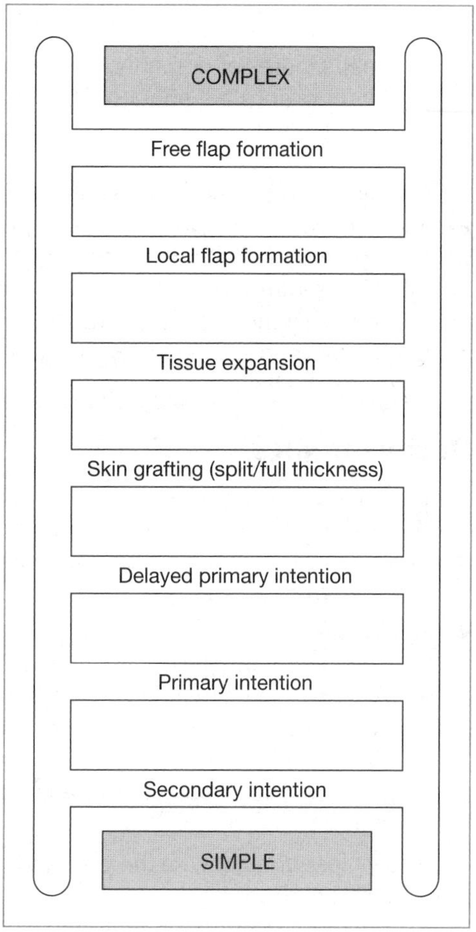

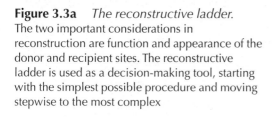

Figure 3.3a *The reconstructive ladder.* The two important considerations in reconstruction are function and appearance of the donor and recipient sites. The reconstructive ladder is used as a decision-making tool, starting with the simplest possible procedure and moving stepwise to the most complex

- Obvious donor-site scarring
- May cause contractures and limit function around joints

Full-thickness grafts (epidermal + dermal components)

The recipient site may have suffered full-thickness tissue loss requiring a full-thickness graft from a donor site. These are usually only used on the face.

Advantages of full-thickness grafts

- Grow with the patient (good for children)
- Better cosmesis
  - Undergo less contracture than split-skin grafts
  - Better colour matching
  - Thinner scars
  - Hair follicles can be transferred (eg in eyebrow replacement)

Disadvantages of full-thickness grafts

- Small ellipses of skin only can be harvested from donor regions
- Donor regions are only used once; they are less painful as can be closed directly
- Need a good vascular supply to take

A donor graft can be 'meshed' using a machine which cuts holes in the graft allowing it to expand to cover an increased area. The perforations allow fluid, blood, and pus to escape which improves the adherence of the graft to the wound. The grafted cells derive nutrients initially from serum at the recipient site and fibrin starts to adhere the graft to the surface of the wound. Alignment of capillaries in the wound and graft ('inosculation') occurs over about 48 hours and subsequently the graft obtains its nutrients via blood flow. This process is called graft 'taking'.

Recipient sites

Recipient sites must be:

- Vascular (avascular structures, such as tendons, cartilage and cortical bone, will not take a graft)
- Free of infection
  - Commensal organisms are allowed
  - Wounds can be treated with antiseptic creams eg silver sulfadiazine
  - Best indication of wound infection comes from wound biopsy rather than a superficial wound swab
  - β-haemolytic *Streptococcus* and large amounts of *Pseudomonas* may lead to graft failure
- Allow close contact with the graft and minimise shearing forces
  - Debride dead tissue
  - Haemostasis is important to prevent haematoma formation
  - Pressure dressings may aid close contact (leave the graft for 5–7 days before removing the dressing)
  - Immobilise the graft while it revascularises

If the skin damage is extensive and there are insufficient donor sites to allow for skin grafting there are other options:

- Donor skin can be stored at 4° C for 1 month, allowing use at a later date
- Cadaveric skin (frozen or preserved with glycerol) is used as a temporary measure and biological dressing; the recipient will eventually reject the transplanted skin but it acts as an aid to future grafts
- Artificial skin is essentially a layered dressing containing collagen fibres and cultured fibroblasts (again it is used to buy time and allow some regeneration of the dermis before definitive grafting can take place)

Research continues into finding methods for culture of autologous cells and production of improved sheets of skin.

Tissue expansion

Can be used to fill defects left by congenital abnormality, surgery, or trauma.

A silastic tissue expander is surgically inserted under fascia or muscle layer on a solid base. The expander is progressively enlarged by injection of saline through an injection port into a reservoir located just under the skin.

Expansion of the skin occurs via skin growth and an increase in epidermal mitotic activity. All other overlying tissues stretch and therefore become thinner. When there is sufficient expansion in the skin and tissues the expander can be removed and the skin mobilised to a local or distant site.

Expanders are available in various volumes ranging from a few mL to several litres. The size of the expander must be large enough to provide the required expansive forces necessary to achieve the desired tissue augmentation.

The shape of the expander depends primarily on the site of expansion and the reconstructive needs. The standard shapes are round, rectangular, or crescent.

Advantages of tissue expansion

- Increases availability of full-thickness skin
- Can be used locally by advancing expanded skin into the defect (an 'advancement flap') often minimising scarring
- Near-perfect matching of colour and texture
- Skin retains its capacity for hair growth (good for covering scalp defects)
- Retains its own vascular and nerve supply

Disadvantages of tissue expansion

- Slow (it takes time for the skin to expand ie 2–4 months)
- Visible bulge of the expander (of benefit in breast reconstruction but very noticeable if used on the scalp, for example)
- Requires repeated visits to inject saline into the reservoir
- Inherent risks of infection around the expander

Flap reconstruction

A flap retains its blood supply through a pedicle of vessels – unlike a graft that generates a new blood supply at the recipient site. Flaps may be local, rotated around their pedicle to a nearby site, or detached and used at a distant site – the 'free flap'. The secondary defect left by raising the flap is often able to be closed by primary intention.

Local flaps

Most small flaps are not designed around a dedicated vessel. Their blood supply is haphazard, supplied by a network of sub-dermal vessels beneath the skin. These are therefore referred to as random pattern flaps. The length of the flap must be shorter than the width of the base of the flap in order to preserve its vascularity and survival.

Z-plasty

This technique overcomes linear shortening or scarring (improves function and cosmesis). Incisions are made as shown in the diagram. As the vertical line of the scar is broken it also becomes cosmetically less obvious.

Z-plasty is used:

- To break up scars forming contractures
- To improve cosmesis by hiding some of the Z-shape in natural lines (eg nasolabial fold)

Transposition flaps

These flaps can be taken at any angle and locally rotated around their base to fill a deficit. They are used to prevent tension or distortion of a wound where there is little spare skin, borrowing the skin to close the deficit from an area nearby where there is excess skin or the scar can be hidden. These are often used in facial reconstruction after trauma or excision of skin cancer.

Axial pattern flaps

Flaps whose base is supplied by a recognised vessel may be significantly longer than the width of that base and still survive. These flaps can be composed of a combination of any tissue supplied by the designated vessel. These flaps may be used locally by rotation around their vascular pedicle, or detached and used as free flaps (eg latissimus dorsi myocutaneous flap is based on the thoracodorsal artery and vein and can be rotated to cover defects of the shoulder, neck and anterior thoracic wall). The pectoralis and rectus abdominus are also used as axial pattern flaps. Large flat muscles are used for transposition as the blood supply is usually from a single named vessel entering the muscle from the periphery.

Free flaps

An axial pattern flap can be detached at its vascular pedicle and transferred to a distant area of the body where its blood supply is reconstructed by microvascular anastomosis to another pedicle. Free flaps are a good alternative to local flaps if there is insufficient tissue locally to fill the deficit, or if using local tissue would further compromise function. Nerve, tendon and bone can be transferred along with muscle and skin to restore function to distant parts of the body (eg radial forearm myocutaneous flaps to reconstruct the mandible).

Successful free-flap reconstruction requires skilled surgeons and experienced nursing care in an ITU setting to monitor flap perfusion and viability.

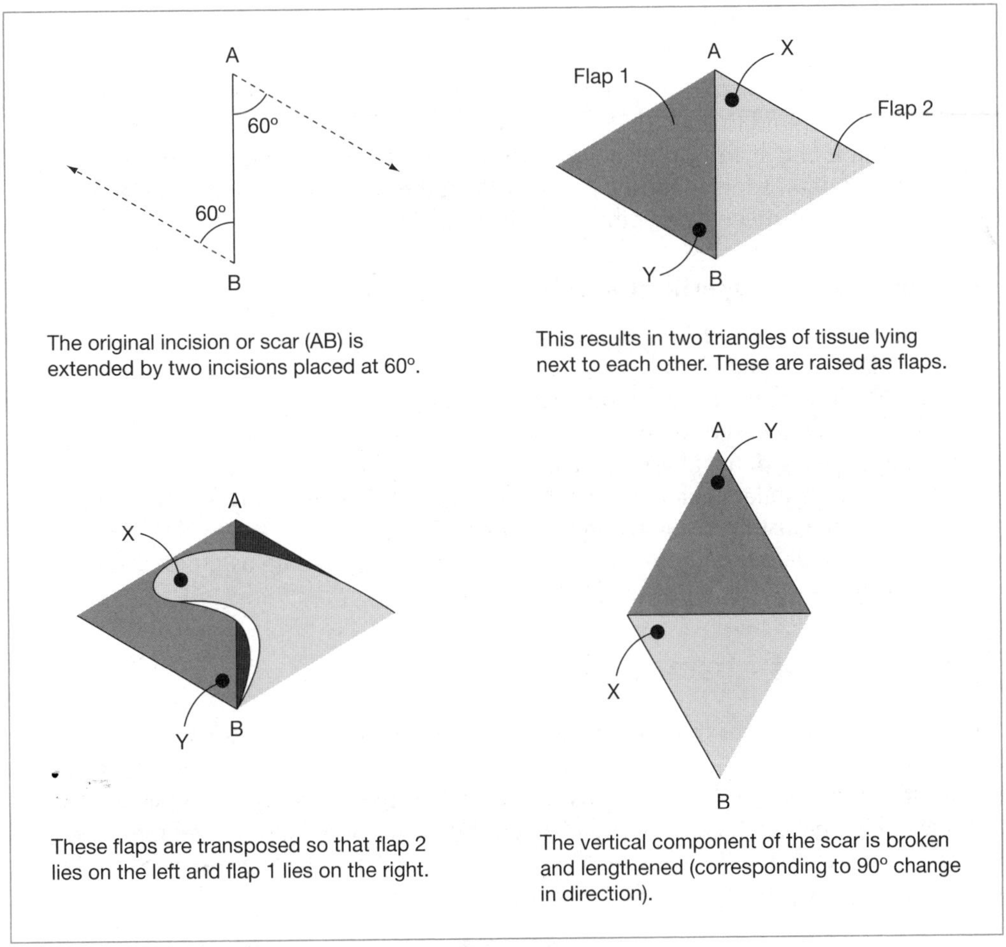
A
60°
60°
B
The original incision or scar (AB) is extended by two incisions placed at 60°.
A
X
Flap 1
Flap 2
Y
B
This results in two triangles of tissue lying next to each other. These are raised as flaps.
A
X
Y
B
These flaps are transposed so that flap 2 lies on the left and flap 1 lies on the right.
A
Y
X
B
The vertical component of the scar is broken and lengthened (corresponding to 90° change in direction).

Figure 3.3b *Z-plasty*

3.4 ABSCESS DRAINAGE

In a nutshell ...

An abscess is a localised collection of pus in a cavity. The cavity may be naturally occurring or caused by tissue destruction or displacement.

If there is pus about, let it out!

Diagnosis of abscesses

Abscess may be difficult to distinguish from cellulitis. The former require surgical drainage, the latter may respond to antibiotics. Abscess may be inferred if the area is pointing or the centre is fluctuant. If in doubt, needle aspiration or US may help. Left alone, many abscesses will drain spontaneously. Pus may track through tissue planes causing the base of the abscess to be much deeper than initially thought.

Common sites for superficial abscesses

- Infection of a pre-existing sebaceous cyst
- Axillary
  - Exclude hidradenitis suppurativa
  - Exclude breast disease
- Anorectal (eg perianal, ischiorectal)
  - Exclude inflammatory bowel disease by rigid sigmoidoscopy +/– biopsy
  - Exclude fistula in ano by proctoscopy
- Groin (beware the femoral pseudoaneurysm masquerading as groin abscess in IV drug users – get an ultrasound before incising it!)

Treatment of abscesses

Superficial skin abscesses may be lanced. Local anaesthetics do not work satisfactorily in inflamed tissue (as the injection is more painful, there is a risk that the needle track will spread the infection, and inflamed tissue has a low pH reducing the dissociation and binding of the anaesthetic compound). Deeper abscesses under the skin require a surgical procedure under GA. Abscesses deep in body cavities may be drained percutaneously under radiological guidance or at open surgery.

Procedure box: Superficial abscess drainage

Indications

Area of fluctuance
Pointing of an abscess
Identification of a superficial collection of pus by imaging
Region (axilla, anorectal, groin)

Patient position

Anaesthetic: the skin may be frozen with ethyl chloride spray or the patient placed under GA
Anorectal abscesses should only be drained under GA as they require thorough colorectal investigation for underlying cause

Positioning should be appropriate to the site of the abscess, thus:

- Perianal and ischiorectal abscesses require the patient to be placed in the lithotomy position
- Axillary abscesses require elevation of the arm

Procedure

Make a cruciate incision over the point of greatest fluctuance (this should be extended into a circular incision once the cavity is defined to de-roof the abscess and allow easier packing)

Release pus (and send for microbiological analysis; targeted antibiotics can then be started if cellulitis persists)

The cavity may be irrigated or curetted down to the base (removes dead tissue)

Gently pack the cavity (eg with gauze ribbon soaked in Betadine™)

NB: Packs are changed frequently until the cavity closes and this is performed initially on the ward and then by the district nurse – it is essential that the incision allows for this to be done with ease. The cavity will granulate from the base regardless of its size but the abscess will recur if its 'roof' (ie the skin) closes before the cavity has healed. Antibiotics are not usually indicated.

Risks

Inadequate drainage (especially loculated abscesses)

Recurrence

Persistent cellulitis (may require antibiotics)

Hazards

Consider the relationship to nearby important structures, for example:

- Anal sphincters in anorectal abscesses
- Cervical and mandibular branches of facial nerve around the jaw
- Femoral vessels in the groin

For a detailed discussion of anorectal abscess, incision and drainage see *Abdomen* chapter in Book 2.

Special cases

- Neck abscesses may be due to simple abscess, furuncle, infected epidermal cysts or branchial cysts, abscess in lymph node, dental abscesses, actinomycosis, or TB (cold abscess). See *Ear, Nose, Throat, Head and Neck* chapter in Book 2. They should be operated on by a suitably experienced surgeon
- Perianal abscesses are usually infection in the anal glands (other causes include fistulas, Crohn's, tumours and HIV). See *Abdomen* chapter in Book 2. An on-table rigid sigmoidoscopy should always be performed

- Breast or axillary abscesses are occasionally related to underlying malignancy. See *Breast* chapter in Book 2. A biopsy should always be sent and follow-up should always be arranged in a breast clinic
- Groin abscesses may be due to suppurating lymph nodes, TB, or psoas abscess (tracking down from the kidney or lumbar spine). An ultrasound scan should be done on anyone at risk of an infected femoral artery aneurysm (such as drug addicts) before incision

3.5 MINIMAL ACCESS SURGERY

In a nutshell ...

Minimal access surgery

Refers to procedures performed through incisions or via orifices, smaller than, or remote from those required for conventional surgery

Conducted by remote manipulation

Carried out within the closed confines of body cavities (laparoscopy, thoracoscopy); lumens of hollow organs (endoluminal or endoscopy) or joint cavities (arthroscopy)

Performed under visual control via telescopes which incorporate the Hopkin's rod–lens system linked to charge-couple device cameras

Types of minimal access surgery

Minimal access surgery includes laparoscopy, endoluminal and arthroscopic approaches.

TYPES OF MINIMAL ACCESS SURGERY WITH EXAMPLES

Laparoscopic	Endoluminal
Lower GI • Rectopexy • Appendicectomy • Hernia repair • Right, left or subtotal colectomy • Anterior resection of rectum • Abdominoperineal resection of rectum and anus	**Vascular** • Angioplasty • Stenting **Upper GI** • ERCP • Stenting strictures of oesophagus or duodenum • Banding varices • Haemostasis of ulcers

TYPES OF MINIMAL ACCESS SURGERY WITH EXAMPLES continued

Laparoscopic	Endoluminal
Gynaecology	**Lower GI**
• Sterilisation	• Colonic stenting
• Investigative laparoscopy	• Polypectomy
Urology	• Banding of haemorrhoids
• Nephrectomy	• TEMS
Upper GI	**Urology**
• Fundoplication	• TURP
• Gastric bypass	• Cytoscopic procedures
• Staging	• Stenting

Advantages and disadvantages of minimal access surgery

Advantages of minimal access surgery

- Less trauma to tissues (smaller wounds, no damage from retraction)
- Reduced post-op pain leading to:
  - Increased mobility (↓ DVT)
  - Improved respiration (↓ chest infections)
  - Reduced need for post-op analgesia (↑ respiration, ↑ bowel function)
  - Decrease in post-op lethargy/mental debilitation
- Decreased cooling and drying of the bowel which may decrease intestinal function and threaten anastomosis; more marked in elderly and children
- Decreased retraction and handling which causes iatrogenic injury and tissue compression leading to decreased perfusion and bowel function
- Reduced adhesions
- Fewer wound complications (eg infection, dehiscence, hernia formation)
- Reduced risk of Hep B and AIDS transmission
- Improved cosmesis
- Better view on monitors for teaching purposes
- Short hospital stay (laparoscopia cholecystectomies can be done as a day case, laparoscopic bowel resections can be discharged on day 4)
- Quicker return to normal activities/shorter rehabilitation

Disadvantages of minimal access surgery

- Lack of tactile feedback
- Problems controlling bleeding
- Needs more technical expertise and thus longer learning curve
- Longer operation times in some cases
- Significant increase in iatrogenic injuries to other organs (may not be seen) eg CBD in lap cholecystectomy
- Difficulty removing bulky organs

- Expensive to buy and maintain cameras, monitors, laparoscopic instruments and disposables
- May be impractical due to previous adhesions or contraindications

Contraindications to laparoscopic surgery

Contraindications for laparoscopy

- Patient refusal
- Unsuitable for GA
- Uncontrollable haemorrhagic shock
- Surgical inexperience
- Gross ascites

Increased risk during laparoscopic surgery*

- Gross obesity
- Pregnancy
- Multiple previous abdominal surgery with adhesions
- Organomegaly (eg spleen or liver)
- Abdominal aortic aneurysm
- Peritonitis
- Bowel distension
- Bleeding disorders

*It used to be thought that the conditions listed here were contraindications to laparoscopy. However, with increasing expertise and use of laparoscopic techniques, many of these patients can be safely operated on by an experienced laparoscopic surgeon.

Equipment for minimal access surgery

All laparoscopic procedures require:

- **Imaging system**
  - Video monitor
  - Light source
  - Camera system
  - At least one video monitor should be positioned for ease of viewing by the surgeon, surgical assistant and the scrub nurse. This may be linked to a method for recording the procedure either by means of photographic images or video. A second or 'slave' monitor is often helpful for the assistant who may be positioned opposite the surgeon
- **Insufflation device**
  - Insufflates the abdominal cavity from a compressed gas cylinder
  - Maximum rate of insufflation and end intra-abdominal pressure can be set by the surgeon (these settings are maintained by the machine throughout the procedure)

- **Gas**
  - Gas used in most abdominal laparoscopic surgery is carbon dioxide (CO_2) although it can lead to hypercardia and acidosis in those with chronic lung disease
  - Helium is a rarely used alternative
- **Energy source**
- **Specialised instruments**

Principles of minimal access surgery

Establishing a pneumoperitoneum

Procedure box: How to establish a pneumoperitoneum

There are two accepted methods: open (Hassan) or closed (Verress). The open method is preferred by the Royal College. The Verress method is safe in experienced hands.

Indications
Abdominal laparoscopic surgery

Patient preparation and position
Supine patient; usually GA and muscle relaxation
Prep and drape anterior abdominal wall for open surgery

Procedure
Small sub-umbilical incision with scalpel through the skin, then:

EITHER: Open (Hassan) method

- Dissect to the linea alba and incise it
- Grasp the peritoneum with forceps and incise it to reveal the peritoneal cavity
- Insert a port using a blunt trocar through the hole
- Pass a camera into the port to confirm the peritoneal cavity has been entered
- Insufflate with 2–3 litres of CO_2 to a final pressure of 15 mmHg
- Subsequent ports can be inserted with a sharp trocar under camera vision

OR: Closed (Verress) method

- Introduce Verress needle (spring-loaded needle with blunt probe) through tented abdominal wall (you will feel two characteristic 'pops' as it passes through the fascia and then the peritoneum)
- Confirm position by aspirating on the needle and then flushing the needle with normal saline. Place a drop of saline on the end of the needle and elevate the abdominal wall (when abdominal wall is lifted this creates decreased intra-abdominal pressure sucking the saline into the intra-abdominal cavity)

- Insufflate with 2–3 litres of CO_2 to a final pressure of 15 mmHg
- Place the first port now by introducing a sharp trocar blindly through a small skin incision assuming that the pneumoperitoneum will have established a safe distance between the internal organs and the abdominal wall
- After inserting the camera, subsequent ports can be inserted with a sharp trocar under camera vision

Risks

Early risks

- Iatrogenic damage to intra-abdominal organs or vessels (rates ~ 0.05% visceral injury and < 0.01% vascular injury)
- Venous gas embolism (rare)
- Conversion to open procedure

Late risks

- Post-op abdominal or shoulder tip pain (minimised by meticulous irrigation and evacuation of gas from the peritoneal cavity – carbonic acid is formed by combination of the CO_2 and water and acts as an irritant)
- Port-site herniation (mid-line most common)

Hazards

- Placement of ports
- Avoid known intra-abdominal hazards (eg pregnant uterus, previous scars or adhesions, aortic aneurysm, hepatomegaly)
- Avoid vessels of the anterior abdominal wall. The inferior epigastric artery runs from the mid inguinal point upwards and medially to a point 2 cm infero-lateral to the umbilicus (see Fig. 3.5a in Chapter 1 of Book 2) and should be avoided when placing iliac fossa ports

Physiological consequences of a pneumoperitoneum

Laparoscopic surgery induces multiple physiological responses in the patient due to:

- Mechanical effects of elevated intra-abdominal pressure due to insufflation of gas (eg decreased venous return)
- Positioning of the patient to extreme positions (eg head down)
- Absorption of CO_2 and biochemical changes

Physiological changes include:

- ↑ or ↓ changes in cardiac output
- ↑ systemic and pulmonary vascular resistance
- ↑ mean arterial pressure (MAP)

- ↑ central venous pressure (CVP)
- ↑ or ↓ venous return
- ↑ or ↓ heart rate
- ↑ partial pressure of CO_2 (pCO_2)
- ↑ peak inspiratory pressure (due to increased intra-thoracic pressure)
- ↓ urine output

Prolonged pneumoperitoneum may cause large volumes of CO_2 to be absorbed, and this overwhelms the buffering capacity of the blood – causing acidosis. If severe the pneumoperitoneum must be evacuated to allow the CO_2 to wash out of the system. Arrhythmias are relatively common although there is more likely to be a problem in those with less cardiovascular reserve (eg elderly patients) and in very prolonged procedures. There is a degree of venous stasis in the lower limbs induced by the elevated intra-abdominal pressure and so DVT prophylaxis is essential.

Placement of laparoscopic ports

Fig. 3.5a shows a few examples of typical placement of laparoscopic ports, however these vary from surgeon to surgeon – there is no 'correct' position. The basic principles are:

- There should be as few ports as possible to do the procedure safely
- Positioning should allow triangulation of the instruments at the operating site. In practice this means that the ports should form a diamond with the target organ at one apex and the camera at the other and one instrument port either side for optimum triangulation and minimum fatigue and contortion; the surgeons' operating hands should be about 10 cm apart with the camera between and behind them, and the table should be low enough to avoid elevating the surgeon's elbows
- Patient positioning should allow a good view of all the areas that need to be inspected (eg tilted head down to view pelvic organs in female appendicectomy, tilted head up and with the right side elevated for cholecystectomy); using gravity in this way reduces the requirement for intra-abdominal retractors which may otherwise necessitate being placed out of the camera view (increasing the risk of iatrogenic damage)
- A 5-mm port should be used if possible although some 10 mm ports are necessary – usually for the camera, removal of organs (eg the gall bladder) or certain larger instruments
- Placement should avoid known hazards (see Procedure box above)

Closure of laparoscopic port sites

Many surgeons will require that 10-mm ports are closed in layers, including closure of the rectus sheath/linea alba with slowly absorbable or non-absorbable interrupted sutures. This prevents port-site hernias. Skin hooks can be used to facilitate a good view of the fascial defect through the small incision. Skin can be closed with skin staples, non-absorbable or absorbable sutures, glue or Steri-strips™. 5-mm port sites usually only require skin closure.

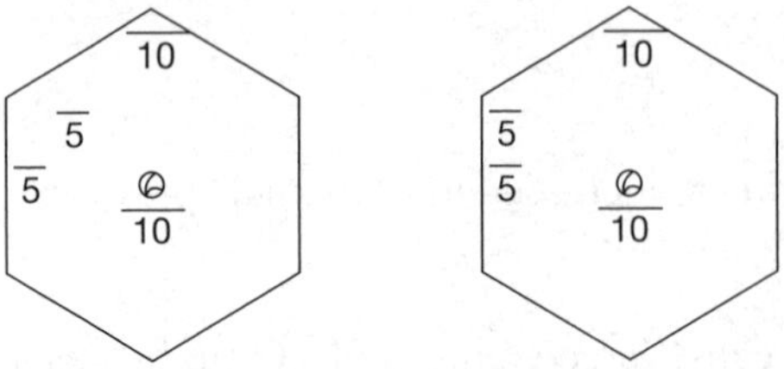

Europe technique

Laparoscopic cholecystectomy: the 10-mm port is inserted in the epigastrium and under the umbilicus for the camera. The placement of 5-mm ports varies with individual preference (common siting shown).

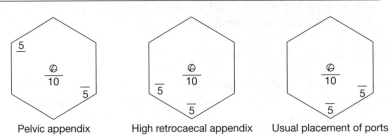

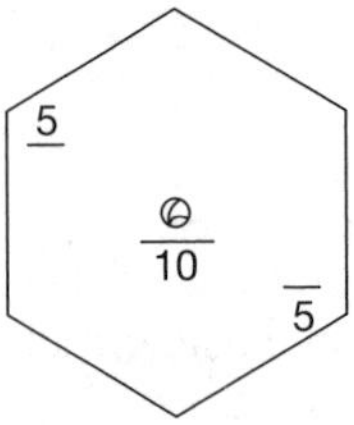

Pelvic appendix

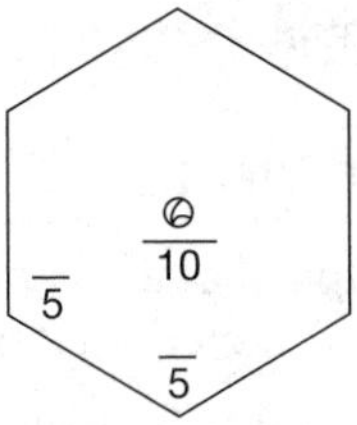

High retrocaecal appendix

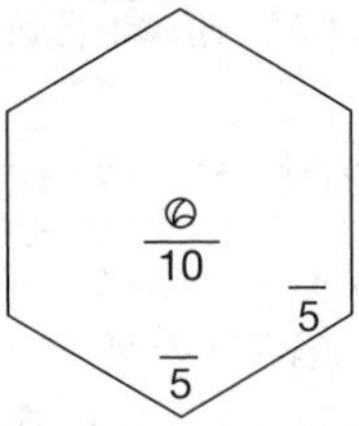

Usual placement of ports

Laparoscopic appendicectomy: the 10-mm port is inserted under the umbilicus for the camera. The first 5-mm port is inserted in the left iliac fossa or the suprapubic region and is used to retract the bowel and allow visualisation of the inflamed appendix. The second 5-mm port is inserted in the right upper quadrant (for pelvic appendix) or in the right iliac fossa (for high retrocaecal appendix). Again, placement of ports varies with the surgery.

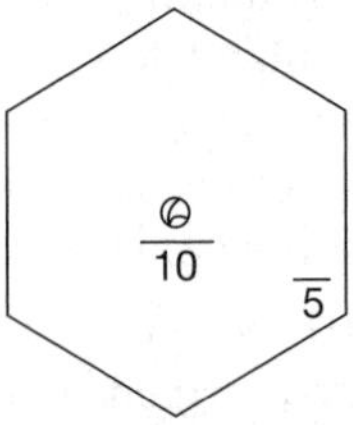

Pelvic diagnostic laparoscopy

Diagnostic laparoscopy: the 10-mm port is inserted under the umbilicus for the camera and a 5-mm port may be sited in the left iliac fossa for the use of instruments to aid organ retraction. A full systematic intra-abdominal inspection must be completed. Further ports can be sited appropriately if pathology is identified.

Figure 3.5a *Port-site insertion for laparoscopic surgery*

Section 4
Tumours and lesions of the skin and subcutaneous tissues

In a nutshell ...

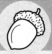

Tumours of the skin can be categorised as follows:

Benign conditions
- Cysts
- Fibroma
- Papilloma
- Haemangioma
- Moles and naevi
- Hidradenitis suppurativa

Pre-malignant conditions
- Keratocanthoma
- Intra-epidermal neoplasia

Malignant tumours
- BCC
- SCC
- Malignant melanoma

4.1 BENIGN SKIN LESIONS

Cysts

- All age groups (rare in children)
- Slow growing and usually asymptomatic (may be unsightly or catch on the hairbrush when in the scalp)
- Become enlarged, red, painful and can discharge offensive purulent contents when infected

Types of cyst

- Epidermal or sebaceous cysts
- Trichilemmal cysts
- Pilar cysts
- Dermoid cysts
  - Congenital dermoid cysts
  - Acquired/implantation dermoid cysts

Epidermal cysts or sebaceous cysts

- Found in the hair-bearing parts of the body (especially scalp, scrotum, neck, shoulders and back)
- Occur wherever there are sebaceous glands (so not the palms of the hands or soles of the feet)
- Vary from a few mm to > 4 cm in diameter
- Arise from infundibular portion of hair follicles
- Histologically comprised of keratinous debris lined by keratinising squamous epithelium with a granular layer

Complications of epidermal cysts

- Infection
- Discharge of foul smelling, cheesy contents
- Malignant change has been reported but is extremely rare
- Multiple cysts occur in Gardener's syndrome

Treatment of epidermal cysts

- Complete surgical removal of entire cyst and its contents intact with an ellipse of overlying skin
- Recurrence occurs if even a small portion of the cyst lining is left behind

Trichilemmal cysts

- Clinically identical to epidermal cysts but not as common
- Genetic predisposition (autosomal dominant)
- 90% on scalp; 70% multiple

Pathology of trichilemmal cysts

- Derived from hair follicle epithelium
- Lined by epithelial cells (do not have the granular layer which characterises epidermal cysts)

Treatment is as for epidermal cyst.

They can be complicated by calcification (not seen in epidermal cysts).

Pilar cysts (pilar tumours)

- Proliferation of epithelium lining cyst
- Ulceration and proliferation: may resemble SCC (Pott's peculiar tumour)
- Malignant transformation is reported but rare
- Treatment is as for epidermal cyst

Dermoid cysts

These are cysts, deep to the skin, that are lined by skin. Skin can become trapped in the subcutaneous tissues either during fetal development (congenital dermoid cyst) or following an injury that forces skin into the deeper subcutaneous tissues (acquired/implantation dermoid cyst). Lined by stratified squamous epithelium but unlike epidermal (sebaceous) cysts, the wall also contains functioning epidermal appendages such as hair follicles, sweat and sebaceous glands.

Congenital dermoid cysts

Occur at sites of fusion of skin dermatomes, typically:

- Lateral and medial ends of the eyebrow (external and internal angular dermoid)
- Mid-line of the nose (nasal dermoid)
- Sublingually
- Mid-line of the neck
- Any point in the mid-line of the trunk (typically the perineum and sacrum)

Complications:

- May create a bony depression
- May penetrate down to the dura
- A nasal dermoid may look like a small superficial pit but may be an extensive cyst that passes between the nasal bones towards the sphenoid sinus

Treatment:

- Rarely troublesome and rarely get infected so can be left alone
- Need experienced surgeon in case of deep extension

Acquired/implantation dermoid cysts

- Occur in areas subject to repeated trauma (eg fingers)
- Commonly confused with a sebaceous cyst (note presence of a scar and history of an old injury)
- Tend to be troublesome, interfere with function, and can become painful and tender
- Rarely infected
- Management: excision

Fibromata

Dermatofibroma

Also called fibrous histiocytoma or sclerosing haemangioma.

- Can occur in any adult but more common in young and middle-aged women
- More common on the limbs
- Benign neoplasm of the fibroblasts of the dermis with normal overlying epidermis
- Histologically some are cellular (histiocytes), some are fibrous (fibroblasts and collagen), some are angiomatous
- Histiocytomata are covered in normal epidermis but can become pigmented to a brown colour due to haemosiderin deposition. May also be pink
- Treatment: do not resolve spontaneously; treated by excision

Neurofibroma

- Benign tumour containing a mixture of neural (ectodermal) and fibrous (mesodermal) elements
- They are hamartomas (overgrowth of cell types normally found in that organ) and are often multiple
- Symptoms: most neurofibromata cause no discomfort; subcutaneous neurofibromata related to a nerve trunk may be tender and may lead to parasthesia or dysasthesia in the distribution of the affected nerve
- Complications: nerve damage (including spinal cord and cranial nerves, typically the acoustic nerve)
- Malignant transformation in von Recklinhausen's disease (below)
- Treatment: excision is tricky due to the non-encapsulated diffuse nature of the lesions, the risk of bleeding and problems with nerve involvement; re-growth is common

Von Recklinghausen's disease

Autosomal dominant condition defined as multiple congenital familial neurofibromatosis. Most of the neurofibromata are present at birth but they increase in size and number during life. Associated with:

- Fibroepithelial skin tags
- Café-au-lait patches (light brown skin discoloration) – six or more of > 1.5 cm in diameter is pathognomic but 30% of von Recklinhausen's disease will have no café-au-lait spots
- Neuromas on major nerves especially acoustic neuromas and dumb-bell neuromas on the sensory roots of the spinal nerves
- Malignant change (neurofibrosarcoma) in 5–13% of von Recklinhausen patients but not generally seen in spontaneous neurofibromata; usually arises from large nerve trunks and carries a poor prognosis
- Phaeochromocytoma
- Scoliosis, intracranial anomalies and mental retardation

Plexiform neurofibroma

- Extremely rare condition involving excessive overgrowth of neural tissue in the subcutaneous fat
- Looks like oedema but the lymphatics are normal
- Called elephantitis neurofibromatosis due to the gross deformity, often of the hand or foot

Papilloma

Papilloma is a broad term that encapsulates several pathologies including skin tags, seborrhoeic keratosis and warts.

Benign papilloma

- Simple overgrowth of all layers of the skin – it is not a benign neoplasm – it is a skin tag
- Can be single, pigmented or sessile
- Can occur at any age but more frequent with advancing age
- Also known as fibroepithelial papilloma or soft fibroma
- Complications: can catch on clothes, and may become injured, infected, red, swollen, ulcerated or infarct (spontaneous ulceration rare)
- Treatment is simple excision with a pair of sharp scissors under a LA (occasionally a single suture is needed to control bleeding from the feeding vessel)

Seborrhoeic keratosis

Also known as senile wart, seborrhoeic wart, verruca senilis, basal cell papilloma.

- Benign overgrowth of the basal layer of the epidermis containing an excess of small, dark staining basal cells
- Occur in both sexes and are more common in the elderly (almost ubiquitous in those aged > 70)
- Become more prominent and are often multiple if the skin is not regularly and firmly washed (hence they are common in inaccessible areas such as the backs of elderly patients)
- Colour varies from normal skin colour to grey or brown
- Appear as raised plates of hypertrophic greasy skin with a distinct edge and a rough, papilleforous surface; the distinguishing feature is that they can be picked or scraped off leaving a pale pink patch of skin which may bleed
- Generally do not need treatment but if they catch on clothes or become a nuisance they are easily scraped off; if infected they can look like a pyogenic granuloma, epithelioma, or malignant melanoma

Warts

- Patches of hyperkeratotic overgrown skin (growth has been stimulated by the presence of a papilloma virus)
- Commonest in children and young adults and may be present for months
- Most typically on hands or feet (verrucas) but also occur on the knees, face and arms
- Greyish brown, hemispherical, only a few mm in diameter and frequently multiple
- They have a rough, hyperkeratotic surface and are hard and non-compressible
- Verrucas (plantar warts) look slightly different because they are pushed into the skin, causing a 'punched out' appearance of a pit containing a wart, surrounded by hardened, thickened, tender skin

Haemangioma

Haemangioma are hamartomas – an overgrowth of a cell type normally found in that organ. A haemangioma (or vascular naevus) is an abnormal proliferation of the embryonic vascular network. Most display arterial, venous and lymphatic elements. Angiogenic and hormonal factors may be responsible.

They are more common in females. They occur in 1–2.6% of newborns, 20% of whom have more than one lesion. All types may ulcerate and induce hyperkeratosis in the overlying stratum corneum. They hardly ever undergo malignant change.

Types of haemangioma

Strawberry naevus

Also known as congenital intradermal haemangioma or cavernous haemangioma. A bright red, lobulated lesion which stands proud of the skin and does, indeed, look like a strawberry. Formed by a capillary network of capillaries radiating from an artery. Present at birth, they often regress spontaneously within months or years. It is not associated with any other congenital vascular malformation apart from other haemangiomata.

Pyogenic granuloma

Common benign tumours arising from the skin vasculature often at the site of trauma. Found most commonly on the palmar surface of the fingers. May also be seen occasionally at the edges of slowly healing surgical wounds.

Port wine stain

Also known as naevus vingus or intradermal haemangioma. A congenital extensive collection of dilated venules and capillaries just below the epidermis. It is similar in histology to the strawberry naevus but does not stick out from the surface of the skin. It also does not tend to regress as the baby grows, but may fade in colour. Common on the face and at the junction between the limbs and the trunk and are very noticeable and disfiguring due to the deep purple-red colour. Occasionally, small vessels within the stain become prominent and bleed. It may present as part of a more extensive vascular abnormality or a syndrome such as the Sturge–Weber syndrome. Sturge–Weber syndrome is a port wine stain in the distribution of the 1st +/– 2nd division of the trigeminal nerve associated with ipsilateral intracranial haemangiomata and a history of epilepsy and/or mental retardation. In general, however, there are never any associated neurological abnormalities and the main symptom is deformity.

Vin rose patch

Also known as salmon patch or naevus flammeus neanatorum. Another congenital intradermal haemangioma in which mild dilatation of the subpapillary dermal plexus gives the skin a pale pink colour. It is often associated with other vascular abnormalities such as extensive haemangiomata, giant limbs due to arteriovenous fistulae, and lymphoedema. The vin rose patch can occur anywhere and causes no symptoms. Unlike the port wine stain it is not dark enough to be disfiguring and has often been accepted by the patient as a birthmark and forgotten about.

Spider naevus

A solitary dilated skin arteriole feeding a number of small branches which leave it in a radial manner. It is an acquired condition and is often associated with a pathological condition such as liver disease. In general > 5 are pathological.

Telangiectasis

A dilation of normal capillaries. Tends to arise after irradiation. Occurs on internal mucosal surfaces as well as the skin, and can lead to GI haemorrhage, epistaxis, haematuria and intracerebral haemorrhage.

Hereditary haemorrhagic telangiectasia (Osler–Weber–Rendu syndrome)

A Mendelian dominant genetic condition with incomplete penetrance affecting 1–2 per 100 000. Tiny capillary haemangiomas scattered over mucus membranes and skin give rise to bleeding (haematemesis, melena, haematuria) and iron-deficiency anaemia. The patient has telangiectasia on the face, around the mouth, on the lips and tongue, the fingers, and the buccal and nasal mucosa. In some variants pulmonary arteriovenous aneurysms are common and increase in frequency with age (as do the telangiectases). Telangiectasia of the face also occurs in the CREST syndrome of calcinosis, Raynaud's syndrome, oesophagitis, sclerodactyly and telangiectasia.

Campbell de Morgan spot

Very common, well defined, uniformly brilliantly red capillary naevus of 2–3 mm in diameter. Develops on the trunk in middle age. No clinical significance.

Treatment of haemangioma

Apart from the strawberry naevus and the port wine stain, patients with the haemangiomata described above do not often seek treatment.

Reassurance and awaiting natural regression is the best line of management initially for the strawberry naevus, as premature treatment may lead to scarring that natural regression will not. Large, ulcerating or persistent lesions may need treatment which is difficult and controversial. Cryotherapy, laser photocoagulation, radiotherapy, sclerosants, electrolysis, steroids and excision with reconstruction have all been used. The port wine stain may fade but does not tend to regress, and many of the above methods have been used, with laser therapy currently the treatment of choice for most specialists. It is usually combined with conservative methods like camouflage creams.

Moles and naevi

There are several pathologies causing a brown blemish on the skin.

- **Freckle:** normal number of melanocytes in their normal position, each producing excess melanin
- **Lentigo:** increased number of melanocytes in their normal position, each producing normal quantities of melanin
- **Mole/pigmented naevus:** increased number of melanocytes in abnormal clusters at the dermo-epidermal junction, each producing normal or excess quantities of melanin. There are four microscopic types of pigmented naevus:
  - Intradermal melanoma or naevus: common mole; light or dark; flat or warty; hairy mole is nearly always intradermal; found everywhere except palm of hand, sole of foot or scrotal skin
  - Compound melanoma or naevus: clinically indistinguishable from intradermal naevus but histologically it has junctional elements which make it potentially malignant
  - Juvenile melanoma: melanomas before puberty are relatively unusual; microscopically they may be indistinguishable from malignant melanoma but usually pursue benign course
  - Junctional melanoma or naevus: pigmented variably light brown to black; flat, smooth, and hairless; may occur anywhere, including (unlike intradermal) palm, sole and genitalia; histologically, naevus cells seen in basal layers of the epidermis as well as in dermis; only a small percentage of junctional naevi undergo malignant change, but it is from this group that the vast majority of malignant melanomas arise
- **Dysplastic naevus:** a pigmented naevus with nuclear abnormalities but no invasion

- **Malignant melanoma:** a mole with signs of abnormal and excessive multiplication or invasion of adjacent tissues
- **Café-au-lait patches:** see neurofibromatosis
- **Circumoral moles:** of Peutz–Jeghers syndrome

Types of mole

There are several clinical varieties of mole.

- **Hairy mole:** always intradermal naevi; contain sebaceous glands which may become infected
- **Non-hairy mole:** may be intradermal, junctional or compound naevi
- **Blue naevus:** uncommon mole deep in the dermis with smooth overlying skin; seen in children
- **Hutchinson lentigo:** a large area of pigmentation that commonly appears in those aged > 60 on the face and neck and is slow growing; mainly smooth, but may develop rough areas of junctional activity which are at increased risk of malignant change
- **Congenital giant naevus**
- **Spitz naevus:** also called juvenile melanoma and can be difficult to distinguish from malignant melanoma; seen as a pink nodule often on the cheek; may grow quickly, persist and become indolent or regress

Treatment of moles

Most Caucasians have 15–20 moles. They do not need excision unless they are disfiguring, a nuisance in some way (eg catching on clothes) pre-malignant (eg Hutchinson lentigo, congenital giant naevus) or develop any suspicious changes (see *Malignant melanoma* in section 4.7).

Signs of malignant change in a mole

Increase or irregularity in size or pigmentation
Bleeding or ulceration
Itching, pain or altered sensation
Spread of pigment from the edge of the tumour
Formation of daughter nodules
Enlarged regional lymph nodes or distant metastases

Hidradenitis suppurativa

An infection of the apocrine sweat glands seen most often in the axillae and groins of Caucasians living in tropical countries. Can be associated with an underlying systemic disease such as diabetes. The condition is chronic and recurring. Many are sterile on culture. The severity of the disease varies from a single abscess which responds to incision and drainage to widespread watering-can sinuses that necessitate radical excision and skin grafting. Despite often having a negative culture, long-term oral metronidazole is commonly used to control flare-ups.

Related conditions include:

- Acne conglobata: affects back, buttocks and chest
- Perifolliculitis capitis: affects the scalp
- Hyperhydrosis: covered in Chapter 9 *Vascular*

Hidradenoma

Hidradenoma is a benign tumour of a sweat gland, which is rare, occurring from middle-age onwards, and frequently multiple and disfiguring (known as a turban tumour); they are soft and non-tender and feel like cysts but do not fluctuate as they are solid; malignant change is rare.

4.2 EXCISION OF BENIGN SKIN LESIONS

In a nutshell ...

Many skin and subcutaneous lumps can be left alone. Reasons for consideration of excision are:

- Diagnosis (when histology required; eg risk of malignancy)
- Pain
- Enlargement (small lesions are easier to excise than large)
- Infection (eg in-growing toenail)
- Cosmesis

Excision techniques

Many skin and subcutaneous lumps can be removed using LA. Skin lesions are best excised with elliptical incisions around the lesion. Subcutaneous lesions may be excised through linear incisions over the lesion. (Remember that epidermal cysts are skin lesions and are best excised with elliptical incisions including the punctum.) Incisions should be along or parallel to Langer's lines, tension lines, or skin creases.

Benign lesions can be excised with small margins of about 1 mm. Malignant lesions require bigger margins of 5–10 mm for basal cell carcinomata or squamous cell carcinomata, depending on the site. Margins for excision of malignant melanomata are discussed in section 4.7. It is sometimes necessary to excise superficial melanoma with a margin of 2–3 mm, and be prepared to return for wider excision depending on the histology and thickness of the lesion.

Closure can be with subcuticular, continuous or interrupted suture, or with glue or Steri-strips™. Closure may be easier if the edges are undermined to relieve tension or if a long thin elliptical incision is used. Infected wounds (eg after infected sebaceous cyst) may be left open, or closure delayed.

Complications of excision

- Incomplete excision (may lead to recurrence)
- Infection
- Dehiscence
- Scarring (including hypertrophic scars and keloid)
- Damage to surrounding structures (especially nerves with a subcutaneous course) – BEWARE
    - Facial nerve (area of the parotid)
    - Mandibular branch of facial nerve (area of the submandibular gland and jaw line)
    - Greater auricular nerve (area of parotid gland)
    - Lateral popliteal nerve (area of neck of the fibula)
    - Spinal accessory nerve (posterior triangle of the neck)

Diagnosis of a suspicious skin lesion

Any changing or new lesion not diagnosed clinically should be referred for a specialist opinion, or an excision biopsy should be performed for histopathological examination. The excision biopsy should always involve complete excision of the lesion, including full thickness of the skin with a 2-mm lateral clearance margin. Incomplete, wedge, or incision biopsies may be tempting in large lesions in cosmetically difficult areas but should never be carried out by a non-specialist because they may miss malignant foci in the lesion and because important diagnostic features involving the margins of the lesion are not available to the pathologist in these specimens.

Special considerations for excision of any lesion

- **Specialist referral:** if the histology turns out to be malignant, specialist opinion should be sought for several reasons:
    - The scar must be excised with adequate margins, which may need reconstructive surgery
    - Lymph node dissection may be necessary (eg in clinically node-positive patients and in some clinically node-negative patients such as men with intermediate-thickness lesions of the trunk, or young patients with tumours that are 1–2-mm thick)
    - Radiotherapy may be required (eg in desmoplastic melanomas or as an option for local BCC)
    - Appropriate follow-up and management of any recurrence must be arranged

- Lesions in difficult anatomic positions may need specialist techniques. For example:
  - Lesions close to the eye by ophthalmic surgeons
  - Lesions on the face by plastic surgeons
- Children may require GA

4.3 CURETTAGE AND CRYOSURGERY

In a nutshell ...

Curettage is a process by which a lesion is scraped off the surrounding skin.

Cryosurgery is a process by which extremes of temperature are applied to a lesion to produce targeted cell death.

Curettage

The lesion is infiltrated with LA and then shaved off using a metal curette (shaped like a shallow spoon with sharp edges). It can be applied to skin lesions that are either softer than the surrounding tissue or that have a natural plane between the lesion and the skin.

Curettage shavings should be sent for histology. This method gives no information as to the completion of the excision. It results in a shallow wound which is often additionally cauterised to kill tumour cells. There is typically less scarring than by surgical excision.

It is suitable for:

- Seborrhoeic keratoses
- Viral warts
- Bowen's disease (in-situ SCC)
- Pyogenic granuloma
- Solar keratoses
- BCCs
- Keratoacanthoma
- Skin tags

Cryosurgery

Cryosurgery is the use of the freezing process to produce targeted cell death. Cell damage occurs by direct freezing of the tissue, disruption of small vessels causing local ischaemia and osmotic change that causes cell lysis during thawing.

It may be used for superficial skin lesions including superficial tumours (eg BCC) and warts, and also for tumours inside the body cavity (eg liver).

Cryotherapy using liquid nitrogen (temperature – 196° C) involves the use of a cryospray, cryoprobe or a cotton-tipped applicator. The nitrogen is applied to the skin lesion for a few seconds, depending on the desired diameter and depth of freeze. A cryoprobe will form an ice ball which reaches – 35° C. The treatment is repeated in some cases, once thawing has completed. This is known as a 'double freeze–thaw' and is usually reserved for skin cancers or resistant viral warts.

Carbon dioxide cryotherapy involves making a cylinder of frozen carbon dioxide snow (–78.5° C) or a slush combined with acetone. It is applied directly to the skin lesion.

Advantages of cryosurgery

- Cheap and quick
- Minimal scarring
- Repeated treatments are possible

Disadvantages of cryosurgery

- Painful
- Causes blistering, swelling and redness of the treated area
- Pigment changes common
- Tissue obliterated so histology unavailable

Complications of cryosurgery in body cavities

- Warm blood flow protects cells (so not suitable for treatment near large vessels)
- Leakage of liquid nitrogen from cracked probes can cause air embolism

4.4 PRE-MALIGNANT SKIN CONDITIONS

In a nutshell ...

Pre-malignant skin conditions include:

Keratocanthoma

Intra-epithelial neoplasia: Bowen's disease, squamous carcinoma in situ (solar keratosis)

Keratocanthoma

Also known as adenoma sebaceum, molluscum pseudocarcinomatosum, molluscum sebaceum.

- **Definition:** a self-limiting overgrowth of hair follicle cells producing a central plug of keratin with subsequent spontaneous regression. Cause unknown – may be self-limiting benign neoplasm or an unusual response to infection
- **Epidemiology:** occurs in adults. Takes 2–4 weeks to grow, 2–3 months to regress. Normally single lesions. More common in males
- **Presentation:** usually occurs on the face. The central core is hard and eventually separates. The lump collapses leaving a deep indrawn scar. Often mistaken for SCC (unlike a keratoacanthoma, SCC grows slower, does not have a dead central core, and gradually becomes an ulcer)
- **Treatment:** should be excised to confirm diagnosis and to prevent depressed scar. Rarely undergoes transformation to SCC

Intra-epithelial neoplasia

Bowen's disease (carcinoma in situ)

A pre-malignant intra-epidermal carcinoma. Appears as slow-growing, thickened brown or pink well-defined plaque. Flat papular clusters covered with crusts. It can look like eczema, and can occur on any part of the body especially the trunk. It is not usually associated with sun damage. A small proportion progress to SCC. Microscopically it is full-thickness dysplasia of the epidermis. Erythroplasia of Queyrat is Bowen's disease of the glans penis. Treatment is excision with a minimum 0.5-cm margin.

Solar keratosis (squamous cell carcinoma in situ)

Resulting from solar damage to the skin and hyperkeratosis of the skin. Usually found in old weather-beaten men (eg farmers) on the backs of fingers and hands, face and helix of the ears. The skin is usually yellow, grey or has brown crusty patches from which arise protruding plaques of horny skin. 25% progress to SCC if untreated. Histologically there is hyperkeratosis and epidermal dysplasia. Unlike Bowen's disease there is dermal collagen damage. The treatment is excision, shaving, cryotherapy or topical application of 5-FU chemotherapy. Developing tethering, fixity, or regional enlarged lymph nodes are worrying features.

Chronic radiation dermatitis may also progress to SCC.

4.5 BASAL CELL CARCINOMA (BCC)

In a nutshell ...

BCC is a common slow-growing malignant epidermal tumour that rarely metastasises.

The major aetiological factor is sunlight

There are several morphological variants with the classical appearance having a rolled everted edge and a pearly white sheen

The prognosis is good if excised with an adequate margin

Epidemiology of BCC

Most common skin cancer. May arise on any part of the skin including the anal margin, but 90% occur on the face above a line joining the angle of the mouth to the external auditory meatus. They are especially common around the eye, nasolabial folds and hairline of the scalp. Twice as likely in males as in females.

Aetiology of BCC

Sunlight, X-rays, arsenic, immunosuppressed patients, basal cell naevus syndrome (dominantly inherited associated with multiple BCCs), and people with inherited defects such as xeroderma pigmentosum.

Pathology of BCC

Macroscopically raised rolled (not everted) edges. Pearly nodules with visible fine blood vessels. Slow growing over years with central ulceration and scabbing.

There are several variations:

- **Multifocal:** emerge from epidermis and spread over several cms
- **Nodular lesions:** grow deep into dermis as cords and islands
- **Flesh coloured:** commonest
- **Scarring, cystic or pigmented** (less common)

Microscopically, solid sheets of uniform, dark-staining cells arising from the basal layers of the skin. Histologically similar to basal cell layer of epidermis. No prickle cells. No epithelial pearls (seen in SCC).

Spread of BCC

Slow but steady local infiltration and destruction of surrounding tissues including skull, face, nose and eye. Hence the term 'rodent ulcer'. Lymphatic and blood spread are extremely rare.

Treatment of BCC

Excision has low recurrence rate if adequate. If advanced, extensive or invading nearby structures, radiotherapy gives good results. The prognosis is good.

4.6 SQUAMOUS CELL CARCINOMA (SCC)

In a nutshell ...

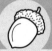

SCC is a common invasive malignant epidermal tumour with a low but significant potential for metastasis.

The major aetiological factors are sun-exposure and chronic ulceration.

SCC spreads via the lymphatics and may metastasise.

Epidemiology of SCC

Very common. Usually in elderly male especially in sun-exposed areas (face, back of hands). More common in men than women.

Aetiology of SCC

Predisposing factors include:

- Exposure to sunshine or irradiation
- Carcinogens (pitch, tar, soot, betel nuts, papilloma virus)
- Lupus vulgaris
- Immunosuppressive drugs
- Chronic ulceration eg Marjolin's ulcer is malignant change in a longstanding scar, ulcer or sinus – typically chronic varicose ulcer, unhealed burn, sinus of chronic osteomyelitis

Marjolin's ulcers tend to be slow growing, painless, and spread to the lymphatics later than classical SCCs, and the edge is not always raised and everted; other features may be masked by the pre-existing ulcer/scar; unusual nodules or changes in a chronic non-healing ulcer or scar should be viewed with suspicion and biopsied early; despite being less invasive and slower growing than a spontaneous SCC it should be treated as vigorously.

Pathology of SCC

Macroscopically a typical carcinomatous ulcer with raised everted edges and a central scab. 'In situ' SCC is where the lesion has not invaded through the basement membrane of the dermo-epidermal junction. Microscopically, solid columns of epithelial cells growing into dermis with epithelial pearls of central keratin surrounded by prickle cells.

Spread of SCC

Local infiltration and lymphatics. Rarely haematological.

Clinical presentation of SCC

Hyperkeratotic and crusty on sun-damaged skin (eg pinna). Ulcerating if on lips or genitals. Friable or papilliferous varieties may occur.

Treatment of SCC

Surgical excision as for BCC with a wider margin required in less well differentiated lesion. Regional node spread is treated by surgical block dissection, or radiotherapy, or both.

Prognosis of SCC

Local recurrence rate is twice that of BCC. Metastasis to local lymph nodes occurs in 5–10% of SCCs if left untreated – less in those arising in sun-damaged skin (0.5%) and more in tumours arising in mucosal surfaces, irradiated areas or Marjolin's ulcers (see above).

4.7 MALIGNANT MELANOMA

In a nutshell ...

Malignant melanoma

Malignant melanoma is an invasive malignant epidermal tumour of melanocytes with significant metastatic potential. The incidence of melanoma is increasing due to behavioural factors (cheap holidays in sunny parts of the world, sunbed use).

Prognosis is related to melanoma size, depth of invasion (Breslow thickness), tumour free excision margins and status of the regional nodes.

Regular follow-up is advised as recurrent disease may present some years later.

Epidemiology of malignant melanoma

10 per 100 000 in the UK, 42 per 100 000 in Australia. Mostly cutaneous but also occur in mucous membrane of nose, mouth, anus, conjunctiva, choroid and pigmented layer of retina. Rare in coloured races, increasingly common in white people. Black people tend to get them on the non-pigmented sole of the foot.

Clinical aspects of malignant melanoma

There are five common clinical types which differ significantly in appearance.

- **Superficial spreading melanoma** (64%): most common type; may occur on any part of the body, usually palpable, but thin with irregular edge and variegated colour
- **Nodular melanoma** (27%): thick, protruding, with a smooth surface and regular outline; may become ulcerated and bleeding
- **Lentigo maligna melanoma** (7%): a malignant melanoma arising in a Hutchinson's lentigo; the malignant areas are thicker than the surrounding pigmented skin, usually darker in colour but seldom ulcerate
- **Acral lentiginous melanoma** (1%) (including subungual melanoma): a rare type, that can present as a chronic paronychia or sub-ungual haematoma; it is an irregular expanding area of brown or black pigmentation on the palm, sole or beneath a nail (beneath the nail is the most common presentation in Afro–Caribbean people)
- **Amelanotic** (1%): least common, with poor prognosis; presents with lymph node involvement

Aetiology of malignant melanoma

Predisposing factors include:

- **Sunlight** (predominantly UVA, but UVB implicated)
  - Childhood exposure is linked with future development of melanoma
  - Recreational exposure (eg holidays) more closely associated with melanoma than regular exposure (eg working outdoors)
  - Sunbeds and tanning lamps carry a potential risk
  - Higher risk for people with fair skins, red hair, albinism, and xeroderma pigmentosum
- **Genetic inheritance** of multiple primary melanomas accounts for a small number of cases (2% of all melanomas have a significant family history, and mutations on chromosomes 1,6,9,10 and 11 have been implicated) but overall familial melanoma is rare
- **Giant congenital naevi** (of > 20 cm maximum diameter at term) have increased risk of malignant change, which may occur in the first 10 years of life; risks/benefits of excision vs observation is a difficult clinical decision

Pathology of malignant melanoma

Half of malignant melanoma cases arise de novo in previously clear skin. Half arise in pre-existing junctional naevi from the melanoblasts in the basal layer of the epidermis (originating from neural crest cells embryologically). Some melanoblasts contain no pigment but all have a positive DOPA reaction (converting dihydroxyphenylalanine (DOPA) into melanin). Initially starts as horizontal melanoma or 'primary cutaneous melanoma' that grows radially. Develops into vertical melanoma that grows into the dermis and is associated with metastasis. May cease to grow or regress naturally due to immune response. Antibodies may be seen early in disease but not in metastatic disease.

Histopathology reporting of malignant melanoma

The four essential components of the report (apart from patient details and site) are:

- Diagnosis of melanoma
- Maximum tumour thickness according to Breslow's method to the nearest 0.1 mm
- Completeness of excision
- Microscopic margins of excision

Other useful information includes histological classification, level of invasion (Clark), vascular invasion, lymphocytic infiltration, horizontal or vertical growth, and predominant cell type, etc.

Classification of malignant melanoma

A modified version of the American Joint Committee on Cancer/Union Internationale Contre le Cancer (AJCC/UICC) staging system is the most widely used.

AJCC staging

pTx	Primary tumour cannot be assessed
pT0	No evidence of primary tumour
Clark level I	pTis: Melanoma in situ (intra-epidermal)
Clark level II	pT1: < 0.75 mm thick and invades the papillary dermis
Clark level III	pT2: 0.75–1.5 mm thick +/– invades to papillary–reticular dermis interface
Clark level IV	pT3: 1.5–4 mm thick +/– invades reticular dermis
pT3a	1.5–3 mm thick
pT3b	3–4 mm thick
pT4	> 4 mm thick

TNM system

Stage I	pT1/T2: N0, M0
Stage II	pT3/T4: N0, M0
Stage III	Any pT: N1–2, M0
Stage IV	Any pT: any N, M1

Treatment of malignant melanoma

Management of the primary tumour

Excision margins depends on the maximum tumour thickness according to Breslow's method (available from the histology report). Remember, an excision biopsy is inadequate for melanoma, as its margins are 2 mm, so the scar must be excised.

Margins for excision

Melanoma in situ	5 mm margin
0.1–1.5 mm thick (pT1–2)	10 mm margin
1.6–4 mm thick (pT3)	10–20 mm margin
> 4 mm thick (pT4)	20–30 mm margin

This protocol is considered acceptable by John Kenealy, Chairman of the Regional Cancer Organisation Expert Tumour Panel on Skin Cancer, Consultant Plastic Surgeon at Frenchay Hospital, Bristol (Kenealy 1999). Historically, very wide margins (up to 5 cm) were recommended, and the evidence is still controversial.

Management of regional lymph nodes

If no clinical lymph nodes are detectable, only certain subgroups are thought suitable for elective lymph node dissection. If node involvement is suspected clinically, surgical clearance after FNA confirmation is indicated.

Sentinel node biopsy may be used to determine regional nodal involvement. (The 'sentinel' node is identified by injecting blue dye or radioactive tracers around the site of the primary tumour). The nodes draining this region can then be identified at the time of surgery by detection of the marker. The node with the most marker is the 'sentinel' – ie that which is most likely to be involved in any metastasis. These nodes can be sent for histology without requirement for complete nodal clearance at the primary surgery. This technique may be difficult in the axilla and head and neck. It may also produce a false-negative result if there is a skip lesion.

Chemotherapy is generally used only for metastatic disease and radiotherapy only for certain types of melanoma (eg desmoplastic tumours). Interferon-β has been used in the past for node-positive patients, but its benefit is unclear.

Regular follow-up is advisable, especially for thicker melanomas (at least 5 years) and recurrent disease.

Metastatic spread: lungs, liver and brain are the commonest blood-borne sites.

Prognosis of malignant melanoma

This relates most closely to Breslow thickness, nodal involvement, and metastasis. Few patients with three or more nodes or disseminated disease survive for 5 years. Nodal recurrence during pregnancy has a worse prognosis.

TUMOUR THICKNESS AND 10-YEAR SURVIVAL RATES

Tumour thickness (mm)	Approximate 10-year survival
< 0.76	> 95%
1.5–2.5	70%
4–7.99	50%
> 8	30%

Other prognostic factors include anatomical site (trunk and scalp worse prognosis than peripheral lesion), and type of growth (superficial spreading better than penetrating, ulcerating lesion).

Chapter 2

Infection and Inflammation

Catherine Sargent and Claire Ritchie Chalmers

Section 1
Inflammatory processes

Chapter 2

In a nutshell ...

Inflammation is a stereotyped response of living tissue to localised injury. It may be acute or progress to chronicity. It is not the same thing as infection (which is a cause of inflammation). There is a spectrum of inflammation ranging through:

Acute inflammation
Characterised by dilated and leaky vessels
Mediated by neutrophils and multiple chemical mediators

Chronic inflammation
Mediated by T-helper cells
Recruits other cells of the immune system such as B cells, macrophages and eosinophils
Cells involved in repair (fibroblasts and angioblasts) are involved

1.1 ACUTE INFLAMMATION

In a nutshell ...

Acute inflammation is a stereotyped response to local injury and essential component of wound repair. It occurs by combination of:
Changes in microcirculation (vasodilation and increased vascular permeability)
Recruitment and activation of phagocytic cells (mediated by neutrophils)

These events are mediated by the release of **chemical mediators**:
- Complement
- Kinins
- Arachadonic acid derivatives (prostaglandins, leukotrienes)
- Histamine
- Serotonin (5-HT)

- Interleukins, cytokines and monokines
- Platelet activating factor (PAF)

Acute inflammation results in resolution, regeneration, abscess formation, scarring or chronic inflammation.

Causes of acute inflammation

Inflammation is the essential response of living tissue to trauma. It destroys and limits the injury and is intimately related to the process of repair. It is therefore an integral component of the body's defence mechanisms, and without it there would be no defence against foreign organisms and no wound healing.

Acute inflammation is usually beneficial, although it can occasionally be harmful (eg anaphylaxis, acute lung injury, systemic inflammatory response syndrome).

Causes of acute inflammation include:

- Trauma (mechanical, thermal, radiation, chemical – includes stomach acid, bile and blood when free in the peritoneal cavity)
- Infection (bacteria, virus, parasite, fungus)
- Ischaemic injury
- Immunological attack (autoimmunity, graft vs host disease)
- Foreign body response (eg mesh in hernia repair)

Mechanism of acute inflammation

Vasodilation and vascular permeability

After the initial injury there is a rapid and transient arteriolar vasoconstriction (reduces blood loss in case of vascular injury). Damage to the vasculature results in a collection of blood and activation of the clotting cascade. The resulting clot fills the wound and consists of a mesh-like fibrin plug in which are trapped a number of activated platelets. Activation of the platelets results in the release of a number of inflammatory mediators. Platelet activation may also activate the complement cascade.

The plasma contains four interlinked enzyme cascades – **the clotting cascade**, **the fibrinolysis cascade**, **complement cascade** and the **kinin system**. These cascades are interrelated and can be activated by each others products. They are discussed in detail in Chapter 4 *Haematology*.

Important inflammatory mediators released by platelets

Prostaglandins (PGs)
Leukotrienes
Histamine
Serotonin (5-HT)

The release of prostaglandins (PGs) and nitric oxide results in persistent arteriolar smooth muscle relaxation and therefore increased local blood flow ('rubor' and 'calor'). 5-HT, histamine, leukotrienes and complement proteins (C3a and C5a) cause activation of the endothelium resulting in increased vascular permeability and exudation of fluid and plasma proteins. Increased oncotic pressure in the interstitial fluid draws water out from the vessels and causes tissue oedema – 'tumour'.

Vessel permeability is due to three different responses

- The immediate-transient response begins at once, peaks at 5–10 minutes, and is over by 30 minutes. It is due to chemical mediators (prostaglandins, histamine, 5-HT). It involves only the venules and is due to contraction and separation of endothelial cells
- The immediate-prolonged reaction is seen only when the injury is severe enough to cause direct endothelial cell damage (eg trauma to the blood vessel). It persists until the clotting cascade ends it
- The delayed-prolonged leakage phenomenon is seen only after hours or days. Venules and capillaries exude protein because their junctions separate due to apoptosis of the endothelial cells

In addition, endothelial cells are damaged as the leucocytes squeeze through the capillary walls and there is a degree of endothelial cell apoptosis. As the tissues heal, new blood vessels are formed which are, in themselves, leaky. This leakage of fluid from the vessels causes sludging, or stasis, in the capillary blood flow as there is a relative increase in the viscosity (thus the application of plasma viscosity measurement in inflammatory states).

Cellular events in acute inflammation

Initially neutrophils, and later macrophages, rapidly migrate to the injured area. Their subsequent activities involve the steps as shown in the shaded box.

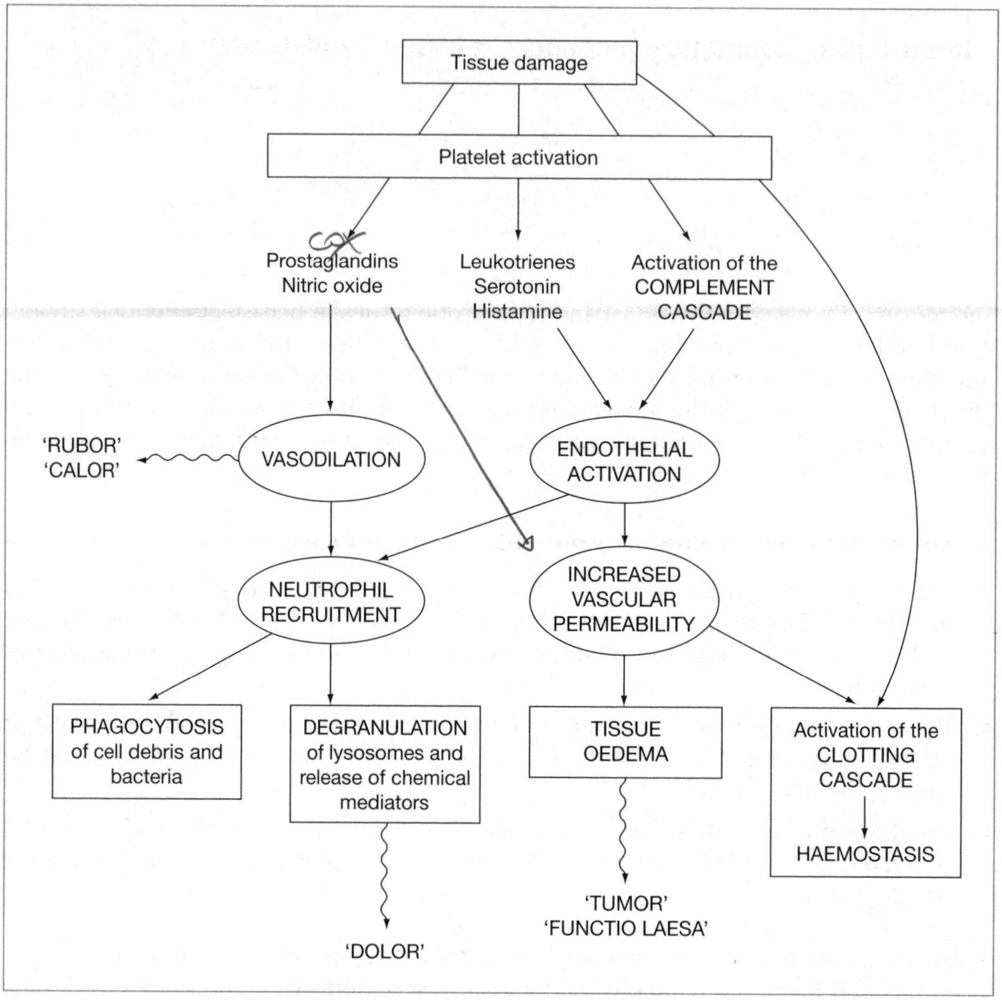

Figure 1.1a *Acute inflammation*

Recruitment of inflammatory cells

Margination: as blood flow decreases, leucocytes move from the centre of the vessel to lie against the endothelium.

Pavementing: adhesion molecules on leucocytes (eg integrins) bind to corresponding molecules on the endothelium (eg ICAM-1; see below); expression of these adhesion molecules is upregulated by specific inflammatory mediators (C5a, IL-1, TNF) in the locality of the inflammation.

Diapedesis or emigration: adherent leucocytes pass through inter-endothelial junctions into the extravascular space; neutrophils are the predominant cell type in the first 24 hours, after which monocytes predominate.

Chemotaxis: leucocytes move to the injury site along a chemical gradient assisted by chemotactic factors (bacterial components, complement factors, leukotriene (LT) B4).

Phagocytosis and intracellular degradation: opsonised bacteria (opsonins IgG and C3b) attach via Fc and C3b receptors to the surface of neutrophils and macrophages; the bacteria/foreign particle is then engulfed to create a phagosome, which then fuses with lysosomal granules to form a phagolysosome, and the contents of the lysosome degrade the ingested particle.

ICAM-1, ICAM-2 and integrins

ICAM-1 and ICAM-2 are cell adhesion molecules belonging to the Ig gene super-family. They are expressed on endothelial cells (upregulated by inflammatory mediators) and act as receptors for β2-integrin (expressed on neutrophils, eosinophils, and T cells). The integrin 'hooks on' to the ICAM molecule and this interaction allows the leucocyte to adhere to the endothelium and emigrate into the tissue from the bloodstream. Integrins thus allow cell–cell interactions and cell–extracellular matrix interactions.

The ICAM family is upregulated in certain disease states such as allergy (eg atopic asthma, allergic alveolitis), autoimmunity (eg IDDM, SLE, MS), certain cancers (eg bladder, melanoma), and infection (eg HIV, malaria, TB) allowing increased leucocyte infiltration of non-inflamed tissue. Reduction in the numbers of cellular adhesion molecules occurs in disease (eg diabetes, alcoholism, steroid treatment) and results in a reduced immune response to bacterial infection.

Cellular components of the inflammatory infiltrate

The neutrophils are the predominant cell type in the inflammatory phase in the first 24 h. They degranulate, releasing their lysosomal contents, and also initiate phagocytosis of bacteria and cell debris. Phagocytosis requires that the particle be recognized and attach to the neutrophil. Most particles must be coated (opsonised) by IgG or complement protein C3b. There are receptors for both on the neutrophil surface. The particle will then be engulfed and a lysosome membrane fused with the phagosome membrane, causing digestion within the phagolysosome. Macrophages become the predominant cell type after 48 h. They continue the process of phagocytosis and secrete growth factors (cytokines) which are instrumental in ECM production. Macrophages are also responsible for fibrosis, and heavy or prolonged inflammatory infiltrates are associated with severe scarring.

Inflammatory mediators in acute inflammation

The inflammatory response to trauma is mediated by chemical factors present in the plasma and produced by the inflammatory cells, as shown in the following table.

MEDIATORS OF THE INFLAMMATORY RESPONSE

Plasma	Cells
Complement system	Vasoactive amines (eg histamine, serotonin)
Kinin system	Lysosomal enzymes
Coagulation pathway	Arachidonic acid derivatives
Fibrinolytic system	Cytokines (eg TNF-α, interleukins)
	Free radicals

Important cytokines responsible for chemotaxis

- Transforming growth factor (TGF-β)
- Basic fibroblast growth factor (bFGF)
- Platelet factor-4 (PF-4)
- β-Thromboglobulin (β-TG)
- Vascular endothelial growth factor (VEGF)
- Platelet-derived growth factor (PDGF)
- Monocyte chemotactic protein-1 (MCP-1)
- Keratinocyte growth factor (KGF)
- Epidermal growth factor (EGF)
- Fibroblast growth factor (FGF)

Complement system

The complement system consists of over 20 component proteins.

- The classic pathway is initiated by antigen–antibody complexes
- The alternative pathway is activated by endotoxins, complex polysaccharides, and aggregated immunoglobulins

Both pathways convert C3 to C3a and C3b.

- C3b initiates the lytic pathway that produces the membrane attack complex (MAC), which forms destructive pores in the membranes of target cells
- C3a and C5a increase vascular permeability by causing release of histamine from granulocytes, mast cells and platelets. C5a is also chemotactic

The biological functions of complement are as follows:

- It yields particles which coat micro-organisms and function as adhesion molecules for neutrophils and macrophages (opsonins)
- It leads to lysis of bacterial cell membranes via the MAC
- It yields biologically active fragments that influence capillary permeability and chemotaxis

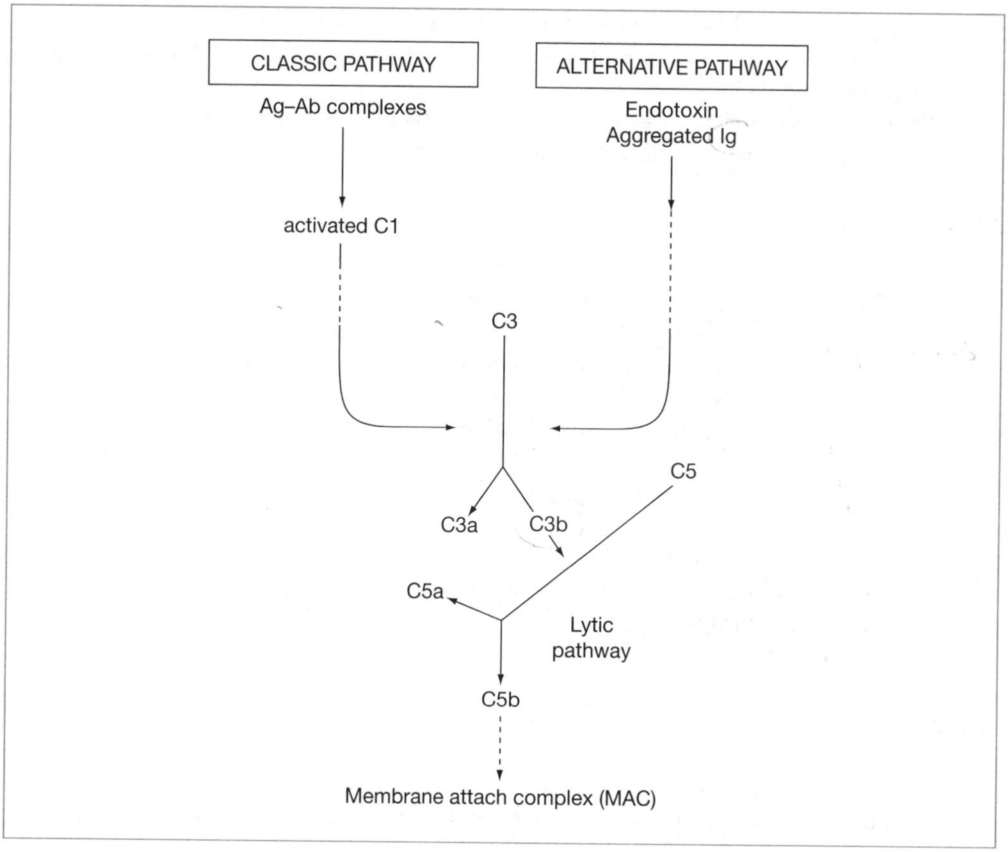

Figure 1.1b *Activation of the complement pathways – classical and alternative*

Kinin system

Activation of coagulation factor XII produces factor XIIa. This converts pre-kallikrein into the active enzyme kallikrein, which produces bradykinin from high-molecular-weight kininogen. Bradykinin is a potent vasodilator and increases vascular permeability.

Coagulation and fibrinolysis

The clotting cascade and fibrinolysis are discussed in detail in Chapter 4 *Haematology*.

Vasoactive amines

Histamine and serotonin

- Mast cells, basophils and platelets contain the amines histamine and 5-HT
- Release from mast cells granules is stimulated by C3a and C5a, IgE immunological reactions and IL-1
- Release from platelets is caused by contact with collagen, thrombin, ADP and by PAF
- Both amines cause vasodilatation and increased vascular permeability

Nitric oxide (NO)

- Found to be of increasing importance in health and disease
- Synthesised by nitric oxide synthase (NOS) during oxidation of arginine to citrulline
- Produced by three NOS genes in neurones, endothelial cells, and the immune system
- Acts to reduce intracellular calcium (smooth muscle dilation, decreased cardiac contractility, reduced platelet and inflammatory cell activation)
- Appears to have protective beneficial effects when produced in neurones and endothelial cells, but pathological activity in inflammatory states
- Has multiple actions in inflammation
  - Local vasodilator
  - Bacteriocidal activity
  - Downregulatory effects on neutrophil function
  - Prolongs neutrophil lifespan
  - Causes apoptosis in macrophages

Lysosomal enzymes

Leucocytes degranulate at the site of infection setting up a cycle of bacterial phagocytosis, tissue destruction, and recruitment of increasing numbers of immune cells.

- Cationic proteins: increase vascular permeability and act as chemotactants
- Acid proteases: most active at about pH 3
- Neutral proteases: degrade extracellular matrix

Arachidonic acid metabolism

Arachidonic acid is a 20-carbon polyunsaturated fatty acid present in cell membranes. Following activation, arachidonic acid is released from the membrane by phospholipases. It is then metabolised via two main pathways: the cyclo-oxygenase (COX) pathway and the lipoxygenase pathway.

COX pathway → prostaglandins PGE2 and PGI2

- Cause vasodilatation and increased vascular permeability
- E-series prostaglandins are hyperalgesic

Lipoxygenase pathway → leukotrienes (LTs)

- Produced by all of the inflammatory cells except lymphocytes
- LT-C4 (plus products D4 and E4) increase vascular permeability and constrict smooth muscle
- LT-B4 makes neutrophils adhere to endothelium and is a potent chemotactic agent

See section 1.4 for a discussion of anti-inflammatory pharmacology.

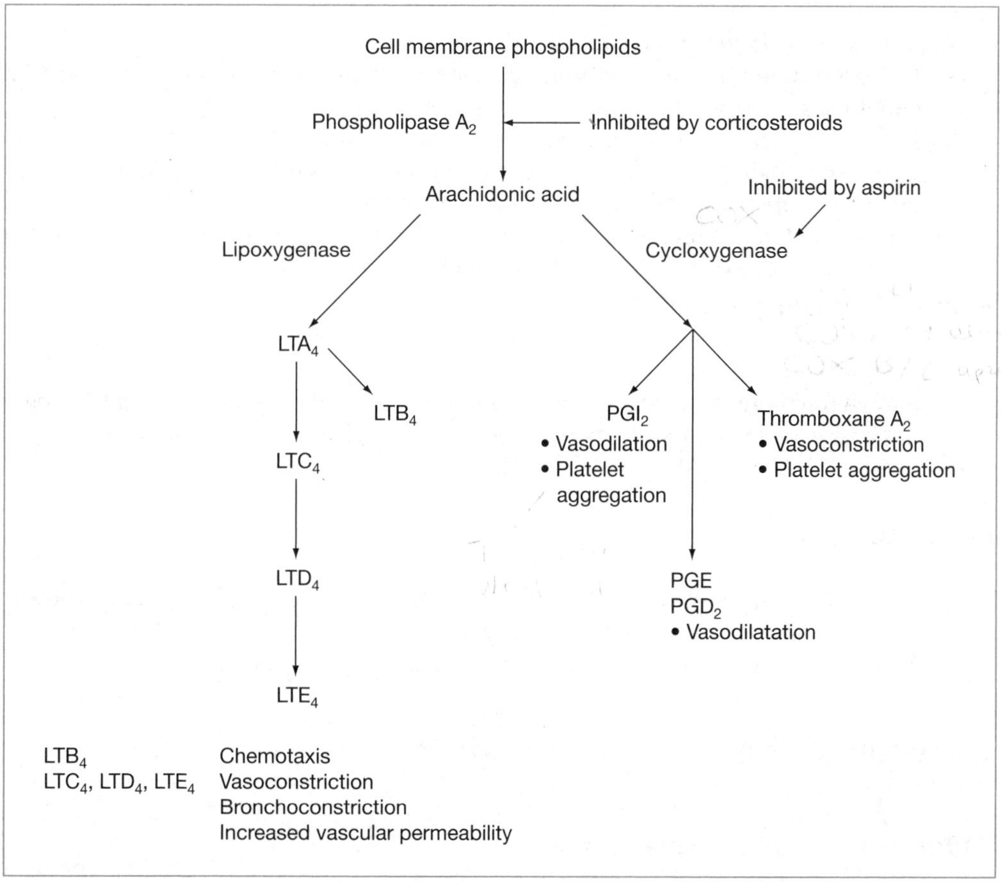

Figure 1.1c *Arachidonic acid metabolism*

Interleukins, cytokines and monokines

- **Polypeptides:** produced by activated monocytes (monokines), lymphocyte (lymphokines), and other inflammatory cells
- **Interferons:** viral infection induces the synthesis and secretion of interferons; they confer an antiviral state on uninfected cells
- **Interleukins**
  - Interleukin-8 is a chemokine produced by monocytes, T lymphocytes, endothelial cells and platelets, which mediates the rapid accumulation of neutrophils in inflamed tissues
  - Interleukin-1 is secreted by numerous cell types (monocytes, macrophages, neutrophils, endothelial cells); it promotes T-cell and B-cell proliferation, tissue catabolism and the acute phase response, and also acts as a pyrogen (see section 2 *The immune system*)
- **Tumour necrosis factor-α (TNF-α)**
  - Produced by monocytes and macrophages, particularly if stimulated by bacterial endotoxins
  - Plays an important part in host defence against Gram-negative sepsis
  - When endotoxin present at a low dose TNF-α enhances macrophage killing, activation of B white blood cells and cytokine production
  - When endotoxin is present at a high dose TNF-α is an extremely potent mediator in the pathogenesis of endotoxin-related shock
- **Platelet-activating factor (PAF)**
  - A wide variety of cells produce PAF, including mast cells, neutrophils, platelets and macrophages
  - It has a multitude of effects and increases vascular permeability, leucocyte aggregation and exudation, smooth muscle constriction and cellular degranulation
  - Research into anti-PAF agents is on-going

Free radicals

- Neutrophils release collagenase, alkaline phosphatase, elastase, myeloperoxidase, acid hydrolases, α1-anti-trypsin and lysosyme
- Monocytes produce acid hydrolases, collagenase, and elastase

Outcomes of acute inflammation

Outcomes of acute inflammation

Resolution
Abscess and pus formation
Scarring and fibrosis
Chronic inflammation

Resolution

Resolution occurs when no structural tissue component has been lost, with restoration of normal cellular and tissue function.

Abscesses and pus formation

- Pus is a body fluid containing neutrophils and necrotic debris
- Chemicals and enzymes released by inflammatory cells damage surrounding tissue and may even cause liquefication necrosis – the mediators released by neutrophils are the worst offenders (predominantly these are proteases and free radicals)
- Collections of pus tend to find their own way out through tissue planes as the pressure inside the abscess builds; there is an increase in osmotic pressure due to the increasing number of molecular products being generated by the continuous action of proteases (eg formation of sinuses in osteomyelitis)

Scarring and fibrosis

Scarring means laying down of dense (type I) collagen in chronic inflammation +/– wound healing. Degree of scarring is determined by repair vs regeneration.

- Repair occurs by laying down of fibrous tissue (fibroblasts produce ground substance, fibronectin and initially type III collagen which is replaced with type I collagen as the scar matures)
- Regeneration can only occur in certain cell types:
  - Labile cells are continuous replicators (eg intestinal mucosa, hair follicles)
  - Stable cells are discontinuous replicators and can divide when required to do so (eg fibroblasts and endothelial cells)
  - Permanent cells are non-replicators and can not divide (eg neurons)

1.2 CHRONIC INFLAMMATION

In a nutshell ...

Chronic inflammation is characterised by three features:

- **Infiltration of tissue with mononuclear inflammatory cells** (monocytes, lymphocyte, +/– plasma cells)
- **Ongoing tissue destruction**
- **Evidence of healing** (scarring, fibroblast proliferation, angioblast proliferation, angiogenesis)

It may be non-specific, autoimmune or granulomatous. Granulomatous disease includes TB, syphilis, leprosy, and schistosomiasis.

Chronic inflammation results from:

- Persistence of the acute inflammatory stimulus (eg cholangitis leading to chronic liver abscess)
- Deranged inflammatory response (eg autoimmune conditions such as rheumatoid arthritis or SLE)
- Recurrent episodes of acute inflammation (eg recurrent cholecystitis or pancreatitis resulting in pseudocyst formation)

Non-specific chronic inflammation

This is when acute inflammation fails to end in resolution or repair, as a result of:

- Persistence of injurious agent (eg chronic osteomyelitis, peptic ulcer due to *Helicobacter pylori*)
- Failure of removal of pus and foreign material (eg undrained abscess)
- Inadequate blood supply or drainage (eg ischaemic or venous ulceration)
- Inadequate drainage of an exocrine gland (eg chronic sialoadenitis)

Pathology of non-specific chronic inflammation

- Tissue macrophages are almost all recruited directly from bloodstream monocytes
- T-helper cells activate B lymphocytes to produce plasma cells (via IL-4)
- Plasma cells produce antibodies against the persistent antigen or the altered tissue components; they divide under the influence of IL-1 from macrophages
- Some degree of scarring always occurs in chronic inflammation; IL-1 also activates fibroblasts resulting in scarring
- Fibrosis is stimulated by TGF-β

Cellular response to chronic inflammation

The predominant cell in the inflammatory infiltrate may vary according to the cause of inflammation.

- **Neutrophils** predominate in inflammation caused by common bacteria
- **Lymphocytes** predominate in viral infections and autoimmune diseases
- **Plasma cells** predominate in spirochaetal diseases (syphilis and Lyme disease)
- **Macrophages** predominate in typhoid fever, TB, and fungal infections (except candidiasis)
- **Eosinophils** predominate in inflammation secondary to allergic reactions, parasites (ie worms) and in most inflammations of the gut

Autoimmune chronic inflammation

Autoimmune diseases are characterised by the production of antibodies against 'self'. These antibodies cause chronic tissue damage, necrosis and may be deposited as antibody complexes. This feeds a state of chronic inflammation. In autoimmune diseases the primary immune cell in the inflammatory infiltrate is the lymphocyte.

Autoimmunity is discussed in detail in section 2.3 of this chapter.

Granulomatous chronic inflammation

This is characterised by small collections (granulomas) of modified macrophages called 'epithelioid cells'. T-helper cells are stimulated by the persistent antigen to produce activating cytokines, which recruit and activate macrophages (eg by IFN-α, TNF-α, etc). Persistence of the causative organism or substance causes the macrophages to surround the offending particle, effectively walling it off. These are then termed epithelioid cells. Epithelioid cells may fuse over several days to form giant multinucleated cells (Langerhans or foreign-body giant cells).

Granulomatous inflammation may be associated with suppuration (pus-filled cavity), caseation, or a central foreign body. It is usually a low-grade smouldering response, occurring in the settings listed in the shaded box.

Causes of granulomatous inflammation

Persistent infection

- Mycobacterium (TB, syphilis, leprosy)
- Atypical fungi

Prolonged exposure to non-degradable substances

- Pulmonary asbestosis
- Silicosis
- Talc

Immune reactions

- Autoimmune disorders (eg rheumatoid arthritis)
- Wegener's granulomatosis
- Sarcoidosis
- Reactions to tumours (eg lymphomas and seminomas)

Tuberculosis (TB)

Organism

Mycobacterium tuberculosis hominis or *Mycobacterium bovis*.

- Identified as acid-fast bacilli (AFBs) in sputum or pus smears by Ziehl–Neelson stain
  - Needs special growth conditions (grow very slowly) so must be specifically requested
  - Three consecutive samples required (bacteria often sparse)
  - Early morning samples best (sputum or urine)
- Waxy, hard to kill, and resistant to drying (they remain infectious)

Transmitted commonly by droplet inhalation or dust containing dried sputum; also can be ingested.

Demographics of TB

Incidence increasing worldwide (increased drug resistance; HIV; non-compliance with treatment). WHO data shows that TB is common in southeast Asia (33% of cases) but is increasing in sub-Saharan Africa (secondary to HIV causing highest mortality per capita). There is an increased risk in populations who are malnourished, overcrowded and economically deprived, in those who have HIV and are immunosuppressed (eg steroids), and in alcoholism.

- **Bacille Calmette–Guerin (BCG)** vaccination (live-attenuated virus) is used in some countries and is most effective in protecting children from TB meningitis
- **Tuberculin (or Mantoux/Heaf) tests** for infection or previous effective immunisation. Intracutaneous injection or topical application of purified tuberculin protein causes a type IV hypersensitivity reaction if there has been previous exposure. (NB: Very immunosuppressed patients cannot mount this response and so the test may be negative despite florid TB.) The interpretation of the result of these tests also depends upon whether the patient in question has been immunised with BCG

Symptoms and signs of TB

TB is a multisystem disease, with the following signs and symptoms:

- **General:** weight loss, night sweats, fever, malaise, 'consumption'
- **Pulmonary:** caseating cavities, empyema, progressive lung destruction, miliary form; cough, haemoptysis (CXR: granulomas and thickening of pleura in upper lobes; diffuse shadowing in miliary form)
- **Gastrointestinal:** commonly ileocaecal; features similar to Crohn's disease +/– RLQ mass
- **Adrenal:** usually bilateral. Tissue destruction can lead to Addison's disease
- **Peritoneal:** primary peritonitis
- **Urinary:** sterile pyuria, renal involvement, predisposes to TCC in bladder

- **Hepatic:** miliary involvement
- **Skin:** may look like carcinoma
- **Bone:** Pott's disease is vertebral TB (+/– neurological compromise); joints (commonly knee and hip)
- **CNS:** meningeal pattern involving base of brain (cranial nerve signs)
- **Lymph node:** lymphadenitis of the cervical nodes (scrofula)
- **Cardiovascular:** usually pericarditis

Primary TB

- Often occurs in childhood
- Caseating granuloma surrounds primary infective focus (often subpleural); associated hilar lymphadenopathy and the initial granuloma together are referred to as the Ghon complex
- Disease may resolve, calcify, or remain dormant and reactivate later in life (often due to subsequent immunocompromise)
- Rarely florid

Secondary TB

- Seen commonly in adults (re-infection/re-activation when bacilli escape the walled-off Ghon focus)
- Commonly at apex of lung
- Active florid infection with spread throughout the pulmonary tree and sequelae such as haemoptysis, erosion into bronchioles and 'open infection'

'Cold abscess'

- Develops slowly so very little associated inflammation (ie 'cold')
- Becomes painful when pressure develops on surrounding areas
- Often affects musculoskeletal tissues
- Pus may track down tissue planes and present as a swelling some distance away
- Can be drained by percutaneous catheter or surgically

Treatment of TB

- Multiple drug therapy (rifampicin, isoniazid, pyrazinamide, ethambutanol) given as triple or quadruple therapy initially
- Requires directly observed therapy to ensure compliance
- Should also give pyridoxine to avoid isoniazid-induced neuropathy

Syphilis

Organism

- *Treponema pallidum*
- Transmitted: sexually (bacterium is fragile and moves from open genital sore to skin/mucus membrane of recipient); vertically (transplacental); via blood transfusion
- Risks: increases risk of transmitting HIV 3–5-fold; teratogenicity

Symptoms of syphilis

These are divided into primary, secondary and tertiary stages.

- **Primary syphilis**
  - Ulceration at site (chancre) within 2–6 weeks
  - May occur on genitalia, lips, tongue or cervix
  - Chancre disappears after a few weeks regardless of treatment
  - 30% progress to chronicity
- **Secondary syphilis**
  - Skin rash (large brown sores) on palms and soles of feet
  - Fever, headache, sore throat, lymphadenopathy
  - Lasts for a few weeks and may recur over next 1–2 years
- **Tertiary syphilis**
  - Damage to heart, eyes, brain, nervous system, bones and joints
  - Development of gummas (granulomas with coagulative necrosis; often in liver, testes, bridge of the nose)

Diagnosis of syphilis

- In early stages the disease mimics many others (called 'the great imitator')
- Diagnosed by two separate blood tests on different occasions (VDRL test)

Treatment of syphilis

- Penicillin IV

Leprosy (Hansen's disease)

Organism

- *Mycobacterium leprae*
- Multiplies very slowly (difficult to culture)

Demographics of leprosy

- WHO data shows 90% of cases are in Brazil, Madagascar, Ethiopia, Mozambique, Tanzania and Nepal
- Transmission probably involves respiratory droplet infection

Symptoms of leprosy

- Disfiguring skin lesions, peripheral nerve damage (sensory loss and muscle weakness), loss of sweating and progressive debilitation (loss of sensation results in repeated injury and damage to hands and feet)
- Predisposes to amyloidosis A

Diagnosis of leprosy

- Classical appearance
- Skin scraping for AFBs

Classification of leprosy

- **Paucibacillary leprosy:** mild with hypopigmented skin papules
- **Multibacillary leprosy:** symmetrical skin lesions, nodules, plaques and thickened dermis, nerve damage and disability
- **Tuberculoid form leprosy:** infection is controlled by the patient's T cells forming granulomas similar to TB (especially in nerve sheaths → leading to damage)
- **Lepromatous form leprosy:** the patient's T cells are unable to control the infection and lesions become diffuse with large disfiguring lesions and bacterial invasion of supporting cells of the nervous system

Treatment of leprosy

- Multidrug therapy (eg rifampicin, dapsone, ethionamide)
- Early treatment reduces infectivity and minimises debilitation

Granulomas and exposure to non-degradable substances

Persistence of any non-degradable substance may lead to granuloma formation as the body 'walls it off'. Granulomas may form around the deposition of endogenous substances (such as in-grown hairs or ruptured epidermoid cysts) or around foreign-bodies (such as asbestos fibres and schistosome eggs). Any foreign body may result in granuloma formation.

Asbestosis

- Asbestosis results from prolonged heavy exposure to asbestos fibres or dust (usually occupational)
- The asbestos fibre is long and pierces through the lung tissue coming to lie near the pleura
- Pathology: There is marked peribronchiolar and alveolar interstitial fibrosis. Granulomas form early in involved areas, and undergo fibrosis as the disease progresses
- Asbestos exposure is also associated with bronchial carcinoma and mesothelioma

Schistosomiasis

- Granuloma formation in GI and urinary tracts due to reaction instigated by deposition of schistosomal ova (fluke)
- Sequelae include bleeding, fibrosis and stricture
- Commonly causes liver involvement and portal hypertension

Immune reactions and granulomas

Granulomas form as a result of immune reactions, typically:

- Type IV hypersensitivity reactions
- Unusual immune reactions: Wegener's granulomatosis, sarcoidosis, Crohn's disease, primary biliary cirrhosis
- Immune reactions to tumours: usually those affecting lymph nodes such as lymphoma or seminoma

Wegener's granulomatosis

Wegener's is a granulomatous vasculitis. Any organ may be involved and granuloma is commonly seen in the respiratory tract. Also commonly causes glomerulonephritis and generalized arteritis. See discussion of vasculitides in the chapter on *Vascular Surgery*.

Sarcoidosis

Sarcoidosis is characterised by non-caseating granulomata of unknown cause. It primarily affects young adults of African or Caribbean descent with a female preponderance. It is commonly found in the chest causing bilateral hilar lymphadenopathy. Extrathoracic disease is more serious and may affect a number of organ systems:

- **Respiratory:** bilateral hilar lymphadenopathy +/– cough, fever, malaise, arthralgia and erythema nodosum. May eventually lead to pulmonary fibrosis
- **CNS:** uveitis (may cause blindness), cranial nerve palsies, diffuse CNS disease or space occupying lesions, granulomatous meningitis
- **Renal:** nephropathy and renal calculi (due to hypercalcaemia)
- **Cardiovascular:** sudden death, tachyarrhythmias, cardiomyopathy, pericardial effusion

It is diagnosed by biopsy and characteristic granulomatous histology. Steroids are used to prevent pulmonary fibrosis, blindness and nephropathy.

1.3 CLINICAL INDICATORS OF INFLAMMATION

Examination findings

The cardinal signs of acute inflammation are 'rubor' (redness), 'calor' (heat), 'dolor' (pain), 'tumour' (swelling) and 'functio laesa' (reduction in function). Increased blood flow due to vasodilation causes redness and heat. Increased vascular permeability results in tissue oedema and swelling with loss of functional capacity. The presence of inflammatory mediators from the complement cascade, neutrophil lysosomal contents, and those released from injured tissue cause pain.

Pyrexia may also be a feature and is a central nervous system response to circulating inflammatory mediators.

Generalised inflammation or the systemic inflammatory response syndrome (SIRS) is discussed in Chapter 7 *Critical Care*.

Investigations for inflammation

Leukocytosis

Leukocytosis in inflammation is predominantly a neutrophilia (ie increase in neutrophils). Initially circulating neutrophils are attracted to the site of inflammation. Subsequently cytokines cause increased release of immature neutrophils from the bone marrow and there are increases in the overall circulating level of neutrophils (called a 'left shift' after the position of columns on the old haematologists counting pad).

Erythrocyte sedimentation rate (ESR)

ESR increases as a result of increased plasma viscosity in inflammatory conditions. It is less useful in sepsis as values rise slowly (more useful in chronic inflammatory states). ESR is fairly non-specific test but can be used to monitor inflammatory states over a period of days to years.

- Value is higher in women than in men, in the elderly, during pregnancy, in anaemia and in obesity
- Values also high in widespread malignancy

Acute-phase proteins

These are about 40 different plasma proteins synthesised in the liver in response to the inflammatory state – referred to as the acute phase response.

- Include clotting proteins, complement factors, transport proteins, and anti-proteases
- Many can be measured as serial markers in acute and chronic disease

C-reactive protein (CRP)

CRP is produced by the liver. It binds to molecules exposed during cell death or on surface of pathogens, and it:

- Acts as an opsonin (aiding phagocytosis)
- Activates classical complement pathway
- Upregulates adhesion molecules
- Increases release of pro-inflammatory cytokines

CRP plasma levels:

- Normal range 0–10 mg/mL
- Levels of > 300 mg/mL are an independently poor prognostic sign
- Levels are sensitive and respond rapidly (can be used < 24 hours so good for acute inflammatory states like sepsis)
- Mildly elevated levels are associated with increased risk of atherosclerosis and colon cancer
- Elevated levels are a common response to surgical trauma (so interpret with care in the first 24 hours post-operatively)

Fibrinogen

Component of the clotting cascade. Leaks out of vessels during inflammation and acts as a framework for:

- Trapping blood cells to form clot
- Confining inflammatory cells to site of inflammation
- Trapping bacteria, so impeding dissemination around body
- Subsequent scar formation

Plasma levels increase with inflammatory stimuli (normal 200–400 mg/dL).

1.4 ANTI-INFLAMMATORY PHARMACOLOGY

Steroids

Glucocorticoids inhibit expression of many of the genes involved in inflammatory and immune responses (include those encoding cytokines, chemokines, cell-surface receptors, adhesion molecules, tissue factor, degradative proteinases, COX-2, and inducible NOS). They bind to a glucocorticoid receptor (GR) in the cell and this interacts directly with DNA at glucocorticoid response elements (GREs) to activate or inhibit transcription of the factors outlined above.

Side effects of steroids

> **Side effects of steroids**
>
> **Mineralocorticoid effects**
> Hypertension
> Fluid retention
>
> **Glucocorticoid effects**
> Diabetes
> Osteoporosis
> Mental disturbance and psychosis
> Muscle wasting (proximal myopathy)
> Peptic ulceration
> Adiposity (altered distribution)
> Thin skin

Adrenal suppression

Withdrawal after long periods causes acute adrenal insufficiency (see *Endocrine Surgery* in Book 2). Steroids must be weaned gradually or replaced with equivalent IV supply if they have been taken long term (approximate equivalent doses to 5 mg prednisolone are 750 μg dexamethasone, 20 mg hydrocortisone, 4 mg methylprednisolone). Patients on long-term steroids will require IV replacement if they become acutely unwell or require surgery.

Cushing syndrome

Signs include moon face, striae, abnormal fat distribution (buffalo hump, supraclavicular fossae), acne, and hypertension. Remember that Cushing's 'syndrome' refers to excessive glucocorticoids and may be iatrogenic. Cushing's 'disease' is due to ACTH secretion by pituitary tumour (see *Endocrine Surgery* in Book 2).

Non-steroidal anti-inflammatory drugs (NSAIDs)

Types of NSAIDs

The differences in anti-inflammatory activity of the different NSAIDs are small but individual patients show considerable variation in their tolerance and response to different NSAIDs.

- Aspirin (salicylate hydrolysed in the body to salycilic acid)
- Indomethacin
- Diclofenac sodium

- Naproxen
- Ibuprofen
- Ketorolac (for post-op pain)
- Celecoxib, rofecoxib, valdecoxib and etoricoxib (arthritidies)

The side effects of the NSAIDs vary, and the newer NSAIDs (eg COX-2 inhibitors) have been developed with improvement in the GI safety profile in mind. However, there have been recent concerns about the cardiovascular safety of the COX-2 inhibitors.

Pharmacology of the NSAIDs

All NSAIDs have similar pharmacology:

- Absorbed passively in stomach and small intestine
- Detectable in plasma at 30–45 minutes. Peak levels occur in inflamed tissue slowly but the compounds persist in inflammatory exudates long after they have been removed from the plasma (ie delayed onset but prolonged action)
- Activity occurs mainly in the peripheral nervous system although they do have some CNS effects
- Ceiling to their analgesic effect
- Can be used to reduce or eliminate requirement for steroid use
- Variability between individuals in response (thought to have a genetic basis)

There are two components to their mechanism of action.

1. The drug molecule inserts into the cell lipid bilayer (more lipophilic at low pH as seen in inflamed tissue). This disrupts cellular signals so, for example, in neutrophils this reduces aggregation and enzyme release.
2. The drug acts on the COX pathway, targeting the iso-enzymes COX-1 and COX-2. This suppresses production of PGE_2 and PGI_2 therefore these drugs act as antipyretic, analgesic and anti-inflammatory agents. This effect does not prevent inflammation itself but acts to suppress the positive feedback of continued prostaglandin production.

- **COX-1** is constitutively expressed and produces prostaglandins important for mucosal integrity in the GI tract and for renal perfusion in the kidney
- **COX-2** is the inducible form. Production is dramatically upregulated by cytokines, mitogens and inflammation. The currently available NSAIDs vary in their potency as inhibitors of COX-2, but virtually all are far more potent inhibitors of COX-1 than COX-2. COX-2-selective drugs have been developed (eg rofecoxib, celecoxib, valdecoxib, parecoxib) which have an improved GI safety profile – although recent evidence suggests that there may be an increase in thromboembolic complications in patients taking long-term COX-2 inhibitors. It is unclear how much the prostaglandins produced by COX-1 may contribute to pain and inflammation; it is also possible that COX-2 produces some beneficial prostaglandins

Side effects of NSAIDs

Side effects of the NSAIDs are:

- GI toxicity (duodenal or gastric ulceration, nausea, dyspepsia)
- Renal toxicity
- Fluid retention and hypertension
- Hypersensitivity reactions (especially bronchospasm in asthmatics)
- Tinnitus

Section 2

The immune system

In a nutshell ...

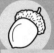

The primary function of the immune system is to eliminate infectious agents and to minimise the damage they cause.

The immune system consists of non-specific defences and specific (acquired) immunity.

Non-specific defences

- Skin and mucus membranes
- Commensal organisms
- Bactericidal body fluids (gastric acid)
- Complement system
- Phagocytes: neutrophils, PMNs and NK cells
- Inflammatory cells: eosinophils, basophils and mast cells

Characteristics
Antigen-independent
Immediate maximal response
No immunological memory

Specific (acquired) immunity

- Lymphocytes: special features include specificity, adaptation, memory

Characteristics
Antigen-dependant
Lag time between exposure and response
Immunological memory

2.1 NON-SPECIFIC MECHANISMS OF IMMUNITY

Skin and mucus membranes

Physical barrier to penetration by bacteria. Often contain an outpost of the immune system for early antigen recognition (mucosa-associated lymphoid tissue; MALT) eg Peyer's patches, intra-epithelial T cells. May employ movement to flush out bacteria (eg intestinal peristalsis, bronchopulmonary mucociliary escalator, urinary voiding).

Commensal organisms

Normal commensals may be overwhelmed by a pathogen due to the use of antibiotics or changes in their growth environment (eg pH). A common example is the loss of normal gut flora with broad-spectrum antibiotics and an increase in colonisation with *Clostridium difficile*.

Bacteriocidal body fluids

Bactericidal activity is due to:

- pH – often due to this (eg stomach acid, vaginal secretions)
- Enzymatic action eg lysosyme in lacrimal secretions
- Thiocyanate in saliva
- Low-molecular-weight fatty acids in the bowel
- Bile acids

Complement system

Components of the complement system are the pharmacological mediators of inflammation. The system is concerned with the initial elimination of foreign micro-organisms, involving opsonisation and chemotaxis.

Phagocytes

All phagocytes have receptors for a variety of molecules: IgG Fc, complement, IFN, TNF and some ubiquitous bacterial proteins. Target cells and organisms become coated in these molecules and the phagocyte is stimulated to engulf the target. Bacteria produce *N* -formyl-methionine which acts as a phagocyte chemoattractant.

Neutrophils

- Neutrophils are polymorphonuclear cells (PMNs)
- Seen as large abundant lymphocytes with a lobed nucleus and multiple cytoplasmic granules (lysosomes)
- Immature neutrophils contain primary azurophilic granules with proteases
- Mature neutrophils contain secondary granules

Mononuclear phagocytes

- Have smooth nuclei and also contain granules in the cytoplasm
- Cells include:
  - Monocytes in circulation
  - Tissue histiocytes
  - Microglial cells (brain)

- Kupffer cells (liver)
- Macrophages (serous cavities and lymphoid organs)

Natural killer (NK) cells

- Class of cytotoxic lymphocytes that carry marker CD16 but no unique receptors for antigenic targets
- Lyse virus-infected cells and tumour-derived cells by recognising Fc fragments
- Release perforins which punch holes in infected cells (causing cell lysis or a channel for the injection of protease enzymes)
- Use a dual receptor system to lyse cells that do not express MHC class I molecules (downregulated in cancer and viral infections) or that express stress-related proteins (infection and tumours produce MICA and MICB)
- Have no immunological memory
- Actions are enhanced by IFNs and IL-2

Bone-marrow-derived inflammatory cells

- Eosinophils, basophils and mast cells release inflammatory mediators in response to infection (prostaglandins, vasoactive amines, leukotrienes and signalling proteins such as cytokines)

2.2 SPECIFIC MECHANISMS OF IMMUNITY

The immune system is adaptive. When a new antigen is encountered cells undergo genetic rearrangements to generate a subgroup of cells capable of attacking the source. These undergo clonal expansion. After resolution, the system retains some of these cells as memory cells. The memory cells provide a background production of specific immunoglobulins and a population of T cells that can be reactivated quickly. This leads to a reduction in subsequent susceptibility to that disease in the future.

This acquisition of increased resistance to a specific infectious agent is known as acquired specific immunity, and forms the basis to many immunisation programmes.

Acquired specific immunity provides the ability to:

- Recognise the difference between self and non-self
- Mount a response that is specific to foreign material
- Remember previous responses so that a subsequent response to previously encountered foreign material will be faster and larger

Cell-mediated immunity (CMI) has distinct roles.

Role of CMI in bacterial infection

- Specific recognition of antigen by T cells
- Non-specific lymphokine production, which upregulates macrophages and activates cytotoxic T cells and B cells

Role of CMI in viral infection

- Upregulation of macrophages and killer cells for cell killing
- Producing interferons

All class I antigens and most of the class II antigens evoke the formation of the antibodies in genetically non-identical individuals.

Antigen presentation

An antigen is a substance capable of inducing a specific immune response. When a host encounters an antigen two things may occur:

- Proliferation of T lymphocytes
- Antibody formation by plasma cells

Dendritic cells and macrophages process antigens and present peptide fragments in association with MHC molecules on the cell surface. These can then be recognised by receptors on T cells. Antigen-presenting cells (APCs) are located in the lymphoid system and in all organs. They present antigens to the rest of the immune system in a manner dependant on the source of the antigen:

- **Endogenous proteins** (or viral proteins) are processed and presented bound to MHC class I molecules (and this combination is then recognised by CD8+ T cells)
- **Exogenous proteins** (taken up by phagocytosis or pinocytosis) are processed and presented bound to MHC class II molecules (and this combination is recognised by CD4+ T-helper cells)

Major histocompatibility complex (MHC)

This important set of genes is on the short arm of chromosome 6. The genes code for the human leucocyte antigens (HLA) which are present on cell membranes and are specific to each individual.

They consist of α and β chains which combine to provide a peptide-binding cleft in which the antigen fragment is displayed. The HLA system is the most polymorphic genetic system in humans (> 1000 alleles) which contributes to a huge array of different possible peptide binding clefts.

The recognition by the recipient's immune system of human leucocyte antigens on the surface of donor cells forms the basis of rejection following organ transplant.

MHC gene products

Based on their structure, distribution and function, the MHC gene products are classified into three groups.

Class I antigens

- Found on all nucleated cells and platelets as cell-surface molecules
- Coded by three loci designated HLA-A, HLA-B and HLA-C

Class II antigens

- Found on dendritic cells, macrophages, B lymphocytes and activated T cells
- Coded for in a region known as HLA-D
- Antigens are HLA-DR, HLA-DQ and HLA-DP
- These are proteins involved in antigen processing

Class III proteins

- Components of the complement system coded for within the MHC (includes C4 and heat shock protein, HSP)

Role of T lymphocytes

T lymphocytes recognise the combination of antigen and MHC molecule via their specialised receptor, the TCR. The TCR is also composed of α and β chains. During T cell development the gene segments encoding these chains are re-arranged, generating a huge diversity in their capacity to recognise peptide fragments.

The CD4 or CD8 molecule is associated with the TCR and its distal portion recognises either MHC class I or class II, respectively. This ensures that the correct type of T cell is brought into contact with the source of the antigen (see below).

Cytotoxic T lymphocytes

CD8+ cells are cytotoxic T lymphocytes that:

- Recognise antigen + MHC class I
- Kill cells infected with viruses or intracellular bacteria
- Memory cytotoxic T cells persist after recovery.

Helper T lymphocytes

These CD4+ cells recognise antigen + MHC class II.

They produce these soluble mediators:

- IFN-γ activates macrophages
- IL-2 stimulates proliferation of B and T cells
- IL-4 promotes differentiation of CD4+ T cells and B cells
- IL-5 stimulates activation of eosinophils
- IL-6 promotes differentiation of B and T cells
- IL-10 suppresses pro-inflammatory cytokine
- production by macrophages
- IL-12 promotes cytotoxic action of T cells and NK cells

Role of B lymphocytes

The B cell receptor for antigen is the antibody molecule. Activated B cells differentiate into plasma cells which secrete immunoglobulins. B cells have a unique ability to produce an almost endless array of antibodies to an enormous number of antigens.

- T-helper cells promote immunoglobulin production
- All have similar monomeric structure except IgM (pentameric structure)

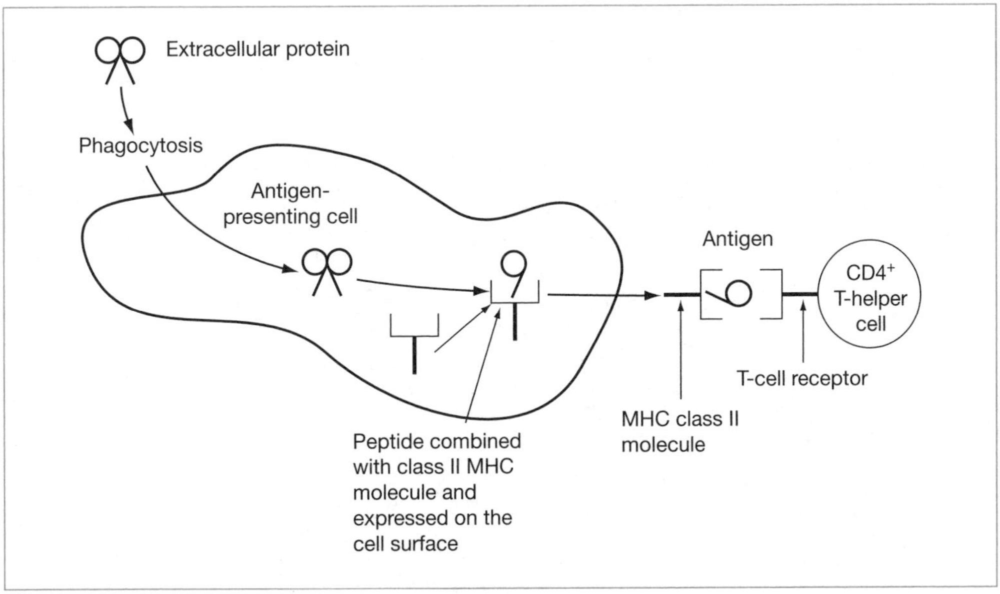

Figure 2.2a *Activation of CD4+ T lymphocytes*

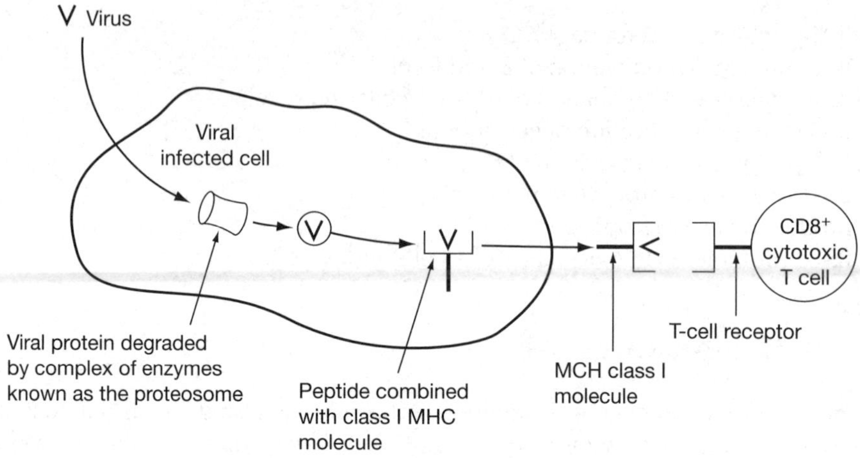

Figure 2.2b *Activation of CD8⁺ T lymphocytes*

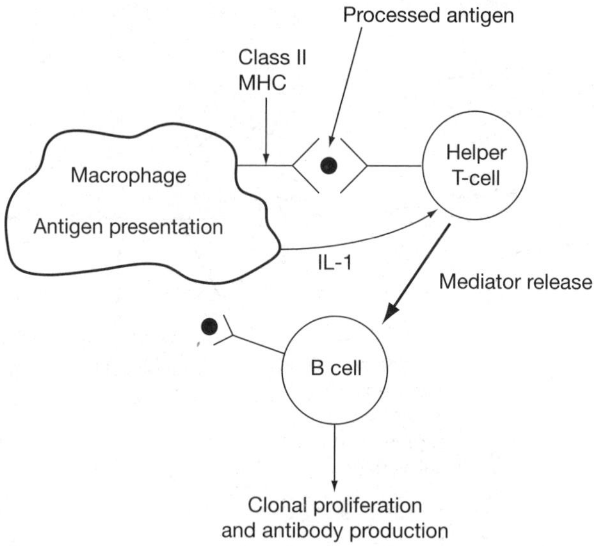

Figure 2.2c *T and B cell interaction*

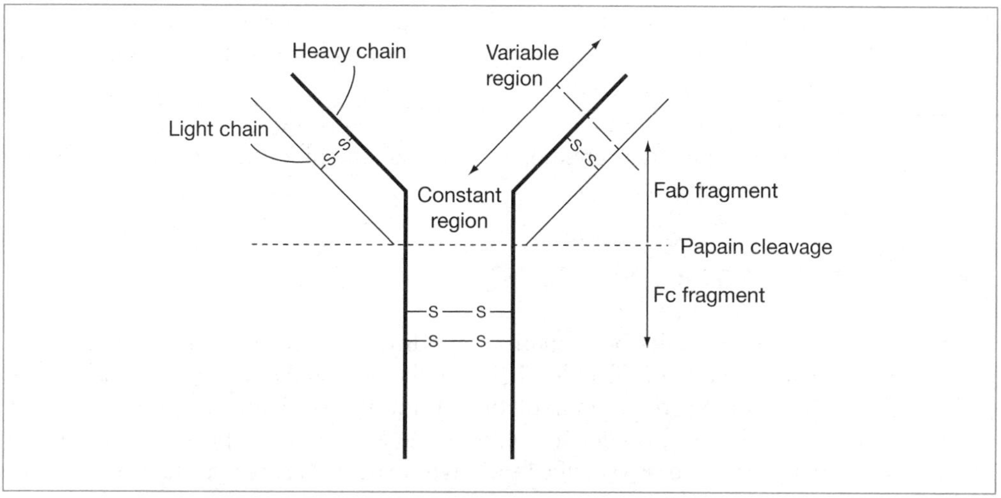

Figure 2.2d *Antibody structure*

An immunoglobulin molecule is a 4-polypeptide chain structure with two heavy and two light chains linked covalently by disulfide bonds (S–S). Digestion with papain produces antigen-binding fragments (Fab) and one Fc fragment, which is involved with complement and macrophage binding.

Light chains are either kappa (κ) or lambda (λ).

There are five main classes of immunoglobulin, based on the Fc fragment of the heavy chain. These are IgG (gamma), IgM (mu), IgA (alpha), IgD (delta), IgE (epsilon).

Antibodies binding to antigen lead to:

- Agglutination and lysis of bacteria (IgM)
- Opsonisation of such organisms
- Initiation of the classical complement pathway
- Blocking of the entry passage of micro-organisms from the respiratory tract, gut, eyes and urinary tract into deeper tissues
- Killing of the infected cell by antibody-dependent cell-mediated cytotoxicity
- Neutralising bacterial toxins and products

Functions of macrophages

Macrophages are generated from blood monocytes and present in most tissues. Functions include:

- **Antigen presentation:** macrophages present antigen to T lymphocytes as processed peptides associated with class II MHC molecules

- **Phagocytosis:** macrophages ingest bacteria opsonised by immunoglobulin +/– complement; this leads to the release of toxic molecules into the phagosome and death of the micro-organism
- **Secretion:** activated macrophages secrete numerous factors including neutral proteases, lysosyme, cytokines, chemotactic factors, arachidonic acid metabolites and complement components

Immune tolerance

As immune cells develop in the bone marrow and thymus they are exposed to self-antigens. Cells expressing receptor molecules that have the potential to recognise self-antigens are deleted to prevent the development of autoimmunity. Some antigens, those in immunologically privileged sites (such as the testis and eye) are not represented during this process and damage to these areas later in life will expose these antigens to the mature immune system for the first time.

2.3 DISORDERS OF IMMUNITY

In a nutshell ...

Hypersensitivity: tissue damage results from an inappropriate immune response to an exogenous antigen

Autoimmunity: immune response against the host's own antigens

Immune deficiency: inadequate immune response (may be due to a congenital or acquired defect)

Neoplastic proliferations: uncontrolled production of various elements of the immune system is a haematopoietic neoplasm

Transplant specific problems: implantation of transplanted material may result in rejection or graft vs host disease

Hypersensitivity reactions: Gell and Coombs' classification

Type I (anaphylactic or immediate)

Exposure to allergen leads to formation of IgE. IgE binds to mast cells and basophils, and then re-exposure to allergen leads to release of mediators from mast cells and basophils.

- Mediators include:
  - Histamine (causes bronchial constriction, increased vascular permeability and increased mucous gland secretion)
  - Leukotrienes (LT-C4, LT-D4, LT-E4 are 1000 times more potent than histamine)
  - Eosinophil and neutrophil chemotactic factors
  - Neutral proteases
  - PAF
- Examples: asthma and peanut allergy, anaphylactic shock

If you have a patient with a suspected anaphylactic reaction it is useful to send a blood sample to immunology 30 minutes after the reaction begins for tryptase enzyme levels. This can confirm anaphylaxis. Sodium cromoglycate and steroids are thought to inhibit mediator release by stabilising lysosomal membranes.

Type II (cytotoxic)

Mediated by antibodies against intrinsic or extrinsic antigens absorbed on the cell surface or on other components. Tissue damage results from complement-dependent reactions and antibody-dependent cell-mediated cytotoxicity.

Complement-dependent reactions

- Antibody complexes with antigen present on the cell surface activate the complement system. The cell then becomes susceptible to phagocytosis by the antibody or C3b present on the cell surface. In addition, cellular damage may be secondary to the formation of the MAC
- Examples: transfusion reaction, autoimmune thrombocytopenia, drug reactions

Antibody-dependent cell-mediated cytotoxicity

- Cells complexed with antibody are lysed by non-sensitised cells (NK cells, neutrophils, and monocytes)
- Examples: parasitic infections, graft rejection

Type III (immune complex-mediated)

- Mediated by immune complexes (antigen–antibody) formed either in the circulation or at extravascular sites. Immune complex leads to complement activation and thence to neutrophil activation with release of lysosomal enzymes, resulting in tissue damage
- Examples: SLE, acute glomerulonephritis, serum sickness

Type IV (cell-mediated/delayed)

- Mediated by sensitised T lymphocytes. Sensitised T cells lead to cytotoxic T cell activation plus release of lymphokines from T-helper cells, and thence to recruitment and activation of macrophages and monocytes, resulting in cell damage
- Examples: TB Mantoux test, transplant rejection

Type V (stimulatory)

- Anti-receptor antibodies lead to stimulation of cell function
- Examples: Graves' disease, myasthenia gravis

Autoimmunity

Autoimmune disorders result from a defect in self-tolerance. Autoimmunity may be tissue-specific or systemic. It is usually a relapsing and remitting condition.

Mechanisms of development of autoimmunity are unclear but may result from:

- Defects in suppressor cell number or function
- Micro-organisms eliciting antibodies that cross-react with self-antigens (molecular mimicry)
- Alteration of self-antigens by drugs or micro-organisms, exposing new antigenic sites
- T cell-independent emergence of B cells that are capable of mounting an autoimmune response

Major autoimmune diseases

Disease	Autoantibodies present against
Organ-specific disease	
Hashimoto's thyroiditis	Thyroglobulin, thyroid microsomes
Graves disease	TSH receptor (thyroid-stimulating Igs)
Atrophic gastritis	Parietal cells
Pernicious anaemia	Intrinsic factor
Goodpasture syndrome	Basement membrane (lungs and kidneys)
Myasthenia gravis	Acetylcholine receptor
Non-organ-specific disease	
SLE	Antinuclear antigen (ANA), DNA, smooth muscle
Rheumatoid arthritis	Rheumatoid factor
Scleroderma	Centromere

Individual diseases are typically linked to a specific class I or class II HLA-antigen (but not both). Diseases linked to class I locations are more common in men eg ankylosing spondylitis and Reiter syndrome (HLA-B27), psoriasis (HLA-Cw6), and those linked to class II are more common in women eg pernicious anaemia and Hashimoto's (HLA-DR5) and rheumatoid arthritis (HLA-DR4).

Monozygotic twins of patients are at increased risk of developing an autoimmune disease (around 25%) and siblings have a slightly increased risk (as they have a slightly different arrangement of HLA-alleles).

Autoantibodies

These should only be requested after discussion with an immunologist when a certain diagnosis is in mind.

- ANA (antinuclear antibody) should be requested only if SLE or Sjögren's is suspected. ANA is sensitive and SLE is unlikely in the absence of a positive ANA
- Anti-Ro and anti-La (associated with Sjögren's)
- Anti-centromere (associated with CREST syndrome)
- Anti-Scl70 (associated with scleroderma)

In general, older patients, even when healthy, will have higher autoantibody levels.

Important autoimmune diseases

See other sections for discussions of:

- Hashimoto's thyroiditis and Graves' disease (*Endocrine Surgery* in Book 2)
- Atrophic gastritis and pernicious anaemia (*Abdomen* in Book 2)
- Rheumatoid arthritis (*Orthopaedics* in Book 2)

Systemic lupus erythematosus (SLE)

Often affects young women. More common in Africa, the Caribbean and SE Asia.

The aetiology of SLE is unclear. There are many theories but it appears to be due to autoantibodies against a variety of normal cell nuclear constituents. These also form complexes that are deposited in other organs causing chronic inflammation. 'Lupus anticoagulant' is an autoantibody generated against membrane phospholipids. It is prothrombotic (it affects the intrinsic clotting cascade) and results in CVAs, multiple miscarriages, DVTs and PEs. Lupus anticoagulant is positive in a third of lupus patients.

SLE is a multisystem disease. It commonly presents with a number of symptoms (eg a 23-year-old woman from Thailand presenting with urticarial rash, mucosal ulceration, arthralgia, alopecia, pleuritic chest pain, fever and weight loss) of the following systems:

- **Dermatological:** may manifest with many types of rash; classically butterfly or lupoid skin rash/discoid rash, and/or photosensitivity

- **Mucous membranes:** ulceration, serositis
- **Cardiovascular:** acute necrotising vasculitis, endocarditis, pericarditis
- **Respiratory:** pleuritis
- **Renal:** immune complexes deposited in the glomeruli (chronic renal failure), ARF
- **Joint:** arthritis/arthralgia
- **Haematological:** anaemia, thrombocytopenia, neutropenia
- **CNS:** mental changes, psychosis, convulsions, CVA

Management should be by specialist only. It is steroid based (causing immunosuppression).

Sjögren syndrome

Mild illness due to autoimmune damage to joints and glandular structures (predominantly salivary and lacrimal but occasionally vulval glands and renal tubules).

Scleroderma

Slowly progressive disorder characterised by a vasculitis and excessive fibrosis. It affects multiple organ systems (skin changes and Raynauds; GI tract and replacement of the smooth muscle with collagen; synovitis; renal damage).

CREST syndrome is a variant: **C**alcinosis, **R**aynaud's, o**E**sophageal dysfunction, **S**clerodactyly and **T**elangiectasia.

Immune deficiency

May affect specific immunity (eg a T cell or B cell problem) or non-specific immunity (eg NK cells or complement). Classification is into primary and secondary disorders.

- **Primary immune deficiencies:** hereditary disorders that typically manifest between 6 months and 2 years of age as maternal antibody protection is lost (eg an 18-month-old boy presenting with recurrent pneumonia, several episodes of otitis media and sinusitis over the last year, failure to thrive; chest X-ray reveals bronchiectasis and serum Igs reveal hypogammaglobulinaemia)
- **Secondary immune deficiencies:** altered immune response secondary to malnutrition, ageing, infection, irradiation, splenectomy, medication (chemotherapy, steroids) or immunosuppression – recurrent, persistent or atypical infections suggest an immune deficiency disorder

Examples of immune deficiency include

IgA deficiency

Common disorder (1 in 600 people affected)
Congenital or acquired following viral infection
Usually asymptomatic
Recurrent pulmonary and GI infections
40% have antibodies to IgA

Common variable immune deficiency

Congenital
Hypogammaglobulinaemia (especially IgG)
May include disorder of T cell regulation in addition to B cell function
Typically presents after the first decade of life with recurrent pyogenic infections
Prone to autoimmune diseases and lymphoid malignancies

X-linked agammaglobulinaemia of Bruton

X-linked primary immunodeficiency disorder
Lack of mature B cells and nearly no immunoglobulin
T cell function and numbers are normal
Recurrent bacterial infections
Most viral and fungal infections are handled appropriately

di George syndrome

Congenital disorder due to fetal damage to the 3rd and 4th pharyngeal pouches
Syndrome involves thymic hypoplasia/aplasia, parathyroid hypoplasia, congenital heart disease and dysmorphic facies
T cell deficiency (prone to viral and parasitic infections)
B cells and Ig levels are normal

Severe combined immunodeficiency disease (SCID)

Group of autosomal or X-linked recessive disorders
Characterised by lymphopenia and defects in T and B cell function
Death usually occurs within 1 year from opportunistic infection (unless treated by bone marrow transplantation)

Complement factor deficiencies

C3 deficiency predisposes to bacterial infections
C2 deficiency increases risk of autoimmune connective tissue disorders
C5–8 defects lead to recurrent *Neisseria* infections (eg recurrent meningitis)

Acquired immunodeficiency syndrome (AIDS) (see section 3.2)

2.4 MANAGEMENT OF THE IMMUNOCOMPROMISED PATIENT

In a nutshell ...

- A patient may be immunocompromised due to a congenital or acquired cause
- The trauma of surgery itself may cause the patient to be immunocompromised
- Immunocompromised patients may exhibit attenuated signs of infection
- Patterns of susceptibility to infection depend on the immunological defect (may be truly pathogenic organisms or opportunists)

The immunocompromised patient may exhibit attenuated signs of infection, whereby the patient:

- May not be pyrexial
- May not generate a haematological response (raised lymphocyte count)
- May not generate localised inflammation (and consequently may have poor wound healing)
- May have masking of clinical signs (eg corticosteroid treatment often masks acute abdominal pain)

The pattern of infection depends on the defect in the immune system:

Generalised immune dysfunction

- Drugs (eg ciclosporin, corticosteroids)
- Trauma, burns, surgical stress
- Blood transfusion

Cell-mediated immunity dysfunction

- Specific B and T cell defects
- Widespread malignancy impairs T and B cell functions
- Haematological malignancy impairs cell-mediated immunity
- Malnutrition is associated with decreased lymphocyte function

Non-specific immunity dysfunction

- Diabetes impairs neutrophil activity
- Vitamin deficiency affects natural killer cells
- Immunoglobulin and complement deficiencies affect phagocytosis (eg splenectomy predisposes to encapsulated bacteria)

Immunocompromised patients are susceptible to two forms of infection:

- The same bugs that cause infection in everyone
- Opportunistic infections (less virulent organisms, viruses and fungal infection)

All infections in the immunocompromised may cause:

- Chest infection
- Urine infection
- Line infection
- Wound infection – macrophage dysfunction predisposes to wound infection (impaired phagocytosis of debris, etc)

Management of immunocompromised patients

Prophylactic pre-op antibiotics
Aggressive treatment of any pre-op infection
Consider diagnoses that may be masked by immunocompromise
Some immunosuppressive medication may be required throughout the operative period (eg transplant recipients, long-term steroid use)
Good surgical technique
Early identification of post-op problems (sepsis screen if pyrexial, requires careful wound management)

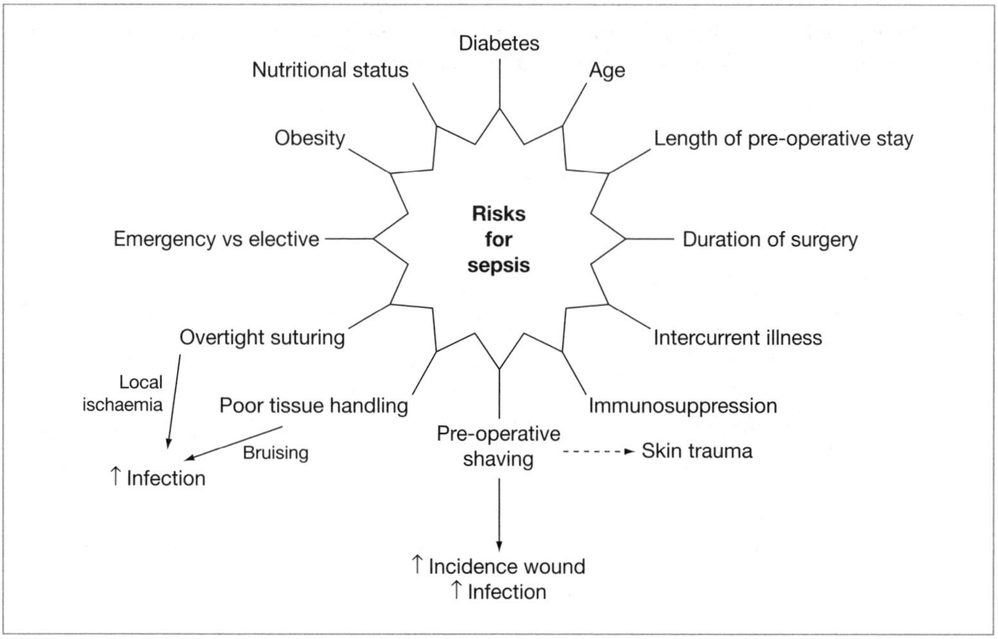

Figure 2.4a *Risks for sepsis*

Splenectomy

Splenectomy results in immunocompromise. Patients are particularly vulnerable to encapsulated organisms. Splenectomy is discussed in the *Abdomen* chapter of Book 2.

Overwhelming post-splenectomy infection

Caused by infection by one of the encapsulated organisms normally destroyed by the spleen. These are *Streptococcus pneumoniae, Neisseria meningitidis* and *Haemophilus influenzae.* Infection with these pathogens can lead to overwhelming sepsis with a mortality of 50–90%. Incidence is about 2% in children and 0.5% in adults, the highest incidence being in those undergoing splenectomy for lymphoreticular malignancy. All patients should have prophylaxis following splenectomy. Interestingly there are some reports that the risk of infection is lower if splenectomy is performed for trauma due to seeding of cells from the damaged spleen around the peritoneal cavity.

Current guidelines for post-splenectomy prophylaxis

The following should be carried out:

- Explanation of risk to patient, with card to carry
- Vaccination with Pneumovax™, HiB and meningococcal vaccines (at least 2 weeks before elective splenectomy or a few weeks after emergency surgery; remember boosters at 5–10 years)
- Antibiotic prophylaxis with penicillin V (or erythromycin) until age 15 only – lifelong prophylaxis should be offered but is particularly important for the first 2 years
- Patients should commence amoxil at first sign of febrile illness

Section 3
Disease-causing organisms

In a nutshell ...

Infection may be due to:
- Pathogenic organisms
- Infection with normal body commensals
- Infection with saprophytic organisms from soil, plants, etc

The pathogenicity of surgical infections depends on the:
- Virulence of the pathogen
- Level of host defence
- Nature of the infection

- **Conventional infections** affect previously healthy individuals
- **Opportunistic infections** affect immunosuppressed hosts
- **Colonisation** refers to a bacterial carrier without clinical symptoms or signs of infection
- **Infection** refers to a bacterial carrier with clinical symptoms and signs of infection
- **Bacteraemia** is the presence of bacteria in the bloodstream
- **Septicaemia** is the presence of bacterial products in the bloodstream (eg toxins) causing a clinical syndrome of septic shock. This term has been superceded by the more accurate terms 'sepsis', 'septic syndrome' and 'septic shock'

3.1 BACTERIA

Mechanisms of bacterial virulence

Exotoxins

- Usually Gram-positive bacteria (eg *Clostridium*)
- Highly toxic, highly antigenic polypeptides
- Specific target sites
- Excreted by living bacteria
- Neutralised by anti-toxins
- Include enterotoxins (eg *Staphylococcus aureus, Escherichia coli*)

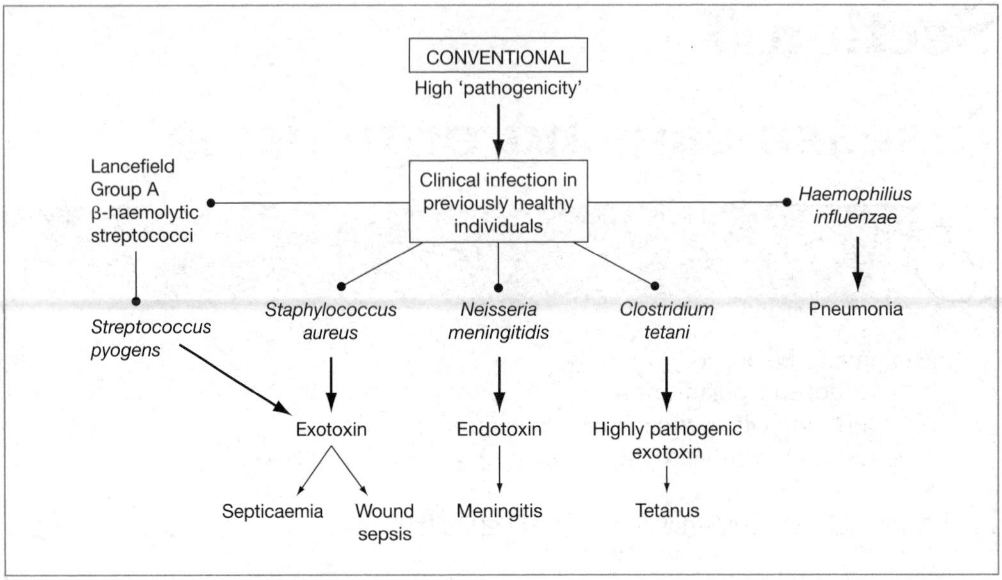

Figure 3.1a *Disease-causing organisms – conventional pathogens*

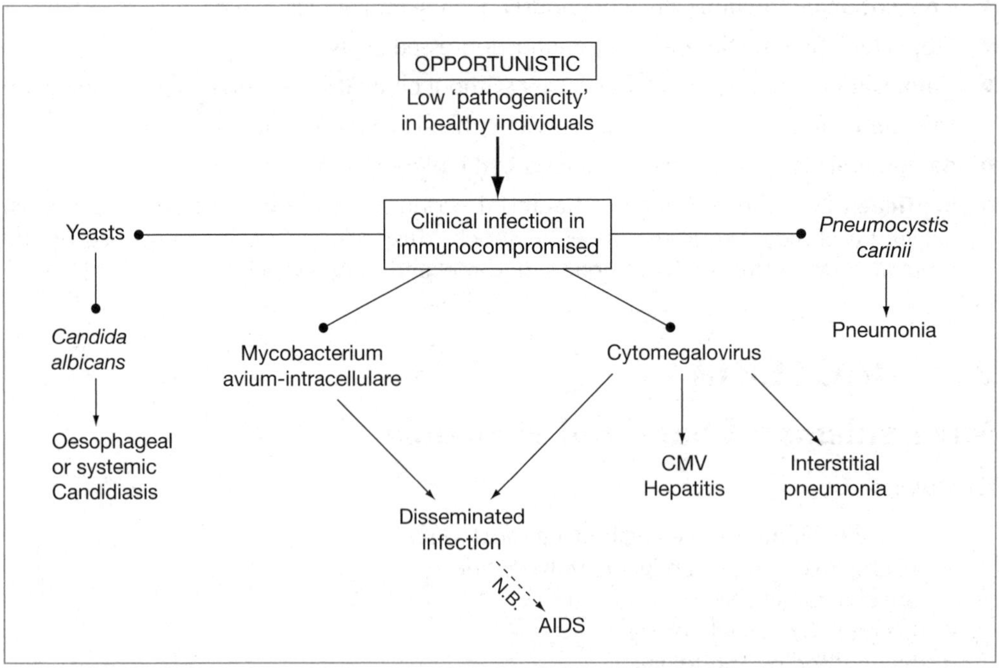

Figure 3.1b *Disease-causing organisms – opportunistic pathogens*

Endotoxins

- Lipopolysaccharide molecules in outer layer of Gram-negative cell walls
- Stimulate non-specific release of mediators from inflammatory cells
- Severe endotoxaemia is life-threatening

Capsules

- Capsule enhances invasiveness
- Increased resistance to phagocytosis
- Reduced effectiveness of bacterial killing within macrophages and polymorphs

Damage to tissues

- Fast-growing bacteria deprive host tissues of nutrients and lower tissue pH
- Secretion of exotoxins
- Destruction of cell walls produce endotoxins (cause systemic response, fever, increased capillary permeability, shock and even DIC)
- Some bacteria express 'super-antigens' which activate all of the B or T cells (some *S. aureus* eg as in toxic shock syndrome; some *Streptococcus*)
- Activation of phagocytosis causes systemic release of mediators from cells

Gram-positive bacteria

Stain blue/purple/black.

Gram-positive cocci

Aerobic cocci

- Staphylococci (clusters): presence of coagulase enzyme = virulence factor:
  - Coagulase-positive *S. aureus*
  - Coagulase-negative skin flora (eg *S. epidermidis*)
- Streptococci (chains/pairs): virulence (ability to lyse RBCs)
  - α-Haemolytic streptococci: partial lysis of RBCs; altered haemoglobin causes green colour around each colony on blood agar (eg *S. pneumoniae* = diplococcus; *S. viridans* group)
  - β-Haemolytic streptococci: complete lysis of RBCs around each colony
- Lancefield grouping
- Used mainly for β-haemolytic streptococci
  - Based on specific polysaccharide antigen extracted from streptococcal cell walls
  - Lancefield group A (eg *S. pyogenes*)
  - Lancefield group B (eg *S. faecalis*)
  - Other Lancefield groups (C and G)
  - γ-haemolytic streptococci: no lysis of RBCs (eg *S. faecalis* (most common) and *S. bovis*)

Chapter 2

Anaerobic cocci

- Anaerobic streptococci
  - Gut flora
  - *Enterococcus faecalis*

Gram-positive bacilli

Aerobic bacilli

- Diphtheroides
  - *Corynebacterium diphtheriae*
  - *Listeria monocytogenes*
  - *Bacillus* spp.

Anaerobic bacilli

- *Clostridium* species (spore-forming)
  - *C. botulinum* (botulism)
  - *C. perfringens* (gas gangrene)
  - *C. tetani* (tetanus)
  - *C. difficile* (pseudomembranous colitis)
- *Actinomycetes* (non-spore-forming; 'sulfur granules')
  - *Actinomyces israelii* (actinomycosis: cervicofacial, pulmonary, pelvic)

Gram-negative bacteria

Stain pink/red.

Gram-negative cocci

Aerobic cocci

- *Neisseria* (pairs)
  - *N. meningitidis*: meningococcus (meningitis and septicaemia)
  - *N. gonorrhoeae*: gonococcus (gonorrhoea)
- *Moraxella*: *M. catarrhalis* (atypical pneumonia)

Gram-negative bacilli

This is a large group.

Aerobic bacilli

- *Pseudomonas (P. aeruginosa)*: immunocompromised host, hospital-acquired infection, associated with respirators, drainage tubes, catheters
- *Vibrio* spp. (*V. cholerae*)
- *Campylobacter* (*C. jejuni*): human infection of small bowel
- Parvobacteria
  - *Haemophilus influenzae*

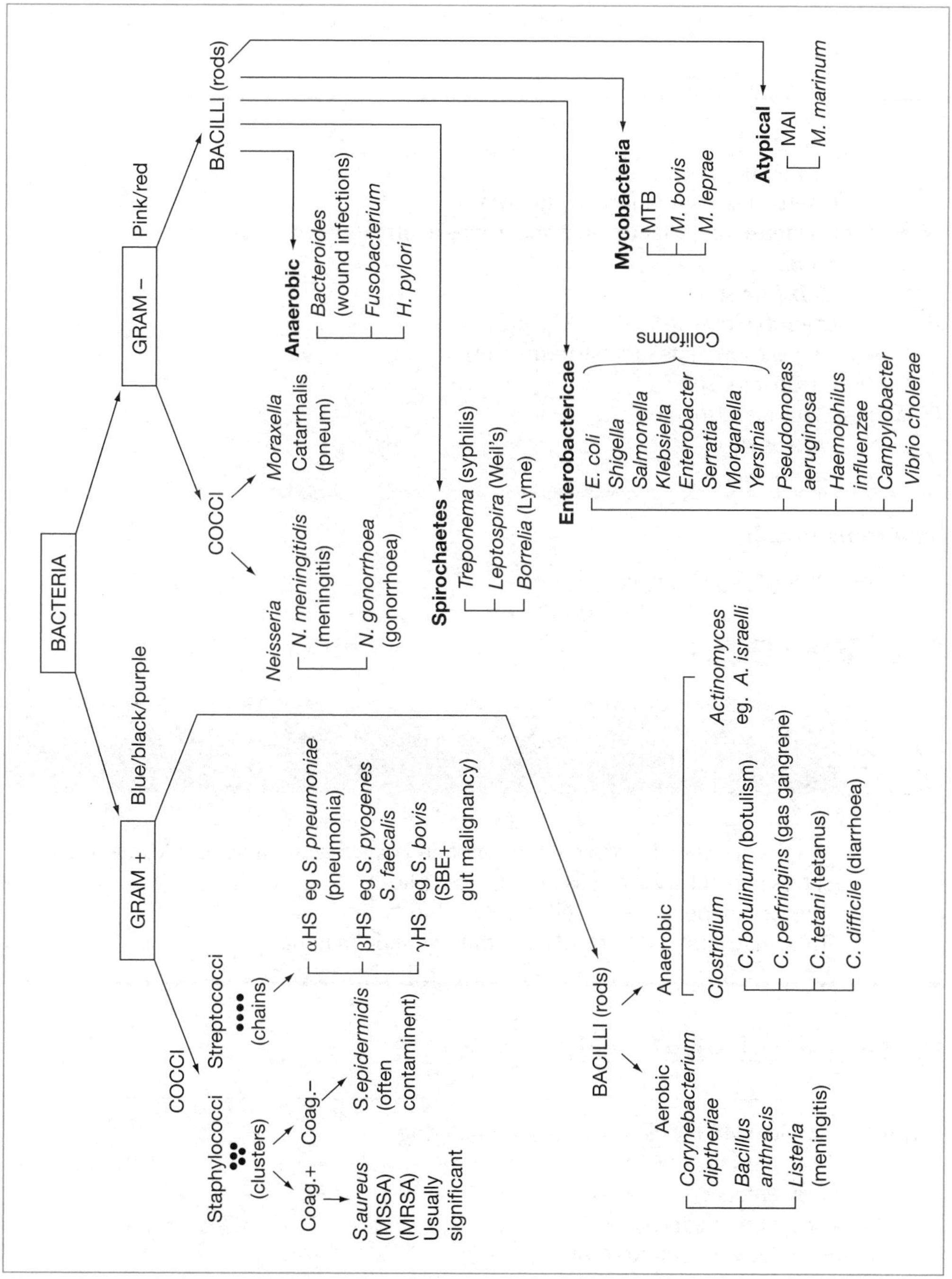

Figure 3.1c *Classification of bacteria*

  - *Yersinia enterocolitica* (gastroenteritis) and *Y. pseudotuberculosis* (mesenteric adenitis)
  - *Bordetella pertussis*
  - *Brucella* spp.
- *Legionella*
  - *L. pneumophilia*
  - Enterobacteria (coliforms; gut flora)
- Lactose fermenters 'facultative anaerobes' (can grow without oxygen)
  - *E. coli*
  - *Klebsiella* spp.
  - *Enterobacter* spp.
  - *Shigella* spp. (late lactose fermenter)
  - *Citrobacter* spp.
- Non-lactose fermenters
  - *Proteus* spp.
  - *Salmonella* spp.

Anaerobic bacilli

- Bacteroides (eg *B. fragilis*)

3.2 VIRUSES

In a nutshell ...

- Viruses are genetic material with protein coats that are able to integrate themselves into eukaryotic cells in order to replicate
- They are dependant on cells for their life cycle
- They may carry DNA or RNA as their genetic material

Pathological viral cycle

The pathological viral cycle involves the following:
- Virion particle attaches to the cell
- Virion enters cell
- Loses protein capsule
- Integrates with cell RNA or DNA
- Virus replicates genetic material
- Virions are produced using host cell's own materials
- Virions are released into the surrounding tissues and blood cells

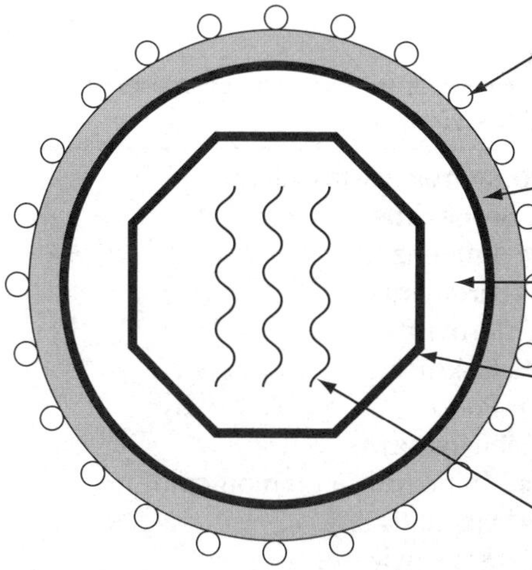

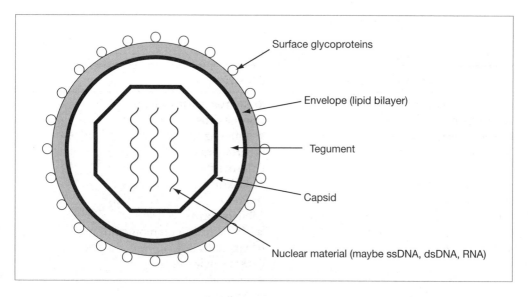

Figure 3.2a *The virion*

Some viruses integrate into the cell genome (becoming a 'pro-virus'). These are often DNA viruses. Others remain in the cytoplasm (most RNA viruses except those with reverse transcriptase). The virus replicates with the cell or hijacks cellular machinery to produce multiple copies of its own genetic material. Viral inclusions (aggregates of viral proteins) become visible in the nucleus or cytoplasm of infected cells. Virions are released from the cell (often by cellular lysis) so shedding multiple copies into surrounding tissues and the bloodstream.

Pathological effects of viruses

Pathological effects occur by:

- Death of the host cell by lysis to release virions
- Rendering infected cells less or non-functional
- Stimulating cell-mediated immunity which kills infected cells
- Stimulating cell proliferation (which may result in carcinogenesis and neoplasia eg EBV)

Viruses usually resolve without treatment unless the patient is immunocompromised. Topical applications exist for localised infection (eg aciclovir cream for herpes virus eruptions). Intravenous treatments are reserved for systemic infections in the immunocompromised.

Intravenous treatments commonly include:

- Nucleoside analogues
- Reverse transcriptase inhibitors (against HIV eg lamivudine and AZT)
- Protease inhibitors
- Interferons

Classification of viruses

CLASSIFICATION OF DNA AND RNA VIRUSES

Double-stranded DNA viruses	RNA viruses
Adenovirus family	**Rotavirus** (gastroenteritis)
Hepatitis B	**Coronavirus**
Herpes viruses	• Influenza
• CMV	**Picornavirus**
• EBV	**Enteroviruses**
• Herpes simplex	• Coxsackie
• Herpes zoster	• Polio
Pox viruses	**Echoviruses**
• Molluscum contagiosum	• Rhinovirus (common cold)
• Smallpox	• Hepatitis A
	Paramyxoviruses
	• Measles
	• Mumps
	• RSV
	Retroviruses
	• HIV-1
	• HIV-2
	• HTLV
	Togaviruses
	• Rubella
	• Hepatitis C
	• Hepatitis G

Immune responses to viruses

Three parts of the immune response to viruses

- Humoral response (neutralising antibodies, produced during vaccination or initial exposure)
- Interferon production
- Cellular response (T cell response for destruction of infected cells)

Specific important viruses

Influenza viruses

- A, B, and C strains
- Symptoms 1–2 days after exposure (fever, myalgia, headache)
- New strains are appearing and periodically cause severe outbreaks (eg avian flu) with large numbers of fatalities (often secondary to pneumonitis)
- Vaccine is available and is useful in the young, but less so in the elderly

Coxsackie viruses

- Coxsackie A causes sore throat with blistering, hand, foot and mouth disease
- Coxsackie B causes pleurisy, myocarditis

Morbillivirus (measles)

- Incubation period 14 days after droplet infection
- Starts as a cold followed by conjunctivitis, Koplik's spots, lymphoid hyperplasia, and rash
- Complications can be severe: pneumonitis, autoimmune encephalitis (may cause brain damage)
- Vaccine included in the MMR (measles, mumps, rubella) triple vaccine given in the 1st year in many countries. There has been an increased incidence of measles and mumps in recent years as a result of reduced uptake in the MMR vaccine amongst parents (after publication of a single spurious paper finding a link to autism). The result was devastating as many children and immunocompromised individuals have been infected with these preventable illnesses. In some cases the results are fatal

Mumps virus

- Mumps usually occurs in childhood: usually with inflammation of salivary glands +/– mild meningitis
- Adults may also get orchitis and infertility, oophoritis and pancreatitis
- Vaccine included in the MMR

Rubella (german measles)

- Mild illness transmitted by droplet infection
- Causes rash, arthritis and is teratogenic (can cause congenital blindness, deafness, heart defects, hepatospenomegaly, and thrombocytopenia in Gregg syndrome)
- Vaccine included in the MMR

Herpes viruses

Herpes viruses types 1–8 are DNA viruses that integrate into the human genome and periodically reactivate throughout life.

- **Herpes simplex 1 (HSV-1):** persists in nervous tissue causing cold sores (reactivated by sunlight, intercurrent illness, and stress). In the immunocompromised host it can also cause fulminant pneumonitis and encephalitis
- **Herpes simplex 2 (HSV-2):** causes genital herpes. It is sexually transmitted. The infection is fulminant if passed to a newborn during birth or to an immunocompromised person
- **Varicella zoster or herpes (chickenpox virus):** is spread by droplet infection and often contracted in childhood. It causes a vesicular rash and can cause pneumonitis and encephalitis in immunocompromised people. It resides in a nerve root and may reactivate as shingles later in life with a vesicular rash on the corresponding skin dermatome, paraesthesia or hyperaesthesia and pain. May also involve the cornea (serious complication). A vaccine is available but not commonly used in Europe (there is increasing use in the USA). Contraction of the disease in the first trimester can cause foetal abnormalities and pregnant women who have not previously had chickenpox must consider treatment with VZV antibodies if exposed to the disease
- **Epstein–Barr virus (EBV) (herpes 4):** EBV infects the B cells and integrates into the genome. Infected cells are eventually eliminated by the T cells of the immune system. EBV causes infectious mononucleosis (also called glandular fever or 'the kissing disease' as it passes via saliva from teenager to teenager). It is also common in gay men. The incubation period is around 6 weeks and the disease features fever, malaise and generalised lymphadenopathy. There may be a mild hepatitis and thrombocytopenia. EBV is also linked to lymphoma (especially Burkitt's and lymphomas of the brain, SCC of the throat, and salivary gland cancers). There may also be a link to MS
- **Cytomegalovirus (CMV) (herpes 5):** a very common infection, often acquired in utero or infancy. It can also be acquired from sexual activity, blood transfusion or transplantation. 80% of adults have positive serology
  - May cause a mononucleosis-type infection initially
  - Remains latent until immunosuppression occurs
  - May cause pneumonia, GI tract perforation, chorioretinitis (in AIDS), or encephalitis, and is the most common precipitating factor for Guillaine–Barré syndrome (commonly in the immunocompromised such as AIDS)
  - May cause fetal abnormalities
  - CMV status of donor and recipient is important in organ transplantation. CMV positive organs are generally not given to CMV negative recipients. Post-transplant immunosuppression may re-activate the virus resulting in the conditions listed above
- **Herpes 8:** Kaposi's sarcoma virus is caused by herpes 8 virus

Hepatitis viruses

The first hepatitis virus was isolated in 1969 and six major viruses are now known (hepatitis viruses A–G). Other common viruses also affect the liver (eg CMV, mumps, rubella).

- **Hepatitis A:** an RNA virus transmitted by the faecal–oral route. It is often picked up through travel. After 6 weeks it causes jaundice, weakness, fever, and flu-like symptoms with tender lymphadenopathy. The disease usually resolves spontaneously, and is occasionally fulminant. It may relapse. Vaccination with IgG is effective
- **Hepatitis B:** a DNA virus with many subtypes. It is transmitted parenterally, vertically, or sexually. Acute illness resolves within a few weeks. Fulminant hepatitis may occur in < 1% cases. The disease progresses to chronicity in 5% of cases. Chronic hepatitis B may cause an active hepatitis with eventual cirrhosis. Treatments for chronic hepatitis B include IFN and lamivudine but these have limited efficacy. Three-stage vaccination is mandatory for healthcare workers and for anyone likely to be exposed to the virus (eg homosexual men). Hepatitis B immunoglobulins (HBIG) can be given in cases of emergency exposure (eg newborn from infected mother; needlestick injury)
- **Hepatitis C:** a single-stranded RNA virus. Risk factors for transmission include exposure to blood (transfusion, needlestick injury), IV drug use, tattoos and body piercings, and multiple sexual partners. Often there are no risk factors identified. The acute phase occurs 6 weeks after infection with flu-like illness +/– jaundice. Chronicity occurs in 50–60%; the disease may progress to chronicity with no symptoms until end-stage liver disease. IFN and ribavirin combination therapy may be given under the care of an experienced hepatology team; transplantation may be required for end-stage disease
- **Hepatitis D:** a co-infection that occurs with hepatitis B infection and is usually associated with parenteral transmission
- **Hepatitis E:** similar to hepatitis A and causes acute but not chronic illness
- **Hepatitis G:** very similar to hepatitis C but does not seem to be pathogenic in humans

Human immunodeficiency viruses (HIV) and AIDS

Pathophysiology of AIDS

AIDS is caused by the human immunodeficiency virus (HIV) – a retrovirus. There are two classes:

- HIV-1 is responsible for the global pandemic
- HIV-2 is less virulent

There are various subtypes of HIV-1 (types A–O) with different geographical distributions. The HIV membrane contains the glycoprotein gp120, which has a high affinity for the CD4 antigen on T-helper cells, monocytes, and macrophages. There is also a molecule called gp41 which stimulates fusion of the HIV virion to the target cell membrane. HIV complexes with the target cell, the virus invades cell, its single-stranded RNA genome is copied as double-stranded DNA by the viral reverse transcriptase system, and viral DNA integrates into the host genome.

Key genes in HIV

Env codes for the production and processing of envelope proteins (gp120 and gp41)
Gag forms matrix protein and proteins of the core capsid and nucleocapsid
Pol directs synthesis of the enzymes (integrase, protease, reverse transcriptase)
Nef is a virulence factor

Viral propagation occurs (via the viral protease system) with subsequent T cell activation. There is an extremely high degree of viral turnover (20% per day) throughout the course of infection, including the latent period. The virus often changes its capsid through mutation producing different strains (even in the same patient) and so development of a vaccine is difficult. Most anti-HIV drugs inhibit either reverse transcriptase or protease synthesis.

CD4+ T-cell depletion increases susceptibility to opportunistic infections and malignancies.

Transmission of HIV

Sexual transmission occurs when the presence of other sexually transmitted diseases aids transmission of the virus (due to ulceration and inflammation of mucosa).

Vertical transmission occurs from mother to child transplacentally (risk is about 25% without prophylaxis) or via breast milk (risk is 5–15%). This risk is reduced with anti-retroviral treatments.

Parenteral transmission is through exposure to infected blood products (transfusion, contaminated needles, etc).

Demographics of HIV infection

Up-to-date information on the incidence and prevalance of HIV in different countries can be accessed via the World Health Organization website (http://www.who.int/hiv).

There is new evidence that adult HIV infection rates have decreased in certain countries and that changes in behaviour to prevent infection – such as increased use of condoms, delay of first sexual experience, and fewer sexual partners – have played a key part in these declines. This predominantly relates to the situation in Africa – 40% HIV infection prevalance in South Africa (higher in sub-Saharan Africa); incidence rates in Kenya have fallen from 10% in 2003 to 7% in 2005 and a similar pattern has been seen in Zimbabwe and some Caribbean countries.

Overall trends in HIV transmission are still increasing, and far greater HIV prevention efforts are needed to slow the epidemic. Increasing incidence of infection has been documented in south-east Asia and eastern Europe. Additionally, the incidence of HIV infection in young heterosexual women in the UK has doubled in the past 5 years. The incidence of HIV in the USA is also increasing – 50% of heroin users in New York, USA are HIV-positive and 1.5% women of childbearing age in the USA are HIV-positive.

1% of cases have occurred in haemophiliacs who received infected blood (majority of cases occurred prior to the advent of routine screening of blood products in the 1980s and most of these patients have now died).

HIV testing

The routine HIV test is ELISA, which detects antibody directed towards HIV. In the early stages (before seroconversion ie in the first 12 weeks or so) the test may be negative but the patient is highly infectious. All patients should give informed consent and be counselled before and after HIV testing.

Clinical symptoms of HIV infection

HIV infection is initially asymptomatic. AIDS is essentially a syndrome, and is characterised by:

- **Vulnerability to infections** by opportunistic micro-organisms (ie those that do not produce severe disease in humans with a normal immune system)
- **Systemic features:** generalised lymphadenopathy (cervical, occipital, epitrochlear and submental); fever; weight loss (accelerates in the terminal phases)
- **Tumours** (Kaposi's sarcoma and non-Hodgkin's B cell lymphoma)
- Variable degree of **nervous system damage** (attacks the brain, spinal cord, and peripheral nerves) causing PML (progressive multifocal leucoencephalopathy)

Opportunistic infections in HIV infection

Respiratory tract infection

- *Pneumocystis carinii*: causes pneumonia; rarely disseminates outside the lung. Symptoms include fever, non-productive cough, and dyspnoea. CXR shows peri-hilar infiltrates and diffuse shadowing. Diagnosed on BAL
- *Mycoplasma tuberculosis*: TB is common in HIV patients. Causes pulmonary infection (commonly miliary form but may present atypically). May also cause extra-pulmonary TB (joints, bone and GI tract). Multidrug resistance is a problem. *Mycobacterium avium complex* (MAC) infection is pathognomic for HIV
- *CMV*: Once a common opportunistic infection seen in AIDS. Often disseminated. Causes pneumonitis, GI and CNS disease (including retinitis and blindness). Fortunately with HAART these are rarely seen now in developed countries

CNS infection

- *Toxoplasmosis gondii*: commonest CNS problem in AIDS; causes multiple brain abscesses visible as ring-enhancing lesions on CT/MRI

- *Cryptococcus neoformans*: causes insidious meningitis in advanced disease; Treat with fluconazole (may need lifelong secondary preventative treatment)
- *Herpes simplex*: causes encephalitis and blistering of mucosal areas

GI tract infection

- *Candida albicans*: causes irritation and ulceration in the mouth and oesophagus during advanced disease. Treated with nystatin or amphotericin orally (or fluconazole systemically)
- *Cryptosporidium*: causes diarrhoea (advise patients to boil water)
- *HIV enteropathy*: small bowel enteropathy caused by the virus itself; causes villous atrophy with malabsorption

Autoimmune phenomena

The HIV virus causes an increase in autoimmune phenomena, possibly due to effects on B cells (eg pancreatic damage leading to diabetes).

Surgical conditions in HIV

Essentially these are infections and tumours, as shown in the shaded box.

Surgical conditions in HIV/AIDS

Infections

Abscesses
Empyema
Peritonitis
Perianal disease
Osteomyelitis

Tumours

Non-Hodgkin's lymphoma: usually high-grade B cell lymphoma; 2% get cerebral lymphoma. Often have EBV as an additional aetiological agent

Kaposi's sarcoma: there are nodules of abnormal vessels and spindle-shaped cells in the dermis. This sarcoma is aggressive and infiltrates other organs (lungs, body cavities and GI system). Caused by herpes virus 8

Natural history of HIV disease

Up-to-date information about the natural history of HIV can be found on the WHO website (http://www.who.int).

Clinical staging is for use where HIV infection has been confirmed (ie there is serological and or virological evidence of HIV infection). The clinical stage is useful for assessment at baseline (first diagnosis of HIV infection) or entry into HIV care. It is also useful in the follow-up of patients in care and treatment programmes.

Clinical staging of HIV infection

Primary HIV infection

- Asymptomatic
- Acute retroviral syndrome

Clinical stage 1 (asymptomatic established HIV)

- Asymptomatic
- Persistent generalised lymphadenopathy

Clinical stage 2 (mild symptoms)

- Moderate unexplained weight loss (< 10% of presumed or measured body weight)
- Recurrent respiratory tract infections (sinusitis, tonsillitis, bronchitis, otitis media, pharyngitis)
- Herpes zoster
- Angular cheilitis
- Recurrent oral ulceration
- Papular pruritic eruptions
- Seborrhoeic dermatitis
- Fungal nail infections

Clinical stage 3 (advanced symptoms)

- Unexplained severe weight loss (> 10% of presumed or measured body weight)
- Unexplained chronic diarrhoea for longer than 1 month
- Unexplained persistent fever (intermittent or constant for longer than 1 month)
- Persistent oral *Candida*
- Oral hairy leukoplakia
- Pulmonary tuberculosis
- Severe presumed bacterial infections (eg pneumonia, empyema, pyomyositis, bone or joint infection, meningitis, bacteraemia, excluding pneumonia)
- Acute necrotising ulcerative stomatitis, gingivitis, or periodontitis
- Unexplained anaemia (< 8 g/dL), neutropenia (< 500/mm^3) and or chronic thrombocytopenia (< 50 000/mm^3)

Clinical stage 4 (severe/very advanced symptoms)

- HIV-wasting syndrome
- Pneumocystis pneumonia
- Recurrent severe presumed bacterial pneumonia

Chapter 2

Chronic herpes simplex infection (orolabial, genital, or anorectal of more than 1 month's duration or visceral at any site)
Oesophageal candidiasis (or *Candida* of trachea, bronchi or lungs)
Extrapulmonary tuberculosis
Kaposi's sarcoma
Cytomegalovirus infection (retinitis or infection of other organs)
Central nervous system toxoplasmosis
HIV encephalopathy
Extrapulmonary cryptococcosis including meningitis
Disseminated non-tuberculous mycobacteria infection
Progressive multifocal leukoencephalopathy
Chronic cryptosporidiosis
Chronic isosporiasis
Disseminated mycosis (extrapulmonary histoplasmosis, coccidiomycosis, penicilliosis)
Recurrent septicaemia (including non-typhoidal salmonella)
Lymphoma (cerebral or B-cell non-Hodgkin's)
Invasive cervical carcinoma
Atypical disseminated leishmaniasis

CD4 counts

The pathogenesis of HIV virus infection is largely attributable to the decrease in the number of T cells (a specific type of lymphocyte) that bear the CD4 receptor. The immunological status of the HIV infected infant, child adolescent or adult can be assessed by measurement of absolute number or percentage of T cells expressing CD4 cells, and this is regarded as the standard way to define the severity of HIV-related immunodeficiency. Progressive depletion of CD4+ T cells is associated with progression of HIV, and an increased likelihood of opportunistic infections and other clinical events associated with HIV.

- At a **CD4 count of 200–350** $\times 10^6$/L infections with common organisms begin to occur (particularly *S. pneumoniae, H. influenzae, M. tuberculosis* and *Candida*); patients may present with weight loss, diarrhoea, fever, fatigue and myalgia
- At a **CD4 count of < 200** $\times 10^6$/L there is increased risk of opportunist infections and tumours (commonly *P. carinii* pneumonia (incidence decreasing with use of prophylaxis), cerebral toxoplasmosis, Kaposi's sarcoma, and candidiasis)
- At a **CD4 count of < 50** $\times 10^6$/L multiple, concurrent infections with organisms of low virulence are common (commonly atypical mycobacterial infections, systematic fungal infections, CMV infection, AIDS dementia complex and lymphoma)

Prognosis in HIV infection

The course of infection depends on viral and host factors, and more recently on treatment options. The mean time from infection with HIV to diagnosis of a major opportunistic infection or tumour is 11.2 years; the mean time to death is around 18–24 months after this (without treatment). With HAART (Highly Active Anti-Retroviral Therapy) patients can expect to have a much longer life expectancy (50–60 years or maybe longer).

Anti-viral treatments for HIV/AIDS

In affluent countries, the progression of HIV disease has been markedly slowed by the use of HAART. This refers to combined therapy with three or more drugs, usually two that target the reverse transcriptase and one that targets the viral protease.

Reverse transcriptase inhibitors

- **Nucleoside analogues:** by mimicking a nucleoside these drugs become incorporated into the growing DNA strand by the viral reverse transcriptase. This then halts further DNA synthesis. Examples include zidovudine (AZT; Retrovir™), lamivudine (Epivir™), and didanosine (Videx™)

Other anti-HIV drugs

- **Protease inhibitors:** these block the viral protease so that the proteins needed for assembly of new viruses cannot be cleaved from the large protein precursor. Examples include indinavir (Crixivan™), saquinavir (Invirase™), ritonavir (Norvir™)
- **Fusion inhibitors:** the viral protein gp41 penetrates the host plasma membrane by a process involving non-covalent binding between two segments of its chain (HR1 and HR2). Fusion inhibitors (eg enfuvirtide, Fuzeon™) act as a competitive inhibitor, binding to HR1 and thus preventing binding of HR2
- **Integrase inhibitors:** a drug that inhibits the HIV-1 integrase has been shown to slow disease progression in experimental animals (monkeys)

Problems with drug treatment

Drug treatment has been shown to slow the progression of the disease, transiently reverse the symptoms of the late stages of the disease and reduce vertical transmission, preventing the infection of babies born to infected mothers. However, the problems with drug therapy include:

- Expense (£5 000 to £10 000/year/patient)
- Side effects (eg nausea, diarrhoea, hepatic damage)
- Complicated dosing regimen
- Resistance: drug treatment selects for the emergence of drug-resistant virions in the patient. This is particularly serious because of the speed at which mutations occur in HIV

3.3 FUNGI

In a nutshell ...

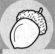

Fungal infections

Fungi can be categorised as:

- Yeasts (eg *Candida, Cryptococcus*)
- Moulds (eg *Aspergillus*)
- Dimorphic fungi (eg *Histoplasmosis*)

They cause different types of disease:

- Local superficial (eg ringworm, tinea versicolor, tinea pedis)
- Subcutaneous (eg sporotrichosis)
- Systemic infections (mycoses; occur in immunocompromised people)

Fungal species

Most fungi are opportunists. They are capable of causing systemic disease in immunocompromised hosts/people.

Candida spp.

- Most common human fungal disease
- *Candida albicans* is a normal commensal
- Overgrowth occurs when the host has:
  - Normal flora eradicated by antibiotics
  - Hyperglycaemia (in diabetes; vaginally during pregnancy)
  - Wet skin (eg groin creases in the obese)
  - Immune dysfunction
- It occurs as white patch +/– ulceration on mucosal surfaces
- Oesophageal candidiasis is a sign of serious underlying immune compromise

Cryptococcus

- Yeast with a polysaccharide coating
- Responsible for meningitis, pneumonia and GI infections
- Any organ can be involved

Aspergillus (aspergillosis)

- Invasive fungus (Aspergillus fumigatus or A. niger)
- Filamentous with septate branching hyphae
- Produces aflatoxin (carcinogen)
- Forms balls of fungus in the lungs (aspergilloma)
- Capable of invading blood vessels
- Causes allergic aspergillosis (asthmatic reaction to airborne spores)
- Causes invasive aspergillosis (systemic; often fatal in the immunosuppressed)

Histoplasma (histoplasmosis)

- Tiny non-encapsulated yeast
- Spores are inhaled from soil, bird or bat droppings
- Spores lodge in the lungs, causing mild fever and symptoms of a cold ('primary histoplasmosis')
- Chronic reactivated histoplasmosis causes pulmonary cavities and granulomas – very similar to TB pattern
- Systemic histoplasmosis is often fatal in immunocompromised people/hosts

Sporothrix (sporotrichosis)

- Occurs while gardening or from rose-thorn injury
- May be superficial or deep and spreading

Pneumocystis carinii

- Described as a fungus or a protozoan
- Usually harmless in immunocompetent adults
- Increasingly seen in immunocompromise (especially AIDS)
- Organisms damage pneumocytes and alveolar spaces fill with organisms and dead cells producing pneumonia (PCP)
- Treatment with co-trimoxazole

Treatment of fungi

Options for treatment of fungal infection include:

- **Polyene antifungals:** not absorbed orally and are used to treat infections such as *Candida albicans* topically (eg nystatin). Amphotericin is used for systemic infections and is given parenterally
- **Imidazole antifungals:** used for vaginal candidiasis and local oral infections (eg ketoconazole, miconazole)
- **Triazole antifungals:** well absorbed and achieve good penetrance into the tissues including the CNS (eg fluconazole)

3.4 PARASITES

In a nutshell ...

Parasitic infections

Protozoa may be:

- Luminal (amoebiasis, cryptosporidosis, giardiasis, trichomoniasis)
- Blood-borne (malaria, trypanosomiasis)
- Intracellular (Chagas' disease, leishmaniasis, toxoplasmosis)

Helminths (worms) may be:

- Platyhelminths (flatworms)
- Cestodes (tapeworms) eg *Echinococcus* (hydatid disease)
- Trematodes (flukes) eg *Schistosoma*, the liver flukes
- Nematodes (roundworms) eg *Ascaris*

Amoeba (eg Entamoeba histolytica)

- *E. histolytica* causes colonic inflammation and diarrhoea
- May be commensal
- Acquired by ingestion of cysts
- Affects right side of the colon (amoeba penetrate the mucosa through the crypts and spread out underneath it causing ulceration and eventually sloughing; occasionally the bowel perforates)
- May cause extra-intestinal disease, predominantly in the liver with formation of abscesses (see *Abdomen* chapter in Book 2) and may also spread to the heart, lungs and brain
- Treatment with metronidazole

Giardia lamblia

- Usually acquired by ingestion
- Accumulates in the duodenum; cysts excreted in the stool
- May be asymptomatic or cause diarrhoea and malabsorption
- Treatment with metronidazole

Cryptosporidium

- Lodges in the brush border of the villi
- Common cause of diarrhoea in children
- Increasingly common in AIDS patients

Trichomonas (trichomoniasis)

- Flagellate organism transmitted sexually
- May be asymptomatic or cause discharge from vaginitis, urethritis and prostatitis

Plasmodium spp. (malaria)

- Four *Plasmodium* species: *P. malariae, P. ovale, P. vivax, P. falciparum*
- Intracellular parasites carried by female mosquitos (humans are intermediate hosts)
- Parasites travel from subcutaneous region to the liver where they multiply and enter RBCs; further parasite multiplication occurs here and then the cells undergo lysis to release the organism (life cycle of 24 hours)
- Symptoms depend on *Plasmodium* type and those from *P. falciparum* include:
  - Pyrexia and rigors
  - Massive haemolysis
  - Hepatosplenomegaly
  - Raised ICP in cerebral malaria
- 'Blackwater fever' (*P. falciparum*) is due to haemoglobinuria which precipitates renal failure and diffuse thrombotic events

Trypanosoma (trypanosomiasis)

- Flagellate parasites
- Responsible for african sleeping sickness and Chagas' disease
- Carried by tsetse flies
- Results in damage to the brain and organ dilatation (megacolon, cardiac dilatation, mega-oesophagus) possibly by an autoimmune process

Leishmania (leishmaniasis)

- Variety of syndromes caused by tiny protozoa
- Found in Africa and South America
- Causes cutaneous (spontaneous healing sores) or mucocutaneous leishmaniasis (non-healing ulceration)

Toxoplasma (toxoplasmosis)

- Intracellular parasite associated with cat faeces
- 50% people have positive serology
- Dangerous for fetuses and immunocompromised people

Helminths

Nematodes (roundworms)

- Eggs are ingested and larvae hatch in the stomach; they pass through the lungs and are coughed up and re-swallowed to settle in the gut
- Can grow to great lengths (up to 30 cm)
- Balls of worms can cause intestinal obstruction or perforation

Cestodes (tapeworms)

- Found in uncooked food
- Worm attaches to the bowel wall
- Uses up vitamin B12 and may cause vitamin deficiency and weight loss

Trematodes (flukes)

- *Schistosoma* (schistosomiasis): lives in the bloodstream, but pathology is from tissue reaction where eggs are laid (500 per day!). Acquired from infected water (eg Lake Malawi). Symptoms depend on affected tissue:
  - Hepatic fibrosis and cirrhosis
  - Urothelium causing SCC and renal failure
- Treatment with praziquantel 40–60 mg/kg; three doses over 1 day is effective
- *Filaria* (filariasis; elephantiasis): larvae carried by mosquitoes and mature worms plug the lymphatics causing obstruction and eventual fibrosis

Treatment of helminth infections is typically with mebendazole (100–200 mg three times daily, for 3–5 days) or with albendazole.

Section 4
Surgical infections

In a nutshell ...

You will come across infections that are due to:

- Primary conditions (eg any surgical condition ending in -itis)
- Community acquired (eg UTI, gastroenteritis)
- Hospital acquired (nosocomial)

Always attempt to identify the organism in order to tailor antibiotic treatment ie send specimens before starting empirical treatment.

Do not delay onset of treatment if clinically septic (ie treat with a 'best guess' antibiotic after sending specimens).

Take advice from microbiologists. This is essential in the immunocompromised and patients previously treated with multiple antibiotics.

4.1 RECOGNITION OF A SEPTIC PATIENT

Definitions of 'sepsis'

- **Sepsis:** clinical evidence of infection
- **Sepsis syndrome:** clinical evidence of infection plus evidence of altered organ perfusion
- **Septic shock:** septic syndrome plus evidence of decreased blood pressure unresponsive to fluid therapy

Clinical indicators of infection

Consider sepsis as a diagnosis in cases of:

- Changes in core temperature
  - Fever: > 37.8 °C
  - Hypothermia: < 36 °C (especially in the elderly)
- Unexplained hypotension

- Oliguria
- Confusion

Patients should be thoroughly examined and a septic screen performed.

Examination for sepsis

Possible foci of infection

Abdominal examination
- Bowel: eg Inflammatory bowel disease, perforation, anastomotic leak, abscess
- Hepatobiliary: eg cholecystitis, cholangitis, hepatitis
- Genito-urinary: eg UTI, pyelonephritis

Respiratory examination (eg pneumonia)
Cardiovascular examination (eg endocarditis)
Skin: surgical wound inspection, percutaneous lines including venflons, abscesses
Joints: Septic arthritis, prosthetic infection
CNS: meningitis, encephalitis
Haematological: recent travel (eg malaria)

Septic screen

The nature of the septic screen should be directed by findings at patient examination. In particular, radiological investigation of sepsis should be targeted to the most likely focus.

Septic screen

Blood tests
- Full blood count (for leukocytosis)
- Acute-phase proteins: C-reactive protein, fibrinogen
- Urea, creatinine and electrolytes
- LFTs/amylase
- Clotting
- ABGs for acidosis

Radiology
- CXR
- Abdominal CT
- Cardiac ECHO

Microbiology
- Blood cultures
- Sputum

Urine

Blood tests for sepsis

Leukocytosis

The white cell count (WCC) may be elevated, referred to as 'leukocytosis'. Differential diagnosis of leukocytosis is discussed in Chapter 4 *Haematology*. Features of leukocytosis pertinent to sepsis will be outlined here. Very high WCC may be indicative of abscess formation (> 20). WCC may be low if there is overwhelming sepsis (NB the elderly may exhibit signs of sepsis without a rise in the WCC).

- **Neutrophils:** increases in the neutrophil count are commonly due to bacterial infection. Neutropenia may occur due to underlying conditions (eg immune deficiency, chemotherapy) or due to overwhelming sepsis. Chemical mediators produced by leucocytes cause increased numbers of neutrophils to form in the bone marrow; these are released early into the bloodstream, producing a neutrophilia indicative of an acute inflammatory response
- **Lymphocytes:** low lymphocyte count is indicative of sepsis, high lymphocyte count may indicate viral illness

Acute-phase proteins

CRP is commonly used as a marker for sepsis as levels respond within 24 hours to inflammatory change (compared to the ESR which takes days). The range for CRP is commonly < 8 to > 285 in most labs. Elevated CRP of > 100 is strongly indicative of bacterial infection. CRP is also commonly elevated post-operatively (as an acute response to trauma) so should be interpreted with care. Fibrinogen levels are also elevated post-operatively.

U&Es and LFTs

Urea, creatinine and electrolytes are important to assess renal function (severe sepsis can result in ARF). Renal function is also important in the administration of certain antibiotics (eg gentamicin). Albumin levels fall in acute sepsis and LFTs may become elevated in cholangitis or sepsis syndrome. Elevation in amylase may occur as a result of pancreatitis or inflammation near the pancreas.

Arterial blood gases (ABGs)

ABGs are important to demonstrate acidosis. Metabolic acidosis may occur in sepsis as a result of low BP and poor tissue perfusion.

Clotting screen

There may also be a non-specific thrombocytosis (increased platelet count). It is not clear whether this translates into increased risk of thrombosis. Sepsis may also result in DIC with deranged clotting parameters such as increasing PT and falling platelet count.

Radiology

CXR may show consolidation or demonstrate free intra-abdominal gas (indicative of perforation of a viscus). Remember that changes in the CXR may lag behind clinical signs. Abdominal collections are best demonstrated by CT but can sometimes be seen on USS.

Microbiology

See 4.3 *Specimen collection* below.

4.2 FEVER IN A POST-OPERATIVE PATIENT

Control of body temperature

In a nutshell ...

Body temperature control is essential for optimal functioning of intracellular enzymes. Aberrations in body temperature compromise organ function.

Body temperature is controlled by balancing heat production against heat loss. The body has mechanisms for reducing temperature when it's too hot, and increasing temperature when it's too cold.

'Normal' temperature is actually a range from 36 to 37.5 °C. It oscillates minutely around a 'set point' determined by the hypothalamus.

Pyrexia is temperature > 37.5 °C
Hypothermia is temperature < 36 °C

Physiological control of normal body temperature

The deep tissues of the body or the 'core' remain at a constant temperature (unless there is a febrile illness). The skin and subcutaneous tissues or 'peripheral' tissue rises and falls with the surroundings:

- Climate (hot vs cold; humid vs dry)
- Exercise (mild vs strenuous)

Heat production in the body

Heat is an essential by-product of metabolism, and so the rate of its production is determined by the metabolic rate. Factors affecting the metabolic rate will therefore affect the rate of heat production.

The majority of this heat is produced in the deep tissues of the body, such as the liver, heart, brain and skeletal muscle (for example, fulminant liver failure is often associated with hypothermia).

The production of heat requires oxygen consumption and this is important in the critically ill, particularly in neonates who have difficulty with body heat regulation. The 'thermo-neutral zone' is a temperature at which the oxygen requirement for temperature regulation is at a minimal level. Nursing neonates at this temperature allows the infant to optimise their use of the available oxygen.

Heat loss from the body

Core heat is conducted to the periphery and lost through the skin into the surrounding environment. Two factors predominantly control the rate of this loss.

- **Insulation:** fat conducts heat only one third as well as other tissues and so it acts as an insulator. It allows the temperature of the skin to approach that of the surroundings with no loss of core temperature
- **Cutaneous blood flow:** blood vessels penetrate the fat to lie directly beneath the skin in a continuous venous plexus. This plexus is also supplied directly by small arteries through AV anastomoses. The rate of blood flow (and thus heat exchange) from the core to the periphery can therefore be controlled by sympathetic vasoconstriction or dilation of the vessels (blood flow can vary from zero to 30% of the cardiac output)

Heat loss from the skin is via:

- **Radiation:** this occurs if the ambient temperature is lower than the skin; 60% of total heat loss via infra-red heat rays
- **Conduction:** conduction of heat as motion to the surrounding air molecules causes these heated molecules to move away from the skin as a convection current, replacing the layer of air in contact with the skin with cold air. This occurs if the ambient temperature is lower than that of the skin. Hairs on the skin help to hold a layer of air in place that is heated by the body to form an insulator zone. This is displaced if the air is moving (eg wind chill). The insulator layer cannot form water molecules and so more heat is lost by conduction in cases of submersion
- **Evaporation:** 0.58 kCal is used to allow evaporation of 1 g water from the surface of the skin. This may be insensible loss from the skin and lungs or due to sweat. Sweating is controlled by the autonomic nervous system (stimulation of the anterior hypothalamus by excess heat causes cholinergic sympathetic stimulation of sweat glands). Sweating occurs even if the ambient temperature is the same or higher than that of the skin

Reduction of temperature when the body is hot

This is achieved by:

- Sweating
- Cutaneous vasodilation
- Inhibition of heat-producing mechanisms (eg shivering, chemical thermogenesis)
- Behavioural modification (eg clothing, seeks shade)

Elevation of temperature when the body is cold

This is achieved by:

- Cutaneous vasoconstriction
- Pilo-erection (elevation of body hairs to increase insulating layer of air next to the skin)
- Increased heat production
    - Shivering
    - Sympathetic excitation
    - Thyroxine secretion
    - Brown fat heating
    - Behavioural modification (eg clothing)

The physiology of abnormal body temperature

Pyrexia

Elevation of the body temperature may be caused by:

- **Toxins** that result from:
    - Infection – eg release of bacterial endotoxins
    - Trauma – eg release of cytokines involved in inflammation and repair
- **Damage to thermoregulatory structures in the brain** – eg tumours or surgery in the region of the hypothalamus

Toxins or pyrogens can cause the set point in the hypothalamus to rise. This initially brings heat-conserving mechanisms into play and the body temperature rises to the new set point. This is especially true of IL-1 and IL-6 released by lymphocytes in response to bacterial toxin.

The activation of these heat-conserving mechanisms causes rigors – vasoconstriction, pilo-erection, shivering and chattering teeth occur despite the presence of a high core temperature.

Removal of the causative agent results in re-setting of the hypothalamus and stimulation of heat-loss mechanisms into play. There is vasodilation of the skin and excess sweating to reduce the body temperature back down to the new set point.

Heat stroke occurs if the environmental conditions prevent sufficient heat loss by convection and sweating (ie low air currents and high humidity) The symptoms (dizziness, abdominal pain, loss of consciousness) are exacerbated by a degree of circulatory shock due to fluid loss. Hyper-pyrexia for short periods causes damage and local haemorrhage in all organs but particularly the brain.

Hypothermia

When core temperature falls below 30 °C the ability of the hypothalamus to regulate temperature is lost. The chemical and enzymatic activity within the cells is decreased several fold, reducing heat production still further. Reduced conscious level and coma depress the activity of the CNS and prevent activation of heat-preserving mechanisms such as shivering.

After surgery or trauma patients often have evidence of a pyrexia and their blood picture demonstrates an acute phase response in the first 24 hours. This is due to:

- Tissue damage necrosis and acute inflammatory response
- Basal atelectasis due to general anaesthesia and posture (bed-bound)

Post-operative pyrexia

A low-grade pyrexia post-operatively often doesn't require further investigation. However, if pyrexia persists you should investigate potential foci of infection.

Common post-op infections

Surgical-site infection
Respiratory infection
Urinary tract infection
Line-associated infection

Whilst a patient remains systemically well with stable haemodynamic and respiratory parameters, there is time to perform adequate septic screen investigations and seek microbiological advice in order to define appropriate antibiotic therapy. Patients who are unstable or demonstrating septic syndrome or shock should have microbiological specimens taken and then be treated with a 'best guess' antibiotic (see section 6).

For a discussion of sepsis, systemic inflammatory response syndrome (SIRS) and multiorgan dysfunction (MODS) see Chapter 7 *Critical Care*.

Surgical-site infection

Surgical-site infection includes:

Superficial wound infection
Deep abscess formation

- Intra-abdominal abscess after abdominal surgery
- Intrathoracic abscess after cardiothoracic surgery
- Intracranial abscess after neurosurgery
- Periprosthetic infection/abscess formation (eg around orthopaedic prosthesis or vascular graft)

Implantation of prosthetic materials carries a higher risk of infection, and such infection is often very difficult to eradicate. For detailed discussions of infection in vascular surgery see Chapter 9 *Vascular Surgery*, and for infection in orthopaedic surgery see the *Orthopaedics* chapter in Book 2.

Common organisms in surgical site infection

Organism related to wound type

- Clean wounds – skin commensals (eg *Staphylococcus epidermidis*, *S. aureus*, enterobacteria)
- Contaminated wounds – site-specific organisms (eg from soil, saliva after bites, perforated viscus eg colon)
- Dirty wounds – site-specific organisms
- Necrotising fasciitis – mixed flora or group A *Streptococcus*
- Infected prostheses – may be skin flora or nosocomial
- Burns – *Pseudomonas*
- Nosocomial infection – eg MRSA

Management includes:

- Wound swab +/– blood cultures if indicated
- Empirical treatment with a broad-spectrum agent likely to cover organisms involved (see section 6)
- Pus won't resolve with antibiotics – it needs formal radiological or surgical drainage

NB: Surgical site infections may be due to an organism resistant to the antibiotic administered prophylactically.

Necrotising fasciitis

This is an infection that spreads along fascial planes, secondarily affecting muscle, subcutaneous tissue and skin.

Aetiology of necrotising fasciitis

- Typically polymicrobial (streptococci; haemolytic staphylococci; *Bacteroides*; coliforms)
- Post-op
- Trauma
- Untreated perineal wound
- Contaminated needle

Pathology of necrotising fasciitis

- Appears benign in initial stages
- If untreated: results in massive subcutaneous oedema and dermal gangrene
- Fournier's gangrene is dermal gangrene of scrotum and penis

Management of necrotising fasciitis

- Rapid aggressive resuscitation
- Broad-spectrum antibiotics
- Skin incisions down to fascia
- Massive debridement of soft tissue with excision of necrotic tissue
- Colostomy if perineal area is involved
- Nutritional support
- Mortality is 30%

Respiratory infection

Post-operative respiratory tract infection may be due to nosocomial infection or aspiration (in the critically unwell). Patients are more prone to respiratory infection after surgery due to:

- General anaesthetic and basal atelectasis
- Supine positioning (prevents full expansion of lung bases)
- Immunosuppression (co-morbid conditions)

Common organisms in respiratory infection

- **Community acquired:** *Streptococcus pneumoniae, Haemophilus influenzae, Mycoplasma* pneumoniae
- **Nosocomial:** often aerobic Gram-negative bacteria – includes *Klebsiella, Escherichia coli, Enterobacter, S. aureus*
  - Common in ventilated patients (50% prevalence)
  - May be opportunistic infection in the immunosuppressed (eg *Pneumocystis carinii*)
- **Empyema (pus in thoracic cavity):** commonly due to *S. pneumoniae* but occasionally *Staphylococcus aureus* secondary to:
  - Primary lung infection
  - Haematogenous or lymphatic spread
  - Direct extension from diaphragmatic, mediastinal or cervical foci
  - Inoculation by penetrating trauma
- **Lung abscesses:** result from aspiration (anaerobic organisms) or granulomatous disease (eg TB)

Urinary infection

See also *Urology and Transplantation*.

Common organisms in urinary tract infection

- Community acquired: commonly *E. coli*; may also be due to *Proteus, Klebsiella*
- Abnormalities of the renal tract: *Pseudomonas*
- Catheterisation/instrumentation of the renal tract: *Staphylococcus epidermidis, Enterococcus faecalis*

Line-associated infection

Common organisms in line-associated infection

- *S. aureus*, coagulase-negative *Staphylococcus*, streptococci, enterococci and Gram-negative species
- Incidence increases with length of time since line insertion (keep sites clean, record date of insertion, observe site regularly, change lines before they become infected, re-site if infection documented)

Management includes:

- Change lines if evidence of infection: may require at least 24-hour antibiotic treatment before re-insertion of tunnelled lines. NEVER pass a guidewire through an infected line and insert a new line along the same guidewire
- Take blood cultures from two separate sites (one through the infected line before it is removed and one from a distant peripheral site; label them accordingly)
- Discuss antibiotic choice with on-call microbiologist

Pyrexia of unknown origin (PUO)

PUO is defined as a prolonged fever (of more than 3 weeks) which remains undiagnosed after sufficient hospital investigation (about a week). Management should involve an infectious diseases physician.

Possible causes of pyrexia of unknown origin (PUO)

Infection (23%)

Abscesses (lung, liver, subphrenic, perinephric, pelvic)
Empyema
Endocarditis
Unusual bacterial infection (*Salmonella, Brucella, Borrelia, Leptospirosis*)
TB and other granulomatous diseases (actinomycosis, toxoplasmosis)
Parasites (amoebic liver abscess, malaria, schistosomiasis)
Fungi
HIV

Neoplasia (20%)
Lymphoma
Solid tumour (GI, renal cell)

Connective tissue diseases (22%)
Rheumatoid arthritis
SLE
Stills disease
PAN (polyarteritis nodosa)
Kawasaki's disease

Drugs (3%)

Other causes (14%)
Pulmonary embolisms
Inflammatory bowel disease (Crohn's/ulcerative colitis)
Sarcoid
Amyloid

It is impossible to reach a diagnosis in up to 25% cases.

4.3 SPECIMEN COLLECTION

The microbiological data available from specimens is often related to the manner of collection and should be interpreted in the light of the patient's clinical condition. Most specimens are processed during working hours but specimens that will be processed out of hours in most labs include:

- CSF
- Aspirates of sterile sites (eg intra-abdominal abscess, thoracic cavity, joints, etc)
- Intra-operative specimens from deep surgical infections (eg debridement of osteomyelitis)
- HIV/hepatitis B and C in transplant donors (recipient status usually known)

Skin swabs

- **Wound infections:** overt infections (with pus) can be swabbed for causative organism to tailor therapy. Often the organism is related to the site of surgery (eg bowel flora in abdominal wounds) but swabs may exclude organisms such as MRSA
- **Ulcers:** little value in swabbing ulceration as this only gives an indication of colonising organisms and will not help in tailoring therapy

- **Abscess cavities:** may be of use if taken from deep in the abscess cavity. Remember that abscesses do not respond to antibiotics but require surgical drainage of pus. Surrounding cellulitits may benefit from therapy tailored to the causative organism

Urine samples

- **Mid-stream urine (MSU):** this is optimal as it is a clean catch sample and results may determine antibiotic choice
- **Catheter stream urine (CSU):** urine from catheters may demonstrate colonisation rather than overt infection (particularly if the catheter is long-term). Treat only if the patient is symptomatic

Stool samples

- **Stool culture:** useful in the returning traveller with diarrhoea. Document region of travel and duration of request card
- ***Clostridium difficile* toxin (CDT):** useful in patients who develop diarrhoea on antibiotics. It is a highly sensitive assay. Document antibiotic treatment and specifically request CDT test. The test remains positive after treatment so there is little point in repeating it

Blood cultures

Blood cultures should be taken if the patient is presumed to be septic before the start of empirical treatment. Cultures do not have to be taken during a temperature 'spike' as patients will remain bacteraemic for many hours. Cultures can be sent even if the patient is afebrile but has other features of sepsis and may provide the elusive diagnosis in the elderly.

Taking a blood culture

Use aseptic technique with gloves and swab the skin several times with alcohol before puncture to prevent skin contamination

Try to take 2 sets from different peripheral venepuncture sites (eg antecubital fossa) – groin and line cultures are likely to be contaminated (however cultures can also be taken from intravenous lines (eg arterial lines, CVP lines) and may help in the diagnosis of line infection)

If considering endocarditis 3 sets of cultures should be taken from 3 sites at 3 separate times

Inoculate aerobic and anaerobic bottles with 10 mL of blood each (do not touch the bottle lids)

Label each bottle with the patient details, site of venepuncture, time of sample, any current antibiotic therapy, and current diagnosis. Indicate if the sample is high risk (eg hepatitis, HIV, etc)

Processing of blood cultures

Once in the lab:

- Specimens are placed in an oscillating incubator
- Bacteria present produce CO_2 which reacts with a disc at the bottom of the bottle producing a colour change which is detected by the machine, flagging the sample up as being positive
- Blood is aspirated from positive bottles for Gram staining (positive or negative) and microscopy (rods or cocci)
- Blood is inoculated onto agar plates with discs impregnated with common antibiotics
- After 24 hours bacterial growth has occurred apart from in the region of antibiotics to which the organism is sensitive
- Additional tests may be employed to identify the organism
- The microbiologists phone positive results and antibiotic sensitivities to the ward (so it is important to correctly identify this on the request form)

Common results from blood cultures

Growth in both bottles

- *Staphylococcus*: in the face of sepsis this is likely to be a significant finding. In a hospital setting this may represent MRSA bacteraemia and so microbiological advice may include a dose of vancomycin
- Coliforms: almost always significant. Consider GI and urosepsis. Will require tailored antibiotic therapy

Growth in one bottle

- May represent contamination and should be interpreted in the light of the clinical context
- May therefore require repeat sample

Joint aspirates

Joint aspiration technique is discussed in *Orthopaedics* (Book 2). It should be performed using aseptic technique to produce a sterile specimen.

Sputum

These are poor quality specimens and usually represent oral flora. For this reason many labs do not process these. Specimens obtained by bronchoalveolar lavage however are of much higher quality and can be used to tailor antibiotic therapy (eg in a critical-care setting).

Advice from your microbiologist

To get the best advice and answers to questions such as *Which antibiotic?* or *How long should we continue antibiotics for?* the microbiologist will want to know:

- Patient age, gender and occupation
- Date of admission
- Pre-morbid conditions (eg diabetes, malignancy, steroid or other immunosuppressant, elderly, pregnant)
- Date and details of surgery or injury
- Current and previous antibiotic therapy
- Results or outstanding microbiological samples
- MRSA status
- Details of current clinical condition: examination findings (temperature, haemodynamic status, chest/abdo/cardiovascular exam)
- Results of septic screen (blood results with WCC differential)
- Allergies (confirmed or suspected)

Section 5
Prevention and control of infection

5.1 INFECTION CONTROL

Identify patients at risk

All patients need careful thought and planning to prevent infection. Some are at increased risk if they have or undergo:

- Trauma (including major surgery itself)
- Burns
- Shock
- Pre-existing sepsis syndrome
- Co-existing metabolic disease (diabetes mellitus, renal failure, liver failure)
- Haematological problems
- Nutritional state problems (malnutrition, obesity)
- Malignancy
- Chemotherapy and/or radiotherapy
- Immunosuppression (steroids, previous splenectomy, transplant, congenital or acquired immune deficiency)

Infection control teams and hospital policy

Infection control teams are multidisciplinary and should include:

- A consultant microbiologist
- Infection control nurses
- Representatives from medical and surgical specialities
- Occupational health personnel
- Management personnel

The infection control team should:

- Meet regularly
- Perform audit evaluations of current hospital status, by:
  - Surveillance of nosocomial infection rates
  - Comparison with published countrywide rates

  - Implementation of alterations to policy
- Advise and implement hospital policy

Patient isolation and ward discipline

Patient isolation

Patients may be isolated because they are:

- Infectious (and require barrier nursing to protect others from the spread of transmissible infection)
- At increased risk of infection (and require 'reverse' barrier nursing to protect them from the spread of transmissible infection. Barrier nursing and reverse-barrier nursing are essentially the same – they use barrier methods to prevent the spread of infection eg gloves, plastic aprons, filtered air and masks to prevent droplet infections)

Ward discipline

- After examining every patient always wash your hands or use an alcohol rub
- Always wear gloves to handle or change dressings, take blood, etc
- Observe isolation procedures
- For MRSA positive patients always wear gloves and an apron and spray stethoscope with alcohol after examining
- Contact infection control team if there are any doubts

5.2 SKIN PREPARATION

In a nutshell ...

Preparation of the patient
Skin (shaving, skin disinfection, adhesive wound drapes)
Bowel (laxatives/enemas)

Preparation of the theatre
Cleanliness, airflow issues, personnel movements

Preparation of the surgical team
Scrubbing up, caps, gowns, gloves, masks, shoes

Pre-op skin preparation

Antiseptics

- Include Betadine™ (iodine based) and chlorhexidine (colourless)
- Should be applied to the skin in circular or sweeping motion (friction on the skin removes some bacterial colonisation)
- Apply several times to high-risk areas:
  - Perineum
  - Groin
  - Axilla
- There is no evidence that Betadine™ placed in the wound during closure reduces the rate of wound infection
- Alcoholic antiseptics are much more effective than aqueous preparations but pooled areas on the skin may ignite if using diathermy

Pre-op shaving

- Causes skin abrasion
- Disrupts deeper flora layers; increased bacterial count on skin surface
- Increased tendency to post-op wound sepsis
- Therefore shave immediately pre-operatively with surgical clippers or use depilatory cream before theatre

Adhesive wound drapes

- Do not prevent infection
- Reported to reduce wound contamination by 50% BUT no decrease in wound infection
- Trapped bacteria may multiply

Preparation of theatre

Theatre design

Theatre design is discussed in Chapter 6 *Peri-operative Care*.

Control of air quality

- Aim: to decrease number of airborne particles carrying bacteria from skin flora
- Positive pressure filtered ventilation (PPFV) prevents bacteria gaining entry to the air
- Laminar flow plus ultraclean air systems give two-fold reduction in post-op wound infections

Greater numbers of people in theatre and movement through doors have been correlated with infection rates.

Preparation of the surgical team

Scrub-up

- Aim: to decrease bacterial skin count
- Chlorhexidine gluconate or povidone–iodine solutions: stiff brushes damage the epidermis; use on fingernails only
- One nail-scrub at beginning of operating list is sufficient

Clothing

- Cotton gowns reduce the bacterial count in the air by only 30%
- Bacteria-impermeable fabrics may reduce bacterial air counts by 40–70%. There is no evidence of reduced wound infection

Caps

- Useful because *S. aureus* can be carried on the scalp
- Prevents hair from falling in the wound

Masks

- Deflect forceful expirations such as coughs and sneezes that carry bacteria (normal speech does not expel bacteria)
- May rub off bacteria-carrying skin squames from the face
- No effect on infection rates
- Prudent use in implant surgery

Gloves

- Effective hand disinfection before gloving up
- Glove punctures or tears do not affect incidence of wound infection
- Double-glove if implanting prosthesis (eg orthopaedic) or if high-risk patient

Shoes

- Plastic overshoes are not proven to reduce wound infection

5.3 ASEPSIS AND STERILISATION

In a nutshell ...

- **Asepsis** is prevention of the introduction of bacteria to the surgical field.
- **Antisepsis** is destruction of pre-existing bacteria in the surgical field.
- **Sterilisation:** complete destruction of all viable micro-organisms, including spores and viruses by means of heat, chemicals or irradiation. Inanimate objects only (eg not skin because it damages tissue).
- **Disinfection:** treatment of tissue or hard surface in an attempt to decrease the bacterial count.
- **Antiseptics:** disinfectants used in living tissue.
- **Cleaning:** physically removes contamination – does NOT necessarily destroy micro-organisms.

Asepsis

Development of asepsis

In the1860s Joseph Lister introduced carbolic acid as a disinfectant for hands and surgical instruments and to be sprayed into the air. A few years later he published in *The Lancet* a reduction in mortality rates during major amputations of from 45% to 15%.

Principles of asepsis

Principles of asepsis

Skin preparation with disinfectant
Bowel preparation pre-operatively
Draping to surround the sterile field
'Scrubbing up' with disinfectant
Use of sterile gloves and gowns
Use of sterile instrumentation and no-touch technique
Good operative technique

Invasive procedures should always be performed in-line with aseptic techniques (may be incomplete in times of life-threatening emergency).

Sterilisation

Autoclave sterilisation

- Saturated steam at high pressure
- Kills ALL organisms, including TB, viruses, heat-resistant spores
- Holding times depend on temperature and pressure (eg 134°C at 30 lb/in^2 has a 3-minute holding time; 121°C at 15 lb/in^2 has a 15-minute holding time)
- Wrapped instruments: use a porous load autoclave – steam penetration monitored with Bowie–Dick test
- Unwrapped instruments: use a Little Sister II™ portable autoclave
- Fluids: use a bottle autoclave

Dry heat sterilisation

- Hot-air ovens
- For moisture-sensitive instruments (no corrosion), non-stainless metals, surgical instruments with fine cutting edges
- Able to process airtight containers and non-aqueous liquids
- Effective BUT inefficient (160°C for at least 2 hours kills ALL micro-organisms)
- Monitor with Browne's tubes III

Ethylene oxide sterilisation

- Highly penetrative gas
- Kills vegetative bacteria, spores and viruses
- Effective at ambient temperatures and pressures
- Effective as a liquid or a gas
- Efficient for heat-sensitive equipment (eg rubber, plastics, electrical equipment, lenses)
- Used for sutures and single-use items
- Flammable if vapour > 3% volume in air
- Toxic, irritant, mutagenic, carcinogenic
- Limited availability and expensive (predominantly industrial process)

Low-temperature steam and formaldehyde sterilisation

- Physicochemical method
- Kills vegetative bacteria, spores and viruses
- 73°C for heat-sensitive items
- NOT suitable for sealed, oily, or greasy items

Irradiation sterilisation

- Use of gamma rays limited to industry
- Use for large batches of single-use items (catheters, syringes)

Disinfection

Disinfection aims to bring about a reduction in the number of viable organisms. Some viruses and bacterial spores may remain active.

Disinfection of inanimate objects can be carried out with:

- Low-temperature steam
- Boiling water
- Formaldehyde gas

Alcohols

- Broadest spectrum at 70% concentration
- Rapidly effective against Gram-positive and Gram-negative bacteria; some antiviral activity
- No residual activity
- Relatively inactive against spores and fungi
- Denature proteins
- Use of alcohols: skin preparation (NB: ensure dryness before using diathermy – explosions and pooling may irritate sensitive areas such as the groin)

Diguanides

Chlorhexidine

- Good activity against *S. aureus*
- Moderate activity against Gram-negative bacteria
- Some activity against *Pseudomonas aeruginosa*, although may multiply in deteriorating solutions
- Non-toxic to skin and mucous membranes
- Poor activity against spores, fungi and viruses
- Inactivated by pus, soap and some plastics
- Causes bacterial cell-wall disruption
- Uses of chlorhexidine:
  - In local antisepsis
  - 4% chlorhexidine in detergent (Hibiscrub™)
  - Chlorhexidine–cetrimide mixture for some dirty wounds
  - 0.5% chlorhexidine in 70% alcohol

Iodophors and iodine

- Broad spectrum of activity against: bacteria, spores, fungi and viruses (including hepatitis B and HIV)
- Easily inactivated by blood, faeces and pus
- Need optimum freshness, concentration, and pH < 4
- Stains skin and fabrics

- Irritant; may cause local hypersensitivity
- Use of iodophors and iodine:
  - Pre-operative skin disinfection
  - Wound antisepsis

Hydrogen peroxide

- Only weak bactericidal activity

Aldehydes (glutaraldehyde and formaldehyde)

- Rapidly active against vegetative bacteria and viruses (including hepatitis B and HIV)
- Slowly effective against spores
- Only fair activity against tubercle bacilli
- Exposure of at least 3 hours to kill ALL microbes (most bacteria killed in < 10 minutes)
- Toxic, with sensitivity reactions in skin, eyes, and lungs (glutaraldehyde is safer)
- Endoscopes are heat-sensitive – disinfect by immersion in 2% glutaraldehyde between each case

5.4 SURGICAL MEASURES TO REDUCE INFECTION

In a nutshell ...

Surgical infection may be caused by:
Endogenous organisms
Exogenous organisms

Surgical infection can be reduced or prevented by:
Environmental factors
Patient factors
Surgeon factors
Surgical technique
Prophylactic antibiotics

If you become aware of changes in the rate of post-op infections you should contact the infection control team. They will analyse the cases and identify any linking factors. This is often reassuring as cases often only represent a statistical cluster rather than a true increase.

Endogenous infection

This is clinical infection with organisms normally found in the patient as commensals. All surgical procedures result in a transient bacteraemia. Good preparation, surgical technique and prophylactic antibiotics minimise the chance of these becoming a significant problem.

- **Lower GI tract**
  - 'Coliforms' (eg Gram-negative bacilli such as *Escherichia coli, Klebsiella, Proteus*)
  - Enterococci
  - Anaerobes (eg *Bacteroides fragilis*)
  - *Pseudomonas*
  - *Enterobacter*
- **Urogenital tract**
  - Vagina: anaerobes, lactobacilli
  - Urethra: skin flora (eg staphylococci, diphtheroids)
- **Upper respiratory tract:**
  - Streptococci, *Haemophilus, S. aureus,* diphtheroids

Conditional pathogens colonise when use of antimicrobials destroy normal flora – this is known as 'superinfection'.

Prevention of endogenous infection

Patient preparation
- Skin disinfection
- Bowel preparation
- Appropriate antibiotic prophylaxis

Avoid disrupting normal flora (give antibiotics only for specific infection)
Treat sepsis with full course of antibiotics, not prophylaxis (inadequately treated infections encourage bacterial resistance)

Exogenous infection

This is clinical infection acquired from an external source. Incidence is low (2%), affecting:

- Hospital staff
- Hospital environment
- Other patients

Wound sepsis

Asepsis means no organisms are present during surgery. A truly aseptic environment is needed in immunocompromised patients. Antisepsis involves prevention of sepsis. Total abolition of organisms is not achieved

Clean wounds

- Incise through non-inflamed tissue
- Ensure no entry into genito-urinary, GI, or respiratory tracts
- Contamination rate < 2% (exogenous sepsis)

Clean–contaminated wounds

- Entry into a hollow viscus other than the colon, with minimal, controlled contamination
- Contamination rate 8–10%

Contaminated wounds

- Breaching of hollow viscus with more spillage: opening the colon, open fractures, penetrating animal or human bites
- Contamination rate 12–20%

Dirty wounds

- Gross pus, perforated viscus (eg faecal peritonitis), or traumatic wounds of > 4 hours
- Contamination rate > 25%

Prevention of wound sepsis

In exogenous infection
Control of operative conditions
Sterilisation (air and instruments)
Aseptic technique
Good surgical technique
Preparation of patient and surgeon

In clean wounds
No-touch technique
Careful and gentle dissection
Careful haemostasis
Minimisation of operation duration
Skin preparation
Prophylactic antibiotics (only if insertion of prosthetic material)

In clean–contaminated wounds
Measures as for *clean wounds* plus:
Single-shot antibiotic prophylaxis
Minimisation of spillage (swabs, suction)
Saline lavage

In contaminated wounds
Full course of antibiotics
Debridement of devitalised tissues (samples to microbiology for causative organism and sensitivity)
Removal of foreign material
Cleaning of tissues
Lavage

In dirty wounds
Full course of antibiotics
Thorough removal of pus
Wound debridement
Thorough lavage
Simplest shortest operation (life-saving)
Avoidance of anastomosis (eg Hartmann's procedure)
Consideration of delayed primary closure

5.5 VACCINATION

In a nutshell ...

Vaccines act by inducing active or passive immunity. Vaccination is used in groups who are susceptible to certain diseases:

- Children (diseases of childhood)
- Travellers to endemic areas of disease
- Healthcare professionals exposed to high-risk patients

Principles of immunisation

Active vs passive immunisation

Active immunisation stimulates the immune system to produce a response resulting in the formation of immunologic memory and thus protection against subsequent exposure. Antigens used for immunisation:

- Live-attenuated organism (bacterium or virus such as TB (BCG), MMR)
- Dead organism (eg tetanus, *Pneumococcus*, influenza virus)
- Characteristic protein from organism (eg purified viral protein coat)

Passive immunisation involves the transfer of pre-formed antibodies to provide immediate protection against disease exposure. For example:

- Maternal transfer of immunoglobulin in breast milk
- Immunoglobulins eg against hepatitis, tetanus, varicella zoster, hepatitis A, rabies

Reasons for immunisation

- For eradication of dangerous childhood disease
- For those who are immunocompromised or have increased susceptibility (eg splenectomy, extremes of age)
- For healthcare professionals with exposure to infection
- For travel to areas of endemic disease

Immunisation of surgical patients

Consider immunisation in the following surgical patients.

Patients with dirty or soil-contaminated wounds

- Tetanus toxoid (intramuscularly)
- Human tetanus immunoglobulin

Splenectomy patients

- Give haemophilus type B (HiB), meningococcal and pneumococcal vaccines
- Re-immunise every 5–10 years
- Give annual influenza vaccine
- For elective cases give vaccinations at least 2 weeks pre-operatively
- For traumatic cases immunise after a few weeks to maximise immune response

Immunisation of healthcare professionals

The most serious health risks are posed by blood-borne viruses:

- Hepatitis B
- Hepatitis C
- HIV

Infections may be passed in either direction:

- From patients to healthcare staff (many infections may be undiagnosed – adopt universal protective precautions at all times)
- From healthcare staff to patients during exposure-prone procedures when there is a risk of exposure to blood (eg cuts), or accidental injury to hands (eg bony spurs, sharp instruments etc)

Common mode of transmission is exposure to any bodily fluid

Blood (needlestick injury; bleeding eg haematemesis, melaena, epistaxis; invasive procedures; spray from arteries during surgery; bone fragments eg trauma and orthopaedic surgery)
Saliva
Urine and stools
CSF
Semen

Healthcare professionals should be immunised against the following diseases capable of nosocomial transmission:

- Hepatitis B
- Varicella zoster
- +/– Rubella
- +/– Measles
- +/– Mumps

Additional vaccination may be required for workers dealing with outbreaks of disease (eg influenza pandemics, meningococcal C disease) or workers commonly encountering other diseases in endemic countries or among certain patient groups (eg hepatitis A).

The Hospital Infection Control Practices Advisory Committee (HIPAC) guidelines suggest that the following personnel should be vaccinated, or be capable of demonstrating immunity to the diseases listed above (as all may come into contact with needles or bodily fluids):

- Doctors
- Nurses
- Emergency service personnel
- Dental professionals
- Students (medical and nursing)
- Laboratory personnel
- Hospital volunteers
- Housekeeping personnel

5.6 NEEDLESTICK INJURY

Causes of needlestick injury

Needlestick injury may occur in situations involving:

- Syringes and hypodermic needles
- Taking of blood/venous access
- Invasive procedures
- Suturing
- Sharp instruments

It commonly occurs with practices such as:

- Re-sheathing needles
- Transferring body fluids between containers
- Poor disposal of needles (use sharps bins)

In the event of needlestick injury follow hospital protocol, which involves:

- Encouraging bleeding by squeezing the wound
- Washing with water/soap/disinfectant (do not suck the wound)
- Reporting the incident (to on-call microbiologist if out of hours)
- Attending the appropriate department immediately (occupational health, A&E)
- Counselling and testing of recipient and donor (for hepatitis B, hepatitis C and HIV status) if required
- Post-exposure prophylactic treatment (eg triple therapy started immediately in the event of high risk exposure to HIV) – this should be discussed with a microbiologist or ID physician

High-risk patients

NB: Many infectious patients do not exhibit symptoms and signs of the disease so precautions should be taken with all patients (eg wear gloves for taking blood and for cannulation, catheterisation and intubation).

Precautions in hepatitis and HIV patients

Surgeons, anaesthetists, theatre nurses, operating department practitioners and other theatre personnel also need protection from potentially infectious agents, in the following ways:

- Contact (with blood, saliva, urine, tears, CSF, stools)
- Air (eg following use of power tools)
- Inoculation (via needlestick, scalpel or bone fragment injuries)

Universal precautions

These precautions serve to protect theatre staff from infection with all cases (eg surgical gloves, gowns, masks, no-touch surgical technique).

Special precautions

These are used for high-risk surgical patients (eg hepatitis and HIV patients). In an ideal world all procedures would be performed using special precautions, but in practice the level of precaution is limited by expense, time, etc. Precautions include:

- Disposable drapes and gowns
- Double-gloving and 'indicator' glove systems
- Face visors
- Blunt suture needles
- Passing of instruments in a kidney dish
- No-touch technique
- Minimal theatre staff
- Only vital equipment in theatre

Some of the special precautions should be undertaken with all patients (eg high-risk patients or in high-risk areas). Special precautions are also used for infective cases to prevent spread of infection to other patients (eg MRSA).

Section 6

Antibiotic control of infection

6.1 TYPES OF ANTIBIOTIC

In a nutshell ...

Antibiotic action is either:
Bacteriocidal (results in death of current bacterial population), or
Bacteriostatic (prevents bacterial replication)

These actions may be achieved by inhibition of protein synthesis, inhibition of nucleic acid synthesis, or inhibition of membrane functions.

Different classes of antibiotics have different spectrums of activity against different organisms.

Mode of action of antibiotics

Bacteriocidal antibiotics

- Include β-lactams, vancomycin, aminoglycosides, and chloramphenicol
- Indications for bactericidal antibiotics include:
  - Life-threatening sepsis
  - Infective endocarditis
  - Opportunistic infections in immunocompromised patients

Bacteriostatic antibiotics

- Include tetracycline, erythromycin, clindamycin, and chloramphenicol
- Bacteria can multiply again
- Final elimination of pathogens depends on host-defence mechanisms with effective phagocytosis

Mechanisms of action

Inhibition of cell-wall synthesis

Leads to osmotic lysis of bacteria with defective peptidoglycan molecules in the cell wall. Antibiotics with bactericidal action:

- β-lactams (penicillin, ampicillin, cephalosporin)
- Vancomycin

Inhibition of protein synthesis

Occurs at the following stages of the bacteria life cycle:

- Transfer RNA – amino acid attachment (eg by tetracyclines, bacteriostatic agents)
- Translocation (eg by chloramphenicol and erythromycin which are bacteristatic at low concentrations; clindamycin and fusidic acid which are bactericidal at high concentrations)
- mRNA attachment to ribosome (eg by aminoglycosides, bactericidals)

Inhibition of nucleic acid synthesis

Bactericidal mechanisms include:

- Decreased RNA replication, for example by:
  - Sulfonamides
  - Trimethoprim
  - Quinolones (ciprofloxacin, nalidixic acid)
  - Metronidazole
- Decreased mRNA, for example by:
  - Rifampicin

Alteration of cell membrane function

- Antibiotics called ionophores alter the permeability of bacterial cell membranes causing lysis. Polymyxin has bactericidal actions against Gram-negative bacilli

SPECTRUM OF ACTIVITY OF ANTIMICROBIALS

	Gram-negative		Gram-positive		
Drug	**Cocci**	**Bacilli**	**Cocci**	**Bacilli**	**Others**
Beta-lactams Benzylpenicillin Penicillin V 1st generation cephalosporins	*Neisseria meningitides* *N. gonorrhoeae*	Produce beta-lactamases	Streptococci: *S. pyogenes* *S. viridans* Anaerobic cocci	*C. perfringens* *S. pyogenes* *S. viridans* Anaerobic cocci	*T. pallidum*
Anti-staphylococcal penicillins Methicillin Cloxacillin Flucloxacillin			*S. aureus* (produces beta-lactamase)		
Aminoglycosides Gentamicin Tobramycin		*Escherichia coli* *Klebsiella* *Proteus* Coliforms *P. aeruginosa*	*S. aureus* (especially gentamicin)		
Macrolides Erythromycin		*Campylobacter* spp.	Streptococci including *S. pneumoniae* (may produce beta-lactamase)	*C. diphtheriae*	*M. pneumoniae*
Vancomycin			*S. aureus*	*C. difficile*	
Metronidazole (active only against anaerobic protozoa and bacteria)		*Bacteroides* spp.	Anaerobic cocci	*Clostridium* spp.	

BROAD-SPECTRUM ANTIBIOTICS

	Gram-negative		Gram-positive		
Drug	**Cocci**	**Bacilli**	**Cocci**	**Bacilli**	**Others**
Aminopenicillins Amoxycillin Ampicillin Clavulanic acid	*N. meningitides* *N. gonorrhoeae*	*E. coli* and other coliforms (not *Klebsiella*) *H. influenzae*	Streptococci including *S. pneumoniae* (beta-lactamase producing)	*Clostridium* spp.	*T. pallidum*
Broad-spectrum antibiotics Piperacillin		*P. aeruginosa* Coliforms			
Cephalosporins (2nd generation; beta-lactamase stable) Cefuroxime Ceftazidime	*N. gonorrhoeae*	*E. coli* and other coliforms (including *Klebsiella*)	Streptococci Staphylococci	*Clostridium* spp.	
Tetracyclines	*N. gonorrhoeae*	*H. influenzae*	Streptococci Staphylococci	*Clostridium* spp.	*M. pneumoniae* *Chlamydia*
Ciprafloxacin	*N. gonorrhoeae*	*Haemophilus* *P. aeruginosa* Coliforms	*S. aureus* and some streptococci		

Antibiotic classes

β-lactams

- **Penicillins:**
  - Examples: benzylpenicillin, flucloxacillin, ampicillin
  - Bactericidal
  - Good penetrance of tissues and body fluids
  - Renal excretion
  - Hypersensitivity (rash alone) occurs in up to 10% of patients (anaphylaxis in 0.05%) and may occur with other beta-lactams (similar molecular structures). There is a 1 in 10 risk of hypersensitivity to cephalosporins in patients with penicillin hypersensitivity
  - May cause antibiotic-associated colitis
- **Cephalosporins:**
  - Broad-spectrum antibiotics (for septicaemia, pneumonia, meningitis, biliary tract and urinary tract infections)
  - Pharmacology similar to penicillins
  - 10% penicillin-allergic patients will be hypersensitive to cephalosporins
  - 1st generation cephalosporins include cephradine
  - 2nd generation cephalosporins include cefuroxime
  - 3rd generation cephalosporins include cefotaxime, ceftazidime, ceftriaxone
- **Other β-lactam agents:**
  - Carbapenams eg imipenem, meropenem
  - Broad spectrum against anaerobes and aerobic Gram-positive and Gram-negative bacteria

Tetracyclines

- Examples: tetracycline, doxycycline, minocycline
- Work by attacking bacterial ribosomes (NB increasing bacterial resistance)
- Used against *Chlamydia*, *Haemophilus influenzae*, *Rickettsia*, *Brucella* and spirochaetes
- Generally safe but should not be used in pregnancy

Aminoglycosides

- Examples: gentamicin, neomycin, streptomycin
- Active against Gram-negative and some Gram-positive organisms
- Not absorbed from the gut (given IV)
- Excreted via the kidney
- Side effects are dose-related (ototoxicity, nephrotoxicity) – as a general guide you can give a single dose of 5–7 mg/kg if renal function is normal; reduce to 3 mg/kg if there is any compromise in renal function

Macrolides

- Examples: erythromycin, clarithromycin
- Antibacterial spectrum similar to penicillins (used for respiratory infections, *Campylobacter*, Legionnaire's disease, *Chlamydia*)
- Clarithromycin has higher tissue concentrations than erythromycin
- Side effects include nausea, vomiting and diarrhoea

Glycopeptides

- Examples: first line vancomycin, second line teicoplanin
- Anaerobes and aerobes; Gram-positive bacteria – used against MRSA
- Side effects are dose-related (ototoxicity, nephrotoxicity) – dose should be reduced in renal failure

Sulfonamides

- Examples: co-trimoxazole, trimethoprim
- Used for PCP, urinary and respiratory tract infections, and *Salmonella* infection
- Side effects include nausea, vomiting and diarrhoea

Metronidazole

- Effective against anaerobic and protozoal infections

Quinolones

- Examples: ciprofloxacin, norfloxacin
- Ciprofloxacin is particularly active against Gram-negative bacteria
- Used for respiratory tract and biliary infections
- Same bioavailability orally as IV (and much cheaper)
- Side effects include GI disturbance, rash, headache, tendinitis
- Avoid in the elderly and epileptics (lowers seizure threshold)

6.2 EMPIRICAL TREATMENT

Sometimes it is not possible to wait for microbiological results to guide your choice of antibiotics. The following should act as a guide. If in doubt, discuss with your local microbiologist.

Which antibiotic? Narrow-spectrum or broad-spectrum?

Narrow-spectrum antibiotics
These are selected for specific infections. They cause less disturbance of normal flora, and are associated with:

- Reduced risk of superinfection
- Fewer resistant strains

Broad-spectrum antibiotics
Use of these is associated with acquiring *Clostridium difficile* (pseudomembranous colitis).

Wound infection and cellulitis

Wound infection

- Clean wounds: flucloxacillin (to cover skin flora)
- Traumatic or abdominal surgical wounds: intravenous cefuroxime 1.5 g three times daily and metronidazole 400 mg three times daily
- Animal bites: co-amoxiclav

If considering necrotising fasciitis (sepsis, delirium, rapidly progressive pain, systemic upset out of keeping with erythema) seek microbiological advice as this is commonly group A *Streptococcus* – give cefuroxime (or clindamycin) and gentamicin.

Cellulitis
Most likely organisms are *Staph*. and *Strep*.

- If not systemically unwell consider oral clindamycin 300 mg four times daily (oral flucloxacillin is not very effective)
- If systemically unwell consider intravenous flucloxacillin 2 g four times daily

Management of ulceration should include imaging to exclude bony involvement. If systemically unwell can consider intravenous cefuroxime 1.5 g three times daily and metronidazole 400 mg three times daily.

Intra-abdominal sepsis

Most intra-abdominal organisms will be covered by intravenous cefuroxime 1.5 g three times daily and metronidazole 400 mg three times daily. If there is a history of rigors, hypotension, or suspected cholangitis then you should also consider a one-off single dose of gentamicin (5 mg/kg – NB check renal function is normal).

Pneumonia

Community-acquired pneumonia
Treatment should be guided by severity. The CURB criteria are a useful guide:

C onfusion
U rea
R espiratory rate
B lood pressure

For mild pneumonia give oral amoxycillin 500 mg three times daily. For moderate pneumonia (1–2 criteria) give oral amoxycillin 500 mg three times daily, and oral erythromycin 500 mg four times daily. For severe pneumonia (> 2 criteria) give intravenous cefuroxime 1.5 g three times daily and oral erythromycin 1 g four times daily.

Hospital-acquired pneumonia

Usually treated with intravenous cefuroxime 1.5 g three times daily. If there is worsening of respiratory function or fever on cefuroxime then consult microbiology (commonly change to intravenous meropenem 500 mg four times daily or Tazocin™ 4.5 g three times daily).

Urinary tract infection (UTI)

Simple UTI

If there is no systemic upset then consider 3 days of oral treatment. The choice depends on local policy (which reflects resistance patterns):

- Nitrofurantoin 50 mg four times daily
- Trimethoprim 200 mg twice daily
- Ciprofloxacin 100 mg twice daily

Complicated UTI

UTI involving urosepsis or pyelonephritis generally presents with rigors and loin pain. Generally best treated with intravenous cefuroxime 1.5 g three times daily plus a single dose of gentamicin (5 mg/kg – NB check renal function is normal).

Catheter-related sepsis

Treatment is not required for asymptomatic bacterial colonisation. Indications for treatment include urinary symptoms, fever, signs of sepsis or high WCC. When changing chronic indwelling catheters it is advisable to give 1.5 mg gentamicin as a single dose (NB check renal function is normal) or oral ciprofloxacin 500 mg 1 hour before the procedure.

Diarrhoea

Diarrhoea after antibiotic therapy

Send stool for CDT. Treat with metronidazole 400 mg three times daily (commonly for 2 weeks). Failure to respond to metronidazole can give oral vancomycin 125 mg four times daily.

Diarrhoea after food-poisoning

May not require treatment. Travellers diarrhoea (with associated pyrexia) or after food poisoning may respond to oral ciprofloxacin 500 mg twice daily.

Septic arthritis

Obtain an aspirate to guide treatment. It is likely to require joint wash out. Give empirical treatment with intravenous cefuroxime 1.5 g three times daily.

Meningitis

Uncommon unless in neurosurgical setting. Should give intravenous ceftriaxone 2 g twice daily (dose before LP). Guidelines now also give consideration to dexamethasone administration. If the patient is elderly, immunocompromised, or pregnant then consider intravenous ceftriaxone 2 g twice daily with amoxycillin 2 g four times daily (to cover *Listeria*) +/– steroids.

6.3 ANTIBIOTIC PROPHYLAXIS

In a nutshell ...

Prophylactic antibiotics
Reduce surgical site infection
Should be given early (before or just after anaesthetic)
Can be given as a single dose at therapeutic concentration
Must be broad spectrum and appropriate to likely organisms

The most important aspect of good antibiotic prophylaxis is to obtain high levels of systemic antibiotics at the time of the procedure and to maintain this for the duration of surgery. Prophylactic antibiotics should not be continued beyond this. This measure aims to reduce the incidence of surgical-site infection, particularly during implantation of prosthetic material. The aim of antibiotic prophylaxis is to prevent bacteria from multiplying without altering normal flora.

Prophylaxis should be started pre-operatively, ideally within 30 minutes of anaesthesia, and antibiotics should be given IV. Early administration of the antibiotic allows time for levels to accumulate in the tissues before they are disrupted by surgery (eg application of tourniquets, opening hollow organs).

A single dose of the correct antibiotic at its therapeutic concentration is sufficient for most purposes. Prophylaxis may be continued for a set duration (eg 24 hours) as a matter of policy in certain circumstances but it should not be inappropriately prolonged.

Choice of antibiotic may be set by hospital policy or surgeon preference but the prophylaxis chosen must be broad spectrum and must cover the organisms likely to be encountered. Policies for surgical prophylaxis that recommend β-lactam antibiotics as first-line agents should also recommend an alternative for patients with allergy to penicillins or cephalosporins.

Issues for consideration

- Is it needed?
- For what pathogen and where?
- Which route of administration?
- Is the patient immunocompromised?

Indications for antibiotic prophylaxis

- Where procedure commonly leads to infection (eg colectomy)
- In reducing post-op infections from endogenous sources (proven value)
- Where results of sepsis would be devastating, despite low risk of occurrence (eg vascular or other prostheses)

It has no value in clean procedures where the risk of sepsis from an exogenous source is < 2%.

Administration of antibiotic prophylaxis

- Choice of antibiotic: bacteriostatic or bactericidal (if immunocompromised)
- Give short courses < 24 hours
- Dosage
  - Single dose (used if 3–6% post-op infection rate) or
  - Multiple dose (used if 6% post-op infection rate)
- Timing of administration
  - Within 1 hour pre-operatively or at induction (15–20 minutes before skin incision or tourniquet inflation)
  - Second dose if operation > 4 hours to maintain adequate tissue levels

NB: Beware of the following when giving antibiotic prophylaxis:

- Toxicity
- Side effects
- Routes of excretion
- Allergies

Examples of antibiotic prophylaxis

- Upper GI surgery: cefuroxime and metronidazole; ciprofloxacin
- Lower GI surgery: cefuroxime and metronidazole
- Orthopaedic surgery:
  - Open fractures: first-generation cephalosporin plus benzylpenicillin (plus gentamicin if grade III or very heavily contaminated)
  - Joint replacement: cefuroxime
- Vascular surgery: cefuroxime, gentamicin and metronidazole
- Cardiothoracic surgery: flucloxacillin and gentamicin

6.4 MICROBIAL RESISTANCE

In a nutshell ...

Hospital acquired (nosocomial) infection is increasing in incidence (sicker patients, rapid patient turnover etc)
Antibiotic resistance is increasing, acquired by spontaneous mutation, transformation and plasmid transfer
There are clinical measures to help reduce the acquisition of both nosocomial infection and antibiotic resistance

Bacterial antibiotic resistance and multiresistant organisms

Bacterial resistance is increasing. Data from the USA shows that in ITU patients up to 30% of hospital acquired infections are resistant to the preferred antibiotic for treatment. Increasing MRSA incidence has been documented (and use of vancomycin results in emerging *S. aureus* resistance to vancomycin). Resistance results from selective survival pressure on bacteria.

Bacteria acquire resistance genes by three mechanisms

- **Spontaneous mutation:** rapid replication times cause spontaneous mutations to arise in bacterial DNA; some of these mutations may confer resistance.
- **Transformation:** one bacterium takes up DNA from another and splices it into its genome using enzymes called integrases, allowing passage of resistance genes against antibiotics, disinfectants and pollutants.
- **Plasmids:** these are small circles of DNA (like small chromosomes) which can be transmitted from bacterium to bacterium and cross bacterial phylogeny.

Resistance may occur by:

- Alteration of bacterial cell-wall proteins to prevent antibiotic binding (eg penicillin resistance)
- Alteration of ribosome structure to prevent antibiotic binding (eg erythromycin, tetracycline, gentamicin)
- Production of antibiotic-destroying proteins

Resistance is passed on to all subsequent bacterial progeny. Resistance may be conferred against multiple antibiotics.

Potential causes of resistance

- Inappropriate prescription
- Failure to finish the course of antibiotics: microbes which are relatively drug resistant will not be killed in the first few days and will become preferentially selected
- Addition of antibiotics to agricultural feed (entry into the food chain)
- Extensive use of antibiotics in sick patients with multiple organisms may promote resistance and transmission between individuals
- Natural evolution of bacteria

Methicillin-resistant *Staphylococcus aureus* (MRSA)

During the last 20 years the prevalence of MRSA in hospitals has fluctuated – it is now nearly 50% in UK hospitals. β-lactam antibiotics inhibit bacterial cell-wall synthesis by inactivating penicillin-binding proteins (PBP); MRSA strains produce an alternative PBP (*mecA* gene) that allows continued cell-wall synthesis.

Prevention of MRSA transmission

- Use of preventative measures (handwashing, alcohol gels, etc)
- Patient screening (especially important if having elective surgery with prosthetic implants)
- Isolation of carrier or infected patients (barrier nursing)
- Removal of any colonised catheters
- Eradication of carriage (nasal: mupirocin; chlorhexidine hair and body wash; hexachlorophene powder)

Systemic MRSA infections

May require appropriate antibiotics if isolated from sterile site (eg MRSA detected in abdominal cavity or in blood cultures). An antibiotic regimen which includes intravenous vancomycin 1 g twice daily should be considered. If the patient is systemically unwell a single dose of gentamicin 5 mg/kg should act as a holding measure until further cultures are back.

Vancomycin-resistant enterococcus (VRE)

There are two types of vancomycin resistance in enterococci:

- Low-level intrinsic resistance (eg *Enterococcus gallinarum*)
- Acquired resistance by transfer of genes (*vanA*, *vanB*, etc) commonly seen in *E. faecalis*

VRE can be carried in the gut without disease (colonisation) and can be picked up by screening.

Chapter 3

Neoplasia

Amer Aldouri and Claire Ritchie Chalmers

Section 1
Epidemiology of Cancer

1.1 CANCER TERMINOLOGY

In a nutshell ...

Epidemiology is the study of disease frequency in populations.

In cancer epidemiology, useful concepts include:

Measures of incidence
Prevalence: proportion of population with a condition at a given time
Incidence: proportion of population developing a condition in a given time

Measures of risk
Risk factor: an agent or characteristic predisposing to the development of a condition
Relative risk: strength of association between risk factor and condition

Measures of outcome
Disease-free survival: an outcome measure in oncology for the time period from diagnosis to detection of recurrence
Life table: a calculation predicting the cumulative probability of surviving a given number of years (eg 5-year survival rate)
Survival curve: plot of probability of survival against time (eg Kaplan–Meier curve)

1.2 CANCER REGISTRIES

In a nutshell ...

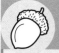

Cancer registries
Monitor levels and changes in different cancers in the population
Collate information from death certificates about deaths from each cancer type

These registries are set up to monitor the incidence and mortality of various cancers in the population, and to determine any changes in these parameters.

Information from death certificates is collated by the National Cancer Registry in England and Wales and is followed up by case-note analysis and post mortem diagnoses, etc. Statistical information from cancer registries should be viewed with caution due to potential errors arising from differences in accuracy of data collection, geographical variations, and in diagnosis rates and post mortem rates, for example.

1.3 CANCER SCREENING

In a nutshell ...

There are criteria for screening programmes and for the screening test used.

Current NHS screening programmes are nationally coordinated and include:

Breast screening
Cervical screening
The English Colorectal Cancer screening pilot

http://www.cancerscreening.nhs.uk/ for further information.

Screening programmes

Criteria for screening programmes

A screening programme needs to fulfil certain criteria (defined by the WHO in 1966). These criteria are:

- The condition is an important health problem
- Its natural history is well understood
- It's recognisable at an early stage
- Treatment is better at an early stage
- A suitable test exists
- An acceptable test exists
- Adequate facilities exist to cope with the abnormalities detected
- Screening is done at repeated intervals when the onset is insidious
- The chance of harm is less than the chance of benefit
- The cost is balanced against benefit

Criteria for screening tests

The screening test must detect the condition at an earlier stage than it would clinically present. This means there should be a detectable latent or pre-clinical phase during which interventional treatment is possible.

The screening test should be:

- Simple and cheap/cost effective
- Continuous
- Highly sensitive (few false negatives)
- Highly specific (few false positives)
- Have a high positive predictive value
- Safe
- Non-invasive
- Acceptable to patients
- Offered to a group agreed to be at high risk
- Easy to perform and analyse

There should also be adequate resources to deal with the workload for both screening and treatment of specific programmes.

Specific UK screening programmes

Breast screening

The WHO's International Agency for Research on Cancer (IARC) concluded that mammography screening for breast cancer reduces mortality. The IARC working group determined that there is a 35% reduction in mortality from breast cancer among screened women aged 50–69 (ie the number needed to screen to save one life is 500). See http://www.cancer-screening.nhs.uk/ for more information.

Women aged 50–64 are routinely invited for breast screening every 3 years. The aim is to extend this to women up to the age of 70. After the upper age limit women are invited to make their own appointments.

There are over 90 breast screening units across the UK, each responsible for an average population of around 45 000 women. These can either be mobile, hospital-based, or permanently based in another convenient location (eg a shopping centre).

The total budget is £52 million (£40 per woman screened).

Cervical screening

This is essentially a smear test, sent for cytology looking for early precursor abnormalities that may be treated to prevent the development of cervical cancer.

All women between the ages of 25 and 64 are invited for a cervical smear test every 3–5 years. The programme is about to change, basing the interval at which screening is offered on patient age.

The total budget (including the cost of treating cervical abnormalities) costs around £150 million a year (£37.50 per woman screened).

Colorectal cancer (CRC) screening

The English CRC screening pilot was recently completed. It assessed the feasibility of CRC screening using the faecal occult blood test for patients aged 50–69. This is positive in about 2% and these people are offered colonoscopy. On this basis, a countrywide screening programme for patients aged 60–90 is being planned (at the time of publication).

1.4 INCIDENCE OF COMMON CANCERS

In a nutshell ...

Cancer is a common disease affecting a third of the population in their lifetime
There are 250 000 new cases diagnosed per year
65% of cancer affects the > 65 age group
Common cancers are different for different age groups (adults, teenagers and children)
Smoking and diet are the main environmental aetiological factors (thought to be responsible for a third of cancer cases each)

Specific clinical information about most common cancers is covered in the other chapters in this book and Book 2.

Cancer incidence by age and gender

Common cancers in adults

50% of adult cancer involves the **big four**: breast, prostate, lung, large bowel.

Remember that the incidence of a cancer is not the same as the death rate from that cancer. Incidence data can be expressed as the number of new cases per 1000 per year or as a percentage.

There is a different incidence of certain cancers in men and women.

COMMON CANCERS ACCORDING TO GENDER (INCIDENCE EXPRESSED AS A PERCENTAGE OF ALL NEWLY DIAGNOSED CASES OF CANCER PER YEAR)

Men			Women		
	Incidence	*Lifetime risk*		*Incidence*	*Lifetime risk*
Prostate	22%	1 in 14	Breast	30%	1 in 9
Lung	17%	1 in 13	Large bowel	12%	1 in 18
large bowel	14%	1 in 18	Lung	11%	1 in 13
Bladder	6%	1 in 30	Ovary	5%	1 in 48
Stomach	4%	1 in 44	Uterus	4%	1 in 73
Head and neck	4%	1 in 44	Non-Hodgkin's lymphoma	3%	1 in 83
Non-Hodgkin's lymphoma	4%	1 in 69	Melanoma	3%	1 in 117
Oesophagus	3%	1 in 75	Pancreas	3%	1 in 96
Kidney	3%	1 in 89	Stomach	2%	1 in 86
Leukaemia	3%	1 in 95	Bladder	2%	1 in 79
Others (individually < 1%)	20%		Others (individually < 1%)	25%	

Common cancers in teenagers

- Testicular cancer
- Brain tumours
- Melanoma
- Leukaemia

Common cancers in children

The risk of cancer in childhood (< 15 years) is 1 in 500 in the UK. For a detailed discussion of oncology in childhood see the *Paediatrics* chapter.

Commonly these cancers are:

- **Haematological:** 25% of childhood cancers are acute lymphocytic leukaemia (ALL). Incidence of Hodgkin's lymphoma peaks in teenagers
- **Brain and spinal cord:** eg astrocytoma and primitive neuroectodermal tumour
- **Embryonal tumours:** occur in different parts of the body and are referred to as ' blastomas' eg medulloblastoma (brain), nephroblastoma (Wilms tumour), retinoblastoma
- **Bone tumours:** osteosarcoma and Ewing's sarcoma. Bone tumour incidence peaks at 14–15 years

Cancer incidence by geographical region

Different cancers have different incidences in different countries and in different ethnic groups.

- **Breast cancer:** much less common in the third world than in developed countries. Its incidence is highest in the west and second-generation immigrants from areas of low incidence (they acquire the elevated risk of their new country)
- **Hepatocellular carcinoma:** most common where hepatitis B infection is common (Far East, sub-Saharan Africa) regardless of race. Iron overload and aflatoxin also contribute in these regions
- **Stomach cancer:** common in Japan and Chile. First-generation immigrants to the west retain this high rate but second-generation immigrants adopt the lower rate of their new country
- **Colon cancer:** westernised countries with low-fibre diets have increased risks of colon cancer
- **Prostate cancer:** highest in Afro–Caribbean people and lowest in Japan
- **Oesophageal cancer:** common in China, USSR and poor nations. The reasons may be dietary
- **Epstein–Barr virus:** ubiquitous around the world, but Burkitt's lymphoma is an African disease, and its distribution corresponds to regions where malaria is endemic. Immigrants to Africa are susceptible, as are the native Black people
- **Skin cancers:** (notably melanomas) are commonest in light-skinned people who have heavy sun exposure at low latitudes and/or high altitudes
- **Cervical cancer:** incidence follows that of STDs (aetiological agent is HPV). It may be less common in areas where men are circumcised
- **Squamous cell carcinoma of the bladder:** caused by schistosomiasis and so is common in endemic areas (eg Egypt)

Changes in cancer incidence in Europe

Factors impacting on incidence of cancer

Behavioural factors

- Women starting to smoke in the 1940s (increase in lung cancer)
- Sunbathing and tanning became fashionable (increase in melanoma)

Environmental exposure

- Asbestos
- Aniline dyes

Diagnostic tests

- Introduction of PSA as a test for occult and asymptomatic prostate cancer

Screening

- May increase incidence (by detection of early tumours)
- May decrease incidence (by detection of pre-cursor lesions that can be treated before the tumour develops eg colorectal polyps, carcinoma in situ of the cervix)

There is a variable lag period before the effects of changes in behaviour or environmental exposure are seen. Implementation of new diagnostic tests or screening programmes may have a much more rapid impact on the incidence figures.

Increasing incidence of cancer in Europe

Data from Europe over the last decade shows increasing incidence in the following cancers:

- Melanoma (54% and 37% increases in incidence in men and women respectively)
- Prostate (60% increase; NB remember introduction of PSA testing)
- Uterus (23% increase in incidence)
- Kidney
- Non-Hodgkin's lymphoma
- Breast
- Leukaemia
- Ovary

Decreasing incidence of cancer in Europe

Incidence is decreasing in the following cancers:

- Large bowel (6–8% decrease)
- Pancreas
- Bladder
- Stomach (28% decrease)
- Lung
- Cervix (24% decrease)

For discussion of survival and mortality rates please refer to the clinical section on individual cancers in Book 2.

Section 2

Molecular basis of cancer

In a nutshell ...

The word ' tumour' literally means 'swelling.' The swelling is either physiological or pathological.

Physiological swelling
eg pregnant uterus

Pathological swelling
Neoplastic
Non-neoplastic (eg pus, inflammatory, bony callus)

Neoplasia is an abnormal mass of tissue, the growth of which is uncoordinated, exceeds that of the normal tissues and persists in the same manner after cessation of the stimuli that evoked the change.

Tumours are **similar** to the organ in which they arose:

- They consist of both parenchymal and stromal elements but come from a single 'cell of origin' in the parent tissue (ie they are clonal)
- They may continue to perform some of the functions of the parent organ (eg mucin production in colorectal tumours; hormone production in endocrine tumours; IgG in myeloma)
- Individual cells look similar to the parent cells and the degree of similarity depends upon the degree of differentiation of the tumour

However, they also **differ** in some ways:

- Deranged histological architecture
- No controlled functional contribution to the body
- Can proliferate rapidly (unlike other differentiated cell groups)
- Can develop metastatic potential

2.1 NORMAL CELL GROWTH

In a nutshell ...

Cells fall into several different categories according to their propensity to divide and their degree of differentiation:

- **Labile cells:** constantly renewed (eg stratified squamous epithelium of the skin)
- **Stable cells:** usually quiescent but can be stimulated to divide (eg hepatocytes)
- **Permanent cells:** do not undergo mitosis in post-natal life (eg neurones, skeletal muscle tissues, glomeruli)

Cells divide as they progress through the cell cycle. There are many regulatory points inherent in the cycle, and disruption of these genes results in uncontrolled replication.

The cell cycle

DNA structure

Deoxyribonucleic acid (DNA) is a strand-like molecule consisting of four building blocks – adenine (A), thymine (T), cytosine (C), and guanine (G). These are paired (A with T and C with G) and their affiliation for each other zips the two strands of DNA into the double helix.

DNA is stored in the cellular nucleus as a folded form called chromatin. This is wrapped around proteins called histones to form complexes called nucleosomes (that look like a bead on a string). Active genes unwrap from the histones opening out the DNA for access by transcriptional proteins. When the cell divides, the nucleosomes become very tightly folded, condensing into chromosomes.

The nucleus of most human cells contains two sets of chromosomes, one set given by each parent. Each set has 23 single chromosomes, 22 autosomes, and a sex chromosome (X or Y). There are therefore 46 chromosomes in each cell.

Phases of the cell cycle

The cell cycle is divided into phases:

G_1 Pre-synthetic
S DNA synthesis (chromosome replication)
G_2 Pre-mitotic
M Mitotic (cell division)
G_0 Quiescent (resting phase)

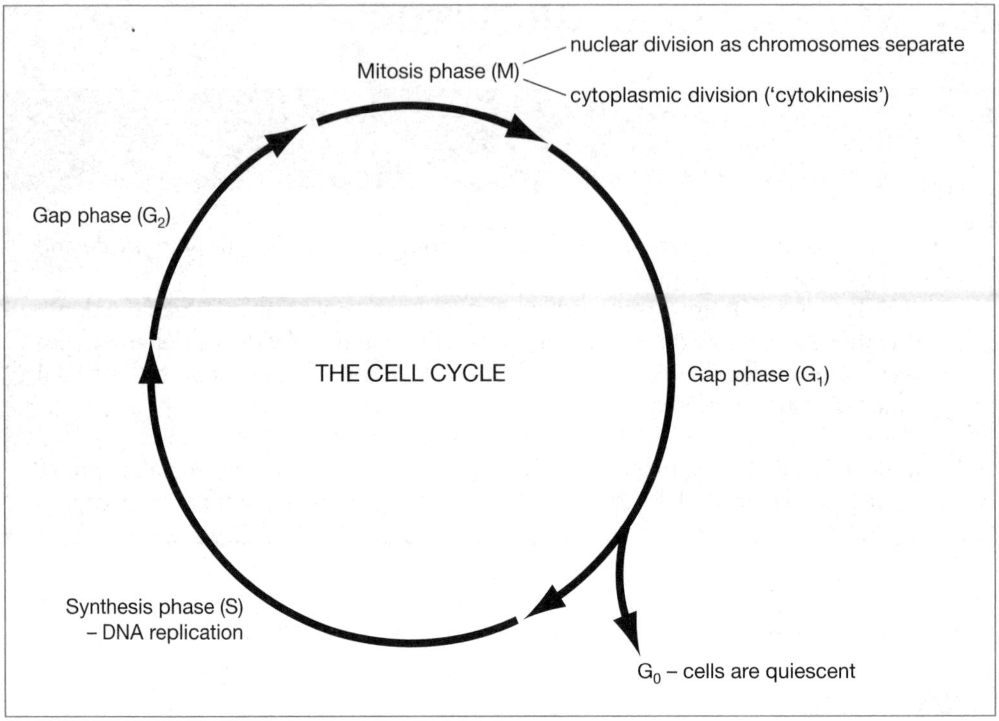

Figure 2.1a *The cell cycle*

Mitosis is divided into several phases:

- **Interphase:** this comprises phases G_1, S, and G_2 of the cell cycle when the cell is in preparation for division. The chromosomes have replicated and there are two copies of each in the cell (ie 92 chromosomes)
- **Prophase:** the chromatin begins to condense and is seen as chromosomes. Centrioles move to opposing ends of the cell and fibres stretch between them forming the mitotic spindle
- **Prometaphase:** the nuclear membrane dissolves and the chromosomes start to move towards the centre of the cell under the control of microtubules
- **Metaphase:** the spindle fibres align with the chromosomes along the metaphase plate (this allows accurate separation of the paired replicated chromosomes to the two cells)
- **Anaphase:** the paired chromosomes separate and are dragged to the opposite sides of the cell by the microtubules
- **Telophase:** the chromatids arrive at the opposite poles of the cell and disperse after new nuclear membranes are formed
- **Cytokinesis:** an actin fibre forms around the centre of the cell and contracts, pinching it into two daughter cells, each with 23 pairs of chromosomes

Control of the cell cycle

There are regulatory points between the different phases of the cell cycle.

Most adult cells are in G_0 (ie outside the cell cycle) and quiescent. The length of the G_1 phase is variable. The length of the S, G_2, and M phases are fairly constant because these processes have a limit as to how quickly they can be performed.

Entry of G_0 cells into the cycle and transition from G_1 to S phase are the two crucial regulatory points of the cell cycle. They are controlled by:

- **Intracellular enzymes:** cyclin-dependant kinases (CDKs) cause cells to move from G_1 to S and also from G_2 to M. They are:
  - Up-regulated by platelet-derived growth factor (PDGF), epidermal growth factor (EGF), and insulin-like growth factor (IGF-1) in the serum
  - Down-regulated by transforming growth factor β (TGF-β)
- **Protein p53:** this protein blocks the cell cycle in G_1 phase if DNA is damaged. This allows for DNA repair or, if the damage is severe, cellular apoptosis. High levels of p53 are seen in damaged cells and loss of p53 activity by gene mutation or deletion is associated with tumour development

Cellular differentiation

This is a complex and incompletely understood process occurring during development of the fetus and occurs continuously in certain systems of the body (eg haematopoiesis).

Definitions relating to differentiation

- **Differentiation:** cell specialisation that occurs at the end of the developmental pathway. Selective genes are activated to produce the differentiated phenotype
- **Stem cell:** a cell from an embryo, fetus, or adult that can reproduce itself for long periods of time and can give rise to specialised cells and tissues
- **Totipotent:** a cell capable of expressing any of the genes of the genome (can give rise to any part of the later embryo or adult). In humans, the fertilised egg is totipotent until the 8-cell stage
- **Pluripotent:** a cell with the potential to generate cell types and tissues from all three primary germ layers of the body
- **Plasticity:** the ability of a stem cell of one tissue type to generate cells from another tissue type
- **Progenitor or precursor cell:** occurs when a stem cell divides into two partially differentiated cells, neither of which can replicate itself but may continue along the path of differentiation

Process of differentiation

Irreversible transition from stem cell to a pre-determined differentiated cell type can take one of two pathways:

- A totipotent or pluripotent stem cell may **proliferate and its daughters progress to terminal differentiation**. As this process progresses these cells loose their ability to divide again. Once committed to this pathway cells cannot change their lineage, resulting in mature differentiated cells that have specific functions and do not divide (eg cells of the blood)
- After trauma some tissues may **selectively replicate to replenish tissues**. This can occur because the stimulus causes some of the cells to de-differentiate, to re-enter the cell cycle, and to replicate rapidly

Regulation of differentiation

There is usually an inverse relationship between cell replication and cell differentiation. Differentiation is complex and is regulated by a number of factors:

Soluble factors

- Hormones (eg glucagons, hydrocortisone)
- Interferon
- Vitamin D
- Calcium ions

Cell–cell interactions

- Effects of high cell density and proximity
- Through gap junctions

Cell–matrix interactions

- Matrix attachments may regulate gene expression

These regulators affect gene expression in the differentiating cell. Gene expression is controlled by a combination of:

- **DNA methylation:** this causes the gene to be silenced
- **Chromatin structure:** regulation of the acetylation of histones causes changes in chromatin configuration that allow genes to be increasingly or decreasingly accessible to transcription

2.2 DISORDERS OF CELL GROWTH

In a nutshell ...

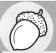

Disorders of growth can be divided into:

Developmental disorders of growth (before an organ reaches maturity)
Hypoplasia
Agenesis
Atresia
Ectopia
Heteroplasia
Hamartoma

Acquired disorders of growth (after an organ reaches maturity)
Hyperplasia
Hypertrophy
Teratoma
Atrophy
Metaplasia
Dysplasia
Neoplasia

When cells become neoplastic they are referred to as 'transformed.'

Developmental disorders of cell growth

- **Hypoplasia:** the organ doesn't reach its full size
- **Agenesis:** vestigial structure only or no development at all
- **Atresia:** failure of canalisation in a hollow lumen causing congenital obstruction (eg GI tract)
- **Ectopia:** location of normal differentiated tissue in an abnormal location (eg thyroid tissue may develop anywhere along the thyroglossal tract)
- **Heteroplasia:** anomalous differentiation of tissues within an organ (eg the presence of sebaceous glands within the mouth) is referred to as heteroplasia
- **Hamartoma:** overgrowth of mature cells that are usually found within the tissue but with disordered architecture (eg haemangioma)

Acquired disorders of cell growth

Hyperplasia

Increase in the number of cells.

The cells mature to normal size and shape. This can occur in response to inflammation, increased workload, excess endocrine drive, or increased metabolic demand, for example:

- Benign prostatic hyperplasia
- Renal hyperplasia (in response to contralateral dysfunction)

Hypertrophy

Increase in cell size but not in number.

This occurs in response to a demand for increased function, for example:

- Increased skeletal muscle volume in athletes
- Increased cardiac muscle volume in hypertension
- Pregnant uterus

NB: Both hyperplasia and hypertrophy can occur simultaneously.

Teratoma

Growth of cells originating from more than one germ cell line.

Teratomas contain a variety of tissues in a variable state of differentiation. They arise in the gonads or the mid-line of the body (eg mediastinum, retroperitoneum, base of skull). They can behave in a benign or malignant manner.

Atrophy

Loss of cell substance causing a reduction in cell size.

These are the different types:

- **Physiological atrophy:** shrinkage of a well differentiated structure when it is no longer required (eg ductus arteriosus after birth)
- **Pathological atrophy:** occurs with age (eg musculature, brain tissue)
- **Local atrophy:** often due to reduced blood flow or neurological input (eg nerve damage) to that region
- **Disuse atrophy:** often musculature due to trauma, immobility, or age

Metaplasia

Reversible replacement of one differentiated cell type with another.

This is an adaptive response and the replacement cells are of the same tissue type. It can be due to chronic irritation or altered cell function. There is greater susceptibility to neoplastic transformation (via dysplasia) but it is not inevitable (eg squamous epithelium changing to gastric type in the distal oesophagus – Barrett's oesophagus).

Dysplasia

Disordered cellular development characterised by increased mitosis and pleomorphism.

This is frequently pre-neoplastic and it may follow metaplasia. May also be called carcinoma in situ, intra-epithelial neoplasia, incipient neoplasia, or pre-cancer.

Neoplasia

'Transformed' is a word that is used to describe the process by which a normal cell becomes neoplastic. The processes involved are called carcinogenesis. Transformed cells adopt the abnormal growth patterns consistent with neoplasia (discussed in section 2.4).

2.3 CARCINOGENESIS

In a nutshell ...

A tumour (neoplasm) is an overgrowth of tissue formed by a clone of cells bearing cumulative genetic injuries. Each of these genetic injuries confers an additional growth advantage to the clone that possesses it (Cole and Nowell 1976).

These mutations can be:

Congenital: already present in the genome (heritable cancers)

Acquired: additional mutations brought about by exposure to a carcinogen (sporadic cancers)

The multistage process of carcinogenesis

Carcinogenesis is a generic term for the acquisition of a series of genetic mutations that lead up to the expression of full malignant potential. As cells undergo carcinogenesis and become neoplastic they become **transformed.**

Cole and Nowell described the multistep process of tumorogenesis in their article in *Science* in 1976. Essentially:

- Neoplasms are monoclonal (they arise from a single cell)
- Neoplasms arise due to cumulative genetic injury
- Neoplasms may develop more aggressive sub-clones as genetic injuries accumulate
- Genetic injuries confer growth advantages:
  - Increased proliferation (failure of control of division)
  - Immortalisation (failure of cell senescence)
  - Loss of apoptotic control
- Genetic injuries may include:
  - Point mutations
  - Amplifications
  - Deletions
  - Changes in control regions (eg gene promoters, enhancer sequences)
  - Translocations of chromosomal material

Carcinogens

In a nutshell ...

Carcinogens can be divided into three types:
- Chemical
- Physical
- Infectious (oncogenic viruses, bacteria, protozoa)

Chemical carcinogens

Chemical carcinogens may act directly to damage DNA (eg alkylating agents) whereas the majority require metabolic conversion from a pro-carcinogen state to become activated (eg polycyclic hydrocarbons (smoke), aromatic amines, amides, and azo dyes, natural plant products, and nitrosamines). The carcinogen is often activated by metabolism via the hepatic P450 mixed function oxidase system of the liver.

Chemical carcinogens can be either **mutagens** (irreversibly directly damage DNA) or **non-mutagens** (reversibly promote cell division). Some heavy metals depolymerise DNA.

The process of **initiation** is exposure to a carcinogen that causes irreversible DNA damage but does not directly lead to a change in phenotype. This is followed by the process of **promotion,** which allows initiated cells to grow into tumours by promoting cell division (eg hormonal influences on tumour growth).

Chemicals are tested for mutagenicity by a variety of in-vitro and in-vivo procedures:

- Production of mutations in bacteria colonies (eg the Ames test), yeast colonies, and in cultured mammalian cells
- Charting unexpected DNA synthesis in cultured mammalian cells
- Use of higher plants to look at chromosome damage

Physical carcinogens

These consist of a wide range of agents:

- Electromagnetic radiation (UV light, ionising radiation)
- Extremes of temperature
- Mechanical trauma
- Foreign bodies and implants

The mechanism of carcinogenesis is thought to be centred around long-term inflammation causing proliferation. There may also be direct DNA damage by radiation. Selection of clones with growth advantages then leads to neoplasia. There are a few reported cases of sarcomatous change around foreign bodies and surgical implants (this is very rare).

Infectious carcinogens

Infection causing persistent inflammation may result in neoplastic transformation (eg bladder schistosomiasis resulting in TCC of the bladder in endemic areas such as Egypt), malaria and Burkitt's lymphoma.

Viral infection may also result in neoplastic transformation. This may be caused by insertion of viral genomic material into the cell (eg EBV incorporation into the genome) or cell lysis due to viral infection stimulating cell turnover and proliferation (eg hepatitis and cirrhosis leading to HCC).

EXAMPLES OF CARCINOGENS (HISTORICAL AND CONTEMPORARY) AND THEIR EFFECTS

Carcinogen	Associated carcinoma	Examples of groups affected
Chemical agents		
B-naphthamine	Bladder carcinoma	Dye workers
Benzopyrene	Lung carcinoma	Painters, printers
Aflatoxin	Hepatocellular carcinoma	Peanut farmers
Asbestos	Mesothelioma	Builders, shippers
Chromium, arsenic, nickel	Lung carcinoma	Miners, smelters
Vinyl chloride monomers	Angiosarcoma of liver	
Diethyl stilbestrol	Adenocarcinoma of the vagina	
Benzol/benzene	Blood and lymphatic cancers	
Nitrates	Gastric cancer	
Physical agents		
UV light	Melanoma (especially UVB) Basal cell carcinoma Squamous cell carcinoma	
Ionising radiation	Leukaemia (blood) Bone Breast Thyroid Skin, tongue, tonsil	Radium workers
Viruses, bacteria and protozoa		
HIV	Leukaemias, lymphomas, Kaposi sarcoma	
Hepatitis B, C	Hepatocellular carcinoma	
EBV	Nasopharyngeal carcinoma, B-cell lymphoma Burkitt's lymphoma, Hodgkin's lymphoma	
HPV 16, HPV 18	Cervical cancer	
Helicobacter pylori	Gastric cancer	
Schistosoma	Squamous cell carcinoma of the bladder	

Genes involved in carcinogenesis

Four classes of genes can be affected to produce a neoplasm:

- Oncogenes
- Tumour suppressor genes
- Anti-apoptotic genes
- DNA mismatch repair genes

Oncogenes

Normal genes involved in cell division are called proto-oncogenes. These genes may become permanently activated by point mutation, translocation, or an increase in the copy number (amplification). This results in permanent up-regulation. Activation of these genes causes cell division and promotes growth in a dominant manner (ie the damaged gene over-rides signals from its undamaged normal counterpart). These genes code for growth factors and their receptors, signal transducing proteins, transcription factors and cell cycle regulators.

Examples of commonly mutated oncogenes include:

- *Ras* oncogene (overexpression of growth factor p21)
- *ERB1* and *ERB2* (overexpression of growth factors)
- Telomerase (important for cellular immortality)

Tumour suppressor genes (anti-oncogenes)

These are normal genes that tell cells when not to divide. They are down-regulated by mutations. They tend to act in a recessive manner (ie usually the malignant phenotype is expressed only when both copies are damaged or missing).

Examples of commonly mutated tumour suppressor genes include:

- *APC* (results in familial adenomatous polyposis, FAP)
- E-cadherin
- *p53* (mutated in up to 50% of tumours)

Anti-apoptotic genes

Normal tissues are subject to genes regulating programmed cell death (apoptosis). Neoplasia is associated with changes in cell senescence and immortalisation of the cell line ie loss of these normal controls results in a reduction in cell death. This occurs when the genes controlling apoptosis are down-regulated by mutation.

Commonly affected apoptosis genes include *bcl-2* (inhibits apoptosis).

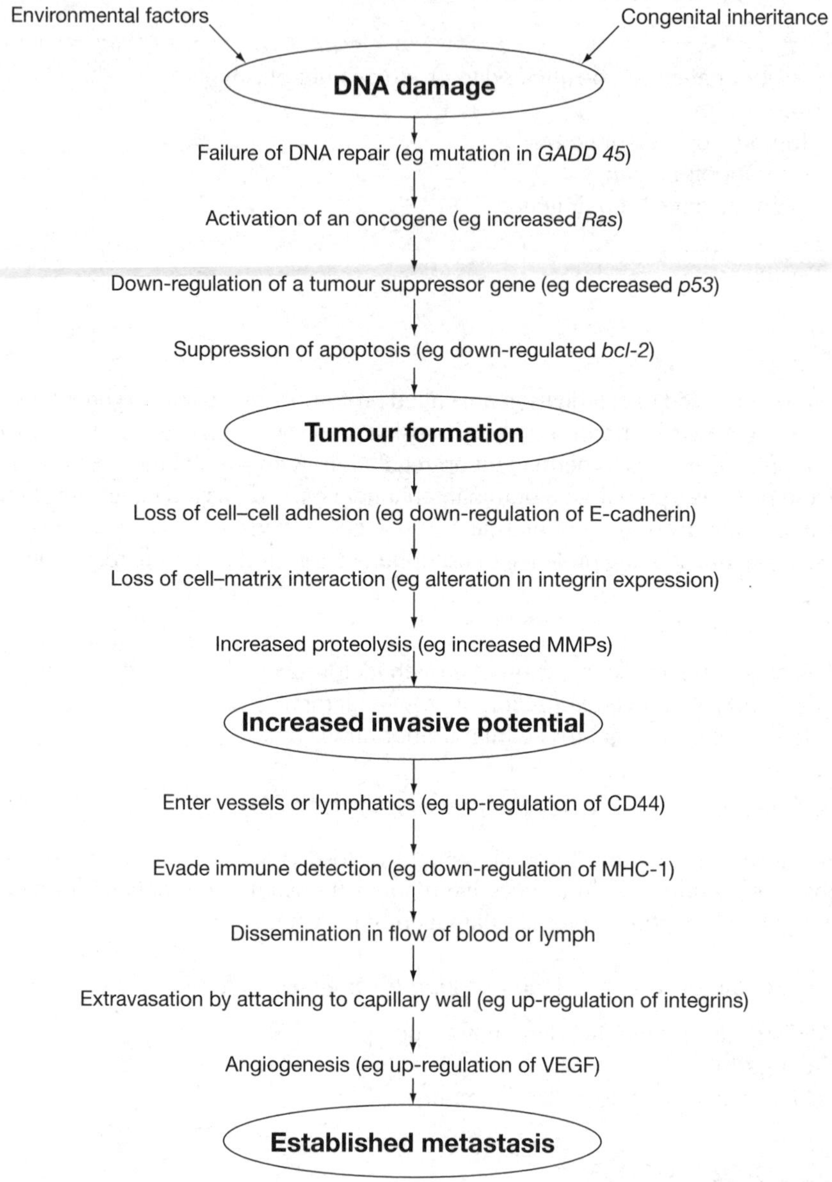

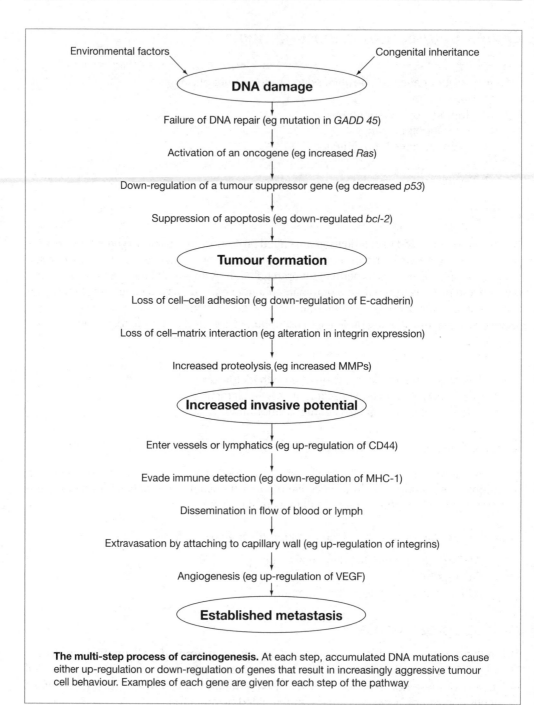

The multi-step process of carcinogenesis. At each step, accumulated DNA mutations cause either up-regulation or down-regulation of genes that result in increasingly aggressive tumour cell behaviour. Examples of each gene are given for each step of the pathway

Figure 2.3a *Overview of carcinogenesis*

DNA mismatch-repair genes

After normal cellular replication, there are genes responsible for recognising and excising mutated gene segments. If the genes themselves undergo mutation they become down-regulated, allowing accumulation of mutations within the cell.

Commonly affected DNA repair genes include *MSH-2*.

There is also a level of interaction between all these gene products, exemplified by the role of p53. This protein is up-regulated by cellular and DNA damage, and high levels can be identified in damaged cells. p53 protein upregulates a CDK inhibitor molecule, causing inhibition of the CDK family. This halts the cell cycle in G1. p53 also upregulates transcription of GADD 45 which is a DNA repair enzyme, and the BAX protein which binds to bcl-2 allowing apoptosis to occur if the DNA is not repaired.

The Knudson two-hit hypothesis

This hypothesis describes the role of recessive genes in tumorogenesis. Both normal alleles of the *Rb* gene on chromosome 13q14 have to be lost before retinoblastoma develops. One may be inherited as a mutated copy, but the tumour will only develop if the second copy undergoes mutation.

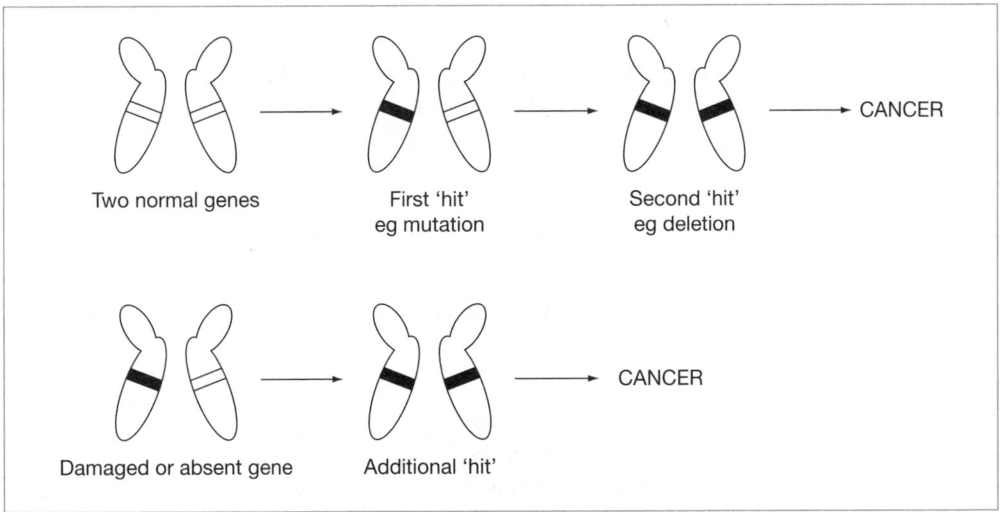

Figure 2.3b *The Knudson two-hit hypothesis*

The Knudson two-hit hypothesis also helps to explain the development of familial cancer.

Familial and sporadic cancers

Familial cancers – congenital mutations

Defective or mutated genes may be inherited via the germ cell line. Patients carrying this defective gene copy are at high risk of developing a tumour. These genes may be either dominant or recessive.

It is estimated that 5–10% of common solid adult tumours may be attributable to an inherited defective gene. The rest (and therefore the majority) are sporadic.

Common genetic mutations in familial cancers

GENES RELATED TO FAMILIAL CANCER SYNDROMES: ALL ARE AVAILABLE FOR GENETIC TESTING

Syndrome	Clinical presentation	Gene
Oncogenes		
Familial malignant melanoma	Melanoma	*CDK 4*
Hereditary GIST syndrome	Stromal tumours of GI tract from oesophagus to rectum	*KIT*
Hereditary papillary renal carcinoma	Bilateral papillary renal carcinoma	*MET*
Multiple endocrine neoplasia type 2	Medullary thyroid carcinoma, phaeochromocytoma Parathyroid adenoma	*RET*
Tumour suppressor genes		
Familial adenomatous polyposis	Multiple colonic adenomas	*APC*
Familial breast and ovarian cancer	Breast cancer Ovarian cancer Prostate cancer Colon cancer	*BRAC 1* *BRAC 2*
Retinoblastoma	Retinoblastoma Osteosarcoma Pinealoma	*Rb1*
Multiple endocrine neoplasia type 1	Parathyroid Pancreas Pituitary	*MEN 1*
Neurofibromatosis	Neurofibromata Schwannomas of cranial nerves	*NF 1* *NF 2*

Von Hippel–Lindau	Haemangioblastoma Renal cell carcinoma Phaeochromocytoma	*VHL*
Li–Fraumeni	Breast cancer Soft tissue sarcoma Leukaemia Osteosarcoma Melanoma Colon cancer Pancreas	*p53*
DNA repair genes		
Hereditary non-polyposis colorectal cancer	Colorectal cancer Endometrial cancer Ovarian cancer Gastric cancer	*MLH 1* *MSH 2* *MSH 3* *PMS 1* *PMS 2*

Clinical aspects of familial tumours

Familial cancers include:

- Breast cancer (+/– ovarian or +/– sarcoma)
- Colorectal cancer
- Ovarian cancer
- Uterine cancer
- Multiple endocrine neoplasia (MEN) syndromes

Suspect a familial cancer if:

Multiple family members are affected
Age of onset is early
Multiple primaries are identified within the same individual
Cancer is bilateral
Cancer is rare form

It is helpful to draw a detailed family tree and mark affected members because this can aid identification of transmission patterns.

Management of familial cancers

Referral to a genetics service should be appropriate to the guidelines for your region. For the purposes of genetics, **close relatives** are considered to be:

- Parent (mother/father)
- Sibling (brother/sister)
- Child (son/daughter)
- Grandparent (grandmother/grandfather)
- Aunt/uncle (NB not by marriage; only consider siblings of the parents)

Guidelines for referral to genetics services

- **Breast cancer**
  - 1 relative (aged < 40 years at diagnosis)
  - 1 relative with bilateral disease
  - 1 male relative
  - 2 relatives (aged < 60 years at diagnosis)
- **Ovarian cancer**
  - 2 relatives (any age at diagnosis)
- **Colorectal cancer**
  - 1 relative (aged < 45 years at diagnosis)
  - 2 relatives (aged < 70 years at diagnosis)
  - 3 relatives with GI, uterine or ovarian cancers
  - Suspected familial adenomatous polyposis (FAP)
- **Multiple primary tumours** in an individual
- **3 close relatives** have had cancers of the GI tract, breast, ovary, prostate, pancreas, thyroid or melanoma

Patients who test positive for a defective gene may require:

- Increased surveillance
  - Watchful waiting
  - Screening (eg mammography, colonoscopy, PSA)
- Prophylactic measures:
  - Lifestyle changes (eg exercise, fat intake)
  - Medical prophylaxis (eg drugs)
  - Surgical prophylaxis (eg mastectomy for *BRCA 1* and *BRCA 2*; total colectomy for FAP)

Sporadic cancers – acquired mutations

Mutations may accumulate with advancing age and with exposure to an environmental mutagen (a carcinogen). Carcinogens act by causing additional genetic mutations within the cell that eventually accumulate sufficiently for the development of neoplasia.

2.4 ABNORMALITIES IN NEOPLASTIC CELL BEHAVIOUR

In a nutshell ...

Neoplastic cells exhibit different behaviour to normal cells in terms of:

- Proliferation
- Differentiation
- Immortality
- Apoptosis
- Karyotype and progression
- Stimulate angiogenesis

For discussion of normal cell behaviour please read section 2.1 first.

Tumour cell proliferation

The rate of cell proliferation within any population of cells depends on three things:

- **The rate of tumour cell division:** tumour cells can be pushed into the cell cycle more easily as there is loss of the regulation that controls movement from one phase of the cycle to the next
- **The fraction of cells within the population undergoing cell division (growth fraction):** this is the proportion of cells within the tumour cell population that are in the replicative pool. Not all cells within a tumour are actively replicating and many are quiescent. The growth fraction is only 20% even in rapidly growing tumours
- **The rate of cell loss from the replicating pool due to differentiation or apoptosis:** overall growth depends on balance between production and loss by apoptosis. In general tumour cells grow faster than they die off

Entry of G0 cells into the cycle and transition from G1 to S phase are the two crucial regulators of the cell cycle. They largely regulate the growth fraction of a cell population. As discussed previously, these points are regulated by CDK which is regulated:

- Positively by PDGF, EGF and IGF-1
- Negatively by TGF-β

Neoplastic cells may:

- Upregulate their receptors
- Mutate intracellular pathways (eg retinoblastoma gene and *p53*) to evade the requirement for these signals

Neoplasms initially grow exponentially and then slow down as they increase in size. This is called **Gompertzian** growth (see Fig. 2.4a). Several mechanisms have been invoked to explain this change in growth rate with larger tumours:

- Decrease in the growth fraction
- Increase in cell loss (eg exfoliation, necrosis)
- Nutritional depletion of tumour cells resulting from outgrowth of available blood supply (under adverse conditions tumours may enter G0 until conditions improve)

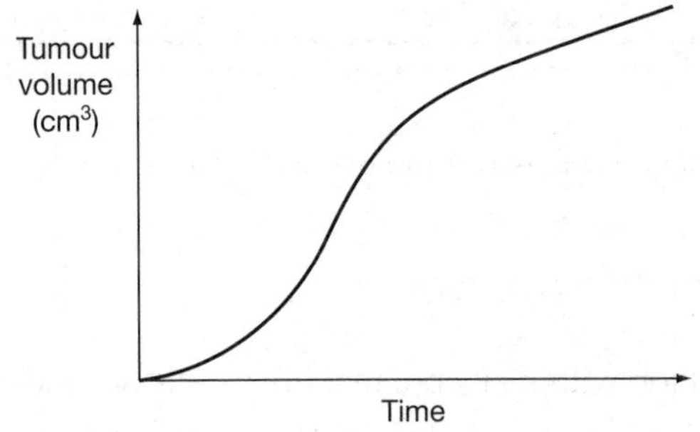

Figure 2.4a *Gompertzian growth curve. Initially growth of a small tumour is exponential but as the tumour enlarges this pattern of growth is unsustainable. Tumour-cell doubling time therefore reduces and overall growth slows*

Latent period: accumulation of cells is slow, therefore it can take several years for a single cell to proliferate into a clinically detectable mass.

Chemotherapy: chemotherapeutics are most effective on cycling cells; tumours with a high growth fraction are more susceptible to antinuclear agents. Debulking tumours or treating with radiation pushes more cells into the cell cycle and therefore increases the number of susceptible cells.

Tumour cell differentiation

Tumour cells may:

- Arise at any stage during the process of differentiation and their progeny can replicate whilst still retaining the characteristics of that stage of differentiation

- Tumour cells lose the inverse relationship between proliferation and differentiation
- Tumour cells may de-differentiate
- Tumour cells may change lineage
- Tumour cells may hypomethylate or hypermethylate genes that would control their replication (eg *p53* is often silenced in this way)

Tumour cell apoptosis

The role of apoptosis

Apoptosis is the process of programmed cell death. It is a controlled sequence of steps that is activated by a number of signals resulting in 'suicide' of the cell. Most importantly it acts to balance mitotic processes within the body. Apoptosis may be physiological or pathological.

Physiological apoptosis

- Development: to create organs of normal size and function (eg creation of web spaces between digits)
- Homeostasis: eg loss of the uterine lining during menstruation or at the tips of the intestinal villi
- Immune function: to recognise antigens that are foreign and not of 'self'

Pathological apoptosis

- Cell damage (eg peeling skin caused by sunburn)
- Cell infection

The process of apoptosis

Apoptosis occurs as a result of activation of one of two pathways.

Intrinsic pathway

- Activated from within the cell as a result of DNA damage or other stress
- Regulated by the **bcl-2** family of proteins (pro-apoptotic and anti-apoptotic members) that stabilise the mitochondrial membrane
- Mitochondria release cytochromes which bind to apoptotic factors and activate cell death via the caspases

Extrinsic pathway

- Activated by apoptotic messages via receptors
- Via **TNF** superfamily of proteins and CD95

Common final apoptotic pathway

Activation of a cascade of proteolytic **caspase enzymes** is the final common pathway to cellular destruction. This manifests as:

- Chromatin condensation
- DNA fragmentation
- Protein cleavage
- Reduction in cellular size and membrane blebbing
- Fragmentation of the cell into membrane-enclosed apoptotic bodies (without release of the cell contents into the surrounding environment)
- Phagocytes engulf and destroy the apoptotic bodies without causing an inflammatory reaction

Loss of the apoptotic pathway is responsible for increased levels of genetic instability and accumulation of genetic mutations. This leads to tumour progression by the expansion of clones with more aggressive phenotypes. It also confers resistance to chemotherapy, radiation, and immune-mediated cell destruction.

The *bcl-2* gene is particularly important in tumours. The products of this gene represent a superfamily which associate with each other by homo- and heterodimerisation. Some dimers are pro-apoptotic and others are anti-apoptotic. The ratio of anti-apoptotic to pro-apoptotic dimers is important for determining resistance of a cell to apoptosis. Mutations causing up-regulation of anti-apoptotic dimers (or loss of pro-apoptotic dimers) result in an overall resistance to apoptosis. Tumours may evade apoptosis by disruption of the control mechanisms for apoptosis, such as mutation of genes like *bcl-2* and *BAX*.

Tumour cell karyotype

The term karyotype refers to the chromosomal arrangement of the genetic material in the cell. Virtually all solid tumours, including the non-Hodgkin's lymphomas, have an abnormal karyotype or chromosomal abnormality. Some of these abnormalities are limited to a given tumour type almost like a 'genetic fingerprint'. A good example of this is the Philadelphia chromosome characteristic of chronic myelocytic leukaemia (CML).

Types of chromosome abnormality

- Gain/loss of whole chromosome (aneuploidy)
- Partial deletion
- Translation from one chromosome to another
- Inversion of a segment of chromosome

Re-arranging genetic material in this fashion has implications for the control of expression of the genes in the abnormal segment. It may place oncogenes in a highly transcriptionally active region of the genome or lead to deletion of tumour suppressor genes.

Tumour angiogenesis

Nutrients can only diffuse to tumour cells over a limited distance, therefore an adequate blood supply is critical for a tumour to grow more than 1–2 mm in diameter. The process by which a tumour recruits and sustains its own blood supply is called angiogenesis.

The majority of endothelial cells in the body are quiescent. Physiological angiogenesis in the adult occurs only as a response to trauma and tissue repair or at certain times (eg the menstrual cycle). Pathological angiogenesis occurs when there is persistent proliferation of endothelial cells in response to a stimulus (eg from a tumour).

The angiogenic switch

Tumours recruit endothelial cells from surrounding vessels and from progenitor cells in the circulation. These cells are stimulated to grow into the tumour from the outside. When this occurs this stage is called 'the angiogenic switch'. The genetic determinant of the angiogenic switch remains unknown. The angiogenic phenotype of a tumour depends on the net balance between pro-angiogenic and anti-angiogenic growth factors in the region of the tumour. These growth factors may be produced by the tumour itself or by stromal or immune cells in the tumour vicinity.

Promoters of angiogenesis

Angiogenic factors are secreted by tumour cells and tumour-associated macrophages. The most important naturally occurring angiogenesis promoters include:

- Fibroblast growth factors (FGFs)
- Vascular endothelial growth factor (VEGF)
- Angiopoietins (Ang-1 and Ang-2; the ratio between them is likely to be important)

Inhibitors of angiogenesis

Naturally occurring proteins:

- Angiostatin
- Endostatin
- Thrombostatin

For discussion of angiogenesis as a target for cancer therapy see section 4.5.

2.5 NEOPLASTIC PROGRESSION – INVASION AND METASTASIS

In a nutshell ...

Neoplastic progression is a term that refers to the generation of sub-clones within the tumour. These sub-clones occur by accumulation of further genetic mutations and have an increasingly aggressive phenotype, allowing invasion and metastasis to distant sites.

Neoplastic invasion

In a nutshell ...

The ability to invade and spread determines the difference between a benign and a malignant phenotype.

Invasion is due to:

Changes in adhesion molecules
- Cell-to-cell interactions
- Cell-to-matrix interactions

Proteolysis

Migration and chemotaxis

Changes in adhesion

Loss of cell-to-cell adhesion

E-cadherin is the major cell adhesion molecule in epithelia; these cell adhesion molecules are down-regulated in several carcinomas.

Loss of cell-to-matrix interactions

Integrins and cadherins bind epithelial cells to the basement membrane; loss of integrins is associated with increased invasive potential. In particular the integrin $\alpha v\beta 3$ mediates adhesion to laminin, fibronectin and fibrinogen. It is overexpressed on the basement membrane of new blood vessels and its activation results in increased cell motility and proteolysis.

Cell adhesion to basement membrane

In normal epithelial cells laminin receptors are expressed on one side of the cell and bind to laminin on the basement membrane; tumour cells have increased numbers of laminin receptors on all sides.

Proteolysis

Degradation of collagen by proteolytic enzymes is a vital step. Up-regulation of proteolytic enzymes groups; the matrix metalloproteinases (MMPs) and plasminogen activators (tPA) correlates with increased invasiveness.

Tumour cell migration

Tumour cells coordinate proteolysis with migration. Migration consists of intermittent and limited attachment and detachment. The direction of migration is stimulated by chemotaxis driven by:

- Host growth factors eg insulin-like growth factors (IGF), HGF, FGF, and TGF-β
- Tumour-secreted factors (called autocrine motility factors)
- Gradient of degraded extracellular matrix components

Neoplastic metastasis

In a nutshell ...

Natural history of a typical malignant tumour:

Neoplastic transformation of a cell
Clonal expansion
Local invasion
Distant spread

Tumour spread may be:

Direct extension (eg direct invasion of bladder from adenocarcinoma of the sigmoid colon)
Transcoelomic (eg ovary)
Lymphatic (eg axillary nodes from carcinoma of the breast)
Haematogenous (eg bone metastases from follicular carcinoma of the thyroid)
Spillage of tumour cells during surgery

Haematogenous metastasis comprises:

Entry to the circulation
Dissemination
Extravasation
Establishment of a distant site
Angiogenesis

Lymphatic metastasis

Basement membranes of the lymphatics do not contain collagen or laminin and so are easier for the tumour cell to invade. This is a common method of metastasis for carcinomas. Cells may become trapped in the filtering lymph nodes draining the site of the primary tumour where they are either destroyed or form deposits and start to grow.

Many primary tumours have well defined regional lymph nodes that are examined for signs of metastasis during resection of the primary. See section 5.2 for discussion of management of these nodes.

Haematogenous metastasis

Entry to the circulation
Tumour cells squeeze through gaps between endothelial cells to enter the circulation in a manner similar to that employed by cells of the immune system in inflammation (remind yourself from Chapter 2 *Infection and Inflammation*). Many of the same molecules have been implicated in this process (eg CD44).

Dissemination in the circulation
Malignant cells avoid detection by decreased expression of MHC-1. They also shed ICAM-I molecules that interact with cytotoxic T-cell receptors, stopping their destruction.

Extravasation
Cells attach to the vessel wall and migrate through it (eg increased expression of integrin VLA-4 in melanoma); reduced expression of the *nm23* gene is associated with increased metastases of breast cancer, but its mechanism of action is unknown.

Establishment of metastasis

This is poorly understood. Traditionally it has been described in the terms of the 'seed and soil hypothesis'. This may also go some way to explain common sites for development of metastasis from specific tumour types. Other common sites for metastasis reflect the vascular drainage of the primary tumour (eg cells shed from a colonic tumour travel via the portal circulation to the liver where they impact in the capillaries). Millions of cells may be shed into the circulation daily, but only a small fraction are successful at initiating colonies. Development of a distant metastasis also requires initiation of an angiogenic process at the chosen site.

Metastasis may be established as an early or late event in the development of the tumour (eg distant spread with no identifiable primary). This may reflect different molecular processes going on in sub-clones within the tumour.

Common patterns of metastasis

Site of metastasis	Possible primary source
Liver	GI Pancreas Lung Breast Genito-urinary Malignant melanoma
Skeletal	Lung Breast Prostate (osteosclerotic) Kidney Thyroid
Brain	Lung Malignant melanoma Breast
Adrenal	Lung Breast
Transcoelomic	Stomach Colon Ovary
Lung	Kidney Breast Colorectal Ovary

2.6 THE IMMUNE SYSTEM AND NEOPLASIA

In a nutshell ...

The immune system and neoplasia

- Malignant transformation is associated with the expression of tumour antigens
- These antigens may be recognised as foreign by the immune system, resulting in destruction of the tumour cell (theory of immune surveillance)
- Tumour cells may practise immune evasion

The theory of immune surveillance

The process of malignant transformation may be associated with the expression of molecules on the cell membrane that can be distinguished as foreign by the immune system. These are called **tumour antigens** and they include:

- Point mutations in normal genes
- Overexpression of self antigens (previously expressed at a low enough level not to induce tolerance)
- Viral antigens
- Products of silent genes not usually expressed as protein (eg *MAGE, BAGE* and *GAGE*)
- Products of fetal proteins (oncofetal antigens)

Tumour antigens may thus be recognised by either arm of the immune system; the cellular and humoral components and the abnormal cells are destroyed before tumours develop. The success of this strategy depends on the immunogenicity of the tumour cells.

This is the **immune surveillance theory**. In particular tumours are targeted by the complement system, IgG and components of the cellular system: cytotoxic T lymphocytes, NK cells and macrophages. Cytotoxic T cells recognise antigens displayed in complexes with MHC class I molecules. Macrophages and dendritic cells engulf tumour cells, presenting their antigens to T-cells in complex with MHC molecules. The T-helper cells respond by secreting cytokines and recruiting other immunological cells. Tumours producing IFN specifically stimulate NK cells which lyse their targets. IFN-α concentration also affects the way that antigens are processed within the cell and this alters their immunogenicity.

Evading the immune system

Tumours may evade the immune system by means of:

- Secretion of anti-inflammatory and immunosuppressive factors such as IL-4, IL-6, IL-10, PGE_2, TGF-β_1 and M-CSF
- Induction of apoptosis in immunological effector cells: tumour cells display Fas ligand which induces apoptosis in the T cell when it binds to its own surface Fas molecule (this exploits the body's system of inducing tolerance)
- Utilisation of immunological ignorance mechanisms
  - Displaying peptides that are not immunogenic
  - Down-regulating MHC class I molecules
  - Shedding large volumes of antigen into the circulation to swamp the T-cell receptors

Section 3
Clinical features of neoplasia

In a nutshell ...

Clinically important effects of a tumour include:

- **Local** clinical features of the tumour
- **Distant** clinical features of the tumour
- **Systemic** features of the tumour
  - Ectopic hormone secretion
  - Cachexia

3.1 DIAGNOSIS OF NEOPLASMS

In a nutshell ...

Diagnosis of a neoplasm be made on characteristic imaging but may be confirmed by cytology or histology.

For discussion of biopsy techniques and procedures see Chapter 1 *Basic Surgical Knowledge and Skills*.

Cytology of tumours

Cytology techniques

- Brushings (eg oesophagus, cervix)
- FNAC
- Fluids:
  - Physiological (eg cells in urine or sputum)
  - Pathological (eg cells in ascites or pleural effusion)

Cytological features of malignancy

- Loss of cellular cohesiveness: nuclei oriented in different directions and are irregularly spaced. Cells become detached from one another
- Pleomorphism: variation in size, shape and number of nucleoli
- Moulding of nuclei: nuclei appear pushed into one another or stacked together like a vertebral column
- Nuclear to cytoplasmic ratio increased
- Chromatin shows irregular clumping and hyperchromasia
- Nuclear membrane is irregular with angular bites
- Abnormal mitoses may be present

Cytology versus histology in the diagnosis of malignancy

- Fine nuclear detail may be lost in formalin fixed histology
- Cohesiveness of cells is more easily evaluated on cytologic material
- Histologic sections provide added information on tissue architecture and relationship of cancer cells to normal structures (depth of invasion, presence of vascular invasion, etc)

Histology of tumours

The architectural features of malignancy are:

- **Invasion of the underlying or surrounding tissue:** extension of tumour beyond the basement membrane for carcinomas and an irregular front penetrating the surrounding tissue for mesenchymal tumours
- **Stromal changes:** the change that occurs in the stroma as tumour invades is called desmoplasia. It is a response to invasion of tissue by malignant tumour cells
- **Loss of normal structure:** as tumours become less and less differentiated, they resemble the tissue of origin less and less
- **New structures:** some tumours will create structures such as glandular structures (colon, endometrium cancers) or papillary structures (thyroid, bladder cancers)
- **Necrosis:** may indicate areas of tumour that have insufficient blood supply
- **Angiogenesis** and **neovasculature**
- **Inflammation:** tumours often cause inflammation and the inflammatory infiltrate is visible
- **Immunostaining:** an antibody is raised against a protein of particular prognostic significance the distribution and concentration of which can then be identified. It can be used for:
  - Identifying poorly differentiated tumours
  - Sub-typing tumours
  - Identifying an unknown primary from a metastatic deposit
  - Assessing tumour microvessel density and angiogenesis

3.2 LOCAL FEATURES OF NEOPLASMS

In a nutshell ...

Local features of neoplasms include:
- Mass
- Pain
- Changes in organ function
- Obstruction in a hollow viscus
- Bleeding
- Infarction

Mass

- May be palpable
- May be a primary tumour or secondary lymphadenopathy
- May be painful or, more commonly, painless (eg breast lump, testicular lump)
- May cause a mass effect:
  - Compression of surrounding structures
  - Raised ICP in intracranial lesions

Pain

This may be a feature of:

- Local compression
- Capsular stretch (eg hepatic, renal)
- Infiltration of regional nerves by the tumour
- Obstruction of a hollow lumen
- Metastasis (eg bone pain)

For discussion of management of malignant pain see section 5.

Changes in organ function

- eg liver metastasis presenting with jaundice

Obstruction in a hollow viscus

- Arising intraluminally (eg embolism of tumour invading large vessel)
- Arising from the vessel wall (eg annular circumferential rectal tumour)
- Arising extraluminally (eg peritoneal deposits obstructing ureters)

Bleeding

- May be effect of local tumour ulceration (eg rectal carcinoma)
- May be result of erosion into large vessel (eg gastric cancer)
- Acute bleed into tumour mass may provoke pain (eg hepatoma)

Infarction

- Torsion and infarction of ovarian masses

3.3 GENERAL CLINICAL FEATURES OF NEOPLASMS

In a nutshell ...

General features of neoplasms include:
Anaemia
Metabolic effects
Exudates
Paraneoplastic syndromes
Cancer cachexia
Ectopic hormone secretion

Distant clinical features of neoplasia

Anaemia

- Occult or overt bleeding
- Poor nutritional state
- Low erythropoietin production

Metabolic effects

- Weight loss
- Anorexia
- Pyrexia
- Altered sensation eg taste

Specific effects of metastasis

- Exudates eg ascites, pleural effusion
- Bone mets and pathological fractures

Paraneoplastic syndromes

Paraneoplastic syndromes refer to non-metastatic systemic symptom complexes that accompany malignant disease. Symptoms may affect any system of the body and occur remotely from the site of the primary tumour of secondary deposits. They may be due to the release of cytokines or autoimmunity generated by cross-reactivity against antibodies produced against the tumour.

Types of paraneoplastic syndrome

Approximately 10% of patients with advanced malignancies have paraneoplastic syndromes. These syndromes are divided into the following categories: miscellaneous (non-specific), rheumatological, renal, gastrointestinal, haematological, cutaneous, endocrine, and neuromuscular.

Paraneoplastic syndromes

Rheumatological

Arthropathies
Scleroderma
SLE
Amyloidosis

Renal

Tumours that can produce ACTH, antidiuretic hormone (ADH), and gut hormones may cause hypokalaemia, hyponatraemia or hypernatraemia, hyperphosphoraemia, and alkalosis/acidosis
Nephrotic syndrome

Gastrointestinal

Malabsorption (especially with tumours that produce prostaglandins eg medullary thyroid)
Diarrhoea

Haematological

Anaemia
Thrombocytosis
Disseminated intravascular coagulation (DIC)
Migrating vascular thrombosis (Trousseau syndrome)

Cutaneous
- Itching
- Herpes zoster
- Alopecia
- Hypertrichosis
- Acanthosis nigricans (blackish pigmentation of the skin occurring in patients with metastatic melanomas or pancreatic tumours)

Endocrine
- Cushing syndrome (excessive ACTH or ACTH-like peptides)
- Hypercalcaemia (osteolysis or calcaemic humoral substances)

Neuromuscular
- Neuromyopathic syndromes such as myasthenia gravis

Management of paraneoplastic syndromes

These may respond to resection of the primary tumour. In some cases, where there are clearly identifiable autoantibodies, immunosuppression is considered.

Cancer cachexia

Cachexia is a wasting syndrome with progressive loss of body fat and severe weakness. Exact cause is unclear but it may be related to the secretion of cytokines by the tumour or as a host response to the tumour. It does not occur in proportion to tumour size (eg can occur dramatically in small oesophageal tumours).

Ectopic hormone secretion and neoplasia

Many tumours that arise from endocrine tissue continue to secrete functional hormones. Some tumours that have no basis in endocrine tissue also secrete peptide molecules that are very similar in structure to active hormones or hormone fragments and these molecules act as analogues.

Most commonly these peptides mimic the CRF–ACTH axis and result in Cushing syndrome. Sometimes ADH may be released and the syndrome of inappropriate ADH is produced.

3.4 TUMOUR TYPING, GRADING AND STAGING

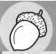

In a nutshell ...

Typing, grading and staging are important for:

Planning of treatment
Type and degree of surgical excision
Consideration of pre-operative radiotherapy or chemotherapy to downsize tumours

To provide accurate prognostic information
For the patient
For the physician

To provide accurate comparison between outcome in different patient groups
Comparisons between treatments
Comparisons between centres

Comparison of features in benign vs malignant tumours

Benign neoplasms

- Expansile, usually slow growing
- Don't metastasise
- Low mitotic rate, little pleomorphism
- Normal chromosome numbers
- Necrosis and haemorrhage unusual
- More likely to be polypoid or papillary (NB not all)

Malignant neoplasms

- Infiltrative, irregular or fast growth rate
- May metastasise
- Pleomorphic, frequent mitotic figures
- Abnormal chromosome numbers
- Necrosis and haemorrhage may occur
- May be fungating or ulcerated

Tumour typing

The first piece of relevant information is the type of tumour. Tumours may be identified by the similarity of their cells to the tissue of origin, if they remain well differentiated. With a poorly differentiated metastatic deposit it may be impossible to identify its source.

Neoplasms are named according to whether they arise from **epithelium** or **stroma**.

Epithelial neoplasms

- **Adenoma:** benign epithelial neoplasm forming a glandular pattern or arising from a gland but not necessarily forming a glandular pattern
- **Papilloma:** benign epithelial neoplasm protruding from a surface which produces finger-like fronds made up of connective tissue processes covered by epithelial cells
- **Cystadenoma:** benign epithelial neoplasm arising from duct or gland epithelium with secretion and distension of the lumen due to lack of drainage
- **Carcinoma:** a malignant epithelial neoplasm

Mesenchymal neoplasms

These are named according to cell type:

- **-oma:** if benign (eg lipoma)
- **-sarcoma:** if malignant (eg osteosarcoma)

Naming of neoplasms

Cells of origin	Benign	Malignant
Epithelium		
Squamous	Squamous cell papilloma	Squamous cell carcinoma
Transitional	Transitional cell papilloma	Transitional cell carcinoma
Columnar	Adenoma or papilloma	Adenocarcinoma
Cystadenocarcinoma or cystadenoma		
Stromal		
Blood vessel	Haemangioma	Haemangiosarcoma
Lymph vessel	Lymphangioma	Lymphangiosarcoma
Fibrous tissue	Fibroma	Fibrosarcoma
Smooth muscle	Leiomyoma	Leiomyosarcoma
Striated muscle	Rhabdomyoma	Rhabdomyosarcoma
Cartilage	Chondroma	Chondrosarcoma
Bone	Osteoma	Osteosarcoma

Cells of origin	Benign	Malignant
Complex cell origin		
Lymphoid		Lymphoma
Haemopoietic cells		Leukaemia
Plasma cells		Multiple myeloma
Embryonic tissue		Blastoma (eg nephroblastoma, hepatoblastoma, retinoblastoma)
Specialised		
Breast	Fibroadenoma	Ductal or lobular carcinoma
Melanocytes	Naevus	Malignant melanoma
Mesothelium	Benign mesothelioma	Malignant mesothelioma
Salivary gland	Pleomorphic adenoma	Carcinoma arising in a pleomorphic adenoma

NB These are just a few examples.

Tumour grading

This is an assessment of the degree of **differentiation** of a tumour and corresponds to the **aggressive behaviour** of the tumour. Tumours are graded as:

- Well differentiated
- Moderately differentiated
- Poorly/undifferentiated/anaplastic

Many different grading systems exist for different tumours that take into consideration growth patterns as well as differentiation status eg Gleason grade for prostate cancer.

Differentiation refers to the degree to which neoplastic cells resemble their tissue of origin. Features of poor differentiation are:

- Increased nuclear pleomorphism
- Atypical mitoses
- Hyperchromatic nuclei
- Increased nuclear to cytoplasmic size ratio
- Giant cells may be present

Tumour grading is important for prediction of tumour behaviour and prognosis. In general, the less differentiated the tumour, the more aggressive its biological behaviour.

Tumour staging

This refers to the size and spread of the neoplasm as assessed by clinician, pathologist or radiologist. Used for decisions on management and prognosis.

Examples:

- Dukes' classification for colorectal carcinoma
- Clarke's classification for malignant melanoma
- TNM (tumour, node, metastasis) system

Staging often requires extensive investigations of the sites most likely to be involved in disease and is aimed at assessing degree of tumour spread to regional nodes and distant sites:

- Blood tests (eg LFTs, tumour markers)
- Cytology or biopsy for histology
- Chest X-ray or CT
- Abdominal USS or CT
- MRI
- Isotope bone scanning
- Positron emission topography (PET)
- Diagnostic or staging laparoscopy
- Full staging may not be possible until after surgery to resect the tumour when regional lymph nodes can be inspected histologically for tumour deposits.
- Failure to identify distant metastasis at the time of staging does not necessarily mean that the patient is free from all tumour cells after resection of the primary. Tumour cells continue to be present in the circulation until the primary is removed and there may be tiny, as yet undetectable, metastatic deposits in other organs or lymph nodes.

TNM staging system

The TNM classification was first developed by the American Joint Committee on Cancer Staging and End Result Reporting and has now been modified for systems for most solid tumours eg breast, colon, thyroid.

The TNM staging system

T = primary tumour

T_0 No primary tumour
T_{is} In situ primary tumour
T_x Unknown primary
T_{1-4} Sizes of primary tumour

N = nodal metastasis

N_0 No nodes
N_1 Few node(s)
N_{2-3} Relates to number, fixity, or distant lymph node group involvement

M = distant metastasis

M_0 No metastasis
M_1 Distant metastasis present

3.5 TUMOUR MARKERS

In a nutshell ...

Tumour markers are substances in the blood whose presence may be useful in monitoring of specific cancers. Markers include:

Epithelial proteins eg prostate specific antigen (PSA)
Hormones eg β-human chorionic gonadotrophin (β-HCG)
Oncofetal antigens eg carcinoembryonic antigen (CEA)

Tumour markers are useful in diagnosis, staging, treatment and detection of recurrence.

PSA (prostate specific antigen)

- A prostatic epithelial protein
- Elevated if > 4 ng/dL (in general)
- Used in conjunction with digital rectal examination, transrectal sonography and needle biopsy for 'screening', diagnosis and monitoring of treatment of prostatic cancer
- It is also elevated in benign prostatic hyperplasia, prostatitis, prostatic infarction, urinary retention, instrumentation and even ejaculation
- Thought *not* to rise significantly following rectal examination
- PSA velocity measures rate of change of PSA with time (> 0.75 ng/dL/year suggests malignancy)
- PSA density compares PSA value with volume of prostate (> 0.15 suggests malignancy)
- Age-related PSA (older patients have a higher 'normal' cut-off)
- Free-total PSA ratio (< 25% suggests malignancy)

CEA (carcinoembryonic antigen)

- An oncofetal antigen, normally expressed in embryonic gut, liver, pancreas
- Elevated in colorectal carcinoma in 60–90% of cases
- May also be elevated in ovarian and breast carcinoma
- Also occasionally elevated in cirrhosis, alcoholic hepatitis, inflammatory bowel disease, pancreatitis
- Not specific or sensitive enough to be used as a screening tool
- Used to monitor efficacy of therapy and detection of recurrence

Alpha-fetoprotein (α-FP)

- An embryonic antigen
- Elevated in carcinoma of liver (also in cirrhosis, chronic hepatitis, normal pregnancy, fetal neural tube defects)
- Also elevated in non-seminomatous germ cell tumours of the testes (NSGCT)

Human chorionic gonadotrophin (β-hCG)

- A hormone
- Elevated in pregnancy
- Elevated in choriocarcinoma, non-small cell germ cell tumour (NSGCT) and in 7% of seminomas where syncytiotrophoblastic elements are present

CA antigens

- CA-125: for non-mucinous ovarian cancers. A high concentration is more likely to be associated with malignancy. Can be used to monitor therapy. Can be raised in other conditions (eg pancreatitis, endometriosis, breast and pancreatic carcinomas)
- CA-15–3: a glycoprotein, occasionally elevated in breast carcinoma
- CA-19–9: a glycoprotein sometimes elevated in pancreatic and advanced colorectal carcinoma

Thyroglobulin

- Elevated in some thyroid carcinomas

Calcitonin

- Elevated in medullary thyroid carcinoma

ACTH/ADH

- Elevated in some small cell lung carcinomas

Section 4
Cancer treatments

In a nutshell ...

The management of cancer patients is usually decided in the context of a multidisciplinary team. Many therapies are combined on the basis of tumour type, grade and stage.

Therapies include:
- Surgery
- Radiotherapy
- Chemotherapy
- Hormonal therapy
- Additional and experimental therapies
- Immunomodulation
- Monoclonal antibodies
- Cryotherapy and radioablation
- Gene therapy
- Anti-angiogenic treatment

4.1 SURGERY

The role of surgery in neoplasia

In a nutshell ...

Surgery is used in diagnosis, staging, treatment and palliation
Surgical design is driven by local invasion and tumour spread (resection en bloc)

Surgery has a diagnostic, staging and therapeutic role in neoplasia. It may be curative or palliative. It forms a primary treatment for many solid tumours.

Surgical design is influenced by the degree of invasion and spread of the tumour. The two most important principles of curative oncological surgery are resection en bloc (ie without surgical disruption of the plane between the tumour and potentially locally infiltrated tissue and without disruption of the lymphatics draining the region of the tumour) and resection margins that are free from tumour cells.

The surgical management of primary tumours, regional lymph nodes and distant metastases is discussed in section 5. Surgical resection of individual tumours is discussed in the relevant chapters.

4.2 RADIOTHERAPY

In a nutshell ...

Radiotherapy

- Radiation may be particulate or electromagnetic
- Radiotherapy kills tumour cells by generating high energy molecular movement
- Tumour susceptibility is related to tumour oxygenation and radiosensitivity of the individual cells
- Radiotherapy may be used as a primary, neoadjuvant, adjuvant or palliative therapy
- It causes damage to normal as well as tumour cells resulting in local and systemic complications

This is the therapeutic use of ionising radiation for the treatment of malignant conditions.

Types of radiation

Particulate: does not penetrate the tissue deeply and is used predominantly to treat cutaneous and subcutaneous conditions.

- Electrons
- Protons
- Neutrons
- α particles
- pi mesons

Electromagnetic: penetrates tissue deeply and is therefore used to treat deep tumour tissue.

- X-rays
- Gamma rays

Mechanism of action

Radiation kills cells by causing high-energy interactions between molecules.

- DNA damage is via release of kinetic energy from free radicals (an oxygen-dependent process)
- Causes deletions and strand breaks within the DNA
- May trigger apoptosis in some cells due to severe DNA damage
- Cells are most sensitive during S phase

Killing cells leads to stimulation of other cells to divide, ie to enter the S phase:

- **Repair:** normal cells take 4 hours to recover (6+ hours for CNS), malignant cells take longer
- **Re-population:** more cells are stimulated to divide due to death of others, after about 3–4 weeks of standard fractionated treatment
- **Re-distribution:** pushes cells into the S phase – more radiosensitive
- **Re-oxygenation:** oxygen is a radiation sensitizer; cell death facilitates re-oxygenation – increases cytotoxicity

The degree of tumour destruction by radiotherapy is related to:

- **Radiosensitivity of tumour**
  - Sensitive: seminoma, Hodgkin's lymphoma,
  - Resistant: tendency to repair DNA damage (eg melanoma)
  - Similar tumour types tend to have similar radiosensitivity (eg all carcinomas)
  - Slow-growing tumours may not respond or respond slowly to radiotherapy
- **Tolerance of normal tissue:** surrounding tissue may be very sensitive to treatment (eg nervous tissue, small bowel), which limits the amount of radiotherapy that can be delivered
- **Tumour size:** larger tumours have areas of low oxygen tension and necrosis and are more resistant. They require more cycles and larger treatment volumes which exposes normal tissue to higher doses of radiation

Administration of radiotherapy

- **Locally** ie the source can be implanted into tissue to be treated (eg brachiotherapy for prostate cancer) or into a cavity eg uterus
- **Systematically** (eg iodine-131 for thyroid cancer)
- **External beam** radiation via linear accelerator

Fractionation describes the number of individual treatments and their time course. The **therapeutic ratio** is the relationship between the amount of radiation tolerated by the normal tissues and that delivered to the tumour.

For radical treatments, aim for maximum possible dose in the smallest volume which will encompass all of the tumour and likely occult spread. This is called the **treatment volume** and it comprises:

- Macroscopic tumour
- Biological margin (0.5–1 cm)
- Technical margin (allows for minute variations in positioning and set up)

The site is accurately localised by imaging and permanent skin markings applied to ensure reproducibility at subsequent sessions.

Complex multifield arrangements divide the tumour into cubes. The radiation is targeted to divide the dose between surrounding normal tissues, because different tissues can tolerate different amounts of radiation (eg liver is more resilient than kidney). It is usually delivered intermittently, allowing normal tissues to recover. This takes at least 4 hours, while malignant tissues take longer.

Improved imaging techniques now allow precise targeting of a tumour shape, which is important if it is located near sensitive structures. Techniques are being refined so that there is an increase in the number of sessions that can be given within a short period of treatment time; this is known as **accelerated radiotherapy** (eg multiple sessions per day for 2 weeks).

Stereotactic radiotherapy is commonly used for brain tumours. The patient's head is placed in a frame and an accurate 3-D image of the tumour is obtained using high-resolution MRI. The beam of radiation is focused on the tumour but rotation of delivery means that the surrounding normal tissues receive minimal doses.

Uses of radiotherapy

Primary treatment

- Sensitive tumours
- Better cosmetic/functional result
- Inoperable or high mortality/morbidity with surgery
- Patient not fit for surgery

Adjuvant radiotherapy

- Post-operative
- Can be given at site of disease (control of margins – mark surgical site with clips for easy identification) or at site of potential metastatic spread

Neoadjuvant radiotherapy

- Pre-operatively, can downstage tumours (eg rectal tumour)
- Can reduce risk of seeding at operation
- Does not cause additional surgical morbidity if performed within 4 weeks of surgery

Palliation

- Palliative radiotherapy aims for symptom relief, from either primary or metastatic disease (eg relief of bone pain, bleeding, dyspnoea, cord compression, superior vena caval obstruction)
- It is given as short courses of treatment, with simple set-ups, to minimise toxicity
- Single fractions are often used to control bone pain

Complications of radiotherapy

Local complications

- Itching and dry skin
- Ulceration
- Bleeding
- Radiation enteritis
- Fibrosis and stricture formation
- Delayed wound healing
- Lymphoedema
- Alopecia
- Osteoradionecrosis

Systemic complications

- Lethargy
- Loss of appetite
- Premature menopause
- Oligospermia
- Acute leukaemia
- Myelosuppression
- Hypothyroidism/renal failure – after many years' treatment

4.3 CHEMOTHERAPY

In a nutshell ...

Chemotherapeutics are drugs that are used to treat cancer by affecting cell proliferation.

They may be used as primary, neoadjuvant or adjuvant therapies.

Chemotherapeutic drugs include:
- Alkylating agents
- Antimetabolites
- Antibiotics
- Vinca alkyloids
- Taxanes
- Topoisomerase inhibitors

Side effects may be acute (related to dose) or chronic (related to duration of treatment).

Tumours may eventually become resistant to individual chemotherapeutics.

Chemotherapeutics are drugs that are used to treat cancer that inhibit the mechanisms of cell proliferation. They are therefore toxic to normally proliferating cells (ie bone marrow, GI epithelium, hair follicles). They can be:

- **Cycle-specific:** effective throughout the cell cycle
- **Phase-specific:** effective during part of the cell cycle

Tumour susceptibility depends on the concentration of drug delivered, on cell sensitivity, and cell cycling of tumour. Drugs are less effective in large solid tumours because of:

- Fall in the growth fraction
- Poor drug penetrance into the centre
- Intrinsic drug resistance of sub-clones

Indications for chemotherapy

Indications for chemotherapy

- **Primary treatment (eg lymphoma)**
- **Neo-adjunctive** treatment to decrease tumour bulk before surgery
- **Adjunctive** treatment for prevention of recurrence
- Advanced disease and **palliation**
- **Maintenance** treatment (eg leukaemia)

Important treatment in:

- Haematological malignancy
- Germ cell tumours
- Ovarian cancer
- Small cell lung cancer
- Breast cancer (locally advanced)

Important neo-adjunct in:

- Colorectal liver metastasis

Important adjunct in:

- Colorectal cancer primaries (Dukes' C stage)
- Breast cancer

Methods of delivering chemotherapy

Methods of delivery for chemotherapeutic agents

Intravenous
Oral
Intra-arterial (eg HCC via the hepatic artery)
Intramuscular
Intrathecal
Intracavitary (eg intravesicular for TCC bladder)
Intralesional

Doses are based on body surface area and are affected by hepatic metabolism and renal excretion.

Efficacy of treatment for different tumours may be improved by:

- Pulsed treatment
- Combinations of drugs with different modes of action (synergy, reduces drug resistance)
- Alternating cycles
- High dose treatment with subsequent replacement of normal tissues (eg bone marrow transplant)
- Scheduling with continuous low dose

Chemotherapeutic agents

Classical alkylating agents

Act by forming covalent bonds with nucleic acids, proteins, nucleotides and amino acids, and so inactivate the enzymes involved in DNA production and protein synthesis.

Side effects of classical alkylating agents

Indications	Side effects
Mustargen Hodgkin's disease Non-Hodgkin's lymphoma Chronic myelocytic leukaemia (CML) Chronic lymphatic leukaemia (CLL)	Very toxic so rarely used Vomiting Bone-marrow depression
Cyclophosphamide Many cancers including: Lymphoma Breast Lung Ovary	Bone-marrow depression Nausea and vomiting (mild unless high dose) Haemorrhagic cystitis (high doses) Pulmonary interstitial fibrosis
Chlorambucil CLL Non-Hodgkin's lymphoma (low grade) Ovary	Bone-marrow suppression Nausea, vomiting, diarrhoea Jaundice, pulmonary fibrosis
Melphalan Multiple myeloma	Bone-marrow depression Nausea and vomiting Diarrhoea Rash Pulmonary fibrosis

Non-classical alkylating agents

Act by causing cross-linkage of DNA strands.

Side effects of non-classical alkylating agents

Indications	Side effects
Cisplatin (C-DDP) (toxic to cycling and resting cells)	
Testis cancer	Renal failure
Ovary cancer	Electrolyte disturbance (hypomagnesia)
Head and neck cancer	Peripheral neuropathy
Bladder cancer	Ototoxicity
Lung cancer	Bone marrow depression
Oesophageal cancer	
Stomach cancer	
Carboplatin	
Ovary cancer Lung cancer Seminoma	Less toxic analogue, but more bone marrow suppression

Anti-metabolites

Act by interfering with purine or pyrimidine synthesis and hence interfere with DNA synthesis.

Side effects of anti-metabolites

Indications	Side effects
Methotrexate (S-phase specific)	
Acute lymphocytic leukaemia (ALL)	Bone marrow depression
Breast cancer	GI symptoms
Lung	Stomatitis
	Renal failure
	Hepatic failure
5-Fluorouracil (5-FU) (toxic to resting and cycling cells)	
Colon	Bone marrow depression
Breast	GI symptoms
Stomach	Alopecia
Oesophagus	Rash
Pancreas	Palmar-plantar syndrome and cardiotoxicity with high-dose infusional treatments

Indications	Side effects
Gemcitabine	
Pancreas Lung	Nausea Flu-like symptoms Oedema

Antibiotics

Act by intercalating between base pairs and prevent RNA production. There are several groups with differing actions.

Anthracycline antibiotics

Complex actions (not fully understood):

- Intercalate into DNA strands
- Bind membranes
- Produce free radicals
- Chelate metals – producing cytotoxic compounds
- Alkylation

Side effects of anthracycline antibiotics

Indications	Side effects
Doxorubicin	
Acute leukaemia Lymphoma Breast cancer Small cell lung cancer Sarcoma Bladder cancer Ovary cancer Wilms' tumour Neuroblastoma	Bone marrow depression Nausea and vomiting Alopecia Cardiac-dose-dependent congestive cardiac failure
Epirubicin	
Breast	Doxorubicin analogue with less cardiac toxicity

Non-anthracycline antibiotics

Act by intercalation, free radical production, and/or alkylation.

Side effects of non-anthracycline antibiotics

Indications	Side effects
Mitozantrone	
Breast cancer	Bone marrow depression Congestive cardiac failure Alopecia Nausea and vomiting
Bleomycin	
Lymphoma Testicular cancer Head and neck cancer	Bone marrow sparing Pneumonitis and pulmonary fibrosis Rash Fever
Mitomycin C	
Breast cancer Bladder cancer (intravesical) Pancreatic cancer Gastric cancer	Bone marrow depression Renal failure (haemolytic-uraemic syndrome with tamoxifen) Stomatitis, rash, alopecia Nausea and vomiting

Vinca alkaloids

Act by inhibiting mitosis, by preventing spindle formation. M-phase specific.

NB: intrathecal administration of vinca alkaloids is fatal!

Side effects of Vinca alkaloids

Indications	Side effects
Vincristine	
Acute leukaemia Lymphoma Neuroblastoma Wilms' tumour Rhabdomyosarcoma	Highly vesicant Neuropathy Bronchospasm

Indications	Side effects
Vinblastine	
Testis	Highly vesicant
Hodgkin's lymphoma	Bone marrow depression
Non-Hodgkin's lymphoma	Bronchospasm
Choriocarcinoma	Abdominal pain and ileus (mimics acute abdomen)
Peripheral neuropathy	
Vinorelbine	
Breast	Highly vesicant
Lung	Bone marrow depression
Abdominal pain and constipation	
Local phlebitis	

Taxanes

Act by inhibiting mitosis through stabilisation of microtubules.

Side effects of taxanes

Indications	Side effects
Docetaxel	
Breast cancer	Allergic reaction
Ovarian cancer	Severe neutropenia
	Alopecia
	Peripheral oedema
	Myalgia
	Peripheral neuropathy
Paclitaxel	
Ovary cancer	Anaphylaxis
Breast cancer	Severe neutropenia
Lung cancer	Sudden total alopecia
	Myalgia
	Peripheral neuropathy

Topoisomerase inhibitors

Inhibit topoisomerase I, an enzyme involved in DNA replication.

Side effects of topoisomerase inhibitors

Indications	Side effects
Irinotecan	
Colorectal cancer	Cholinergic syndrome Profuse diarrhoea (may be life threatening)

Side effects of chemotherapy

Acute complications

- Nausea and vomiting
- Diarrhoea or constipation
- Mucositis
- Alopecia
- BM suppression
- Cystitis
- Phlebitis
- Renal and cardiac toxicity

Chronic complications

- Carcinogenesis (especially alkylating agents which cause leukaemias. Risk proportional to dose)
- Pulmonary fibrosis
- Infertility

Drug resistance in tumours

- Reduced drug uptake
- Increased concentrations of target enzymes to minimise the effects of enzyme inhibition
- DNA repair mechanisms (eg melanoma cells)
- Mutations coding for cell pumps which extrude the drug
- Salvage pathways
- Drug inactivation

4.4 HORMONAL THERAPY

Up to 15% of tumours may have hormone responsive elements.

Prostate tumours

- Subcapsular orchidectomy (bilateral)
- Antiandrogens
- LHRH analogues
- Stilboestrol (oestrogen)

Breast tumours

- **Tamoxifen:** pre- and post-menopausal women if ER- and/or PR-positive
- **Aromatase inhibitors:** prevent oestrogen production from peripheral fat – no effect on ovarian oestrogens, so post-menopausal only. Recent evidence of superior survival in advanced disease compared with tamoxifen for 3rd-generation aromatase inhibitors (eg anastrazole)
- **Progestogens:** now tend to be used 3rd line, as aromatase inhibitors are superior
- **LHRH analogues:** monthly goserelin in pre-menopausal women (3-monthly preparation does not reliably suppress menstruation in all)

Thyroid tumours

- Thyroxine to suppress TSH secretion
- Liothyronine used

4.5 ADDITIONAL AND EXPERIMENTAL THERAPIES

In a nutshell ...

Additional potential therapies include:

Immunomodulation: used in renal cell carcinoma, bladder carcinoma
Monoclonal antibodies
Cryotherapy and radiofrequency ablation

Experimental therapies include:

Gene therapy
Antiangiogenic therapy

Immunomodulation

Renal cancer

- Radioresistant
- Chemoresistant
- Some success with IL-2 and α-interferon

Bladder cancer

- BCG vaccine used intravesically
- Used in treatment of CIS and high-grade (non-invasive) tumours
- May be used long term as 'maintenance therapy'

Monoclonal antibodies

The first two monoclonal antibodies in clinical use are rituximab and trastuzumab.

- **Rituximab** (MabThera™) is a monoclonal antibody that causes lysis of B lymphocytes and is licensed for treatment of relapsed low-grade lymphoma. It is being used earlier in the course of disease in clinical trials
- **Trastuzumab** (Herceptin™) can used in metastatic breast cancer, if the tumour over-expresses human epidermal growth factor receptor-2 (HER-2). 16–18% of patients are likely to be strongly HER-2-positive. Infusion-related side effects are common with both (chills, fever, hypersensitivity reactions)

Both can exacerbate chemotherapy-related cardiotoxicity.

- **Bevacizumab** (Avastin™) binds to VEGF and works as an anti-angiogenic agent. It is used in advanced colorectal cancers

Cryotherapy and radiofrequency ablation

Probe inserted into tumour either percutaneously under radiological control or intra-operatively.

- Freezing temperature causes 'ice ball'
- Mainly used in palliation
- Increasing use in primary treatment for liver tumours

Experimental therapies

Gene therapy

There are on-going trials of gene therapy with glioblastoma.

Anti-angiogenic agents

Most of the endothelial cells in an adult are quiescent during health. Therapies targeting the process of angiogenesis are therefore directed specifically at tumour growth.

Current options include:

1. Targeting endogenous pro-angiogenic factors, such as:
    - Anti-VEGF antibodies (trials in colorectal cancer are on-going in the US)
    - Anti-angiogenic pharmacology (eg COX-2 inhibitors)
2. Administering endogenous anti-angiogenic compounds or molecules eg angiostatin, endostatin

Section 5

Cancer Management

In a nutshell ...

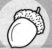

Active treatment modalities for neoplasia include:

Surgery
Radiotherapy
Chemotherapy
Hormonal manipulation
Monoclonal antibodies
Novel approaches

Palliative care, including close attention to adequate pain control, is also a fundamental pillar of management.

5.1 MANAGEMENT OF THE PRIMARY TUMOUR

In a nutshell ...

The primary tumour may be treated by a combination of:

Curative surgery
Functional reconstruction
Surgical palliation or debulking
Radiotherapy
Chemotherapy
Observation and medical palliation (eg presentation at late stage)

Curative surgery

Curative surgery involves removal of the entire tumour with an intact perimeter of normal tissue leaving resection margins free of tumour cells.

It may demand an aggressive approach that has higher risks of post-operative complications. Actual or likely directions of tumour spread must be known in order to clear the surgical field (eg mesorectal excision for rectal cancer). If the regional lymph nodes are involved or suspected and lymph node clearance is planned then this should be performed en bloc (ie without disrupting lymphatic connections between tumour and nodes or between tumour and locally infiltrated tissue).

Functional reconstruction

May be performed at the same time as primary surgery or later. Includes:

- **Reconstruction** or re-modelling (eg closure of soft tissue defects)
- **Restitution** or restoration (eg continuity of the bowel)
- **Replacement** or substitution or (eg free flaps)

Additional management options

- **Neo-adjunctive:** used pre-operatively to downstage or debulk a tumour
- **Adjunctive:** used post-operatively to reduce risks of recurrence or treat micrometastases
- **Palliative:** relieves symptoms whilst being unable to remove entire tumour burden and so is not curative.

5.2 MANAGEMENT OF THE REGIONAL LYMPH NODES

In a nutshell ...

Treatment of the regional lymph nodes may take many forms:
Surgical lymph node sampling to predict involvement (sentinel node biopsy)
Surgical lymph node clearance
Local radiotherapy (primary or adjuvant)

The role of the regional lymph nodes in cancer is still up for discussion. Many believe that these nodes may not act as filters for malignant cells and that fairly large tumour emboli may skip the regional nodes altogether.

These nodes may have an important role in the early immune response to tumours allowing appropriate antigen recognition and prevention of widespread tumour cell dissemination. For many tumours, elective lymph node resection has not shown any survival benefit.

Lymph node sampling

Surgical lymph node sampling as a means of detecting metastatic disease is increasing.

Sentinel node biopsy

Essentially there is a single node through which lymphatic drainage from the primary tumour passes to reach the chain of regional lymph nodes. The node that predominantly drains the site of the primary tumour is identified by the injection of a tracer substance into the area of the primary tumour. This may be a visible blue dye or radioactive substance (eg human albumin nanocolloid).

Sentinel nodes can then be identified either visually or by hand-held gamma probe at open surgery. There is more than one sentinel node in up to 50% of patients. These nodes are excised and sent for histopathology to look for metastatic deposits. The residual nodes are also scanned for evidence of radioactivity (should have a ratio of at least 3 : 1 radioactivity for sentinel node vs other nodes in vivo and 10 : 1 ex vivo).

Following the success of the Almanac trial (Goyal *et al.* 2004), the principle of sentinel node detection for breast cancer has been adopted as a mainstay of staging. This is associated with a significant reduction in post-operative morbidity and loss of function when compared with radical axillary dissection. It is also applied selectively to patients with malignant melanoma.

For further discussion about sentinel node biopsy see *Breast* in Book 2.

Lymph node clearance

Regional lymph node clearance may be indicated for:

- Visible involvement by tumour
- Symptomatic involvement by tumour
- Occult involvement by tumour (eg identified by lymphoscintography above)
- For staging (eg Dukes' stage of colorectal cancer)
- Prophylactically when shown to improve prognosis

It is associated with a higher morbidity eg axillary dissection, radical neck dissection.

It is associated with improved prognosis in certain tumour types (eg malignant melanoma).

Radiotherapy to lymph nodes

This may be undertaken:

As a primary treatment

- Treatment and control of inoperable involved nodes
- Treatment of extracapsular nodal spread

As an adjunct

- For potential regional microscopic disease

5.3 MANAGEMENT OF DISTANT METASTASES

In a nutshell ...

The management of distant metastases may require:
Curative treatment
Maintenance treatment
Palliative treatment

Techniques include:
Surgical resection
Ablative therapy
Chemoradiotherapy
Palliation
Psychological support

Management of metastatic deposits depends on their location and the type of primary tumour.

- **Resectable disease:** some common target organs (eg lung, liver) offer sufficient functional reserve to allow resection of metastatic deposits from certain tumours. Resection of metastatic deposits has been shown to improve survival for liver and lung metastases from colorectal cancer and for regional lymph node resection in malignant melanoma
- **Unresectable secondary tumours:** organs that have little functional reserve (eg brain) or which present a challenge to resection (eg bi-lobar liver disease) may be treated with ablative therapies (eg cryo- or radioablation)
- **Maintenance treatment:** secondaries may require repeated ablation or repeated courses of chemoradiotherapy

- **Palliative management:** distant metastases may require surgery or intervention to bypass obstruction to the bowel or ureters from widespread intraperitoneal disease, radiotherapy in the management of pain from bony deposits or neurological infiltration

5.4 ONCOLOGICAL EMERGENCIES

In a nutshell ...

Oncological emergencies include:
Neutropenia and sepsis
Hypercalcaemia
SVC obstruction
Spinal cord compression

Neutropenia and sepsis

Neutropenia may result from:

- Pancytopenia due to bone marrow replacement with malignant cells
- Treatment resulting in bone marrow suppression

These patients may be complicated and require aggressive antibiotic management. Discuss with microbiology for advice before initiating therapy.

Hypercalcaemia

Often seen in tumours of the breast, bronchus, prostate, myeloma, kidney and thyroid. May be due to bone mets or ectopic PTH secretion.

Presentation of hypercalcaemia in neoplasia
Clinically – 'bones, moans, stones and groans'.

- Malaise
- Nausea and vomiting
- Constipation
- Abdominal pain
- Polyuria/polydipsia
- Bone pain
- Renal stones
- Psychosis

Management of hypercalcaemia in neoplasia

- May resolve with treatment of the primary malignancy
- Optimise fluid balance
- Stop thiazide diuretics
- May use oral phosphates, calcitonin or NSAIDs

SVC obstruction

Typically occurs with lung carcinoma or lymphoma.

Presentation of SVC obstruction in neoplasia

- Plethoric congested facies
- Obstructed dilated neck veins (if the patient elevates their arms then the veins on the affected side do not empty)
- Dizziness on bending forward
- Dyspnoea and pulmonary oedema
- Headache
- Risks of venous thrombosis (stagnation of blood)

Management of SVC obstruction in neoplasia

- Diagnosis of underlying cause
- Local radiotherapy
- Dexamethasome 4 mg every 6 hours may help

Spinal cord compression

Distribution of malignant spinal cord compression is 70% thoracic, 20% lumbosacral and 10% cervical. For further discussion see *Orthopaedics* in Book 2.

Presentation of spinal cord compression in neoplasia

- Back pain (worse on straining or coughing)
- Leg weakness
- Upper motor neurone and sensory signs
- Urinary retention

Management of spinal cord compression in neoplasia

- Emergency MRI scan for diagnosis
- Discuss with neuro-orthopaedics
- Radiotherapy to vertebrae may be helpful
- May require surgery if histological diagnosis unclear or the spine is mechanically unstable
- High-dose steroids may be helpful

Chapter 4

Haematology

Sheila Fraser and Claire Ritchie Chalmers

Section 1
Composition of the blood

1.1 BLOOD COMPOSITION

In a nutshell ...

The total blood volume in an adult is about 5.5 litres.

Blood is divided into **plasma** and **cells**.

There are three main types of blood cells:

- Erythrocytes (red blood cells)
- Leucocytes (white blood cells) which consist of:
  - Neutrophils
  - Eosinophils
  - Basophils
  - Lymphocytes
  - Monocytes
  - Thrombocytes (platelets)

The haematocrit is the percentage of the blood volume formed by erythrocytes.

Plasma

Blood is divided into plasma and cells. Plasma is a protein-rich solution, which carries the blood cells and also transports nutrients, metabolites, antibodies and other molecules between organs.

The haematocrit (or packed cell volume-PCV) is the percentage of the blood volume formed by erythrocytes and is usually 45%. Over 99% of blood cells are erythrocytes, therefore 2.5 litres of blood is formed from erythrocytes and 3 litres from plasma.

Cells

All blood cells originate from pluripotent stem cells in the bone marrow. At birth the marrow of most bones produces blood cells. In adults the red-cell-producing marrow remains only in the axial skeleton, ribs, skull and proximal ends of humerus and femur. Pluripotent stem cells divide early into lymphoid stem cells, which differentiate into lymphoid and myeloid stem cells – the basis for all other blood cells. Cells of the immune system are discussed in Chapter 2.

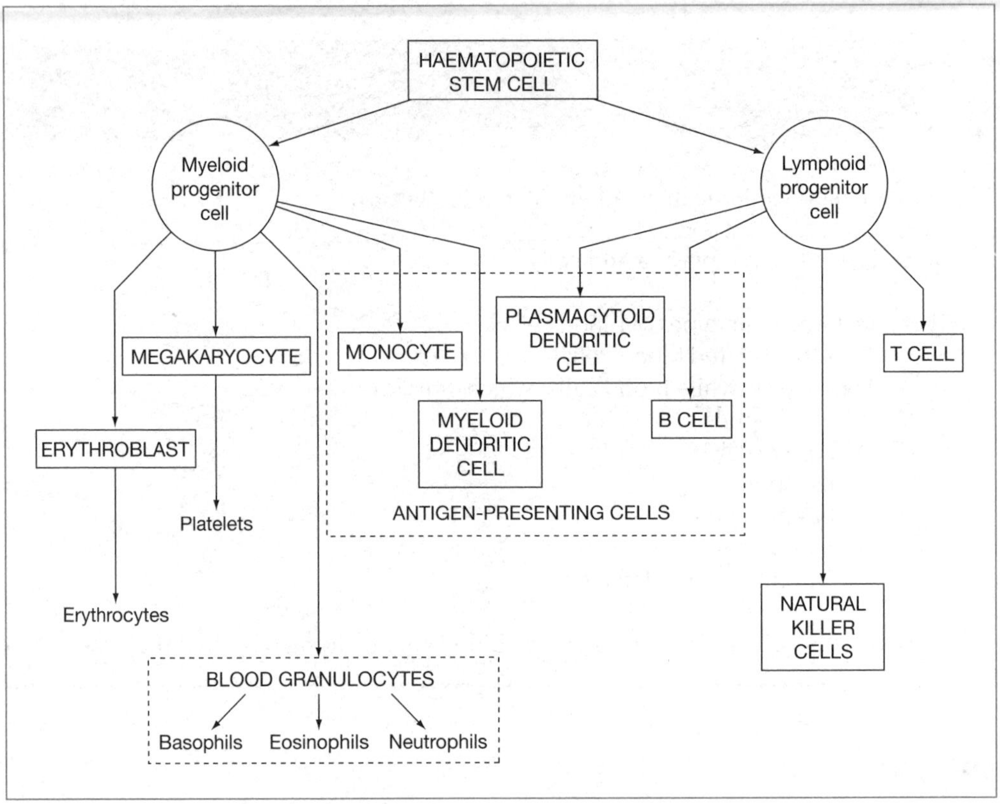

Figure 1.1a *Haematopoiesis (B and T cells are commonly called lymphocytes)*

Erythrocytes

- Transport oxygen via haemoglobin
- Bi-concave disc shape increases surface area to volume ratio and so maximises oxygen exchange
- Contain no nucleus or organelles
- Reticulocytes (immature erythrocytes) contain residual RNA

- Average lifespan is 120 days
- Broken down by macrophages within the spleen, liver and bone marrow
- Synthesis stimulated by erythropoietin production from the kidneys

Leucocytes

- Part of the immunological defence mechanism of the body
- Transported in the blood; most functions take place when cells have left the blood to enter the tissues
- Five main types:
  - Neutrophils
  - Eosinophils
  - Basophils
  - Lymphocytes
  - Monocytes

Together, neutrophils, eosinophils and basophils are known as polymorphonuclear granulocytes due to the presence of cytoplasmic granules and multi-lobed nuclei.

Neutrophils

- Most abundant leucocyte (40–70%)
- Spend 14 days in the bone marrow but have half-life of only 7 hours in the blood
- Major cell in acute inflammation
- Very important role against bacteria
- Migrate from blood to tissues via endothelium

Eosinophils

- Make up 5% of leucocytes
- Important defence against parasitic infections
- Increase in allergic states (eg hay fever, asthma)

Basophils

- Least common leucocyte (0.5%)
- Probable mast cell precursor – similar structure and function
- Initiate immediate hypersensitivity reactions – anaphylaxis via histamine release

Lymphocytes

- Second most common leucocyte (20–50%)
- Important for specific immune response
- Three types of lymphocyte: B cells, T cells and natural killer (NK) cells
- Activated B cells convert into plasma cells and produce antibodies (called the humoral response)

- T cells produce the cell-mediated response. There are three subsets:
  - T-helper cells (activate macrophages and B cells)
  - T-cytotoxic cells (kill target cells)
  - T-suppressor cells (modulate the immune response)
- NK cells perform cell-mediated killing, mainly of viruses and tumour cells

Monocytes

- These account for 15% of leucocytes
- Largest leucocyte, mobile phagocytic cell
- Important in inflammatory reactions
- Located in blood and bone marrow, precursors of macrophages in tissues and lymphoid organs

Thrombocytes (platelets)

- Small, discoid, anuclear cells
- Produced from megakaryocytes, the largest cell in the bone marrow, via cytoplasmic fragmentation
- Circulate for 8–10 days
- Essential for normal haemostasis
- Form a platelet plug in response to loss of endothelium lining blood vessels

Surgery and general haematology

There may be changes in haematology as a response to major surgery, including:

- Leucocytosis (usually due to increase in neutrophil count relative to lymphocytes)
- Relative anaemia
  - Chronic illness
  - Blood loss
  - Impaired erythropoiesis
  - Decreased serum iron
- Relative thrombocytosis
- Increased acute phase reactants including ESR and CRP

1.2 ANAEMIA

In a nutshell ...

Anaemia is the reduction in the concentration of circulating haemoglobin below the expected range for age and sex.

Adult male: < 13 g/dL

Adult female: < 11.5 g/dL

It may be acute or chronic.

Causes of anaemia are:

Decreased production

- Impaired erythrocyte formation
- Impaired erythrocyte function

Increased loss

- Blood loss (acute/chronic)
- Decreased erythrocyte lifespan (eg haemolysis)

Physiological anaemia occurs in pregnancy due to a relative increase in plasma volume.

Anaemia may be classified by cause or by the effects on the cells when viewed as a blood film.

Classification of anaemia

The blood film

Anaemia can be classified according to the morphological appearances of erythrocytes on a blood film.

Look at the mean cell volume (MCV) to determine whether the cells are too small (microcytic), too large (macrocytic), or of the correct size (normocytic).

The intensity of colour of the blood cells as seen on the blood film is also important – cell colour can be decreased with central pallor (hypochromic) or normal (normochromic).

Causes of anaemia

Microcytic hypochromic red cell appearance

- Thalassaemia
- Iron deficiency
  - Malabsorption
  - Chronic blood loss, usually GI or GU tract
  - Decreased dietary intake
  - Increased demand

Normocytic normochromic red cell appearance

- Acute blood loss
- Anaemia of chronic disease
- Endocrine disease
- Malignancy
- Haemolytic anaemia
- Erythrocyte abnormality
  - Spherocytosis
  - Elliptocytosis
  - G-6-PD deficiency
- Haemoglobin abnormality
  - Sickle cell anaemia
- Extrinsic factors
  - DIC
  - Infections
  - Chemical injury
  - Sequestration

Macrocytic red cell appearance

- **Megaloblastic** (interference with DNA synthesis causing morphological abnormalities)
- Folate deficiency
- B_{12} deficiency
  - Pernicious anaemia
  - Gastrectomy
  - Ileal resection
  - Crohn's
- Drugs
  - Azathioprine
  - AZT
  - Hydroxyurea
  - Methotrexate
- Non-megaloblastic anaemia
  - Liver disease
  - Alcohol
  - Pregnancy
  - Hypothyroidism
  - Increased reticulocyte number

Clinical effects of anaemia

Clinically anaemia becomes apparent when the oxygen demands of the tissues cannot be met without some form of compensatory mechanism. A slowly falling haemoglobin level allows for tissue acclimatisation. Compensatory mechanisms include a tachycardia and increased cardiac output, and chronically a reticulocytosis due to increased erythropoiesis and increased oxygen extraction from the blood.

When the patient is relatively anaemic the blood has a lower haematocrit and decreased viscosity. This improves blood flow through the capillaries and so, in cases of critical illness, patients requiring transfusion may not have their anaemia corrected beyond 9–10 g/dL.

Anaemia is not a diagnosis. If a patient presents with low haemoglobin it is important to look for a cause, although emergency surgery should not be delayed. When there is no time for further pre-operative investigation, correction of anaemia (by transfusion) may be required to be part of resuscitation whilst surgical intervention is ongoing.

Reversible causes of anaemia should be corrected before elective surgery. Mildly anaemic patients who are otherwise well may tolerate general anaesthesia and surgery well. More profound anaemia should be treated by consideration of transfusion, iron supplementation, etc.

Investigating anaemia

History

- Acute or chronic blood loss (eg menorrhagia, p.r. bleeding or change in bowel habit)
- Insufficient dietary intake of iron and folate (eg elderly, poverty, anorexia, alcoholic)
- Excessive utilisation of important factors (eg pregnancy, prematurity)
- Malignancy
- Chronic disorders (eg malabsorption states affecting the small bowel)
- Drugs (eg phenytoin antagonises folate)

Further investigation of anaemia

A peripheral blood film will show the morphology of the anaemia and then investigations can be tailored to the particular classification.

It is important to look at low haemoglobin in relation to the leucocyte and platelet counts, to consider a pancytopenia. A reticulocyte count indicates marrow activity.

Tests for haemolysis include serum bilirubin (unconjugated), urinary urobilinogen, haptoglobin and haemosiderinuria. A Schilling's test is undertaken in suspected B_{12} deficiency. A bone marrow biopsy maybe considered and other tests where relevant, such as thyroid function tests, U&Es, G-GT (gamma-glutamyl transferase).

Specific investigations for iron deficiency include blood tests such as ferritin, transferrin and total iron-binding capacity. Vitamin C increases iron absorption by an unknown mechanism. Examine the likely sources of blood loss: GI tract (upper and lower endoscopy); investigation of renal tract (IVU, cystoscopy); menorrhagia, etc. Replacement therapy should comprise 200 mg ferrous sulphate t.d.s.

Folate deficiency (folate found in green vegetables and offal) may be due to insufficient intake or excessive utilisation (eg pregnancy – NB subsequent deficiency of folate causes neural tube defects). Measurement of red cell folate (< 160–640g/L) is more accurate than serum levels. Exclude vitamin B_{12} deficiency, as administration of folate will aggravate neuropathy. Replacement therapy should consist of 5 mg folate once daily. If possible, these investigations should be sent off before commencement of iron or a blood transfusion, which will obscure the results.

1.3 POLYCYTHAEMIA

In a nutshell ...

Polycythaemia is an increase in erythrocyte concentration causing a rise in haemoglobin and PCV (packed cell volume).

It may be primary or secondary and the resulting increase in blood viscosity predisposes to thrombotic pathology.

Treatment usually requires venesection of a unit of blood at set time intervals.

Causes of polycythaemia

Primary polycythaemia – polycythaemia rubra vera (PRV)

- Excess erythrocyte production despite low erythropoietin levels
- Due to a proliferation of pluripotent stem cells with an associated rise in leucocytes and platelets
- Unknown cause and insidious onset
- Diagnosed with Hb > 18 g/dL in males and > 16 g/dL in females

Secondary polycythaemia – increase in erythrocytes only

Appropriate increased erythropoietin production in response to hypoxia

- High altitude
- Cardiac disease
- Pulmonary disease
- Smoking
- Haemoglobinopathy

Inappropriate increase in erythropoietin

- Renal or hepatic carcinoma
- Cerebellar haemangioblastoma
- Renal transplantation
- Large uterine fibroids

Relative (decrease in plasma volume, normal erythrocyte mass)

- Dehydration
- Burns

There is an increase in blood viscosity. Clinically this leads to an increased risk of MI, CVA and PVD and splenomegaly. Haemorrhagic lesions occur in the GI tract and polycythaemia rubra vera is associated with peptic ulceration, although the link is unclear.

Polycythaemia rubra vera may result in acute leukaemia (15%), myelofibrosis (30%) or death via a thrombotic complication (30%).

If possible, surgery should be delayed and a haematologist consulted. In an emergency consider pre-operative venesection and store the blood for an autologous transfusion if required.

1.4 NEUTROPENIA

In a nutshell ...

Neutropenia is a neutrophil count of $< 2 \times 10^9$/L.

Severe neutropenia is a neutrophil count of $< 0.5 \times 10^9$/L.

It may be primary (rare) or secondary due to drugs or leukaemia. The big risk is that of infection.

Causes of neutropenia

Primary causes of neutropenia

- Congenital neutropenias are rare. Most are benign; if severe they are usually fatal at a young age
- Beware of ethnic variations; patients of African ancestry often have low neutrophil counts

Secondary causes of neutropenia

- Drugs
  - Immunosuppressives (eg azathioprine)
  - Antivirals (eg zidovudine)
  - Antibiotics (co-trimoxazole and sulfonamides)
  - Chemotherapy
- Disease:
  - Leukaemia
  - Septicaemia
  - Hypersplenism
  - Bone marrow failure
  - Viral infection
  - RA
  - SLE

Counts of $< 0.5 \times 10^9$/L may result in severe sepsis. Neutropenic infections are usually disseminated with septicaemia, fungaemia and deep abscess formation.

In hospitals prophylactic measures for afebrile neutropenia are undertaken. These consist of isolation, antifungals, antiseptic mouthwash and avoidance of food with a high bacterial load.

Broad-spectrum antibiotics are given in febrile neutropenia. G-CSF (granulocyte-colony stimulating factor) may also be considered, which decreases the number of infective episodes and the duration of neutropenia.

1.5 NEUTROPHILIA

In a nutshell ...

Neutrophilia is usually caused by infection or inflammation.

It may also be a result of metabolic disease, haemorrhage, poisoning, malignancy and changes in physiology.

Causes of neutrophilia

Acute infection

- Bacteria (cocci and bacilli)
- Fungi
- Spirochaetes
- Viruses
- Rickettsiae

Infections such as typhoid fever, parathyroid fever, mumps, measles, and tuberculosis usually are not associated with leukocytosis.

Inflammation

- Burns
- Trauma (eg post-op)
- MI
- Gout
- Glomerulonephritis
- Collagen vascular disorders
- Hypersensitivity reactions

Postoperatively, neutrophilia may occur for between 12 and 36 hours as a result of tissue injury. Leukocytosis also can occur in intestinal obstruction and strangulated hernia.

Metabolic

Neutrophilia commonly occurs in diabetic ketoacidosis, pre-eclampsia, and uraemia, especially with uraemic pericarditis.

Poisoning

- Lead
- Mercury
- Digoxin
- Insect venom

Acute haemorrhage

Acute haemorrhage, especially into body spaces such as the peritoneal cavity, pleural cavity, joint cavity, and intracranial (eg extradural, subdural, or subarachnoid space) cavity is associated with leukocytosis and neutrophilia. This probably is related to the release of adrenal corticosteroids and/or epinephrine secondary to pain and a degree of local inflammation (blood in body cavities is an irritant).

Malignant neoplasms

Neutrophilia can occur in association with rapidly growing neoplasms when the tumour outgrows its blood supply. This is thought to be due to TNF-α

Physiological neutrophilia

- Strenuous exercise
- Adrenaline
- Pregnancy and labour
- Neonates

Other causes

- Cushing's disease and corticosteroids
- Haematological disorders – chronic myelocytic leukaemia, polycythaemia vera, myelofibrosis
- Chronic idiopathic neutrophilia
- Hereditary neutrophilia

The differential white cell count

The differential white cell count can be very helpful in elucidating the diagnosis (eg consider the cause of pyrexia – is it viral or bacterial?). The following table shows causes of changes in the differential white cell count.

THE DIFFERENTIAL WHITE CELL COUNT

Type of cell	Normal range	↓	↑	↑↑↑
Neutrophil	2.0–7.5 × 10^9	Leukaemia Septicaemia Hypersplenism Bone marrow failure Viral infection SLE and RA	Bacterial infection Inflammation Surgery Trauma Burns Haemorrhage Drugs (eg steroids)	Leukaemia Severe infection Disseminated malignancy
Lymphocyte	1.3–3.5 × 10^9	Stress Malnutrition Infections Immuno-suppressants Radiotherapy Primary immuno-deficiency Uraemia Bone marrow failure SLE	Viral infection Chronic lymphocytic leukaemia	EBV infection
Eosinophil	0.04–0.44 × 10^9		Asthma Allergy Parasitic infection Skin diseases (eg pemphigus) Malignant disease	
Monocyte	0.2–0.8 × 10^9		Acute or chronic infection Malignant disease Myelodysplasia	
Basophil	0–0.1 × 10^9		Viral infection Urticaria Myxoedema Haemolysis Polycythaemia Ulcerative colitis Malignancy	

Chapter 4

1.6 LYMPHOPENIA

This is a lymphocyte count of < 1 × 10^9/L. Lymphopenia is associated with opportunistic infections, encapsulated bacterial, fungal and viral infections.

Causes of lymphopenia:

- Stress – trauma, burns, surgery
- Malnutrition
- Infections – TB, HIV, sarcoidosis
- Immunosuppressant drugs eg steroids
- Radiotherapy
- Primary immunodeficiency syndromes (Di George syndrome, primary antibody deficiencies)
- Uraemia
- Bone marrow failure
- SLE

1.7 LYMPHOCYTOSIS

Lymphocytosis is used for a lymphocyte count over 5 × 10^9/L.

Causes of lymphocytosis are:

- Viral infections – especially EBV, CMV, HIV
- Chronic infections – TB, toxoplasmosis
- Haematological malignancy – chronic lymphocytic leukaemia (CLL), lymphoma
- Acute transient response to stress – 24 hours only

1.8 THROMBOCYTOPENIA

In a nutshell ...

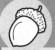

Thrombocytopenia is a platelet number of < 150 × 10^9/L.

Causes include:

Production failure
Decreased thrombocyte survival
Sequestration

Causes of thrombocytopenia

Platelet production failure

- Aplastic anaemia
- Drugs – cytotoxics
- Alcohol
- Viral infections – EBV, CMV
- Marrow infiltration – leukaemia, myelofibrosis, myeloma, metastatic infiltration
- Hereditary thrombocytopenia

Decreased platelet survival

- Idiopathic thrombocytopenic purpura (ITP)
- Drugs – heparin, penicillamine, gold
- Infections –sub-acute bacterial endocarditis (SBE), meningococcus
- Thrombotic thrombocytopenic purpura (TTP)
- DIC
- Blood transfusions – cause dilutional thrombocytopenia
- Haemolytic uraemic syndrome (HUS)
- Extracorporeal bypass – platelets are activated in the extracorporeal circuit, and are therefore ineffective in haemostasis

Sequestration of platelets

- Caused by hypersplenism (see chapter on *Abdomen* in Book 2)
- Counts of $< 70 \times 10^9$/L are inadequate for surgical haemostasis, and spontaneous bleeding may occur with platelet numbers of $< 20 \times 10^9$/L

Clinical conditions in thrombocytopenia

Platelet dysfunction

Excess surgical bleeding may occur with a normal platelet number due to platelet dysfunction. The commonest cause in surgical practice is antiplatelet medications such as aspirin, clopidogrel and warfarin. Patients should be advised to stop these pre-operatively. Aspirin in particular should be stopped 14 days pre-operatively.

Disseminated intravascular coagulation (DIC)

Simultaneous activation of both the coagulation and fibrinolytic systems in the body causes widespread microvascular thrombosis, fibrin deposition, and bleeding due to the consumption of clotting factors and fibrinolysis.

Thrombotic thrombocytopenic purpura (TTP)

This is a condition of unknown cause, usually affecting young adults. Deposition of widespread hyaline thrombi in small vessels causes microangiopathic haemolysis, renal failure and neurological disturbance.

Haemolytic uraemic syndrome (HUS)

Usually this occurs post acute illness, especially URTIs and GI infections. *Escherichia coli* has been implicated. Characteristics include a microangiopathic haemolysis, thrombocytopenia and acute renal failure.

Idiopathic thrombotic purpura (ITP)

Autoimmune destruction of platelets, due to IgG antibody attack. Two types exist:

- Acute (occurs in children; post-viral; usually self limiting; Henoch–Schönlein purpura)
- Chronic (occurs in adults; female predominance; treated with high-dose steroids; rarely requires splenectomy)

1.9 THROMBOCYTOSIS

In a nutshell ...

Thrombocytosis is a rise in the circulating platelet count.

It may be primary or secondary.

Platelets may be numerous but functionally inactive (if functionally active then an antiplatelet agent may be indicated).

Causes of thrombocytosis

Primary thrombocytosis – *essential thrombocythaemia*

- Related to polycythaemia rubra vera
- Platelet count of $> 1000 \times 10^9$/L
- Clinically causes bruising, bleeding and cerebrovascular symptoms
- High platelet count causes splenic atrophy due to recurrent thromboses, after initial hypertrophy

Secondary thrombocytosis

Secondary thrombocytosis is a reaction to:

- Haemorrhage
- Connective tissue disorders
- Surgery
- Splenectomy

- Malignancy
- Myeloproliferative disorders

Patients who have a thrombocytosis and who are at risk of a thrombo-occlusive event (such as those who are immobile, have other risk factors for DVT, or who have vascular grafts or complex vascular anastomoses) often require treatment with an antiplatelet agent.

1.10 PANCYTOPENIA

In a nutshell ...

Pancytopenia is a global reduction in the number of erythrocytes, leucocytes, and platelets.

Causes include drug reactions, bone marrow infiltration, hypersplenism and aplastic anaemia.

Clinically these patients are **anaemic**, **neutropenic** and **thrombocytopenic**.

Causes of pancytopenia

- Drugs
  - Causing bone marrow depression
  - Commonest cause whilst in hospital
  - Includes cytotoxic drugs, immunosuppressants, antiretrovirals
- Bone marrow infiltration
  - Lymphoma, leukaemia, myeloma, myelofibrosis, metastatic infiltration
- Hypersplenism
- Megaloblastic anaemia
- HIV
- Aplastic anaemia
  - Reduction in pluripotent stem cells
  - Congenital (Fanconi's, autosomal recessive, 50% 1-year survival)
  - Idiopathic
  - Secondary (drugs, infections, radiation, paroxysmal nocturnal haemoglobinuria)

Clinical effects of pancytopenia

Anaemia: may require transfusion to maintain Hb. Repeated transfusion may drop the platelet count further.

Neutropenia: pancytopenic patients may require a neutropenic regimen if their neutrophil count is < 0.5 x 10^9/L. They are at risk of neutropenic sepsis.

Thrombocytopenia: a platelet count of < 40 x 10^9/L put patients at risk of traumatic bleeding. Platelet counts < 20 x 10^9/L put the patient at risk of spontaneous bleeding. Transfusion may be required.

1.11 SICKLE CELL DISEASE

In a nutshell ...

Sickle cell disease is a genetic mutation (commonly inherited) causing changes in haemoglobin structure and altered oxygen binding.

It may be homozygous or heterozygous (sickle cell trait).

The disease has predominance in Africa and is found in India and the Middle East.

Clinical problems include:
- Haemolytic anaemia
- Vaso-occlusive crises

Genetics of sickle cell

- At birth the majority of the haemoglobin in the body is fetal haemoglobin – HbF
- By the age of 6 months 80–90% of this is replaced by adult haemoglobin – HbA

Haemoglobin is made up two α and two β chains. An inherited genetic mutation of the β chain leads to the formation of sickle cell haemoglobin, HbS. This is a single amino acid substitution. Glutamine at position six on the β chain is replaced by valine. This changes the oxygen-binding capacity of the molecule.

- Sickle cell haemoglobin can be present as a trait in the heterozygous state – HbAS
- Or as sickle cell disease in the homozygous state – HbSS

The disease usually manifests itself at the age of 6 months, when HbF levels fall.

Clinical aspects of sickle cell disease

De-oxygenated HbS is insoluble and polymerises causing the red blood cells to form rigid, inflexible shapes. Repeated exposure to low oxygen tensions whilst travelling through capillaries causes red blood cells to adopt a rigid sickle shape. This is primarily reversible with reoxygenation (and as such responds to oxygen therapy).

This results in:

- **Haemolytic anaemia** and sequelae such as pigment gallstone formation due to the hyperbilirubinaemia
- **Vaso-occlusive crises**
    - Cause infarction and severe ischaemic pain
    - Commonly seen in the:
        - Bones especially fingers (dactylitis)
        - Chest
        - Kidney
        - Liver
        - Penis (priapism)

In the long term there is an increased susceptibility to infections, especially *Streptococcus pneumoniae* and *Salmonella meningitis*, chronic renal failure and blindness.

Sickle cell disease and surgery

Diagnosis is via FBC, peripheral blood film and sickle solubility test. This is confirmed by Hb electrophoresis.

It is important in surgery to try to avoid precipitating factors. These include hypothermia, hypoxia, infection, hypotension, dehydration and acidosis – all common problems in surgical patients.

Sickle cell trait is usually asymptomatic. Cells do not sickle unless oxygen saturations are below 40%, which is very rare. Anaesthetists should be made aware of patients with the trait pre-operatively in order to avoid any degree of hypoxia.

Many hospitals have a protocol whereby patients from at-risk populations (such as Africans or those of Middle-Eastern descent) have a routine sickle cell test before surgery.

1.12 THALASSAEMIAS

In a nutshell ...

Thalassaemias are inherited disorders of defective synthesis of globin chains in haemoglobin.

They cause haemolysis, anaemia and ineffective erythropoiesis.

They are found mainly in Africa, the Orient, Mediterranean, Asia and the Middle East.

Types include:
- β-thalassaemia major (homozygous)
- β-thalassaemia minor (heterozygous)
- α-thalassaemia

β-Thalassaemia

The most common of the thalassaemias, β-thalassaemia minor, is the heterozygous state. It produces a symptomless microcytosis, which may be accompanied by a mild anaemia.

β-Thalassaemia major is the homozygous form, with either none or a much-reduced number of β chains. It presents as a severe anaemia from 3 months onwards needing regular transfusions. Clinically there is a failure to thrive with recurrent infections. Extramedullary haemopoiesis causes hepatosplenomagaly and bone expansion leading to frontal bossing and a characteristic appearance.

The aim should be to transfuse to an Hb above 10 g/dL, while preventing iron overload with desferrioxamine, an iron-chelating agent. Folate supplements are required. Splenectomy for hypersplenism and bone marrow transplantation can be considered.

α-Thalassaemia

Four genes are responsible for the α chains and the disease is caused by gene deletions. If all four genes are deleted the condition is fatal. A three-gene deletion causes moderate anaemia and splenomegaly – HbH disease. Patients are not usually transfusion dependent. Two-gene deletion causes a microcytosis, which may be associated with a mild anaemia. This is α-thalassaemia trait.

Apart from sickle cell and thalassaemia there are other variants of haemoglobin. The most common are:

- HbC – causes a mild haemolytic anaemia
- HbE – causes a mild microcytic anaemia

Section 2

Haemostasis and coagulation

2.1 PHYSIOLOGY OF HAEMOSTASIS AND COAGULATION

In a nutshell ...

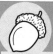

Haemostasis is the physiological cessation of bleeding. It consists of a series of complex interrelated events involving:

- Endothelial cells
- Platelets
- The clotting cascade
- Fibrinolysis

Key events in haemostasis

- Vascular injury with exposure of subendothelial tissue factor and collagen
- Vasoconstriction
- Platelet adherence and aggregation at the injury site (platelet plug)
- Platelet degranulation
- Activation of the coagulation cascade
- Platelet plug stabilised with cross-linked fibrin
- Fibrinolysis and vasodilatation
- Regulatory feedback mechanisms achieve a balance between haemostasis and fibrinolysis

Role of endothelial cells in haemostasis

Endothelial cells form a barrier between their enveloping connective tissues and the blood. They also produce thrombotic and antithrombotic factors.

ENDOTHELIAL CELLS IN HAEMOSTASIS

Factor	Action
Antithrombotic factors	
Prostacyclin (PG-I2)	Inhibitor of platelet aggregation and vasodilator
Thrombomodulin	A glycoprotein bound to the endothelial cell membrane. On complexing with thrombin it activates protein C, (co-factor of protein S), which degrades factors Va and VIIIa. It thus reduces fibrin formation
Nitric oxide	Vasodilator and inhibitor of platelet aggregation and adhesion
Tissue plasminogen activator (tPA)	Regulates fibrinolysis
Thrombotic factors	
von Willebrand's factor (vWF)	Co-factor for platelet adhesion and factor VIII
Platelet activating factor (PAF)	Platelet aggregation and activation
Plasminogen activator inhibitor	tPA inhibitor

Role of platelets in haemostasis

Platelets play a crucial role in haemostasis:

- At sites of vascular injury they bind, via vWF, to subendothelial collagen
- On activation they secrete the contents of their alpha and dense granules: fibrinogen and ADP induce aggregation and thromboxane A_2 causes vasoconstriction
- Aggregation of platelets forms a platelet plug
- Their cell membrane becomes pro-coagulant by providing binding sites for coagulation factors and fibrin
- The platelet plug becomes stabilised with cross-linked fibrin

The clotting cascade

Antithrombin III inactivates thrombin in the presence of heparin. It also inactivates factors VIIa, IXa, Xa, XIa, kallikrein and plasmin. See Fig. 2.1a.

Fibrinolysis

Fibrinolysis occurs in response to vascular injury. Plasminogen is converted to the serine protease plasmin by a number of activators. Plasmin not only cleaves fibrin but also fibrinogen, factors V and VIII. See Fig. 2.1b.

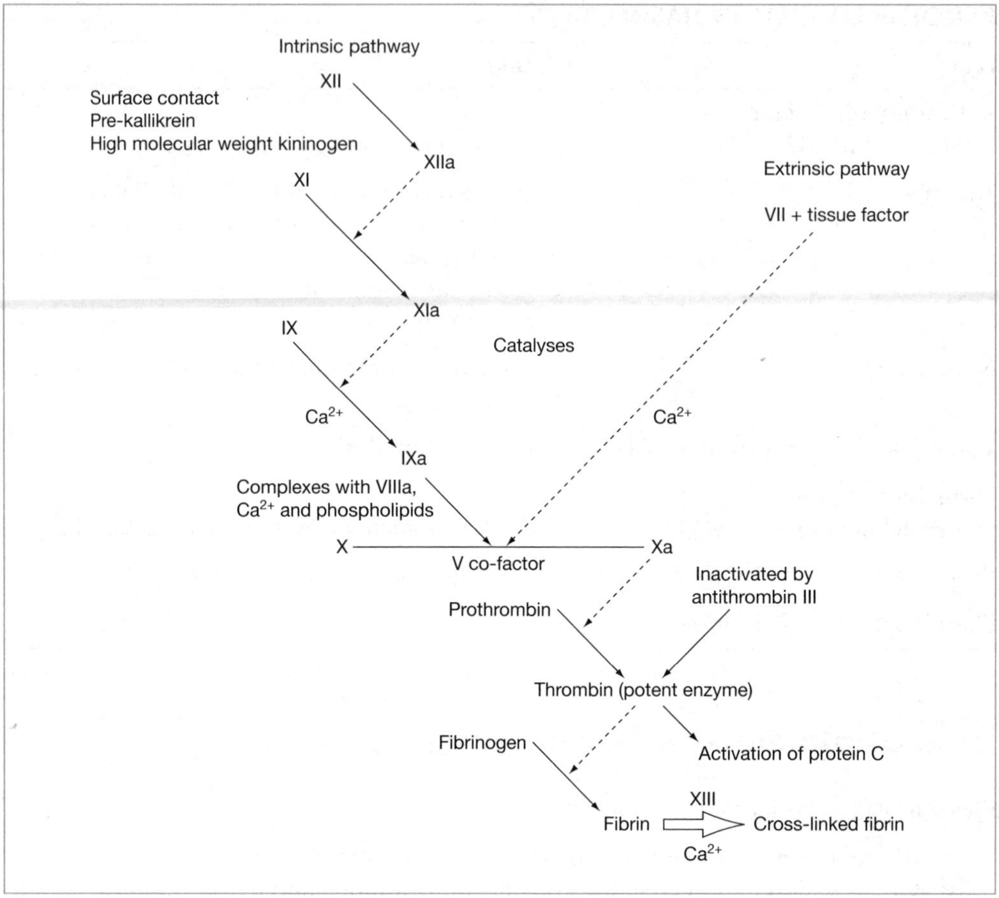

Figure 2.1a *The coagulation system*

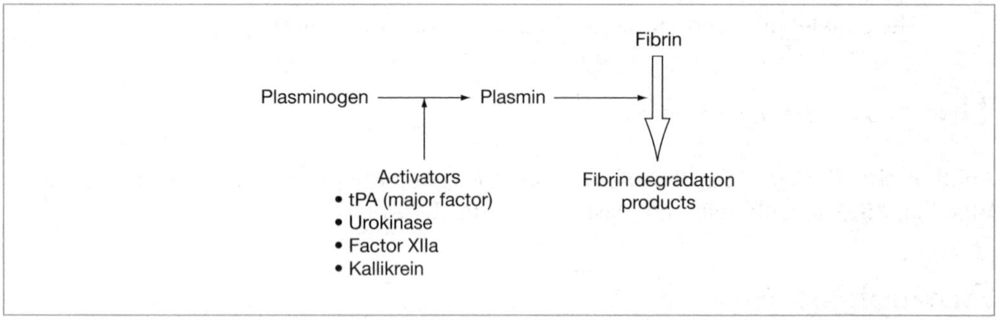

Figure 2.1b *Fibrinolysis. Tissue plasminogen activator (tPA) is released from endothelial cells. Its action is enhanced by the presence of fibrin, hence plasmin formation is localised to the site of the fibrin clot*

2.2 DIAGNOSING DISORDERS OF HAEMOSTASIS AND COAGULATION

In a nutshell ...

The relationship between thrombosis and fibrinolysis is finely balanced. Disorders result from disruption of this equilibrium with over-emphasis or deficiency in one system relative to the other.

Disorders of haemostasis result in a predisposition to haemorrhage (bleeding disorders, section 2.3) or predisposition to thrombosis (thromboembolic disorders, see section 2.4).

In addition to a thorough history and physical examination, a number of simple tests can be employed to assess a patient's haemostatic function.

Screening tests for a clotting disorder

- **Full blood count (FBC) and film:** thrombocytopenia is a common cause of abnormal bleeding. If a patient is suspected of having platelet dysfunction then specific assays can be performed. The bleeding time is a crude assessment of platelet function
- **Activated partial thromboplastin time (APTT):** measures the intrinsic as well as the common pathway factors (X to fibrin). Normal time is about 30–40 seconds
- **Prothrombin time (PT):** assesses the extrinsic system factor (VII) as well as the common pathway factors. It is often expressed as the international normalised ratio (INR)
- **Thrombin time (TT):** this detects deficiencies of fibrinogen or inhibition of thrombin. Normal clotting time is 14–16 seconds
- **Specific coagulation factor tests:** assess genetic disorders of coagulation predisposing to haemorrhage:
  - Haemophilia (factor VIII deficiency)
  - Christmas disease (factor IX deficiency)
- **Fibrinogen and fibrin degradation product (FDP) levels:** are useful for detection of on-going intravascular coagulation (eg DIC)

RESULTS OF BLOOD TESTS IN COMMON BLEEDING DISORDERS

	PT	APTT	TT	Platelet count
Liver disease	↑	↑	N	↓
Warfarin	↑	N	N	N
Heparin	N	↑	↑	N
Factor VII deficiency	↑	N	N	N
Factor VIII deficiency	N	↑	N	N
Factor IX deficiency	N	↑	N	N
DIC	↑	↑	↑	↓

↑ = increased; ↓ = decreased; N = normal.

2.3 BLEEDING DISORDERS

In a nutshell ...

Bleeding disorders may be congenital or acquired.

Congenital
- Haemophilia A and B
- Von Willebrand's disease
- Platelet function disorders

Acquired
- Thrombocytopenia
- Platelet function disorders
- Vitamin K deficiency
- Hepatic failure
- Renal failure
- Acquired vascular defects

Congenital bleeding disorders

Haemophilia A

Haemophilia A is an X-linked recessive disorder that results from a deficiency or an abnormality of the coagulation factor VIII. It affects 1 in 10 000 males (females can also rarely be affected) and up to 30% of cases are due to spontaneous mutations. It is characterised by bleeding into soft tissues, muscles, and weight-bearing joints, the onset of which may be delayed by several hours after the injury. The functional level of factor VIII determines the severity of the disorder:

Severe disease

- < 1% factor VIII
- Frequent bleeding after minor trauma

Moderate disease

- 1–5% factor VIII
- Less frequent bleeding

Mild disease

- 5–25% factor VIII
- Persistent bleeding usually secondary to trauma

The majority of affected individuals have factor VIII levels below 5%. 10–20% of patients develop antibodies to factor VIII. Treatment depends on the severity of the disorder and the proposed surgery. Factor VIII concentrate may have to be given repeatedly or continuously to maintain factor VIII levels. Desmopressin can be used transiently to raise the factor VIII level in patients with mild haemophilia.

Haemophilia B

Haemophilia B, also known as Christmas disease, is an X-linked disorder. It is clinically indistinguishable from haemophilia A. It occurs in 1 in 100 000 male births and is due to a defect or deficiency in factor IX. Treatment involves either prothrombin complex concentrate, which contains all of the vitamin K-dependent clotting factors, or factor IX concentrate.

Von Willebrand's disease

Von Willebrand's disease is the most common of the congenital bleeding disorders, occurring in as many as 1 in 800–1000 individuals. Von Willebrand factor (vWF) is a plasma glycoprotein that has two main functions: it aids platelet adhesion to the sub-endothelium at sites of vascular injury, and it serves as the plasma carrier protein for factor VIII. Three main disease subtypes have been described:

- Type I (most common): autosomal dominant (quantitative reduction of vWF)
- Type II: variably inherited (qualitative defects in vWF)
- Type III (very rare): autosomal recessive (almost no vWF)

Patients with the disease develop mucosal bleeding, petechiae, epistaxis and menorrhagia similar to patients with platelet disorders. Treatment depends on the symptoms and the underlying type of disease. Cryoprecipitate, factor VIII concentrate, or desmopressin can be used.

Congenital platelet function disorders

These are very rare. They include:

- Bernard–Soulier syndrome (defect in platelet plasma membrane)
- Grey platelet syndrome (defect in storage granules)
- Cyclo-oxygenase and thromboxane synthetase deficiency

Acquired bleeding disorders

Thrombocytopenia

- Normal platelet count 150–400 × 10^9/L
- Spontaneous bleeding uncommon 40–100 × 10^9/L
- Spontaneous bleeding often severe < 10 × 10^9/L

Causes of thrombocytopenia include:

- Decreased production (marrow aplasia, marrow infiltration, uraemia and alcoholism)
- Decreased survival (drugs, ITP)
- Increased consumption (DIC, infection, heparin therapy)

Platelet function disorders

These can be caused by:

- NSAIDs
- Heparin
- Alcohol
- Haematological malignancy

Vitamin K deficiency

Vitamin K is a fat-soluble vitamin that is absorbed in the small intestine and stored in the liver. It serves as a co-factor for γ-carboxylase in the production of coagulation factors II, VII, IX, X and protein C and protein S. The normal liver contains a 30-day store of the vitamin, but the acutely ill patient can become deficient in 7–10 days.

Causes of vitamin K deficiency are:

- Inadequate dietary intake
- Malabsorption
- Lack of bile salts
- Hepatocellular disease
- Cephalosporin antibiotics

Parenteral vitamin K produces a correction in clotting times within 8–10 hours. Fresh frozen plasma (FFP) should be administered to patients with ongoing bleeding.

Hepatic failure

Hepatocellular disease is often accompanied by impaired haemostasis.

This is because of:

- Decreased synthesis of coagulation factors (except factor VIII)
- Decreased synthesis of coagulation inhibitors (protein C, protein S and antithrombin III)
- Reduced clearance of activated coagulation factors, which may cause either DIC or systemic fibrinolysis
- Impaired absorption and metabolism of vitamin K
- Splenomegaly and secondary thrombocytopenia

Renal failure

Renal failure causes a decrease in platelet aggregation and adhesion.

Acquired vascular defects

This is a heterogeneous group of conditions characterised by bruising after minor trauma and spontaneous bleeding from small blood vessels. Examples include:

- **Senile purpura:** due to atrophy of perivascular supporting tissues
- **Scurvy:** defective collagen due to vitamin C deficiency
- **Steroid purpura**
- **Henoch–Schönlein syndrome**
- **Ehlers–Danlos syndrome:** hereditary collagen abnormality

2.4 THROMBOEMBOLIC DISORDERS

In a nutshell ...

Thrombophilia refers to conditions predisposing to thrombosis.

Congenital prothrombotic disorders

Factor V Leiden mutation
Antithrombin III deficiency
Protein C and protein S deficiency

Acquired prothrombotic disorders
DIC
Hyperviscosity of any cause

Thrombocytosis refers to a rise in circulating platelet count (see section 1.9). A predisposition to thrombosis increases the risks of DVT, PE and recurrent miscarriage.

Thrombophilia

Investigating thrombophilia

Clinical presentation of thrombophilia is with atypical or recurrent thrombosis. These patients are often young, may have a family history of thrombosis, and present with thrombotic conditions such as DVT/PE, recurrent spontaneous abortion, and mesenteric thrombosis.

Thrombophilia screen

These tests assess genetic disorders of coagulation predisposing to thrombosis:

- Factor V Leiden mutation
- Antithrombin III
- Protein C
- Protein S

Identifying a genetic predisposition to thrombophilia should prompt screening of family members and giving advice about minimising risk factors (eg avoiding use of the OCP).

Congenital prothrombotic disorders

Factor V Leiden mutation

- A genetic mutation in the factor V gene causes a change in the factor V protein making it resistant to inactivation by protein C
- Factor V Leiden is inactivated by activated protein C at a much slower rate, so leading to a thrombophilic state (propensity to clot) by having increased activity of factor V in the blood
- Common in northern European populations (4–7% of the general population is heterozygous for factor V Leiden and 0.06–0.25% of the population is homozygous for factor V Leiden)

Antithrombin III deficiency

- Rare autosomal dominant disorder
- Antithrombin III inactivates thrombin, factors VIIa, IXa, Xa, XIa, kallikrein, and plasmin
- Antithrombin III level is measured by immunological assay
- $< 70\%$ of the normal value increases risk of venous thrombosis

- Deficiency is also associated with liver disease, DIC, nephrotic syndrome and heparin therapy
- Prophylaxis and treatment involves antithrombin III concentrate and anticoagulation

Protein C and protein S deficiencies

- Autosomal dominant disorders with variable penetrance
- Protein C is activated by thrombin binding to thrombomodulin, a glycoprotein bound to the endothelial cell membrane; this causes a reduction in fibrin formation by the degradation of factors Va and VIIIa; protein S acts as a co-factor
- Protein C and protein S levels can be assessed by immunoassay techniques
- Treatment involves replacement of protein C or S and anticoagulation

Acquired prothrombotic disorders

Disseminated intravascular coagulation (DIC)

DIC is a systemic thrombohaemorrhagic disorder. It is the pathological response to many underlying conditions.

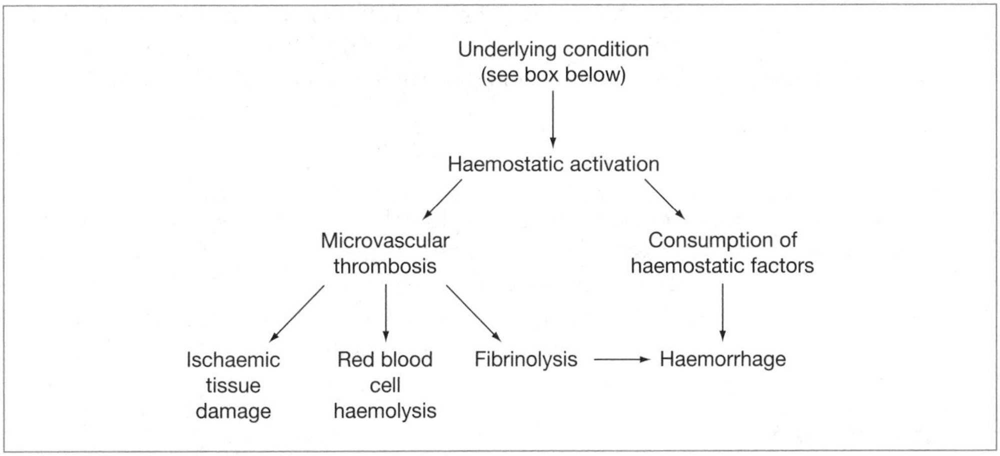

Figure 2.5a *Disseminated intravascular coagulation (DIC)*

Conditions associated with DIC

Malignancy
Massive tissue injury and trauma
Obstetric complications (eg placental abruption, septic abortion, intrauterine fetal death, amniotic fluid embolism)
Infections (especially Gram-negative bacteria)
Miscellaneous (eg acute pancreatitis, drug reactions, transplant rejection, ARDS)

The clinical presentation is extremely variable. Most patients present with easy bruising and haemorrhage from venepuncture and IM injection sites. This may progress to profuse haemorrhage from mucous membranes and shock. Although haemorrhage is the most common presentation, about 10% present with widespread thrombosis and resultant multiorgan failure.

Laboratory features of DIC

- Thrombocytopenia
- Prolonged PT, APTT, TT
- Increased fibrin degradation products (also increased after surgery)
- Reduced fibrinogen level
- Fragmented red blood cells

Management of DIC

- Diagnosis and treatment of the underlying disorder
- Shock exacerbates DIC therefore adequate fluid resuscitation is essential
- Use FFP, cryoprecipitate and platelet concentrates as required; be guided by regular laboratory screening

Use of heparin is controversial; it has been given in an attempt to reduce thrombin formation via antithrombin III activation, but trials have shown little benefit; however, if thrombosis is the predominant feature, heparin should be used at a relatively early stage.

Aetiology of venous thromboembolism

Venous thrombosis occurs in response to factors described by Virchow's triad. The relative importance of these factors to each other is still under debate. Venous thrombosis develops due to activation of coagulation in an area of venous stasis, as an imbalance between thrombogenesis and the circulating inhibitors of coagulation. Thus, prophylactic regimens are based on minimising stasis and providing anticoagulation.

Virchow's triad

Endothelial damage (eg smoking, previous DVT)
Reduced venous flow or stasis (eg immobility, obstruction to flow)
Hypercoaguability (eg heritable coagulopathy, smoking, malignancy)

Clots usually start in the deep veins around cusps or occasionally in larger vessels after direct venous wall trauma. They either:

- Dissolve spontaneously (with or without treatment)
- Propagate proximally (20%)

DVT occurs in 50% of patients undergoing major abdominal or pelvic surgery if no prophylactic measures are taken. It is also common in joint replacement surgery and the elderly.

20% of those with DVT are at risk of developing a PE (the risk of embolus from a below-knee DVT is very small; it increases substantially if the clot extends to above the knee; the risk of subsequent embolism is very high if the ileofemoral segment is involved).

Deep venous thrombosis (DVT)

Venous thrombosis or DVT is common in surgical patients. It can cause pulmonary embolism, which carries a high mortality and therefore should be prevented. It may also cause a post-phlebitic limb with ulceration many years later.

Factors predisposing to deep venous thrombosis

These can be divided into patient factors and factors involving the disease or surgical procedure.

Patient factors

- Age
- Previous DVT or PE
- Immobility
- Obesity
- Pregnancy
- Thrombophilia (eg protein C and protein S deficiencies, lupus anticoagulant and factor V Leiden)
- OCP

PATIENT FACTORS INFLUENCING RELATIVE RISKS OF THROMBOEMBOLISM

Status	Relative risk of venous thrombosis
Normal	1
OCP use	4
Factor V Leiden, heterozygous	6
Factor V Leiden, homozygous	80
Prothrombin gene mutation, heterozygous	3
Prothrombin gene mutation, homozygous	20
Protein C deficiency, heterozygous	7
Protein C deficiency, homozygous	Severe thrombosis at birth
Protein S deficiency, heterozygous	6
Protein S deficiency, homozygous	Severe thrombosis at birth
Antithrombin III deficiency, heterozygous	5
Antithrombin III deficiency, homozygous	Fatal in utero
Homocysteinaemia	3

Factors involving the disease or surgical procedure

- Trauma or surgery, especially of the pelvis and lower limb
- Malignancy, especially pelvic and abdominal
- MI
- Congestive heart failure
- Polycythaemia
- IBD
- Nephrotic syndrome
- Length of operation

Risks of deep venous thrombosis according to procedure

Low risk

Minor surgery (< 30 minutes); no risk factors other than age
Major surgery (> 30 minutes); age < 40; no other risk factors
Minor trauma or medical illness

Moderate risk

Major general, urological, gynaecological, cardiothoracic, vascular or neurological surgery; age > 40 or other risk factors
Major medical illness; heart or lung disease; cancer; IBD
Major trauma or burns
Minor surgery, trauma or illness in patients with previous DVT, PE or thrombophilia

High risk

Fracture or major orthopaedic surgery of pelvis, hip or lower limb
Major pelvic or abdominal surgery for cancer
Major surgery, trauma or illness in patients with previous DVT, PE or thrombophilia
Lower limb paralysis
Major lower limb amputation

INCIDENCE OF DVT AFTER COMMON SURGICAL PROCEDURES

Type of operation	Incidence of DVT (%)
Knee surgery	75
Hip fracture surgery	60
Elective hip surgery	50–55
Retropubic prostatectomy	40
General abdominal surgery	30–35
Gynaecological surgery	25–30
Neurosurgery	20–30
Transurethral resection of prostate	10
Inguinal hernia repair	10

Symptoms of deep venous thrombosis

DVT may be asymptomatic and difficult to diagnose. You must have a high level of suspicion in patients at risk. Symptoms may be a combination of those below:

Below-knee symptoms

- Swelling
- Pain and calf tenderness (from inflammation around the thrombus; can be demonstrated by Homan's sign of increased pain on dorsiflexion of the foot but this is very non-specific)
- May have mild calf erythema
- Grumbling mild pyrexia

Above-knee symptoms

- May be asymptomatic and difficult to diagnose. Again you must have a high level of suspicion in patients at risk
- Swelling
- Pain and tenderness
- Grumbling mild pyrexia
- Phlegmasia caerulia dolens is a painful, purple, congested and oedematous lower limb associated with extensive ileofemoral DVT (there is usually underlying pelvic pathology)

Well's criteria

Well's criteria are used to determine the probability of spontaneous DVT (from a meta-analysis published by Anand *et al* 1998).

Each clinical sign is assigned one point:

Active cancer (Rx within 6 months or palliative)
Paralysis, paresis or recent lower limb POP
Recently bedridden for > 3 days or major surgery within last 4 weeks
Localised calf tenderness
Entire leg swelling
Calf swelling > 3 cm larger than other limb
Pitting oedema (> other limb)
Collateral superficial veins (non-varicose)

A high probability of an alternative diagnosis scores minus 2.

Overall score

High probability of DVT	Scores ≥ 3
Moderate probability of DVT	Scores 1–2
Low probability of DVT	Scores < 1

Chapter 4

Investigating deep venous thrombosis

- Duplex Doppler US
- Ascending contrast venography (gold standard)
- ^{125}I-fibrinogen scanning (research only)

Differential diagnosis of deep venous thrombosis

- Lymphoedema
- Cellulitis
- Ruptured baker's cyst

Complications of deep venous thrombosis

- Pulmonary embolism
- Post-phlebitic limb
- Resolution without complication

Prevention of deep venous thrombosis

The highest risk of thromboembolism occurs at and immediately after surgery. Measures are therefore required to prevent venous thromboembolism in the peri-operative period.

General preventive measures for thromboembolism

Early post-operative mobilisation
Adequate hydration in the peri-operative period
Avoid calf pressure
Stop the oral contraceptive pill 6 weeks pre-operatively (advise alternative contraception)

Specific preventive measures for thromboembolism

Graded elastic compression stockings: these should be well fitting, applied pre-surgery, and left on until patient is mobile, except in cases of peripheral vascular ischaemias (eg patients for femoro-crural bypass)
Intermittent pneumatic calf compression: various devices available
Electrical calf muscle stimulation
Post-operative leg elevation and early ambulation
Heparin prophylaxis: traditional unfractionated heparin, 5000 units SC given 2–4 hours before surgery and continued twice daily until patient is mobile. This has

been largely superceded by low-molecular-weight (LMW) heparin. Various regimens are available. Advantages of LMW heparin are: less propensity to bleeding; longer half-life; only needs once daily administration; lower incidence of heparin-induced thrombocytopenia and heparin-induced osteoporosis. Heparin prophylaxis should be discontinued 24 hours before administration or withdrawal of epidural anaesthesia, to prevent bleeding into the epidural space

Other agents affecting blood coagulability: antiplatelet agents (eg aspirin, dipyridamole, dextran) have been tried. Although they do reduce platelet activity, none is widely used for DVT prophylaxis. Oral anticoagulants (eg warfarin) are not used for surgical DVT prophylaxis because of the unacceptably high risk of haemorrhage

In principle, the method used should be simple to use, acceptable to patients, and have minimal adverse effects.

- All hospital inpatients need to be assessed for clinical risk factors and risk of thromboembolism; should have graded prophylaxis depending on the degree of risk
- Low-risk patients should be mobilised early
- Moderate- and high-risk patients should be mobilised early AND receive specific prophylaxis

In practice, the methods used vary between clinicians and units but it is important that each centre has specific policies regarding prophylaxis.

Pulmonary embolus (PE)

Symptoms and signs of pulmonary embolus

Symptoms and signs of pulmonary embolism depend upon the size and number of emboli. Pulmonary emboli vary from multiple small emboli to solitary large emboli impacting at the bifurcation as a 'saddle' embolism. Small emboli may be completely asymptomatic.

- Shortness of breath
- Increased respiratory rate
- Pleuritic chest pain
- Decreased oxygen saturations
- Sinus tachycardia
- May have small haemoptysis
- Shock and circulatory collapse
- Cardiac arrest with electromechanical dissociation (EMD) or pulseless electrical activity (PEA)

Investigating pulmonary embolism

ECG changes

- Commonly a sinus tachycardia is seen
- May be signs of right-heart strain (eg right-bundle-branch block)
- Classical pattern of S1 Q3 T3 is very rarely seen

CXR changes

- Acutely there may be no changes seen (but alternative diagnoses can be excluded)
- A wedge of pulmonary infarction may be visible in the days following the PE

Arterial blood gases

- Acute hypoxia in the absence of CXR signs should also raise the suspicion of PE, especially in a pre-operative patient

Diagnosis of pulmonary embolism

- Ventilation–perfusion scan
- CT pulmonary angiography
- Pulmonary angiogram
- ECG changes (as above)

Complications of pulmonary embolism

- Pulmonary hypertension (multiple small emboli over a period of time)
- EMD cardiac arrest (eg large saddle embolus) – cause of 10% hospital deaths

Treatment of DVT and PE

- **Analgesia**
- **Graduated compression stocking**
- **Anticoagulation with heparin** (low-molecular-weight is commonly used). Long-term anticoagulation is undertaken with warfarin: the length of anticoagulation after surgery depends upon the underlying cause of the DVT and the continued presence of any risk factors; a simple DVT due to transient immobility usually requires 3 months anticoagulation
- **Caval filter:** to reduce the risk of fatal PE when an extensive DVT is present (eg ileofemoral) or when there have been multiple emboli, a filter may be placed into the IVC (this looks like the bare spokes of an umbrella on imaging)
- **Fibrinolytic agents** may be used in cases of very extensive DVT (NB not after major surgery)

2.5 ANTICOAGULATION

In a nutshell ...

Many surgical patients are pharmacologically anticoagulated because of associated co-morbidity either pre- or post-operatively

In addition some patients have pathological defects in clotting because of their liver disease

Peri-operative management of anticoagulation is important because poor management leads to risks of haemorrhage or of thrombosis

Pharmacological anticoagulants include:
- Antiplatelet agents (eg aspirin, dipyridamole, clopidogrel)
- Heparin (eg unfractionated and low molecular weight)
- Warfarin

Anticoagulants

Many pre-operative elective surgical patients are on some form of anticoagulation. Management depends on the type of anticoagulation and the reason for the anticoagulation.

For elective surgical patients on oral anticoagulation, the challenge is to balance the risk of haemorrhage if the INR is not reduced, against the risk of thrombosis if the INR is reduced for too long or by too great an amount.

Antiplatelet agents

Aspirin

Usually this is given as prophylaxis against cerebrovascular disease, ischaemic heart disease, and peripheral vascular disease.

Low-dose aspirin irreversibly acetylates the enzyme cyclo-oxygenase. Affected platelets are therefore unable to synthesise thromboxane A_2 and become inactivated throughout their 7-day life span. Other NSAIDs cause a reversible effect that lasts 3–4 days.

It is often safe to leave patients on aspirin through the peri-operative period, but in certain procedures where there is a special risk of bleeding (eg thyroidectomy, TURP) it should be stopped. Because of its long half-life it should be stopped 1 week before the proposed date of surgery.

Other antiplatelet agents

Dipyridamole: this may be used as secondary prophylaxis against thrombosis in patients with ischaemic heart disease, TIAs or peripheral vascular disease who are intolerant to, or have suffered side effects from, aspirin.

Clopidogrel: this drug is also used in the prevention of thrombotic events in patients with known ischaemic disease. There may be slight benefit in combining clopidogrel with aspirin but this raises the risk of catastrophic bleeding. This drug must be stopped two weeks or longer before surgery.

Heparin

Heparin is a potent anticoagulant that binds to and activates antithrombin III, thus reducing fibrin formation. Heparin is neutralised with IV protamine (1 mg protamine for every 100 units of heparin). It can only be given parenterally or subcutaneously. The dose is monitored by measuring the ratio of the patient's APTT to control plasma. LMW heparins are given on the basis of the patient's weight and do not require monitoring.

LMW heparin is usually given SC throughout the peri-operative period for DVT prophylaxis. It may be stopped 24 hours before the proposed date of surgery in procedures with special risks of bleeding, or where the use of epidural anaesthesia is anticipated. IV heparin has a more profound anticoagulant effect, but a shorter half-life, and only needs to be discontinued 6 hours before a procedure.

Warfarin

Warfarin blocks the synthesis of vitamin K-dependent factors. It prolongs the PT and may slightly elevate the APTT. It is highly plasma-protein bound, therefore caution must be exercised when giving other drugs because these may potentiate its effects. Treatment of major bleeding consists of the administration of vitamin K and FFP.

The dose is adjusted to maintain the INR (ratio of the patient's PT to that of control plasma) at a level between 1 and 4 according to the degree of anticoagulation required. Warfarin has a more prolonged effect on anticoagulation. It is usually given to patients at special risk of thrombosis, such as those with artificial heart valves, thrombophilia, previous DVT or PE.

Warfarin's effect is monitored by INR measurement:

INR of 0.8–1.2	Normal coagulation
INR of 1.2–2.0	Mild anticoagulation – moderate risk of surgical bleeding
INR of 2.0–3.5	Normal therapeutic range – severe risk of surgical bleeding
INR of > 3.5	Severely anticoagulated – surgery should not be contemplated until INR is reduced

Section 3
Transfusion medicine

In a nutshell ...

Blood products are a scarce and expensive resource, and they are not without risks to the recipient.

- Safety of the blood product supply is maintained by donor selection criteria and screening of all samples
- Compatibility of transfusion is based on the ABO and rhesus D typing

Blood components include:

- Red cell concentrates
- Platelet concentrates
- Granulocytes
- Fresh frozen plasma
- Albumin solutions
- Coagulation factors

Use of blood products can be minimised by:

- Autologous transfusion (eg cell saver)
- Pharmacological methods

Adverse effects of transfusion include:

- Immunological reaction (incompatible red cells, white cells, platelets, granulocytes, plasma antibodies)
- Infection

3.1 BLOOD COLLECTION, GROUPING AND ADMINISTRATION

Blood collection

In the UK, the supply of blood and plasma is based entirely on the good will of voluntary, healthy blood donors. Donation from individuals at high risk of viral transmission is excluded and measures are taken to ensure that samples of blood are collected in a sterile and accountable manner.

See section 3.3 for discussion of risks associated with receipt of transfusion.

Over 90% of donated blood is separated into its various constituents to allow prescription of individual components and preparation of pooled plasma from which specific blood products are manufactured (see section 3.2).

Blood grouping

Red blood cells carry antigens, typically glycoproteins or glycolipids, which are attached to the red cell membrane. Over 400 groups have been identified, the most important of which are the:

- ABO system
- Rhesus system

ABO system

- Consists of A, B, O allelic genes
- A and B control synthesis of enzymes that add carbohydrate residues to the cell surface glycoproteins
- Antibodies occur naturally in the serum appropriate to the missing antigen as shown in the table
- Blood groups, antigens and serum antibodies

Blood group	Antigen on cells	Antibody in plasma
A	A	Anti-B
B	B	Anti-A
AB	A and B	None
O	No A or B antigens	Anti-A and Anti-B

Transfusion of red cells expressing an antigen against which the recipient possesses an antibody causes a massive immune response resulting in clumping and destruction of the donor cells. This causes multisystem failure and is usually fatal.

Transfusion of plasma containing an antibody against an antigen expressed on the red cells of the recipient will also cause an immune response, but of a lesser degree because the antibody concentration is significantly diluted by the recipient's own plasma.

Antibodies to the ABO antigens are naturally occurring, whereas antibodies to other red cell antigens appear only after sensitisation by transfusion or pregnancy. The rhesus system is an example of this.

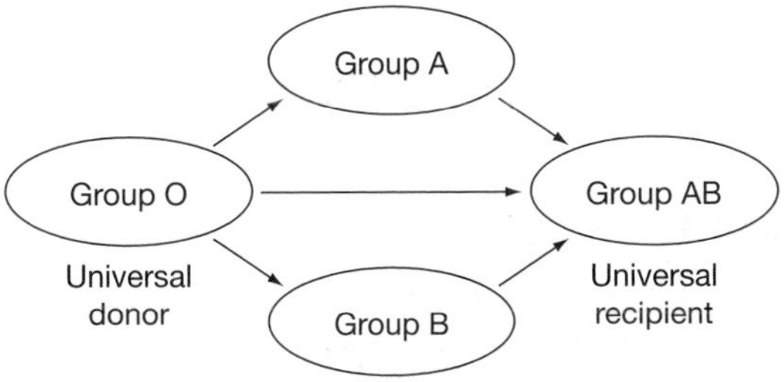

Figure 3.1a *The ABO system. Arrows denote compatible transfusion. Group O is termed the 'universal donor' because it is compatible with all three of the other groups. Group AB is termed the 'universal recipient' as these patients can receive blood from any group*

Rhesus system

Rhesus-positive (Rh+) patients express the rhesus antigen on their red cells. Rhesus-negative (Rh–) patients do not have antibodies to this antigen unless they have previously been exposed to Rh+ blood (due to previous transfusion or birth of an Rh+ child).

85% of people are rhesus positive.

All Rh– females of childbearing age should be given Rh– blood as the development of antibodies to the rhesus antigen will cause haemolytic disease of the newborn in any future Rh+ pregnancies.

Blood compatibility testing

Donor and recipient ABO and rhesus type must be compatible. Subsequent testing is to identify additional antibodies in the recipient's serum which may react with the donors red cells. This can be achieved in one of two ways:

- **Antibody screening:** tests for the presence of antibodies in the recipient's serum to a number of test red cells of the same ABO and rhesus grouping. Agglutination of the test cells indicates the presence of an unusual antibody and this must be characterised further in order to choose compatible red cells for transfusion
- **Cross-matching:** is a direct test of compatibility between donor red cells and the recipient's serum

Administration safety

There are a number of safety measures to ensure that ABO incompatible transfusion does not occur.

Ordering blood products

- Identify the recipient
- Provide adequate information on the request card (name, age, date of birth, hospital number, gender, diagnosis, previous transfusion, pregnancies)
- Ensure adequate labelling of the recipient's blood sample as soon as it is taken to minimise error

When the blood arrives on the ward

- Identify the recipient (name, age, date of birth, hospital number) both verbally, if possible, and by means of the hospital ID bracelet – this must be done by two separate members of staff
- Check that the ABO and rhesus grouping on the front of the unit is compatible with the patient's blood group
- Double check anything you aren't happy about with the laboratory before commencing transfusion

When transfusing blood monitor temperature and pulse every 30 minutes

- A sharp spike of temperature (> 39 °C) at the start of transfusion suggests intravascular haemolysis and the transfusion should be stopped
- Slow elevation of temperature may be due to antibodies against white cells and the infusion should be slowed

If there is any evidence of a severe transfusion reaction

- Stop the infusion
- Re-check patient identity against the unit
- Send the unit back to the blood bank with a fresh sample taken from the patient for comparison
- Supportive management of the patient. Severe reactions may result in cardiovascular collapse

3.2 USE OF BLOOD COMPONENTS

In a nutshell ...

Blood components

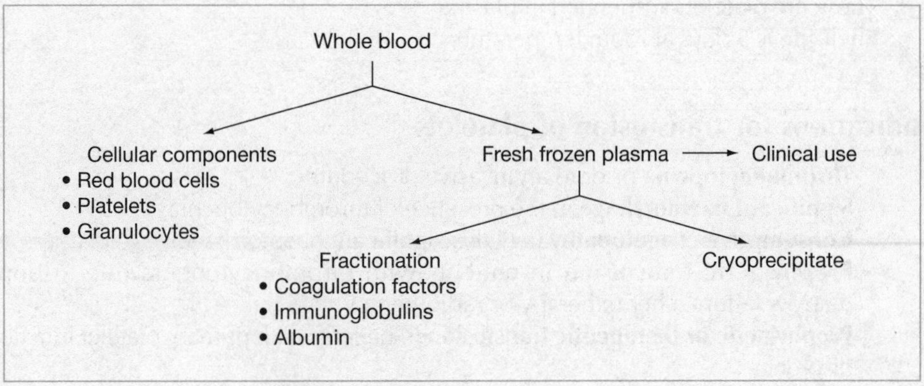

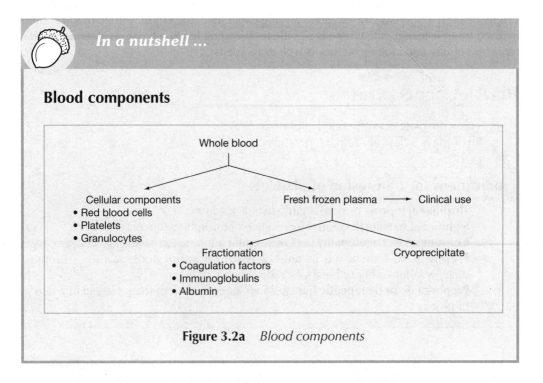

Figure 3.2a *Blood components*

Red blood cell (RBC) concentrates

In whole blood granulocytes and platelets lose function, many coagulation factors lose activity, and aggregates of dead cells, platelets, and other debris are formed unless it is used within a few days.

RBC concentrates or packed cells consist of whole blood from which the plasma has been removed. RBCs are suspended in a solution (SAG-M) containing sodium chloride, adenine, glucose and mannitol. The volume of one unit is 350 mL and its shelf-life is 35 days at 4 °C.

Storage changes include increases in potassium and phosphate concentrations, decreases in pH, haemolysis, micro-aggregation of dead cells, and loss of clotting factor VIII and V activity.

Washed RBCs are used in patients who cannot tolerate granulocyte and platelet debris normally present in RBC concentrates.

Units of **rare blood types** may be stored for up to 3 years at –65 °C in glycerol-containing media.

Transfusion of RBC concentrates may occur when Hb < 7 g/dL (unless severe ischaemic heart disease when transfusion may occur if Hb < 10 g/dL). RBC concentrates should simply be used to increase the oxygen-carrying capacity of the blood. Whole blood should be used for transfusion when there is significant bleeding leading to hypovolaemia, as this replaces volume and clotting factors as well as red cells.

Platelet concentrates

- These are platelets suspended in plasma
- Shelf-life is 5 days at room temperature

Indications for transfusion of platelets

- **Thrombocytopenia** prior to an invasive procedure
- **Significant haemorrhage** in the presence of thrombocytopenia
- **Consumptive coagulopathy** (eg DIC, significant haemorrhage)
- **Prophylactic transfusion** in patients with thrombocytopenia due to bone marrow failure, chemotherapy or radiotherapy
- **Prophylactic or therapeutic transfusion** in patients with primary platelet function disorders

Platelet concentrates should be ABO-group compatible. Anti-D immunoglobulin should be given to pre-menopausal RhD-negative women to prevent sensitisation.

Granulocytes

- Shelf-life is very short – 24 hours at room temperature
- Prepared from a single donor or a pooled collection

Fresh frozen plasma (FFP)

- Prepared by centrifugation of donor whole blood within 6 hours of collection and frozen at –30 °C
- Contains all coagulation factors
- Shelf life is 12 months at –30 °C
- Unit volume is about 250 mL (use at a dose rate of 10–15 mL/kg initially)
- Should be used within 1 hour of thawing
- Also high in sodium, glucose and citrate
- Cryoprecipitate is produced by the slow thawing of FFP; this is rich in factors VIII and XIII, fibrinogen, and vWF
- Individual clotting factors, immunoglobulins, and plasma proteins may be isolated from plasma

Indications for FFP transfusion

- **Prophylaxis or treatment of haemorrhage** in patients with specific coagulation factor deficiencies for which the specific factor is unavailable
- **DIC** – in conjunction with cryoprecipitate and platelets
- **Haemorrhage secondary to over-anticoagulation** with warfarin (treatment with vitamin K or prothrombin complex and factor VII may be more effective)
- **Following replacement of large volumes of blood** (eg > 4 units) where coagulation abnormalities often occur (guided by APTT)
- **Thrombotic thrombocytopenic purpura**
- **Correction of intrinsic clotting disorder** (eg liver coagulopathy) prior to invasive test or surgery

FFP is not indicated in hypovolaemia, plasma exchange, nutritional support and immunodeficiency states.

Group-compatible FFP should be used to prevent Rh immunisation. RhD-compatible FFP should be used in pre-menopausal women.

Albumin solutions

Albumin should not be used as a general purpose plasma volume expander; it has no proven benefit over other colloid solutions. In addition it should not be used as parenteral nutrition, or in impaired protein production or chronic protein loss disorders.

The only proven indication for the administration of 20% albumin is diuretic-resistant oedema in hypoproteinaemic patients.

Coagulation factors

- **Cryoprecipitate:** used in haemorrhagic disorders with a fibrinogen deficiency (eg DIC)
- **Factor VIII concentrate:** for treatment of haemophilia A and von Willebrand's disease
- **Factor IX concentrate:** contains factors IX, X, and XI. It is used in the treatment of haemophilia B and congenital deficiencies of factors X and XI. When combined with factor VII concentrate it is more effective than FFP in the treatment of severe haemorrhage due to excessive warfarinisation and liver disease
- **Other specific coagulation factors**: are available including anticoagulant factors, protein C and antithrombin III

Pharmacological ways to minimise use of blood products

Aprotinin: haemostatic agent; precise mechanism of action unknown; shown to decrease re-operation due to bleeding in cardiac surgery
Tranexamic acid/ε-aminocaproic acid: lysine analogues that inhibit fibrinolysis
Desmopressin (DDAVP): analogue of vasopressin which elevates factor VIII levels and promotes platelet aggregation (NB: can cause vasodilation and hypotension)
Erythropoietin (EPO): renal hormone that induces red cell progenitor proliferation and differentiation; it can be used to raise haematocrit pre-op but there are concerns about thrombotic side effects

Autologous transfusion

Concerns over the potential complications associated with blood transfusions mean that auto-transfusion has become more popular. There are three methods of administering an autologous transfusion:

- **Pre-deposit:** blood is taken from the patient in the weeks prior to admission for elective surgery
- **Haemodilution:** blood is taken immediately prior to surgery and then re-introduced post-operatively
- **Intraoperative:** blood lost during the operation is processed and re-infused immediately (eg cell saver). Contraindications are exposure of the blood to a site of infection, or the possibility of contamination with malignant cells

Autologous transfusion (by the first two methods) is contraindicated in patients with active infection, unstable angina, aortic stenosis, and severe hypertension. Due to patient restriction and high administration costs, auto-transfusion has a limited role in the UK although it is used extensively overseas (especially in areas with high risks of viral transmission).

3.3 ADVERSE EFFECTS OF BLOOD TRANSFUSION

In a nutshell ...

Adverse effects of blood transfusion may be classified by:

Timescale (early vs late)
Volume (complications of large volume transfusion)
Repetition of transfusion

Early complications

- Immunological complications
  - Incompatible red cells (acute haemolytic reaction)
  - Incompatible white cells (pyrexia)
  - Incompatible platelets (purpura)
  - Reaction to plasma (anaphylaxis)
- Fluid overload
- Transfusion related lung injury (TRALI)

Late complications

- Infection
- Delayed hypersensitivity reaction
- Volume complications: the effects of massive transfusion
- Citrate toxicity
- Acidosis
- Hypocalcaemia
- Hyperkalaemia
- Hypothermia
- Clotting abnormalities
- Repetitive transfusion complications
- Iron overload

Early complications of blood transfusion – Immunological complications

Incompatible red cells

The mortality associated with the transfusion of blood products is around 1 per 100 000 units transfused. ABO incompatibility is the most common cause of death and is predominately due to clerical error.

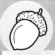

Immediate haemolytic transfusion reactions

- Most severe haemolytic transfusion reactions are due to ABO incompatibility
- 5–10 mL of blood is sufficient to cause a reaction
- Symptoms: rigors, substernal pain, restlessness
- Signs: fever, hypotension, bleeding, haemoglobinuria, oliguria, jaundice
- Rhesus incompatibility does not cause complement activation and is usually milder

Delayed haemolytic transfusion reactions

- Typically occurs 5–10 days after transfusion
- Occurs in approximately 1 in 500 transfusions
- Due to a secondary response; occurs in patients who have been immunised to a foreign antigen by a previous transfusion or pregnancy, but in whom tests prior to the transfusion do not detect the low antibody concentration
- Signs are minimal: unexplained pyrexia, jaundice, unexplained drop in Hb (anaemia), urobilinogenuria
- Management includes:
  - Blood film (shows spherocytosis or reticulocytosis)
  - Direct antiglobulin test
  - Check LFTs, clotting and red cell antibody screens

Incompatible white cells

- Febrile reactions
- Relatively common in patients who have had previous transfusions or have been pregnant
- Symptoms: facial flushing and fever shortly after commencing the transfusion
- Due to the recipient's leucocyte antibodies complexing with donor leucocytes and causing the release of pyrogens from monocytes and granulocytes
- Most reactions respond to slowing the transfusion and giving aspirin or paracetamol

Incompatible platelets

Post-transfusion purpura may occur in patients who have been previously sensitised to a foreign platelet antigen. On subsequent exposure they mount a secondary response which causes destruction of the patient's own platelets.

Adverse reactions to plasma

- Urticaria results from a patient's IgE antibody complexing with a protein present in the donor's plasma; it usually responds to slowing the transfusion rate and administering an antihistamine
- Anaphylactic reactions rarely occur; they are usually due to anti-IgA antibodies in the patient's plasma binding to normal IgA in the donor's plasma; the incidence of anti-IgA individuals is about 1 in 1000

Transfusion-related acute lung injury (TRALI)

This is the result of incompatibility between donor antibodies and recipient granulocytes.

- Clinical picture similar to ARDS
- Can occur 30 minutes to several days following transfusion
- Fever, dyspnoea, cough
- CXR: shadowing in peri-hilar and lower lung fields
- Treat as for ARDS

Late complications of blood transfusion

Infectious complications

Infective risks associated with blood transfusion

- Hepatitis viruses (B and C)
- HIV
- Syphilis
- Variant Creutzfeldt–Jakob disease (vCJD)
- CMV
- Parvovirus
  - Can cause aplastic crisis in a patient with sickle cell anaemia
- Bacteria
  - Very uncommon
  - Incidence less than 1 in 1 million units
  - *Yersinia enterocolitica* and *Pseudomonas* spp. are the most common
  - Usually caused by delayed administration of donated blood (when stored at room temperature, blood is an excellent culture medium)
- Parasites
  - Recent travel to regions where malaria is endemic is a contraindication to blood donation
  - *Plasmodium malariae* has a long incubation period so a few cases of transfusion-related malaria still occur

Screening of donations

- **Anti-HCV and anti-HbsAg:** incidence of hepatitis B transmission is about 1 in 200 000 units transfused; the risk of hepatitis C transmission is between 1 in 150 000 and 1 in 200 000
- **Anti-HIV 1 and anti-HIV 2:** since the 1980s all blood has been screened for HIV. Some patients (eg haemophiliacs) who received regular transfusion before this time have been infected. Risk of transmission is now less than 1 in 2 million units

- **Syphilis**
- **vCJD** is a prion disease and the transmissible element (the prion) has been found in leucocytes. All blood for transfusion from 2000 onwards is now leucocyte depleted

Complications associated with massive transfusion

This is defined as transfusion of the total blood volume in < 24 hours. It can result in:

- Cardiac abnormalities (ventricular arrhythmias) due to low temperature, high potassium concentration and excess citrate with low calcium concentration
- ARDS/acute lung injury
- DIC

Citrate toxicity

- Neonates and hypothermic patients find it difficult to excrete citrate
- Citrate binds ionised calcium and potentially lowers serum calcium levels also
- Need cardiac monitoring

Acidosis

- Lactic acid produced by red cell glycolysis
- Can exacerbate acidosis of the acutely shocked patient
- Transfusion usually improves acidosis due to reversal of hypoxia and improved tissue perfusion

Hypocalcaemia

- Citrate normally rapidly metabolised so effects not normally seen
- Corrected by 10% calcium gluconate if patient has an abnormal ECG

Hyperkalaemia

- Plasma potassium content of blood increases with its storage
- More problematic during massive transfusion

Hypothermia

- From rapid transfusion of stored blood
- Use blood warmers

Clotting abnormalities

- Lack of platelets and clotting factors in stored blood
  - Give FFP during massive transfusions
  - Consider platelets if level < 50×10^9/L
- DIC

Complications associated with repetitive transfusions

When patients undergo repetitive transfusions they may develop antibodies to lesser known blood groups. It is therefore important if the patient has undergone multiple transfusions (either in the past or present admission) to indicate this on the request card so that direct compatibility between donor and recipient blood can be made. This minimises the risks of transfusion reactions. Multiple antibodies can make the patient very difficult to cross-match.

Miscellaneous complications of blood transfusion

- Fluid overload
- Air embolus
- Iron overload
- Immunosuppression. There is some evidence that blood transfusion results in a poorer prognosis in patients with colorectal cancer
- Graft versus host disease (GVHD) – immunodeficient patients at risk

Section 4
Lymphoreticular malignancy

4.1 LEUKAEMIA

In a nutshell ...

Leukaemias are a group of neoplastic disorders of white blood cells. The cells replace the bone marrow and may spill over into the blood or infiltrate other organs. The leukaemias can be divided into:

Myeloid or lymphoid
Acute (blastic) or chronic

	Myeloid	Lymphoid
Acute	**Acute myelogenous leukaemia (AML)** Group of neoplastic disorders of the haematopoietic precursor cells of the bone marrow	**Acute lymphocytic leukaemia (ALL)** Malignant proliferation of lymphoblasts
Chronic	**Chronic myelogenous leukaemia (CML)** Group characterised by an uncontrolled proliferation of granulocytes	**Chronic lymphocytic leukaemia (CLL)** Monoclonal expansion of lymphocytes

Clinical features of leukaemia

Presentation depends on whether the condition is acute or chronic (chronic are often asymptomatic but may have an acute 'blastic' phase or crisis, eg CML). In general there are:

Constitutional symptoms

- Malaise
- Weakness
- Fever
- Polyarthritis

Bone marrow failure causing pancytopenia

- Anaemia
- Infection (neutropenia)
- Oral ulceration and gingival overgrowth
- Bleeding (thrombocytopenia)

Leukaemic infiltration

- Bone pain
- CNS symptoms (eg cranial nerves, cord compression)
- Splenomegaly
- Hepatomegaly
- Lymphadenopathy

Pathology of leukaemia

A clone of malignant cells may arise at any stage of maturation in either the lymphoid, myeloid, or pluripotential stages. Aetiology is thought to be:

- **Genetic:** correlations seen in twin studies and Down syndrome; the Philadelphia chromosome is seen characteristically in CML
- **Environmental**: viruses, radiation exposure, chemicals, drugs (eg alkylating chemotherapeutic agents)

Diagnosis of leukaemia

There are characteristic cells in blood and bone marrow (BM).

- **ALL:** characterised by a homogeneous infiltrate of at least 30% lymphoblasts; usually small with scant cytoplasm, no granules, and indistinct nucleolus
- **AML:** BM aspirate shows blast cells of myeloid origin. Multiple large nucleoli, delicate chromatin, grey-blue cytoplasm, and Auer rods (presence of Auer rods is virtually diagnostic of AML)
- **CLL:** BM infiltration exceeds 30% lymphocytes, which are mature with less than 55% atypical or blast forms. The nuclei are round, cytoplasm is scant, chromatin is compact, nucleoli are inconspicuous, and mitotic figures are rare
- **CML:** BM is hypercellular, with expansion of the myeloid cell line (ie neutrophils, eosinophils, basophils) and its progenitor cells

Specific forms of leukaemia

Acute lymphocytic leukaemia (ALL)

- Predominantly a disease of childhood (occurrence in adults has worse prognosis)
- May be pre-B cell, T cell, or null cell type
- Tends to present with bone pain or pancytopenia due to BM infiltration with malignant cells
- Often there is neutropenia and fever
- Treated with chemotherapy. Remission occurs in 65–85%. Bone marrow transplant is considered for relapsing disease (eg allogeneic sibling donor or unrelated)

Acute myelogenous leukaemia (AML)

- Increasing incidence with age (median 65 years)
- More common in men
- Long-term complication of previous chemotherapy (eg for lymphoma)
- Tends to present with pancytopenia and hepatosplenomegaly
- Treatment with chemotherapy +/– BM transplant

Chronic lymphocytic leukaemia (CLL)

- Usually > 40 years
- 25% leukaemias
- Twice as common in men
- Presents with lymphadenopathy
- 99% are B cell malignancies (1% T cell)
- Staging relates to presence of BM failure and correlates well with survival

Chronic myelogenous leukaemia (CML)

- Commonly occurs age 40–50
- Slight male preponderance
- 15% leukaemias
- Presents with leucocytosis and splenomegaly
- Constitutional symptoms common
- Has three phases: chronic (responsive to treatment), accelerating or transitional (unresponsive to treatment) and blastic phase (pre-terminal)

4.2 LYMPHOMA

In a nutshell ...

Lymphoma is a cancer of the reticuloendothelial system
Lymphoma may be sub-classified into Hodgkin's disease and non-Hodgkin's lymphoma
Hodgkin's disease predominantly affects the young and generally has a good prognosis
Non-Hodgkin's lymphoma generally affects the middle-aged and elderly and has a poor prognosis

Hodgkin's lymphoma (Hodgkin's disease)

Demographics of Hodgkin's lymphoma

- Common in males
- Young adults

Clinical features of Hodgkin's lymphoma

- Painless progressive lymph node enlargement (cervical/supraclavicular)
- Malaise, fever, weight loss, pruritus
- SVC obstruction
- Bone pain (secondaries)
- Splenomegaly, hepatomegaly

Pathology of Hodgkin's lymphoma

- Must have Reed–Sternberg (RS) cells
- Rubbery nodes
- Spreads to bone and liver

Rye classification of Hodgkin's lymphoma

1	Lymphocyte predominant	15%
2	Nodular sclerosing	40%
3	Mixed cellularity	30%
4	Lymphocyte depleted	15%

The prognosis worsens from 1 to 4

Staging of Hodgkin's lymphoma

Based on the Ann Arbour classification:

A Absence of systemic symptoms (ie weight loss, fever, anaemia)
B Presence of above symptoms

I Confined to one lymph node site
II In more than one lymph node site but all on one side of diaphragm
III Nodes above and below diaphragm
IV Spread beyond lymphatic system (eg liver and bone)

Diagnosis of Hodgkin's lymphoma

- Node excision biopsy
- CXR: mediastinal nodes
- IVU: retroperitoneal nodes compress renal calyces
- CT scan

Staging laparotomy is now rarely used due to improved imaging techniques.

Treatment of Hodgkin's lymphoma

- Stage I: radiotherapy
- Stages II–IV: combination chemotherapy

80% cure rate in good prognostic groups (ie lymphocyte-predominant stage I).

Non-Hodgkin's lymphoma (NHL)

NHLs are tumours originating from lymphoid tissues, mainly of lymph nodes. They are a progressive clonal expansion of B cells (85%) or T cells, natural killer (NK) cells or macrophages. This is a very diverse group of conditions, each with distinct and different clinical features.

- Usually present in patients aged > 50 but some aggressive NHLs can be seen in children
- Classification is based on morphology and grade (low, medium, high)
- Staging is based on the Ann Arbour stages discussed above

Treatment consists of chemotherapy +/– radiotherapy of the involved field. BM transplant may be considered for relapse.

Poor prognostic factors include:

- Age > 60 years
- More than one region affected
- Stage > II
- Longer time for response to chemotherapy (eg more than three cycles)

4.3 MULTIPLE MYELOMA

In a nutshell ...

Multiple myeloma is a neoplastic proliferation of plasma cells resulting in gradual replacement of the bone marrow with cancer cells.

It causes pancytopenia, bone symptoms, hypercalcaemia and renal impairment.

Multiple myeloma is a malignant proliferation of monoclonal plasma cells with production of an individual paraprotein. Common in the 65–70 age group with a male to female ratio of 3: 2.

Clinical features of multiple myeloma

- BM replacement with proliferating plasma cells causes pancytopenia (anaemia, bleeding secondary to thrombocytopenia)
- Lytic bone lesions (risks of bone pain, pathological fractures, hypercalcaemia, spinal cord compression)
- Soft tissue masses
- Over-production of antibodies causes:
  - Renal impairment
  - Hyperviscosity
  - Amyloidosis
- Impaired humoral immunity (susceptible to infection with encapsulated organisms)
- Asymptomatic patients may be identified through screening (consider this diagnosis if total protein level is > albumin + globulin)

Pathology of multiple myeloma

Aetiology is thought to be a combination of:

- Genetic factors
- Environmental exposure to chemicals in agriculture
- Radiation exposure

Investigating multiple myeloma

- FBC – normal, or evidence of pancytopenia
- ESR – virtually always high
- U&Es (evidence of renal failure)
- Uric acid (may be normal or raised)
- 24-hour urine collection for Bence–Jones protein (λ light chains)
- Plasma electrophoresis for paraprotein band
- β2-microglobulin and CRP are prognostic indicators
- Skeletal X-rays or targeted MRI (osteoporosis, crush fractures, osteolytic lesions)
- Pepper-pot skull is characteristic

Classification of multiple myeloma

This is based on the monoclonal product

- 55% IgG
- 25% IgA
- 20% light chain disease

Staging of multiple myeloma

- **Stage I** involves *all* of the following:
  - Haemoglobin > 10 g/dL
  - Calcium < 12 mg/dL
  - Radiograph showing normal bones or solitary plasmacytoma
  - Low M protein values (IgG < 5 g/dL, IgA < 3 g/dL, urine < 4 g/24h)
- **Stage III** involves *any one* of the following:
  - Haemoglobin < 8.5 g/dL
  - Calcium level > 12 mg/dL
  - Radiograph showing advanced lytic bone disease
  - High M protein value (IgG > 7 g/dL, IgA > 5 g/dL, urine > 12 g/24 hours)
- **Stage II** is anything in-between

These three stages are subclassified according to renal function (A = normal creatinine; B = elevated creatinine).

Mean survival

- 60 months for stage I
- 42 months for stage II
- 23 months for stage III

Diagnosis of multiple myeloma

- Monoclonal band on plasma electrophoresis
- Bence–Jones protein in urine
- Plasma cells on BM biopsy
- Osteolytic bone lesions

Cannot diagnose on the basis of paraproteinaemia alone.

Treatment of multiple myeloma

- Myeloablative therapy (high-dose radiotherapy and chemotherapy) with autotransplantation of BM stem cells
- Plasmapheresis for renal failure
- Hydration and bisphosphonates for hypercalcaemia
- Radiotherapy for bone pain (myeloma is highly radiosensitive)
- Vaccinate against encapsulated organisms

Chapter 5

Trauma

Claire Ritchie Chalmers

Section 1
Overview of trauma

1.1 HISTORICAL PERSPECTIVE

Trauma care and surgery have been inextricably entwined since the beginnings of society. Battlefield surgeons such as Ambrose Pare (1510–1590) used empiric observation, common sense, and 'hands on' personal experience to improve the treatment of battle wounds during the Napoleonic wars. The plastic surgeon Archibald Hector McIndoe (1900–1960) improved the treatment of burns in RAF pilots during World War II. He noted that those who ditched in the sea had less scarring and infection of their burn sites, leading to the use of saline soaks instead of tannins. Both men found that conventional practice was inadequate and sought to improve care and techniques for the sake of their patients and for the common good.

In 1976 an orthopaedic surgeon crashed his light aircraft in Nebraska, resulting in the death of his wife and injuring his children. The emergency care that he and his family received was inadequate and this became the impetus for the development of the Advanced Trauma Life Support (ATLS) training course.

The Royal College of Surgeons of England was one of the first bodies outside of the USA to implement ATLS training (in November 1988). This system has provided a framework and approach to acute trauma care so that trauma team personnel can communicate and prioritise in a similar way, allowing parallel or simultaneous treatment in the multiple-injury patient, by a co-ordinated team approach. This has increased the speed with which injuries are identified and treated, making the most use of the 'golden hour', in order to improve survival and patient outcome.

1.2 THE TRI-MODAL DISTRIBUTION OF DEATH

In a nutshell ...

Mortality from trauma can be considered in three phases – immediate, early, and late (see Fig. 1.2a). 50% of deaths caused by trauma occur in the first 10 minutes after the accident.

- **Immediate phase death:** these deaths are almost always unpreventable. They include massive brain injuries, or great vessel injuries (eg aortic avulsion associated with a fall from a height), airway occlusion, cord transection or exsanguination
- **Early phase death:** occurs within the first few minutes to hours when the opportunity for prompt and appropriate diagnosis and intervention can prevent loss of life or limb (the so-called 'golden hour'). The ATLS system mainly addresses this phase of care, and emphasises the need for rapid assessment and resuscitation
- **Late phase death:** occurs days to weeks after the injury, during which time deaths can occur due to sepsis and multiple organ system failure, or complications arising as a consequence of the initial injury or surgery. The quality of care in phases 1 and 2 will obviously have an impact on mortality in phase 3, and on overall outcome

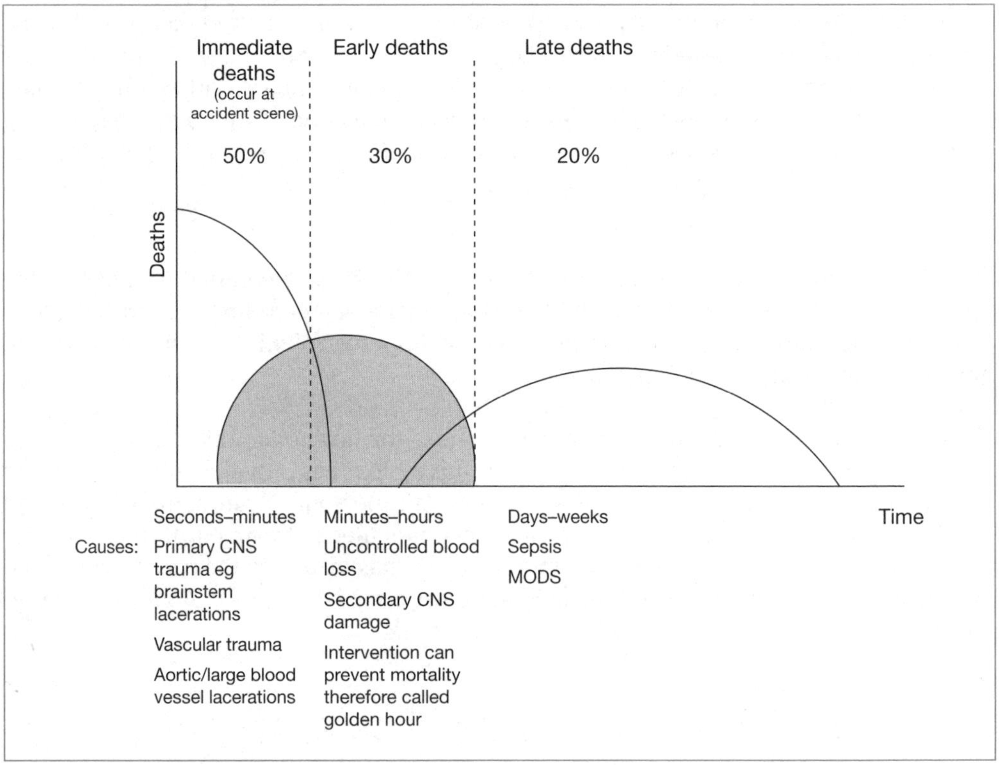

Figure 1.2a *Mortality from trauma – tri-modal distribution*

1.3 PRE-HOSPITAL CARE

In a nutshell ...

The primary role of pre-hospital care is to:
- Temporarily stabilise the patient
- Expedite transport of the severely injured patient to the site of definitive treatment

Pre-hospital treatment is driven by rapid assessment and the principles of ATLS.

Pre-hospital care in the UK is delivered in a variety of ways depending upon illness or injury severity. These include:

- **NHS Direct:** this scheme provides information via the telephone or internet from senior nurses on minor illness or injury with the emphasis on self care. Patients may be diverted to primary care or the ambulance service if necessary
- **Minor injury units:** care is delivered by emergency nurse practitioners and these centres have links with local A&E departments and radiology services
- **Primary care:** general practitioners may manage minor injury
- **Road ambulance service:** the emergency ambulance service usually mobilised by telephone (999) from either the patient or a witness at the scene. Vehicle tracking is used to mobilise the nearest resource, and clinical information is relayed to the ambulance team. Calls are prioritised according to clinical need (A for life-threatening, B for serious but not life-threatening, and C for neither serious nor life-threatening) by computer software used in the ambulance control room. Road ambulances are usually manned by a paramedic and a technician, and an ambulance officer or manager may also be sent to manage the scene at complex incidents. Clinical care at the scene is delivered in accordance with national clinical protocols. Clinical information is relayed by ambulance staff at the scene to the proposed A&E department to allow advance preparation of facilities and staff to receive the patient (eg preparation of the resus room and trauma call). Patients are usually delivered to the nearest A&E department and some may subsequently require secondary transfer to a tertiary referral centre for definitive care
- **Air ambulance:** air ambulances are primarily staffed by suitably trained paramedics and technicians, but in some regions these teams also include trained senior doctors and nurses (eg the Helicopter Emergency Medical Service (HEMS) in London)
- **Mobile medical teams (MMTs):** these teams consist of trained medical personnel, often from the A&E department of the nearest hospital, or doctors trained by organisations such as the British Association for Immediate Care (BASICS). They may be mobilised to entrapments or major incidents. Extrication requires close co-ordination between medical and fire services

The techniques of pre-hospital care vary from country to country. In the US, pre-hospital care personnel are taught to 'scoop and run' with the aim of delivering the patient to the place of definitive care as quickly as possible. This may involve bypass of the local facilities and targeting of tertiary facilities (eg delivery of cardiothoracic injuries direct to a cardiothoracic unit). In France, pre-hospital care involves the mobilisation of intensive care units to the scene with more emphasis on stabilising the patient before transfer.

The value of information obtained from the emergency agencies in the field cannot be underestimated. Detailed and early information allows mobilisation of the trauma team, including laboratory services, porters, and the X-ray department. Advance knowledge of the number of casualties and the type and extent of injuries allows for preparation of the appropriate equipment (such as chest drains, thoracotomy sets and O-negative blood), so they are available as soon as the patient arrives. Ideally, continual updates should be provided by the emergency services so that the receiving team is appropriately prepared.

Principles of immediate care

The principles of immediate care have been outlined by the American College of Surgeons Committee on Trauma (ACS-COT) in a format similar to ATLS. A basic outline is shown below:

- **Assess potential safety issues** at the scene and take steps to make it as safe as possible
- **Quickly assess the patient:** observe vital signs and level of consiousness, determine the nature of accident and likely mechanism of injuries

Indications of potential significant trauma

- **Penetrating injury** to thorax, abdomen or head
- **Major bony injury:** two or more proximal long bone fractures; pelvic fracture; traumatic amputation proximal to wrist or ankle
- **Burns** involving more than 15% of the body surface area or to face and potentially to airway
- **Evidence of high-energy impact:**
  - Fall from a height (more than 6 metres)
  - Pedestrian in a road traffic accident (hit at more than 20 m.p.h. or thrown by impact)
  - Car occupant in a road traffic accident (unrestrained; speed greater than 20 m.p.h.; intrusion into passenger compartment of > 30 cm; ejection of passenger from vehicle; roll-over of vehicle; death of another car occupant; extrication time > 20 minutes)

Pre-hospital resuscitation follows ATLS principles:

- **C-spine immobilisation:** in-line immobilisation with a hard collar, sand-bags and tape
- **Airway management:** can be difficult. Can often be maintained with basic measures. Intubation without anaesthesia and rapid sequence induction is ill advised as it can induce vomiting and raise intracranial pressure
- **Breathing:** give oxygen
- **Circulation:** haemorrhage should be controlled with direct pressure; ensure good venous access before releasing from vehicle. Fluid resuscitation should be given to a systolic blood pressure of 90 mmHg
- **Disability:** fractured limbs should be splinted and the patient prepared for transport
- **Analgesia:** can be achieved with ketamine or Entonox™ (contraindicated if possibility of pneumothorax or basal skull fracture)

Initial hospital care

Most A&E departments in the UK that deal with trauma cases have a designated area for receiving trauma cases. This is obviously essential for rapid access to specialist equipment and services.

The table below indicates the minimum resources that should be readily available in a centre receiving trauma cases.

ESSENTIAL RESOURCES FOR TRAUMA MANAGEMENT

Airway management	Circulatory support	Infrastructure
Laryngoscope	Large bore cannulae	Rapid communication links
ET tubes	Warmed crystalloid solutions	Laboratory support
Fully stocked anaesthetic trolley	O-negative blood	Radiology – immediate access
Suction	Giving sets	Designated trauma team of medical personnel
Oxygen	Blood sampling equipment	

1.4 TRIAGE AND MAJOR INCIDENTS

Triage

In a nutshell ...

'Triage is the sorting of patients based on the need for treatment and the available resources to provide that treatment' (definition from the ATLS manual).

Triage is a system for dealing with a large number of casualties. The aim is to offer the most medical treatment to the largest number of patients, resulting in the best possible outcome.

To be of use triage needs to be **quick**, **efficient**, and **reproducible**. It should involve continual re-assessment of patients by appropriate medical staff, with regular re-adjustment of patient priorities.

There are usually two types of triage.

When there is sufficient treatment capacity to deal with multiple casualties, patients with life threatening and multisystem injuries are treated first. Essentially this sort of triage occurs in the A&E department all the time – as patients present to the department they are rapidly assessed and prioritised by a member of the nursing team. The categories are based on order of priority (eg accidents prioritised 1 to 5; medical emergencies prioritised 1 to 5). All patients in category 1 are seen first, followed by those in category 2, and so on.

When there is insufficient treatment capacity to deal with multiple casualties, patients with the greatest chance of survival are treated first. This form of triage was originally invented by the military to deal with multiple battlefield casualties. Triage in this situation is usually performed by personnel who assess casualties without giving treatment, often by categorising them into life-threatening or limb-threatening, urgent, serious, and minor groups.

Major incidents

All hospitals have a major incident plan (MAJAX) that details management within each department should a major incident occur, such as management in A&E and creating bed space in the ITU. In general, all available personnel are asked to congregate in the A&E department where they will be assigned tasks by the coordinator.

1.5 TRAUMA SEVERITY SCORING

In a nutshell ...

Trauma scoring systems may be used for:

Communication about the status of individual patients
Monitoring improvement or deterioration in an individual
Prognostic information about an individual
Triage of multiple casualties

They include the:

Injury severity score (ISS)
Revised trauma score (RTS)
Trauma score–injury severity score (TRISS)

Injury severity score (ISS)

- Anatomical description
- Score of 0–6 is given to each body region depending on severity of injury; the three highest scores are squared and added together to produce the ISS score
- Disadvantage: the score is static (needs absolute diagnosis before score can be calculated)
- Subjective

Revised trauma score (RTS)

- Physiological description
- Score calculated using the GCS, respiratory rate, and systolic BP
- Flexible (varies with patient's progress)
- Objective (little inter-observer variability)

Trauma score–injury severity score (TRISS)

- Combined ISS and RTS scoring
- Also includes age of patient and mechanism of injury (ie penetrating or blunt)
- Indicator of patient prognosis

Section 2
Injury and shock

2.1 THE BIOMECHANICS OF INJURY

In a nutshell ...

In all cases injury results from a transfer of energy to the tissues.

Trauma may be sustained by means of:
- Blunt trauma
- Penetrating injury
- Blast injury
- Deceleration injury
- Crush injury
- Burn injury
- Hypothermia and hyperthermia
- Barotrauma

In all cases injury results from a transfer of energy to the tissues. This energy travels as a shock wave that travels at different speeds through air, fluid, and tissues of different densities. Maximal disruption occurs at a site of interface between these media due to differential compression and re-expansion. Objects travelling at speed (eg bullets) cause cavitation of tissues as the tissue particles absorb energy and move away from the site of impact.

Blunt trauma

Road-traffic accidents (RTAs) are the most common cause of blunt trauma and are usually associated with simultaneous head and neck (50%), chest (20%) or abdominal and pelvic trauma (25%).

A careful history of the mechanism of injury, combined impact speed, whether a seat belt was worn or an airbag inflated, whether pedestrian or motorcyclist, will enable the trauma surgeon to develop an idea of which areas of the body and underlying organs are at risk. Investigations are useful but should not delay an essential laparotomy, which is necessary in about 10% of blunt trauma patients.

The physical examination should include:

- **Inspection:** bruising, seat belt marks and distension may all denote underlying injury
- **Palpation:** signs of peritonism due to blood, urine or faeces in the peritoneal cavity
- **Percussion:** a crude indicator of the presence of free fluid
- **Auscultation:** essential in evaluating the chest

Penetrating injury

These may be due to blades, glass or metal fragments, shrapnel, bullets and so may be associated with other mechanisms of trauma.

- May be solitary or multiple injuries
- Cause damage only in the direct area (eg stabbing) or in a cone related to explosive force and speed of travel (eg high-velocity vs low-velocity bullets)
- The process of cavitation associated with high-velocity missiles sucks dirt, clothing and skin into the wound, increasing the risk of secondary infection

Blast injury

A blast injury is due to an explosion (eg gas, chemical, bomb) and so has multiple mechanisms of injury:

- **Pressure wave:** travels faster than the speed of sound and can cause rupture of air-filled structures eg tympanic membrane, lungs ('blast-lung syndrome'), bowel
- **Penetrating injury** from shrapnel
- **Falls** (the body may be thrown by the blast wind)
- **Crush injuries** from disruption of the environment eg falling masonry
- **Burns** eg thermal, chemical

Deceleration injury

Occurs on impact in vehicular accidents and falls from a height. Relatively mobile structures avulse from the site at which they are anchored:

- Cervical spine
- Brain
- Main bronchus
- Thoracic aorta
- Renal vessels
- Transverse mesocolon

Crush injury

Initial injury plus sustained compression of the tissues causes ischaemia and muscle necrosis.

Crush syndrome may be a feature of any severe injury, which results in ischaemia of large amounts of soft tissue. Results in fluid loss, DIC, and release of myoglobin from muscle (rhabdomyolysis) and toxins from damaged tissue. Can clog the renal tubules causing ATN and renal failure requiring dialysis. Treat with large volumes of fluid, watch urine output and plasma K^+.

Burn injury

In a nutshell ...

A burn is a coagulative necrosis of variable depth. Burns account for 6% of A&E presentations.

Types of burn

- Thermal: the most common
- Chemical: alkali burns are more severe than acidic burns (acidic burns limit their own extent of damage by producing a coagulated barrier)
- Electrical
- Radiation

Burns are categorised by **depth** and **area**. Remember Wallace's Rule of 9s.

Physiological consequences of burns

Local: coagulative necrosis
General: predominantly related to fluid shifts

Management strategies

Initial resuscitation (ABCs)
IV fluid replacement
Protection of the burnt surface and prevention of infection
Surgical intervention

Classification of burns

Depth of burn

Burns should be clinically judged by their depth. Ultimate classification may not be until operative assessment.

A HELPFUL GUIDE TO BURN CLASSIFICATION

	Superficial burns	Deep dermal burns	Full thickness burns
Appearance	Pink and painful Often blistered	Pink-white with reduced blanching No sensation	Black/white Dull to pinprick
Repair	Takes 14 days to heal Heals from adnexal structures outwards	Takes 3–4 weeks to heal Scarring (+/– pigment changes)	Minimal healing from wound edges only Usually needs grafts to cover the site

Area of burn

Wallace's Rule of 9s is used to estimate area of significant burn. Do not include areas of simple erythema.

Wallace's Rule of 9s

Head 9%
Arms 9% each
Legs 18% each (9% anterior surface, 9% posterior surface)
Trunk 36%
Perineum 1%
Palm of hand 1%

A major burn corresponds to total body surface area (TBSA) affected:

- 15% TBSA in adults
- 10% TBSA in children

Physiology of burns

There is coagulative necrosis of tissues exposed to heat or another injurious source. Capillary beds are disrupted, and these then leak plasma into the surrounding interstitium. Damage equates to the time of exposure to the injurious element and – in the case of

Chapter 5

thermal burns – the actual temperature. Thus lower temperatures with longer exposure may cause the same amount of damage as higher temperatures that are of short duration. Response to a major burn is generalised, with global oedema (not just in the vicinity of the burn itself) and profound hypovolaemic shock due to fluid loss.

Physiological consequences of burn injury

Hypovolaemic shock
Consequent reduction in cardiac output
Increased peripheral vascular resistance

Increased haematocrit
Due to loss of plasma

Increased metabolism
Increased oxygen demand
Increased nitrogen loss

Increased levels of cortisol
Increased catabolism
Increased gluconeogenesis

Management of burns

Initial resuscitation of the patient with burns

Follow the ABCDE protocol. Beware of impending airway compromise with inhalational injury indicated by the following signs:

- Facial or oropharynx burns
- Hoarseness or stridor
- Soot in the nostrils or sputum
- Expiratory bronchi
- Dysphagia
- Epiglottic swelling with drooling

Secure IV access (may require cut-down). IV fluid resuscitation is essential when the burn exceeds 15% TBSA (consider oral rehydration if less than this). Urinary catheterisation and hourly urine output is essential.

- Take routine venous bloods and ABGs
- Baseline CXR
- Appropriate analgesia

Intravenous fluid replacement formulas

Many formulas are available. The Brooke Army Hospital Formula is used commonly, but requirements should be tailored to each patient. In the first 24 hours give:

- Colloid (plasma, plasma substitutes, dextran) – 0.5 mL/kg/% TBSA of burn IV
- Electrolytes (Ringer's lactate) – 1.5 mL/kg/% TBSA of burn IV
- Water (5% dextrose in water) – 2000 mL IV (less for children)

Half of the above volumes are given in the second 24 hours, after which most patients can drink normally.

Like all other formulas, the physiological response of the patient needs to be taken into account (ie urine output, BP and pulse, respiratory rate and peripheral perfusion) and the volume replacement should be adjusted to these values. Hb and HCT (haematocrit) measured regularly can be a helpful guide to rate of resuscitation. Also:

- Consider blood transfusion (1 unit for each 10% of deep burns)
- Remember analgesia (pain increases catecholamine release which increases catabolism)
- Continual reassessment is essential

When to transfer to the burns unit

- Full thickness burns > 10% TBSA (children 5%)
- Burns involving hands, feet, or perineum
- Respiratory system is involved
- Circumferential burns
- Significant electrical or chemical burns

Transfer is safe only when:
Airway is stable (intubation prior to transfer may be indicated)
Fluid resuscitation is instigated

Protection of the surface and prevention of infection

- Blisters will protect the underlying wound and so should be preserved; the epithelium should be removed if they have already burst
- Apply a sterile non-adherent dressing unless it's a difficult area (eg face, perineum) which is left exposed
- Use sterile gloves and antibacterial agents (eg silver sulfadiazine)

Surgical intervention

- **Partial thickness:** expose to allow wound to dry, thus reducing access by organisms and the subsequent risk of infection. Silver sulfadiazine dressing reduces the number of Gram-negative organisms
- **Deep dermal:** clean and dress and leave undisturbed for 2 weeks. Then shave the wound down to healthy tissues in areas which have not healed and graft if necessary
- **Full thickness:** immediate excision (within 1 week improves survival) and grafting is the aim (if the patient is elderly, grafting is kept to an absolute minimum), allowing the wound a delay to see if it will heal unaided

Allografts and xenografts are useful in the short term, for coverage which reduces the need for analgesia and the risk of infection. Escharotomies performed in any areas of full-thickness circumferential burns; otherwise asphyxia (due to trunk burns) and compartment syndrome (due to limb burns) are inevitable.

See Chapter 1 *Basic Surgical Knowledge and Skills* for further discussion of plastic surgical techniques and skin grafting.

Complications of burns

Local complications of burns

- Scarring
- Infection
  - Usually with endogenous organisms
  - Can lead to multiple organ dysfunction syndrome (MODS)
- Damaged local circulation
  - Decreased immune defences
  - Compromised phagocytosis
  - Decreased chemotaxis

General complications of burns

- Fluid shifts
- Electrolyte disturbances
  - Increased K^+
  - Increased Na^+ (inadequate fluid resuscitation)
  - Decreased Na^+ (dilutional, over-enthusiastic resuscitation)
- Respiratory failure
  - Upper respiratory tract damage as direct result of heat
  - Lower respiratory tract damage (oedema)
  - Decreased surfactant
  - Reduced lung compliance
  - Decreased macrophages
  - Lung parenchyma damage (by toxic products)

- Myonecrosis
  - Commonly seen with electrical burns and some deep burns
  - RBC breakdown
  - Results in haemoglobinuria and rhabdomyolysis with consequent renal failure: causes increase in plasma K^+
  - May exacerbate DIC
- Massive increase in catabolism
  - Resultant huge nitrogen losses
  - Stress ulcers common, therefore feed patients early with high-energy diet
- Pancreatitis
- Acalculus cholecystitis
- Increased risk of pulmonary embolism
- Septic thrombophlebitis: often exacerbated by IV access, therefore limit this access to essential access. CVP lines discouraged

Hypothermia

Hypothermia may be accidental (usually due to environmental exposure) or intentional (eg cardiac bypass).

It is associated with the use of alcohol, illicit drugs, overdoses, psychiatric conditions and major trauma. Symptoms may include:

- **Mild hypothermia (32–35 °C):** lethargy, confusion, amnesia, shivering, loss of co-ordination and fine motor skills, dysarthria
- **Moderate hypothermia (28–32 °C):** delirium, stupor, slowed reflexes, bradycardia
- **Severe hypothermia (< 28 °C):** coma, dilated pupils, dyspnoea, arrhythmia or cardiac arrest

The management of hypothermia occurs in two stages: initial pre-hospital care and definitive hospital management by re-warming.

On scene: reduce further heat loss from evaporation, radiation, conduction, or convection. Remove wet clothing, and replace it with dry blankets or sleeping bags. Move the patient to a sheltered environment. Re-warm with heat packs or skin-to-skin contact.

Definitive management: this is by re-warming. It may be undertaken slowly or rapidly. There is some evidence that in severe hypothermia rapid re-warming provides the best prognosis. Options for re-warming include:

- Warmed blankets and heat lamps
- Heated IV fluids such as saline (fluid temperatures up to 65 °C have been used)
- Heated humidified oxygen
- Warmed gastric, thoracic, or peritoneal lavage
- Cardiopulmonary bypass
- Warm water immersion (Hubbard technique)

Management of arrhythmia or cardiac arrest: defibrillation is ineffective at hypothermic core temperatures. Use intravenous bretylium (if available) followed by extended cardiopulmonary resuscitation (CPR) until active re-warming begins and successful defibrillation is more likely. Death can not be declared until the patient is warm.

Hyperthermia

Hyperthermia occurs when the body loses its ability to respond to heat. Inability to respond to heat manifests as a spectrum of illnesses from heat rash, to heat exhaustion and heat stroke. The normal body response to heat is discussed in Chapter 2 *Infection and Inflammation*.

Heat exhaustion is an acute heat injury with hyperthermia caused by dehydration. It occurs when the body no longer can dissipate heat adequately because of extreme environmental conditions or increased endogenous heat production. It may progress to **heat stroke** when the body's thermoregulatory mechanisms become overwhelmed and fail.

Heat stroke is extreme hyperthermia with thermoregulatory failure. The condition is characterised by serious end-organ damage with universal involvement of the CNS. Heat stroke is defined as pyrexia (> 41 °C) associated with anhidrosis and neurological dysfunction. However, these criteria are not absolute. Heat stroke occurs in two forms:

- **Exertional heat stroke:** usually in young fit individuals undertaking strenuous activity in a hot environment for a prolonged period of time. Anhidrosis is not always a factor. Associated with abdominal and muscular cramping, nausea, vomiting, diarrhoea, headache, dizziness, dyspnoea and weakness. Risk factors include preceding viral infection, dehydration, fatigue, obesity, lack of sleep, poor physical fitness and exercise at altitude
- **Non-exertional heat stroke:** an impaired response to temperature seen in the elderly, chronically ill and very young. Associated with confusion, delirium, hallucinations, seizures and coma

Barotrauma

Barotrauma refers to injuries caused by pressure changes. These may be due to explosions or diving injuries and have been reported after deployment of airbags during RTAs. Barotrauma affects regions of the body that contain air, such as the middle ear and the lungs, perhaps leading to rupture of the eardrum or a pneumothorax. Barotrauma sustained from an explosion may be complicated by other mechanisms of trauma, penetrating or crush injuries, burns and smoke inhalation.

2.2 THE PHYSIOLOGY OF SHOCK

In a nutshell ...

Shock occurs when tissue perfusion is insufficient to meet metabolic requirements and leads to disordered physiology. Shock is characterised by hypotension.

Types of shock

- Hypovolaemic
- Neurogenic
- Cardiogenic
- Septic
- Anaphylactic

In trauma cases, hypotension is always assumed to be hypovolaemia due to haemorrhage, until proven otherwise. This leads to a typical picture of a patient who is cold, pale, clammy, anxious or confused, and peripherally 'shut down'.

Monitored variables in types of shock

	HR	CVP/PAOP	CO	SV	SVR
Hypovolaemic	↑	↓	↓	↓	↑
Cardiogenic	↑	↑	↓	↓	↑
Septic	↑	↓	↑	↓	↓
Tamponade	↑	↑↑	↓	↓	↑
Neurogenic	↓	—	↓	—	↓

Hypovolaemic shock

Pathophysiology of hypovolaemic shock

In hypovolaemic shock the reduction in blood flow leads to decreased tissue perfusion, causing hypoxia and lactic acidosis, both of which lead to further circulatory collapse and the result may be multiple organ dysfunction syndrome (MODS). Haemorrhage is the acute loss of circulating blood volume and is the cause of hypovolaemic shock in trauma patients.

This model of hypovolaemic shock hinges on the fact that acidosis leads to actual cellular destruction, which is caused by dysfunction of the cell membrane's Na^+/K^+ pump in the acidotic environment. Normally, intracellular Na^+ is exchanged for extracellular K^+. When this system fails Na^+ accumulates intracellularly, taking water with it, and causing the cell to swell. The intercellular spaces enlarge as the cells pull away from each other, allowing fluid to escape into the interstitium and disrupting the integrity of the individual organs.

In situations where there is inadequate cardiac output despite fluid replacement, inotropes (such as dopamine, dobutamine or adrenaline/epinephrine) may be considered.

Remember

CO = SV × HR (normal value is 6 litres per minute)

SBP = DBP + PP

CO is cardiac output; SV is stroke volume; HR is heart rate; SBP is systolic blood pressure; DBP is diastolic blood pressure; PP is pulse pressure; PVR is peripheral vascular resistance.

This demonstrates that PP, a major determinant of SBP, is governed in part by the PVR which will be raised due to peripheral vasoconstriction following hypovolaemic insult. Therefore the SBP will appear normal in a situation where the cardiac output may be much reduced. This is especially true in the young fit patient, compensating for the blood loss.

PHYSIOLOGICAL RESPONSES TO HYPOVOLAEMIA

	Class I	Class II	Class III	Class IV
Volume loss (mL)	0–750	750–1500	1500–2000	> 2000
Loss (%)	0–15	15–30	30–40	> 40
Pulse (b.p.m.)	< 100	> 100	> 120	> 140
Blood pressure	Unchanged	Unchanged	Decreased	Decreased
Pulse pressure	Unchanged	Decreased	Decreased	Decreased
Urine output (mL/hour)	> 30	20–30	5–15	Anuric
Respiratory rate (breaths/minute)	14–20	20–30	30–40	> 40
Mental state	Restless	Anxious	Anxious/ confused	Confused/ lethargic
Fluid replacement	Crystalloid	Colloid and crystalloid	Colloid and blood	Colloid and blood

These values refer to the 'average' 70 kg man with a blood volume of 5 litres. Values are irrespective of body fat proportions. Calculate fluid replacement in an obese patient to be the same as the predicted weight, to avoid over-filling.

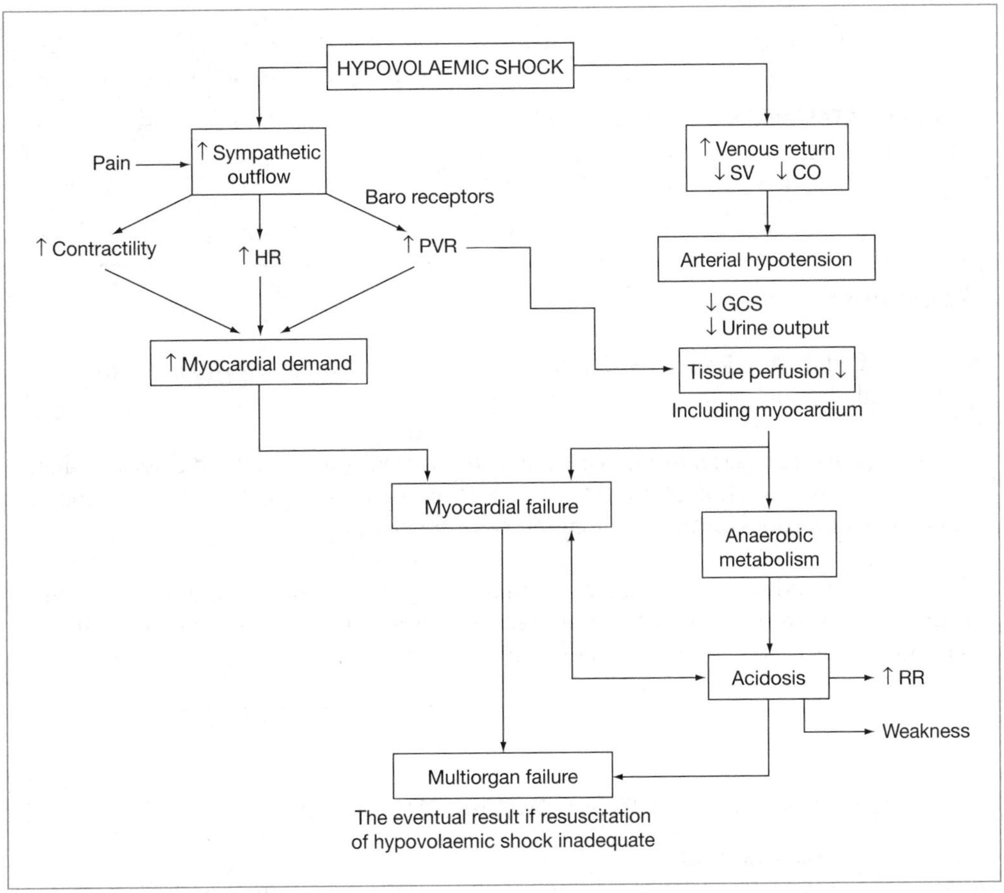

Figure 2.2a *Pathophysiology of hypovolemic shock*

The principles of immediate management of hypovolaemic shock are to stop the bleeding and to replace the volume lost.

1. Control any obvious haemorrhage

Direct pressure
Elevation of injured limb
Head-down tilt

2. Establish IV access

Two 16-gauge cannulae, or if this is not possible:

- Fore-arm antecubital veins
- Cut-down to great saphenous vein
- Intra-osseous access in children (< 6 years) if initial IV access fails

Chapter 5

Central access only after the patient is more stable; this is useful as a guide to fluid replacement after the initial resuscitation but is not an effective route for resuscitation.

3. Follow ATLS guidelines for fluid replacement and identification of cause of hypovolaemia (see sections 3 and 4 of this chapter)

Remember

CVP may be falsely raised in tension pneumothorax, pericardial effusion, air embolus, pericardial effusion, or MI.

Physiological responses may be distorted by β-blockers, coronary heart disease, pacemakers, age, narcotics, anatomical location of injury, pre-hospital fluid replacement, pneumatic anti-shock garment, spinal injury, or head injury.

Transient responders are patients who initially respond favourably to a bolus of fluid with a trend towards normalisation of their physiology but who subsequently deteriorate again. This is an important sign of ongoing blood loss.

Fluid replacement in hypovolaemic shock

Crystalloid versus colloid

There is a great deal of debate about the use of crystalloid or colloid in the initial resuscitation of the patient with hypovolaemic shock. Traditionally in the UK colloid has been used, whereas in the US crystalloid is preferred. The following advice is taken from the ATLS guidelines. Use an initial bolus of 1–2 litres of Ringer's lactate (equivalent to Hartmann's solution). Titrate fluid resuscitation thereafter to response following the initial bolus.

- **Normal saline:** 25% remains in the intravascular compartment. Excess may lead to hyperchloraemic acidosis and sodium overload
- **Haemaccel™, Gelofusine™ and Volplex™** exert greater oncotic pressure than isotonic crystalloid solutions, therefore fluid tends to remain in the intravascular compartment for longer
- **Blood:** if the patient has obviously lost large volumes of blood then blood replacement is indicated, even if the Hb measurement is normal. There is a delay in the fall of serum haemoglobin in acute haemorrhage as it takes time for fluid shifts to occur. Cross-matched blood is rarely available immediately

The patient's response to fluid resuscitation is indicated by improvement of the following signs and evidence of organ perfusion:

- Pulse (see Fig. 2.2b)
- Blood pressure
- Skin colour
- CNS state

Urine output in hypovolaemic shock

This is a sensitive and quantitative indication of progress of resuscitation and reflects end-organ perfusion. A normal urine output reflects that resuscitation has been sufficient to reach the renal autoregulatory threshold, and achieve normal renal blood flow. A urinary catheter can be placed quickly and safely in the trauma patient, in the absence of a urethral injury.

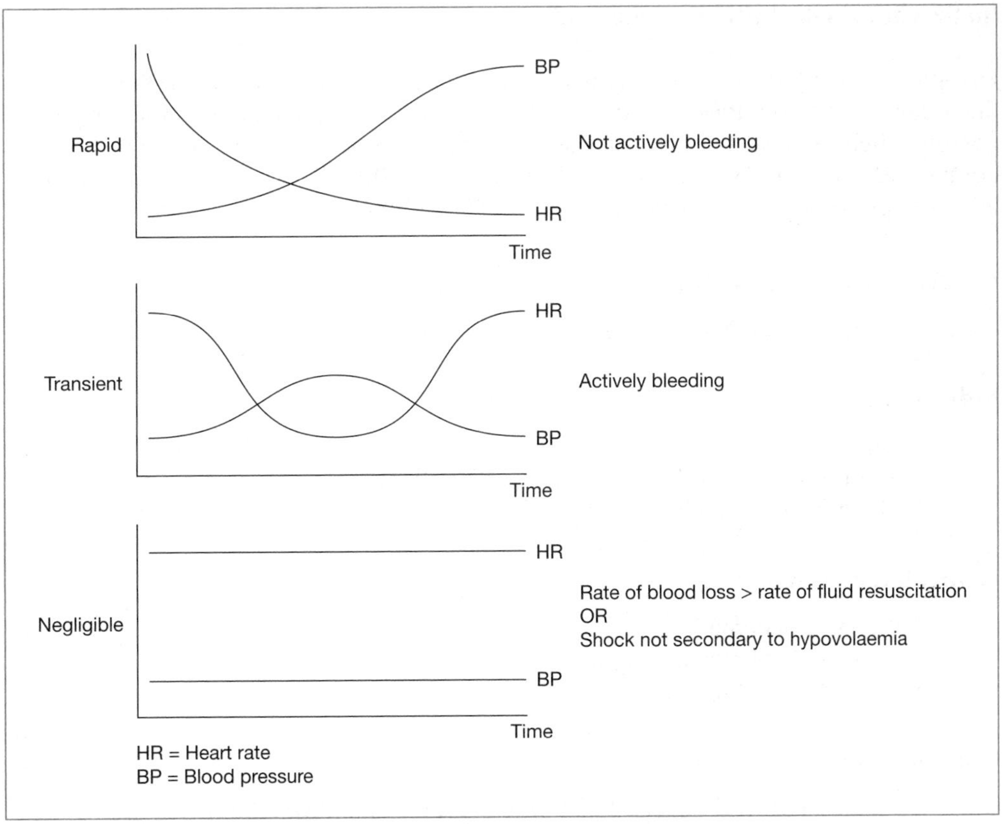

Figure 2.2b *Response to initial fluid resuscitation*

Expect the following values for urine output:

Adult	0.5 mL/kg per hour
Child	1.0 mL/kg per hour
Infant	2.0 mL/kg per hour

Acid–base balance in hypovolaemic shock

Initial respiratory alkalosis occurs due to increased respiratory rate. Later, metabolic acidosis ensues if there is uncompensated tissue hypoperfusion or insufficient fluid replacement leading to anaerobic metabolism. This will be reflected by a lowered pH, a progressive base deficit and low bicarbonate. Adequate fluid resuscitation, oxygen administration and transfusion to maintain adequate oxygen delivery can correct this process.

Occult haemorrhage

'In the chest, in the belly, or on the road'

Possible locations of significant 'hidden haemorrhage' are in the thorax, in the abdomen (including the retroperitoneal space), and pelvic fractures. If there are multiple long bone fractures there may be enough soft tissue haemorrhage to cause hypotensive shock. In compound fractures expect double the blood loss. This illustrates the importance of adequate pre-hospital information and the clinical history.

Pneumatic anti-shock garment (PASG)

For discussion of pelvic fractures see *Orthopaedics* in Book 2.

Indications

- Splinting pelvic fractures with concomitant haemorrhage and hypotension
- Interim support for a shocked patient with abdominal trauma en route to theatre
- Support for lower limb fractures

Contraindications

- Pulmonary oedema
- Suspected diaphragmatic rupture
- Haemorrhage above the PASG

Complications

- Compartment syndrome and skin problems associated with prolonged use
- Deflation accompanied by sudden hypotension (therefore deflate gradually and resuscitate accordingly)

Neurogenic shock

Injury to the descending sympathetic pathways can lead to loss of vasomotor tone with pooling in capacitance vessels and failure to generate a tachycardic response. This results in profound hypotension, which in the trauma setting may mistakenly be attributed to hypovolaemia. Appropriate treatment requires the selective use of inotropic agents, rather than aggressive and inappropriate volume replacement, which may result in pulmonary oedema. Atropine may be necessary to counteract an associated bradycardia.

Other shock syndromes

Shock syndromes all tend to result in hypotension. Hypotension is due to:

- Loss of volume in hypovolaemic shock
- Loss of vasomotor tone in neurogenic shock
- Impaired cardiac function in cardiogenic shock
- Loss of peripheral vascular tone due to vasodilation in septic and anaphylactic shock

Cardiogenic shock is discussed in Chapter 7 *Critical Care* and sepsis and anaphylaxis are discussed in Chapter 2 *Infection and Inflammation*.

The metabolic response to trauma

Trauma results in activation of the sympathetic nervous system, the immune system, and the central nervous system. These systems work in concert to minimise the effects of volume loss and maintain the blood pressure (by raising the heart rate) to conserve fluid volume (by activation of the renin–angiotensin axis and secretion of ADH) and to tackle infection.

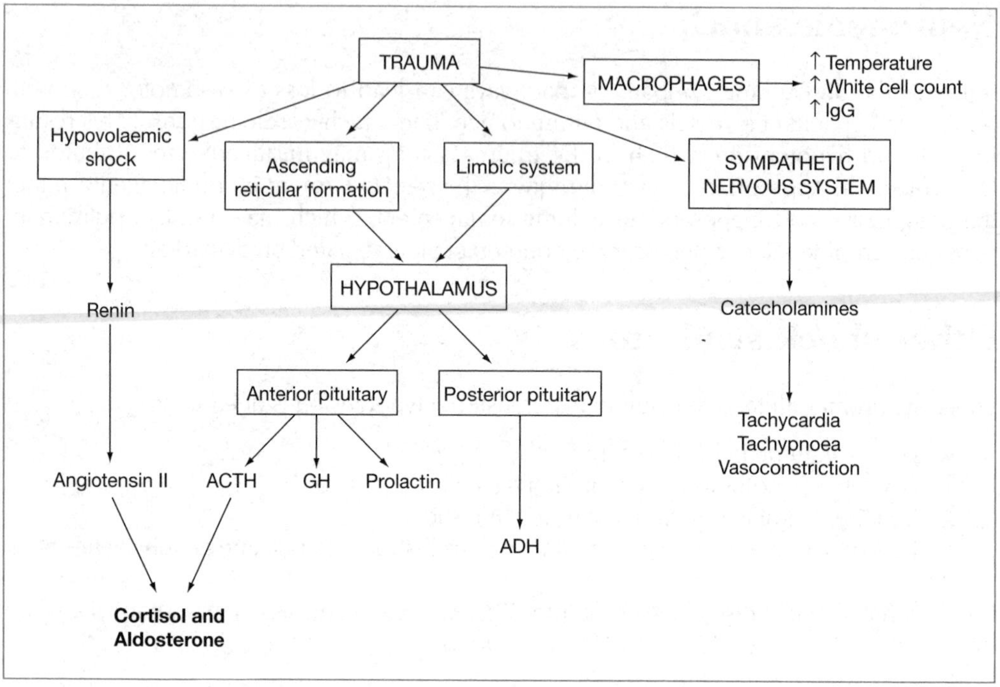

Figure 2.2c *The metabolic response to trauma*

Section 3

Resuscitation: The primary survey

In a nutshell ...

The ABCDE protocol is the standard management of trauma patients.

The aim of this system is to save 'life before limb,' that is to preserve heart, brain and lung oxygenation and circulation. It is based on the ATLS format and involves continuous reassessment and adjustment in response to changing needs.

A (airway)	Check that the airway is patent and protect it. Ensure that the cervical spine is protected, especially in the unconscious patient.
B (breathing)	Check that there is adequate bilateral air entry and that there are no clinical signs of life-threatening chest conditions.
C (circulation)	Detect shock and treat if present. Appropriate access is essential.
D (disability)	Briefly assess the neurological status using the 'AVPU' mnemonic
E (exposure)	Completely undress the patient. Inspect the entire body along guidelines for the secondary survey, including the spine, with a 'log roll'. Keep the patient warm.

The important principles to remember are:

- Always assess a trauma patient in this order (ABCDE)
- If there is an immediately life-threatening problem in A, you cannot proceed to B until the airway is secured. If there is an immediately life-threatening problem in B, you cannot proceed to C unless it is dealt with. In a severely injured patient you may never get to E

3.1 AIRWAY AND C-SPINE

In a nutshell ...

Assessment of the airway in the primary survey

Is the airway compromised?

- No ventilatory effort
- Cyanosis, stridor, use of accessory muscles
- Patient unable to speak although conscious

If so, it must be made safe immediately by one of the following:

- Clear mouth of foreign bodies or secretions
- Chin lift, jaw thrust
- Establish oral or nasopharyngeal airway with bag and mask ventilaton
- Definitive airway (intubation) and ventilation
- Surgical airway and ventilation

Is the airway at risk but currently not compromised?

- Decreased GCS
- Facial trauma
- Burn to face

If so, call for anaesthetic/ENT support and be prepared to provide a definitive airway if needed. Constantly reassess the situation.

Is the airway safe?

- Patient speaking
- Good air movement without stridor

If so, give oxygen and move on to assess breathing.

Control of the C-spine in the primary survey

- In-line survey manual immobilisation (assistant holds patient's head with both hands)

  or

- Hard cervical spine collar with sandbag and tape

The C-spine should be controlled by one of the above methods throughout the primary survey until it is safe to fully assess it clinically and, if necessary, radiologically.

Hypoxia is the quickest killer of trauma patients, therefore maintenance of patent airway and adequate oxygen delivery are essential. Remember that all trauma patients must be assumed to have a cervical spine injury until proved otherwise.

Recognition of a compromised airway

- Risk factors (eg head injury, drugs, alcohol)
- Clinical signs (eg stridor, cyanosis, accessory muscle use)
- If a patient can speak, his airway is patent

Management of a compromised airway

- Chin lift and jaw thrust
- Guedel airway
- Nasopharyngeal airway
- Definitive airway
  - Nasotracheal
  - Orotracheal
  - Cricothyroidotomy
  - Tracheostomy

Remember, if the airway is obstructed you cannot move on to assess breathing until the airway is secured.

Anatomy of the airway

The anatomy of the airways is illustrated in Fig. 3.1a and Fig. 3.1b.

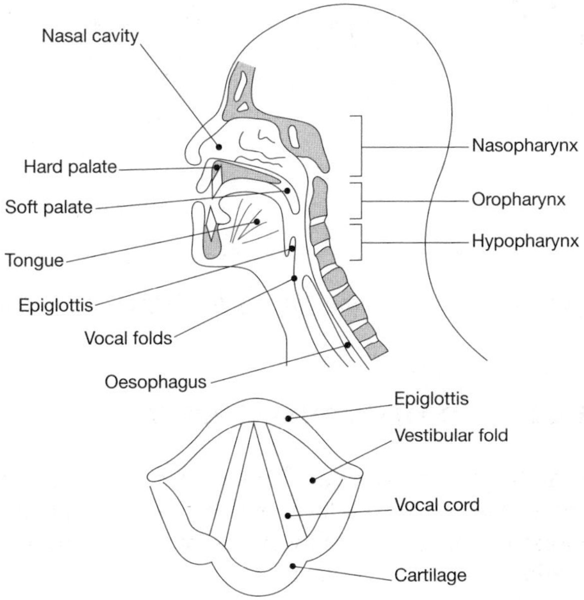

Figure 3.1a *Anatomy of the upper airway*

Chapter 5

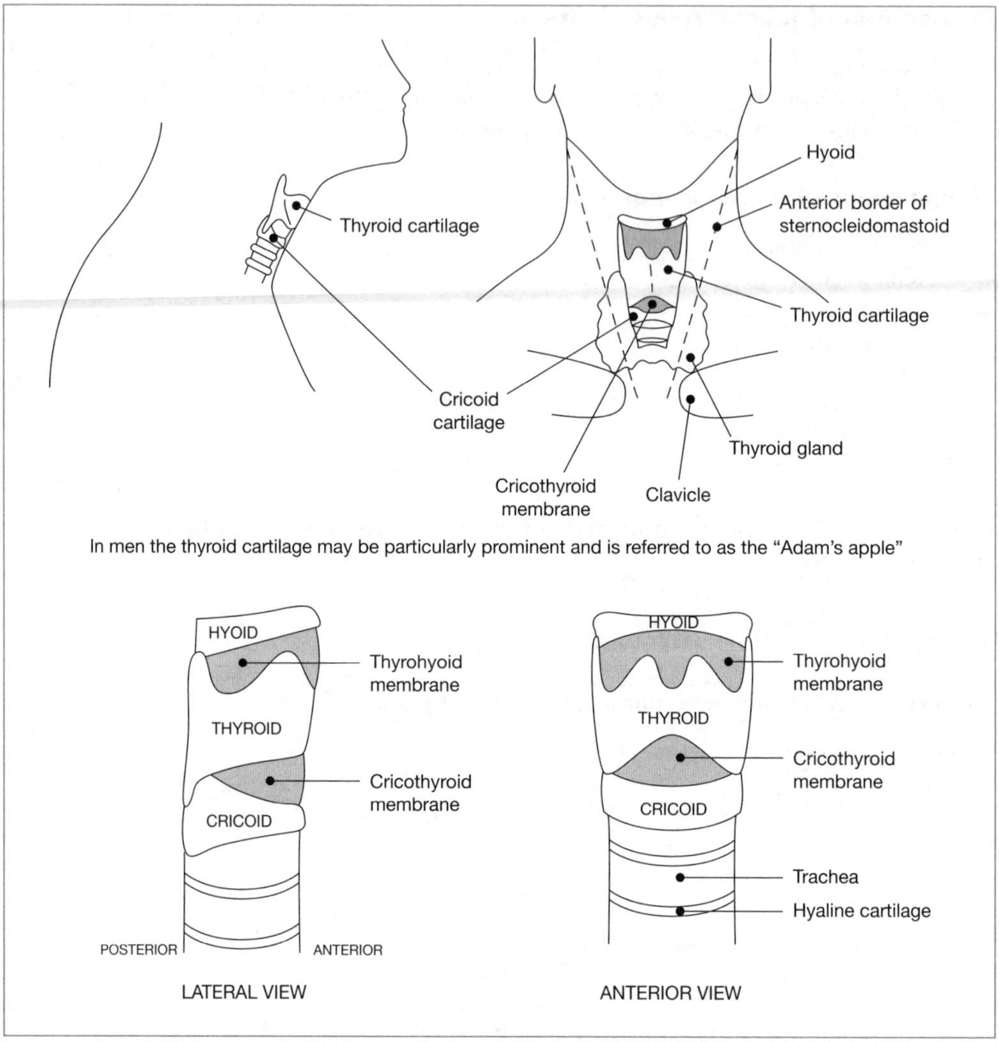

Figure 3.1b *Surface markings of the larynx and trachea*

Recognition of a compromised airway

Airway obstruction can be gradual or sudden and the clinical signs (tachypnoea, cyanosis, and agitation) may be subtle. An altered level of consciousness due to head injury, drugs, alcohol or these factors combined makes airway compromise particularly likely especially from the risk of aspiration of stomach contents.

Vomiting or the presence of stomach contents in the oropharynx requires immediate suction and turning the patient into the lateral 'recovery' position.

Associated chest injuries may reduce ventilation/oxygenation and injuries of the neck may cause airway compromise by pressure from oedema or an expanding haematoma or tracheal perforation.

LOOK	Facial or airway trauma, agitation, cyanosis, use of accessory muscles
LISTEN	Stridor, gurgling, snoring or hoarseness
FEEL	Chest wall movement

Administer supplemental oxygen at 15 litres/minute with reservoir bag.

Management of an obstructed airway

The following must be achieved with simultaneous immobilisation of the cervical spine. In the unconscious patient the airway may be obstructed by vomit, dentures, broken teeth, or the tongue falling backwards. The mouth should be gently opened and inspected. A gloved finger may be used to remove debris and a Yankauer sucker used for secretions.

The 'chin lift' and 'jaw thrust'

See Fig. 3.1c. Both these manoeuvres are aimed at maintaining the patency of the upper airway (eg when the tongue has fallen backwards). To perform a jaw thrust place your hands on either side of the patient's head. Your thumbs should lie on the patient's chin. Find the angle of the mandible with the tips of your index fingers. Maintaining the neutral position of the C-spine, grip the mandible and lift it forwards and upwards. This lifts the base of the tongue away from the airway. This position is sometimes called 'sniffing the morning air'.

- **Advantages:** no additional equipment needed. Holding both sides of the head may be combined with temporary in-line stabilisation of the C-spine. Can be used in a conscious patient
- **Disadvantages:** requires practice to maintain airway. Difficult to maintain for long periods of time

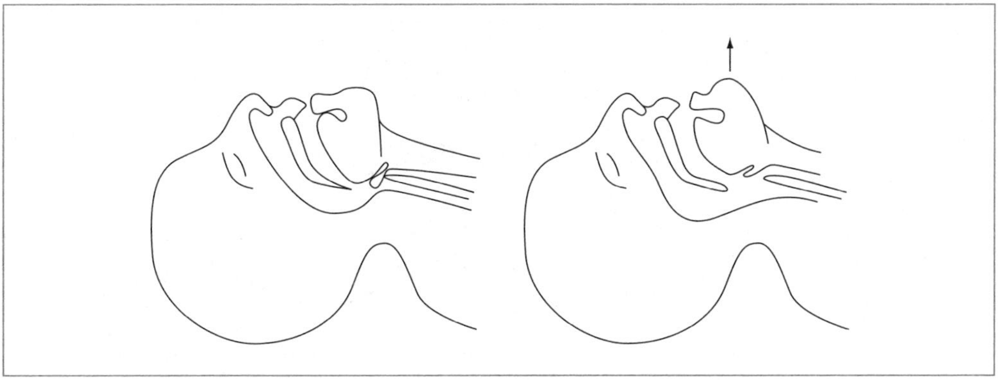

Figure 3.1c *The 'chin lift' and 'jaw thrust'*

Chapter 5

The Guedel airway

See Fig. 3.1d. Used for temporary 'bag and mask' ventilation of the unconscious patient prior to intubation.

- **Advantages:** easy to insert; widely available; various sizes
- **Disadvantages:** sited above vocal cords so does not prevent airway obstruction at this site. Can provoke gag reflex. Does not prevent aspiration of stomach contents

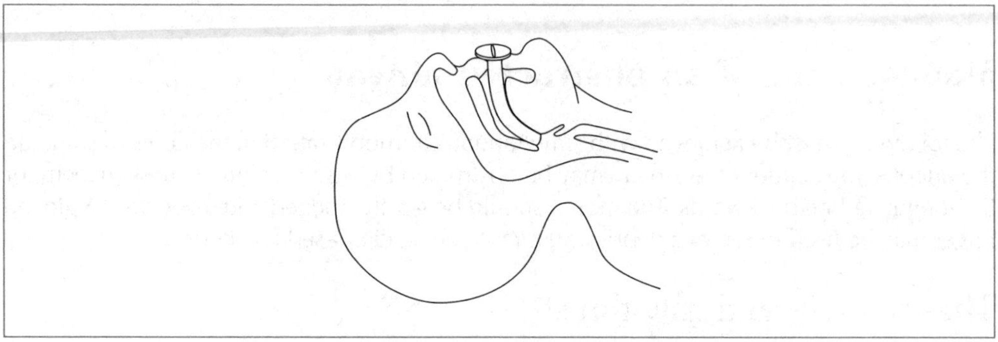

Figure 3.1d *The Guedel airway*

The nasopharyngeal airway

See Fig. 3.1e. Used to prevent upper airway obstruction (eg in a drowsy/still conscious patient).

- **Advantages:** fairly easy to insert; unlikely to stimulate gag reflex in comparison with oropharyngeal (Guedel) airway
- **Disadvantages:** less widely available, uncomfortable for the patient, sited above the vocal cords. Insertion dangerous if facial trauma present. Does not prevent aspiration of stomach contents

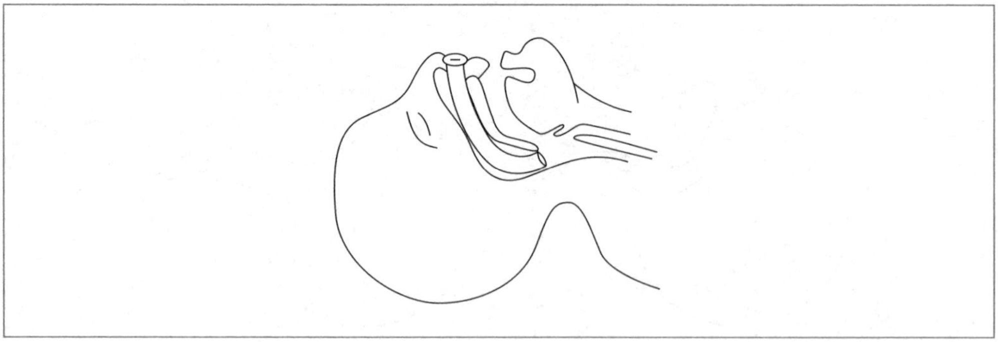

Figure 3.1e *The nasopharyngeal airway*

The definitive airway

If the above measures are insufficient then a definitive airway is indicated. This will ensure free passage of oxygen to the trachea, distal to the vocal cords.

Indications for a definitive airway

- Apnoea
- Hypoxia refractory to oxygen therapy
- Protection from aspiration pneumonitis
- Protection of the airway from impending obstruction due to burns/oedema/facial trauma/seizures
- Inability to maintain an airway by the above simpler measures
- Head injury with a risk of raised ICP
- Vocal cord paralysis

Types of definitive airway

- Orotracheal intubation
- Nasotracheal intubation
- Surgical airway (eg tracheostomy or cricothyroidotomy)

Orotracheal intubation

A definitive airway may be secured by orotracheal intubation using an endotracheal tube (ETT). In cases of oral trauma, nasotracheal intubation may be preferred.

For discussion of nasotracheal and orotracheal intubation see Chapter 7 *Critical Care*.

Surgical cricothyroidotomy

This technique is quick and can be performed without hyperextension of the potentially injured cervical spine. It provides a large calibre airway that can be secured, and it is therefore the technique of choice for a surgical airway in the early management of trauma patients.

Procedure box: Surgical cricothyroidotomy

Indications

May be needle cricothyroidotomy or open surgical cricothyroidotomy. Indication is failed orotracheal intubation due to:

- Severe oedema of the glottis
- Fracture of the larynx
- Severe oropharyngeal haemorrhage obstructing passage of a tube past the vocal cords

Contraindications

(Relative) surgical cricothyroidotomy is not recommended in children aged < 12 in whom the cricoid cartilage provides the only circumferential support for the upper trachea.

Patient positioning

- Supine with neck extended

Procedure

Needle cricothyroidotomy

- Skin preparation with Betadine™ or chlorhexidine
- Identify the relevant landmarks: the cricoid cartilage and thyroid cartilage with the cricothyroid membrane between
- Puncture the skin in the line with a 12 G or 14 G needle attached to the syringe, directly over the cricothyroid membrane. A small incision with a #11 blade may facilitate passage of the needle through the skin
- Direct the needle at a 45° angle inferiorly, while applying negative pressure to the syringe, and carefully insert the needle through the lower half of the cricothyroid membrane
- Aspiration of air signifies entry into the tracheal lumen
- Remove the syringe and withdraw the needle while advancing the catheter downward into position, being careful not to perforate the posterior wall of the trachea
- Attach the oxygen tubing over the catheter needle hub

Intermittent **jet ventilation** can be achieved by occluding an open hole cut into the oxygen tubing with your thumb for 1 second and releasing it for 4 seconds. After releasing your thumb from the hole in the tubing, passive exhalation occurs. This can be used for temporary ventilation (30–40 minutes) until a definitive airway can be established. CO_2 gradually accumulates due to inadequate exhalation and this technique cannot be used with chest trauma. It is not recommended for children.

Open surgical cricothyroidotomy

Skin preparation with Betadine™ or chlorhexidine

Identify the relevant landmarks: the cricoid cartilage and thyroid cartilage with the cricothyroid membrane between

If the patient is conscious the surgical field is infiltrated with 10 mL of LA with adrenaline/epinephrine to reduce haemorrhage

Stabilise the thyroid with the left hand

Make a transverse skin incision over the cricothyroid membrane. Carefully incise through the membrane

Insert the scalpel handle into the incision and rotate it 90° to open the airway or use a pair of artery forceps to dilate the tract

Insert an appropriately sized, cuffed endotracheal tube or tracheotomy tube into the cricothyroid membrane incision, directing the tube distally into the trachea

Inflate the cuff and ventilate the patient

Observe lung inflation and auscultate the chest for adequate ventilation

Hazards

Haemorrhage

Damage to cricoid and thyroid cartilages

Post-procedure instructions

Observe for haemorrhage as clots may obstruct airway.

Complications

This is a temporary airway. A formal tracheostomy is more suited to long-term management.

Tracheostomy

An open surgical tracheostomy is slow, technically more complex, with potential for bleeding, and requires formal operating facilities. It is not appropriate in the acute trauma situation, but is better suited to the long-term management of a ventilated patient. It is performed when a percutaneous tracheostomy would be difficult (eg abnormal or distorted anatomy).

Percutaneous tracheostomy is also time-consuming and requires hyperextension of the neck. In addition the use of a guidewire and multiple dilators make it an unsuitable technique in the acute trauma situation.

For discussion of tracheostomy see Chapter 3 in Book 2 *Ear, Nose, Throat, Head and Neck.*

Cervical spine control

In the first part of the primary survey of a trauma victim cervical spine control is vital. The patient's head should be held with in-line traction immediately if the neck is not immobilised on a spinal board. A hard cervical collar alone is not sufficient to control the cervical spine: sandbags and tape should be used.

3.2 BREATHING

In a nutshell ...

Assessment of breathing in the primary survey

If the airway is safe or has been secured, you can move on to assessing breathing.

- Full examination
- Check saturation and/or arterial blood gases
- Provide supplemental oxygen
- Identify any of the six immediately life-threatening chest injuries and treating them immediately before moving on with the primary survey (the recognition and management of these conditions is covered in section 4.3):
    - Airway obstruction (see section 3.1)
    - Tension pneumothorax
    - Sucking chest wound and/or open pneumothorax
    - Massive haemothorax
    - Flail chest
    - Cardiac tamponade
- Ensure ventilation is adequate before moving on to assess circulation

Supplemental oxygen must be delivered to all trauma patients.

Spontaneous breathing may resume when the airway is protected. If an ET tube has been inserted then intermittent positive pressure ventilation (IPPV) must be commenced as the diameter of the tube dramatically increases the work of breathing.

Ventilatory support may be required:

- Bag and mask assistance
- IPPV

Examine the chest:

- Expose and observe
- Palpate
- Percuss
- Auscultate

Injuries that may compromise ventilation are:

- Thoracic injuries
  - Pneumothorax (simple, open, or tension)
  - Haemothorax
  - Pulmonary contusion
  - Rib fractures and flail chest
- Abdominal injuries: pain causes splinting of the abdominal wall and diaphragm
- Head injuries

Injuries compromising breathing must be dealt with early. This often requires insertion of a chest drain, which is discussed in section 4.3 of this chapter.

3.3 CIRCULATION

In a nutshell ...

Assessment of the circulation in the primary survey

If the airway is safe and ventilation is adequate, you can move on to assessing circulation.

- Assess haemodynamically status
- Identify sites of haemorrhage
- Establish IV access
- Send off blood for cross-matching and other investigations
- Give a bolus of intravenous fluid if the patient is shocked

If the patient is haemodynamically unstable and is losing blood, action must be taken before moving on with the primary survey. This may mean transferring the patient to the operating theatre at this stage of the primary survey if there is uncontrolled internal bleeding.

Assess the patient's haemodynamic status

- Pulse and BP
- Conscious level (cerebral perfusion)
- Skin colour (peripheral perfusion)

Remember to assess the patient's likely pre-morbid condition, bearing in mind AMPLE history (see section 3.6), age group (elderly, child), medication (eg β-blocker), lifestyle (athletic).

Hypotension should be presumed to be secondary to haemorrhage until proved otherwise.

Identify sites of haemorrhage

- External
- Internal (thoracic cavity, abdominal cavity, extremities due to fractures)
- Occult

Establish IV access

Establish IV access with a cannula of sufficient diameter to allow large volume fluid resuscitation:

- Two large gauge (brown or grey) cannulae, one in each antecubital fossa
- Venous cut-down
- Intra-osseous line
- Femoral venous catheterisation

Central lines tend to be of narrow diameter and are not ideal for administering large volumes of fluid quickly.

You can send venous blood for baseline tests as soon as access is established:

- FBC
- Cross-match
- U&Es

Management of the individual traumatic pathologies which can cause haemorrhage are dealt with in sections 4.2–4.6.

Signs and symptoms of class I–IV shock are discussed in section 2.2.

3.4 DISABILITY

In a nutshell ...

Assessment of disability in the primary survey

If the airway is safe, ventilation is adequate, and there is no uncontrolled haemorrhage, you can move on to assessing disability.

- Neurological status (AVPA)
- Pupils

Remember, shock can cause decreased consciousness.

Neurological status

Briefly assess neurological status using the acronym **AVPU**:

A lert
V erbal stimuli (responds to)
P ain (responds to)
U nresponsive

Pupils

Check pupils for:

- Size
- Symmetry
- Response to light

The anatomy, physiology, pathology and management of head injuries are discussed in section 4.2.

3.5 EXPOSURE AND ENVIRONMENT

In a nutshell ...

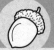

Exposure in the primary survey

If the airway is safe, ventilation is adequate, and there is no uncontrolled haemorrhage or evidence of severe or progressing head injury, you can move on to exposing the patient and attending to his environment.

- Undress fully
- Keep warm
- Prepare for full inspection, log roll and examination in the secondary survey

The patient should be fully exposed in order to look for hidden injuries in the secondary survey. Remember that the patient may already be hypothermic and maintenance of their body temperature is essential:

- Warmed fluids
- Warm resus room
- External warming devices (blankets, bear-hugger, etc)

3.6 MONITORING AND IMPORTANT INVESTIGATIONS

In a nutshell ...

Completing the primary survey: monitoring and investigations

If the airway is safe, ventilation is adequate, there is no uncontrolled haemorrhage, or evidence of severe or progressing head injury, and the patient is exposed with attention to his environment, the time has come to complete the primary survey and move on to the secondary survey. Before this is done you must:

- Take an AMPLE history
- Give analgesia
- Set up:
  - Pulse oximetry
  - ECG leads

- Monitor:
  - Urine output
  - Conscious level
- Send blood investigations if not already done
- Do the three trauma X-rays:
  - AP chest
  - Pelvis
  - C-spine
- Fully re-assess the ABCDEs

You are now ready to progress to the secondary survey.

History

It is important to take a medical history from the patient in the primary survey. Use the mnemonic AMPLE to remind you of each section.

AMPLE mnemonic

A llergies
M edication
P ast medical history
L ast meal
E vents of the injury

Don't forget to consider analgesia for the patient at this point – it does not affect diagnosis of the injury, and it is not ethically acceptable to leave the patient in pain.

Monitoring in the resuscitation room

- Pulse oximetry and ABGs
- ECG leads
- Conscious level
- Urinary output

Initial urgent investigations

- Blood tests (FBC, cross-match, U&Es)
- ABGs
- Imaging: X-rays (AP chest, pelvis, C-spine) are usually performed rapidly and may help in the assessment of injuries

Section 4

Assessment: The secondary survey

In a nutshell ...

The secondary survey starts after the initial resuscitation as the patient begins to stabilise. It is carried out whilst continually reassessing ABC. Immediately life-threatening conditions should already have been detected and treated.

- Obtain a complete medical history
- Perform a sequential thorough examination of the body, starting at the head and working down the body looking for hidden injuries
- Obtain all necessary investigations: bloods, X-rays (of cervical spine, chest and pelvis)
- Perform any special procedures
- Monitor patient's response to treatment

Follow up with 'Fingers and tubes in every orifice'

- p.r.
- p.v.
- Check ENT
- NG tube insertion (if no skull fracture)
- Urinary catheter insertion if no evidence of genito-urinary trauma

4.1 PATIENT OVERVIEW

In a nutshell ...

The role of the secondary survey is to obtain an overview of the patient's injuries and proceed to treat each one. This ensures that minor but potentially problematic injuries are not overlooked in the severely injured patient. The secondary survey should only be attempted on completion of the primary survey when life-threatening injuries have been managed and the patient is stable. Start at the top and systematically work down.

- Head
- Neck
- Thorax
- Abdomen
- Pelvis
- Extremities
- Spine
- Tetanus

Documentation is vital at this stage.

Secondary survey of the head

- Neurological state
  - Full GCS assessment
  - Pupils
  - Eyes
- Examination of the face
  - Check facial bones for stability
  - Loose or absent teeth
- Examination of the scalp
  - Presence of soft tissue injuries/haematoma
  - Signs of skull fracture
  - Periorbital haematoma
  - Scleral haematoma with no posterior margin
  - Battle's sign
  - CSF/blood from ears or nose

Secondary survey of the neck

- Risk factors for cervical spine injury
  - Any injury above the clavicle
  - High-speed RTA
  - Fall from height
- Neck examination
  - Thorough palpation of bony prominences
  - Check for soft tissue swellings
  - Check for muscle spasm
  - X-ray of C-spine

- Exclude:
  - Penetrating injuries of the neck
  - Subcutaneous emphysema
  - Elevated JVP

Secondary survey of the thorax

- Exclude pathology (pneumothorax, haemothorax, rib fractures, mediastinal injury, cardiac contusion)
- Examine the full respiratory system, especially reassessing air entry
- Inspect chest wall (bony or soft tissue injury, subcutaneous emphysema)
- CXR
- ECG
- ABG should be obtained to monitor whether ventilation is adequate

Secondary survey of the abdomen

- Examine thoroughly (abdominal wall injury suggests internal viscus injury)
- Insertion of a NG tube to decompress the stomach is suggested as long as there are no facial fractures or basal skull fractures
- Involve surgeons early if suspect internal injury
- After general resuscitation the main decision to be made in this area is whether a laparotomy is necessary

Secondary survey of the pelvis

- Check for bony instability which indicates significant blood loss
- Identify any genito-urinary system injuries suggested by: high-riding prostate felt p.r.; blood found on p.r. examination; blood found on p.v. examination; blood at external urethral meatus; gross haematuria
- Urethral catheterisation is only performed if there is no evidence of genito-urinary injury

Secondary survey of the extremities

- Examine the full extent of each limb (remember hands and feet including individual fingers and toes)
- Exclude soft tissue injury, bony injury, vascular injury, neurological injury
- Control haemorrhage; elevate limb; apply direct pressure (tourniquets are not favoured)
- Correct any obvious bony deformity as this will decrease: fat emboli; haemorrhage; soft tissue injury; requirement for analgesia; skin tension in dislocations
- Caution: check and document neurovascular supply to limb before and after any manipulation

Secondary survey of the spine

- Examine the spinal column for alignment, stepping and tenderness
- Examine the peripheral and central nervous systems
- Exclude sensory or motor deficits

Tetanus status and prophylaxis

- Check tetanus status, as shown in the table

TETANUS STATUS

Tetanus status	Minor injuries	Major injuries
Unknown or < three doses	Tetanus toxoid only	Tetanus toxoid and tetanus IgG
Full course received with last booster < 10 years ago	No treatment needed	No treatment necessary
Full course received with last booster > 10 years ago	Tetanus IgG	Tetanus IgG

Documentation

Document ABCDE status, observations, history of injury, AMPLE history, and site and nature of all injuries seen. All Accident and Emergency units will have trauma proforma sheets available to assist this.

4.2 HEAD AND FACIAL INJURY

In a nutshell ...

Head injuries may involve skull fracture, focal injury, or diffuse brain injury.

They may be classified according to severity, mechanism of injury or (most usefully) pathology.

The five aims of emergency management are:

- Assessment
- Resuscitation
- Establishing the diagnosis
- Ensuring metabolic needs of the brain are met
- Preventing secondary brain damage

Head injuries account for approximately 10% of A&E attendance in the UK. Around 50% of trauma deaths are associated with head injury.

The anatomy of the brain and skull is discussed in *Elective Neurosurgery and Spinal Surgery* in Book 2.

Classification system for head injuries

Patients with head injuries are a very diverse group and their injuries may be classified in a number of ways.

Severity of injury

- Minor GCS 8–15
- Major GCS < 8

Mechanism of injury

- Blunt
- Penetrating injuries

Pathology of injury

- Focal/diffuse
- Primary/secondary
- Skull/intracranial lesions

- **Primary brain injury** is neurological damage produced by a causative event
- **Secondary brain injury** is neurological damage produced by subsequent insults (eg haemorrhage, hypoxia, hypovolaemia, ischaemia, increased ICP, metabolic imbalance, infection)

The main aim of treatment is to:

- Diagnose a primary brain injury and provide optimum conditions for recovery
- Minimise/prevent secondary brain injury by maintaining brain tissue oxygenation

Mechanisms of brain damage

Hypoxia/ischaemia

Permanent damage occurs within 3–4 minutes.

Contusion

The brain has a soft consistency and is poorly anchored within the cranial cavity. It therefore moves during acceleration/deceleration. Contact with the skull can cause bruising (contusions). The frontal and temporal lobes are particularly vulnerable. Contrecoup injury refers to injury on the opposite side of the brain to the impact (eg damage to frontal lobes after impact on the back of the head). This is due to the mobility of the brain within the skull vault.

Diffuse axonal injury

Axonal tracts may be torn by shearing forces, resulting in a spectrum of damage from reversible to irreversible. The transient LOC (concussion) is due to a mild form of this stretch injury. Severe forms can cause persistent vegetative states. Microscopically this causes 'retraction balls' of neurological tissue.

Mild	Coma lasting 6–12 hours	Concussion
Moderate	Coma lasting > 24 hours	No brainstem dysfunction (mortality 20%)
Severe	Coma lasting > 24 hours	With brainstem dysfunction (mortality 57%)

Intracranial haemorrhage causes destruction of tissue immediately adjacent to the injury and compression of surrounding structures (see below).

Intracranial haemorrhage

Focal injuries

Extradural haematoma
Subdural haematoma
Intracerebral haematoma

Extradural haematoma

This results from trauma – often trivial trauma (eg a blow to the temporal or parietal bone causing rupture of the underlying middle meningeal artery). Children and young adults are more susceptible as the dura becomes more adherent to the skull with advancing age. Initial concussion is typically followed by a 'lucid interval' as the expanding haematoma is accommodated. Rapid decompensation may then follow when the ICP rises as the inner edge of the temporal lobe descends into the tentorial opening (coning).

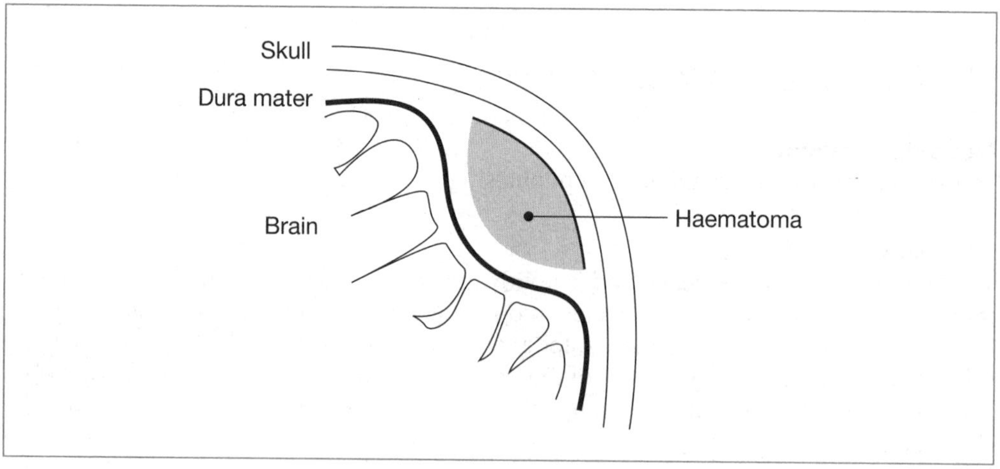

Figure 4.2a *Extradural haematoma*

Acute subdural haematoma

A severe head injury may leave a thin layer of clot over the surface of the brain in the subdural space, either by rupture of a bridging vein due to shearing forces, or due to laceration of brain substance. In either case there is usually severe underlying primary brain damage and deterioration is more rapid than with an extradural haematoma.

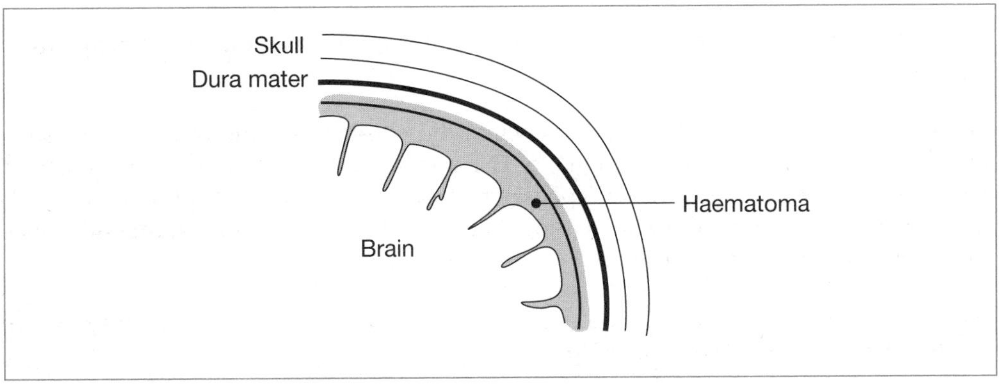

Figure 4.2b *Acute subdural haematoma*

Intracerebral haematoma

These injuries are the least remediable of the compressing intracranial haematomas. They are usually associated with cerebral laceration, contusion, oedema and necrosis, all of which contribute to their compressive effects. Removal of such clots has unpredictable and often disappointing results.

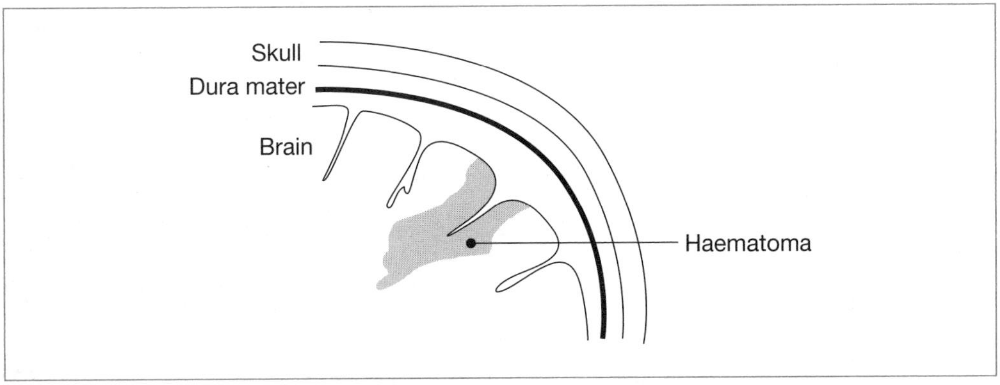

Figure 4.2c *Intracerebral haematoma*

Raised intracranial pressure

Intracranial pressure (ICP)

Normal ICP = 10 mmHg
Abnormal ICP > 20 mmHg

The Monroe–Kellie doctrine explains intracranial compensation for an expanding intracranial mass.

The addition of a mass (eg haematoma) within the constant volume of the skull results initially in extrusion of an equal volume of CSF and venous blood in order to maintain a normal ICP. However, when this compensatory mechanism reaches its limit the ICP will increase exponentially with the increasing volume of the haematoma. Normal ICP does not therefore exclude a mass lesion.

Causes of raised intracranial pressure

Haematoma
Focal oedema secondary to contusion/haematoma
Diffuse cerebral oedema secondary to ischaemia
Obstruction of CSF flow (rare)

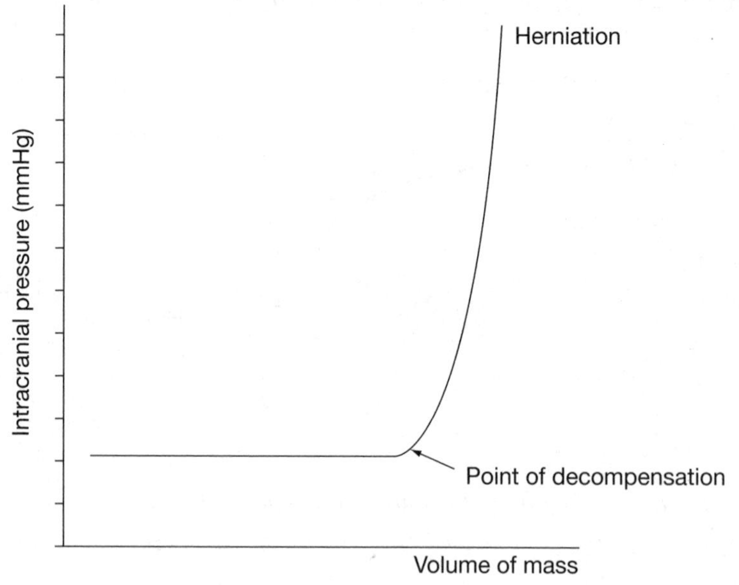

Figure 4.2d *Volume–pressure curve*

Effects of raised intracranial pressure

Tentorial herniation
Pupillary dilatation as a result of 3rd cranial nerve compression
Motor weakness as a result of corticospinal tract compression
Coning results in compression of vital cardiorespiratory centres against the bone as the brainstem is squeezed through the foramen magnum

Rising ICP causes Cushing's response

Respiratory rate decreases
Heart rate decreases
Systolic BP increases
Pulse pressure increases

Death results from respiratory arrest secondary to brainstem infarction/haemorrhage. Direct measurement of ICP has proved more reliable than waiting for clinical signs to develop. ICP can be monitored extradurally, subdurally and intraventricularly.

Cerebral blood flow

CPP = MAP – ICP

CPP is cerebral perfusion pressure, MAP is mean arterial pressure, ICP is intracranial pressure.

Cerebral perfusion pressure is maintained by a phenomenon called autoregulation. Blood flow to the brain (Fig. 4.2e) is increased by:

- Rising CO_2 levels
- Rising extracellular K^+ levels
- Decreased pO_2

Autoregulation is severely disturbed in head injury, and CPP of < 70 mmHg is associated with poor outcome. Therefore the priority with a head injury is to maintain cerebral perfusion, because these patients are susceptible to secondary brain injury due to hypotension.

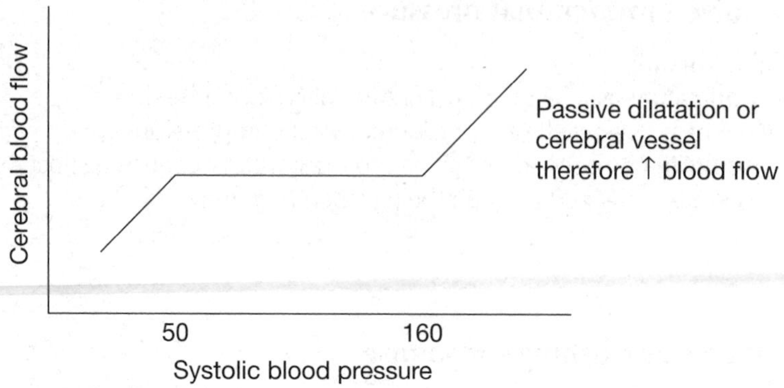

Figure 4.2e *Control of cerebral blood flow*

Management of raised intracranial pressure

- CT scan for diagnosis of underlying cause
- Definitive management of underlying cause if possible

Conservative management

- Sedate and intubate
- Nurse the patient with tilted head up (aids venous drainage)
- Maintain normal or low pCO_2
- Establish monitoring with an ICP bolt and transducer
- Aim to maintain CPP at 60–70 mmHg by:
  - Optimal fluid management
  - Judicious use of inotropes
- Aim to maintain ICP at 10 mmHg by:
  - Mannitol (0.5 g/kg) may result in a transient mild reduction in ICP
  - Hyperventilation to pCO_2 of > 4 kPa
  - Thiopentone infusion (15 mg/kg)
  - Hypothermia
- Emergency burr holes or craniotomy

Burr holes

A burr hole is a small hole through the skull over the site of an intracranial haematoma. The aim is for partial evacuation and reduction in ICP. Only a small volume of haematoma (often gelatinous and clotted) can be evacuated and the hole must be placed directly over the site of the haematoma to have any chance of doing so.

This is an emergency measure, used to buy time. Placement of burr holes should not delay definitive neurosurgical intervention. It should only be performed if training has been received from a neurosurgeon.

Procedure box: Burr holes

Indications

Patients with signs of severe elevated ICP and impending herniation (eg pupil dilatation) due to epidural or subdural haematoma.

Contraindications

Presence of facilities for definitive neurosurgical intervention.

Patient positioning

Supine under GA.

Procedure

- Identify the location of the haematoma (usually frontal or temporal)
- In the absence of a CT scan, place a burr hole on the side of the dilated pupil, 2 fingerwidths anterior to tragus of ear and 3 fingerwidths above
- Perform a straight scalp incision with haemostasis and insert a self-retainer
- Elevate the periosteum with a periosteal elevator
- Drill a hole through the skull to the dura with an automatic perforator or a manual Hudson brace
- Hook the dura up through the hole and open the dura with a cruciate incision
- Slowly decompress the haematoma with gentle suction and irrigation using a Jake's catheter until the returning fluid is clear (this catheter can be left in situ for drainage)
- Close the scalp with clips to skin
- More than one burr hole may be placed to evacuate large haematomas

Post-procedure instructions

- Transfer to neurosurgical care
- Nurse flat for 48 hours and observe drain output
- Re-scan if the patient's GCS deteriorates

Hazards

- Damage to underlying tissues (brain, blood vessels)

Complications

- Bleeding (scalp, bone edges)
- Damage to brain
- Failure to evacuate sufficient haematoma

Monitoring after head injury and surgical interventions

Assessment of conscious level

Consciousness is controlled by the reticular activating system located in the upper portion of the brainstem.

Causes of altered conscious level

Trauma	Infection
Poisons	Psychiatric disorders
Shock	Alcohol
Epilepsy	Raised ICP
Opiates	Metabolic disorders (eg uraemia)

The Glasgow coma scale (GCS)

The GCS offers a reproducible, quantitative measure of the patient's level of consciousness.

GLASGOW COMA SCALE

Best motor response	6	Obeys commands
	5	Localises to pain
	4	Withdraws from pain
	3	Abnormal flexion
	2	Extension
	1	None
Best verbal response	5	Orientated
	4	Confused
	3	Inappropriate
	2	Incomprehensible sounds
	1	None
Best eye-opening response	4	Open spontaneously
	3	Open to speech
	2	Open to pain
	1	None

Pupil size

Assessment of pupil size and symmetry on admission and subsequently every few hours is important. Sudden unilateral pupil dilatation ('blowing a pupil') may be indicative of pressure on the nucleus of the 3rd cranial nerve as it is forced against the bone of the skull at the foramen magnum with impending coning.

Intracranial pressure (ICP) monitoring

Monitoring ICP may be performed as an **invasive** procedure.

- **Cranial hollow screws and bolts:** a catheter is inserted through a small hole drilled in the skull and placed in contact with the brain; this is linked to a pressure transducer
- **Ladd device:** uses fibreoptics to measure ICP
- **Ventricular cannula:** placement of a cannula in the ventricular system is useful in hydrocephalus and allows therapeutic CSF drainage if required
- **Fully implantable devices** may be used as part of a shunt for chronically raised ICP

Increasingly, methods are being developed to monitor ICP **non-invasively**.

- **Transcranial Doppler:** gives estimation of flow in the middle meningeal artery
- **Infrared spectroscopy:** gives estimation of brain tissue oxygenation

ICP monitoring is useful in clinical management. It also provides additional assessment of brain death as cerebral perfusion essentially ceases when the ICP exceeds the diastolic BP.

Problems associated with ICP monitoring include:

- Cost
- Infection
- Haemorrhage

Management of head injuries

Treatment priorities and management decisions depend on whether the head injury is minor or major.

Minor head injuries

The management aim is to detect those at risk of developing an intracranial haematoma.

RISK OF HAEMATOMA FOLLOWING MINOR HEAD INJURY

	Skull fracture	No skull fracture
Fully conscious	1 in 45	1 in 7900
Confused	1 in 5	1 in 180
Coma	1 in 4	1 in 27

Criteria for skull X-ray after recent head injury

Loss of consciousness or amnesia at any time
Neurological symptoms or signs
Suspected penetrating injury
CSF or blood from the nose or ear
Large scalp haematoma/laceration
History of high-velocity injury
Difficulty in assessing the patient
Alcohol intoxication; young age; epilepsy

The skull X-ray is a useful adjunct to clinical examination (simple scalp laceration is not a criterion for skull X-ray).

Criteria for admission of the patient with a head injury

- Loss of consciousness lasting more than 5 minutes (or amnesia)
- Confusion or decreased GCS
- Skull fracture
- Neurological symptoms and signs
- Worsening headache, nausea, or vomiting
- Extensive laceration
- Difficulty in assessment (eg in alcohol intoxication)
- No responsible adult at home
- Other medical conditions (eg clotting abnormalities)

Note the following:

- Post-traumatic amnesia with full recovery is not an indication for admission
- Patients who are sent home should be discharged in the care of a responsible adult, and given written instructions about possible complications and appropriate actions should their condition deteriorate

Major head injuries

The aim of management is prevention of secondary cerebral damage. Major head injuries often have concomitant cervical spine injury.

Management of major head injury

Maintain ventilation with $PaO_2 > 13$ and $PaCO_2 < 5.3$ kPa

Intubation is appropriate when gag reflex is absent, or $PaO_2 < 9$, $PaCO_2 > 5.3$
Use rapid sequence intubation
Exclude any pneumothoraces before ventilation
Remember that a talking patient indicates a reduced risk of complications as this is indicative of a patent airway

Maintain adequate MAP

NB: CPP = MAP – ICP

Mannitol

0.5–1 g/kg over 10–30 minutes to help reduce ICP

Antibiotics

Penicillin V 6-hourly if any signs of open fracture of the skull

Analgesia

Criteria for consultation with a neurosurgical unit

- Fractured skull in combination with any abnormal neurology
- Confusion or other neurological disturbance that persists for more than 12 hours
- Coma that continues after resuscitation
- Suspected open injury of the vault or the base of the skull
- Depressed fracture of the skull
- Deterioration of the patient's GCS

Note: Before assuming that the deterioration is due to CNS neurological damage, exclude possible hypoxia and metabolic causes (eg hypoglycaemia).

Facial injuries

In a nutshell ...

An appreciation of the anatomy of the face is needed.

Initial management of facial injury

History of injury

Mechanism of injury
Loss of consciousness
Visual disturbance (flashes of light, photophobia, diplopia, blurry vision, pain, or change in vision present with eye movement)
Hearing (tinnitus or vertigo)
Difficulty moving the jaw
Areas of facial numbness

Examination

ABCDE

Inspect for:

Asymmetry
Abrasions and cuts
Bruising
Missing tissue
Teeth and bite for fracture and mal-occlusion

Palpate for bony injury (tenderness, crepitus and step-off) especially orbital rims, zygomatic arch, medial orbital area, nasal bones, mandibular length and teeth

Place one hand on the anterior maxillary teeth and the other on the nasal bridge: movement of only the teeth indicates a Le Fort I fracture; movement at the nasal bridge indicates a Le Fort II or III fracture
Ear canal examination: look for discharge, Battle's sign, integrity of the tympanic membrane, and lacerations
Eye examination (see below)
Cranial nerve exam

Maxillofacial surgery is a speciality not covered in this text. A basic knowledge of the bones, soft tissues, blood supply and nerve supply of the face should be appreciated. The muscles and nerve supply of the face are discussed in Book 2 (Chapter 3 E*ar, Nose, Throat, Head and Neck*). The bones and blood supply of the face are described below.

Bones of the face

The bones of the face include:

- Facial skeleton
- Naso-orbital complex
- Bones of the orbit (see the *Eye* section of *Ear, Nose, Throat, Head and Neck* in Book 2)
- Temporal bone
- Temporomandibular joint
- Zygomatic arch
- Pterion
- Mandible
- Hard palate

Facial skeleton

The bones of the face are shown in Fig. 4.2f. The face can be divided into three zones:

- **Upper zone:** the frontal bone
- **Mid zone:** between the frontal bone and mandible, including the orbit, nasal cavity, maxillary and ethmoid
- **Lower zone:** mandible

Naso-orbital complex

This consists of the:

- Nasal bones (right and left)
- Lacrimal bones (right and left)
- Maxillary bones (right and left)
- Ethmoid bone

These bones are important because fracturing them may damage the nasal septum, ethmoidal sinuses, or the cribiform plate.

Temporal bone

The temporal bone contributes structurally to the cranial vault. It is one of the most complex bones of the body. It consists of five parts: the squamous, the mastoid, the tympanic, the zygomatic, and the petrous segments. It is intimately related to the dura of the middle and posterior fossa. Anteriorly, it communicates with the middle ear. Many important structures are found within or passing through the bone:

- Part of the carotid artery
- Jugular venous drainage system
- Middle ear
- Vestibulocochlear end organs
- Facial nerve

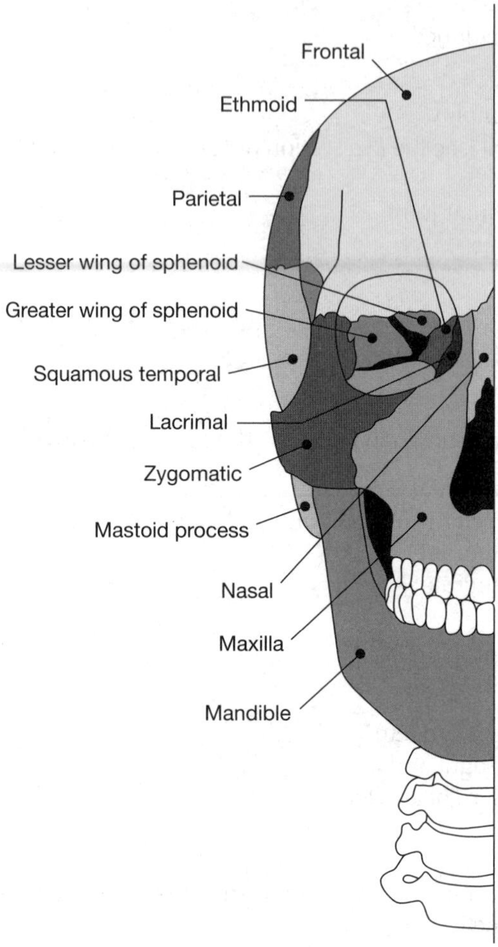

Figure 4.2f *Bones of the face*

Temporomandibular joint (TMJ)

The TMJ is a sliding joint, formed by the condyle of the mandible and the squamous part of the temporal bone. The articular surface of the temporal bone consists of a convex articular eminence anteriorly and a concave articular fossa posteriorly. The articular surface of the mandible consists of the top of the condyle. The articular surfaces of the mandible and temporal bone are separated by an articular disc, which divides the joint cavity into two small spaces.

Zygomatic arch

This is made up of the zygomatic processes of the:

- Temporal bone
- Malar (zygoma)
- Maxilla

The zygomatic branch of the facial nerve runs along the mid-portion of the arch where it is susceptible to damage by fractures (causing inability to close the eyelid by denervation of the orbicular is oculi).

Pterion

This is the name of an area where three bones meet. These are the:

- Greater wing of the sphenoid
- Squamous temporal bone
- Parietal bone

Mandible

This has several parts, namely the:

- **Symphysis:** the bone of the chin, extending back bilaterally to an imaginary line drawn vertically at the base of the canine teeth
- **Body:** the bone between the angle and symphysis
- **Ramus:** the bone between the coronoid, the condyle and the mandibular angle
- **Mandibular angle** (see Fig. 4.2g)
- **Alveolar ridge:** the horseshoe of bone directly beneath the teeth
- **Coronoid process**
- **Condyle of temporomandibular joint**

The inferior alveolar nerve provides sensation to the lower gums, lower lip, and the skin of the chin.

Blood supply of the face

The facial artery is a branch of the external carotid artery. It passes the side wall of the pharynx, upper surface of the submandibular gland, and inferior border of the masseter towards the medial angle of the eye, giving off superior and inferior arteries among other branches. Other arteries that supply the face include:

- **The superficial temporal artery** (from the external carotid)
- **The supraorbital and supratrochlear** branches of the ophthalmic artery (from internal carotid)

The venous drainage of the face is into the internal and external jugular veins. There is a communication with the cavernous sinus via the ophthalmic veins.

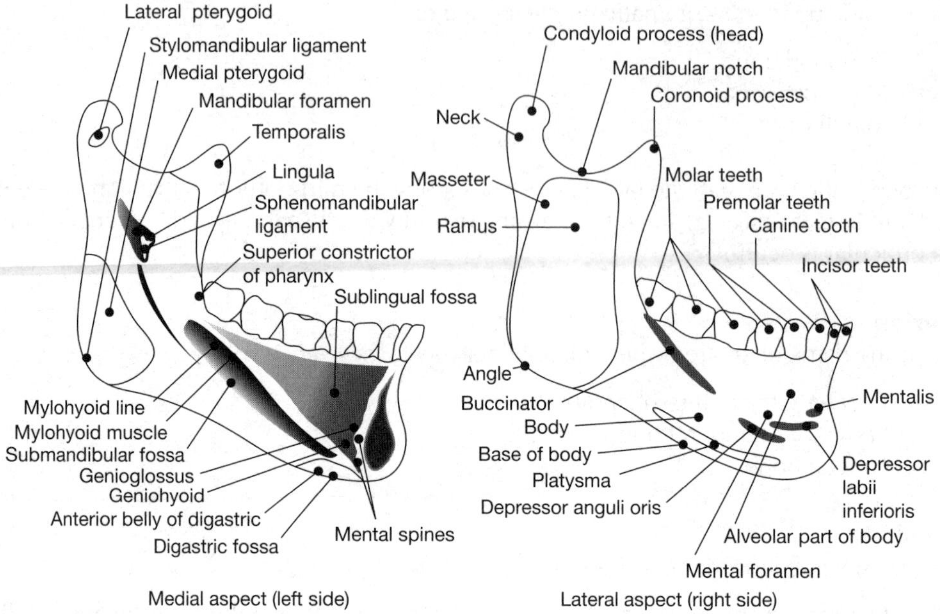

Figure 4.2g *Anatomy of the mandible and the teeth*

Bony facial injury

Frontal bone fractures

The frontal bone is very thick and fractures result from a great deal of force with direct impact to the forehead (so are often associated with other injuries). The patency of the nasofrontal duct is of great importance (because blockage can cause abscess formation). Anterior sinus wall fractures require fixation if they are displaced. Posterior sinus wall fractures are examined for dural tears and CSF leakage.

Nasal bone fractures

Trauma to the nose

May result in:

- Epistaxis
- Fractured nasal bones
- Septal fracture or dislocation
- Septal haematoma

Fractured nasal bones

A broken nose should only be treated if there is deformity. Initial simple manipulation may be sufficient to straighten the nose. Otherwise refer the patient for plastic surgery 7–10 days after the injury (time for the swelling to reduce) with a recent pre-injury photo. The nasal bones can be reduced under GA, or a formal rhinoplasty may be required.

Septal injury

Deviation of the septum may cause:

- Airway obstruction
- Septal haematoma (must be drained urgently as can lead to septal abscess and saddlenose deformity)

Naso-ethmoidal fractures

These extend from the nose to the ethmoid bone and can result in damage to the medial canthus, lacrimal apparatus, or nasofrontal duct. They also can result in a dural tear at the cribriform plate. Fractures with associated dural tears require neurosurgical review, and patients should be admitted for observation and IV antibiotics.

Temporal bone fractures

- Tend to be managed several weeks after presentation
- Fractures can be longitudinal (80%) or transverse (20%)

Signs of longitudinal fractures

- Swollen external auditory canal
- Tear of the tympanic membrane
- Bleeding from the ear
- CSF otorrhoea
- Facial nerve palsy (less commonly)

Signs of transverse fractures

- Haemotympanum
- 50% have facial nerve palsy
- Sensorineural hearing loss
- Vertigo
- Nystagmus
- IX, X, XII nerve palsies

Management of temporal bone fracture

- Hearing test
- EMG (if facial nerve palsy)
- Surgical decompression and grafting of facial nerve (may be indicated)

Temperomandibular joint (TMJ) dislocation

Most cases of dislocation occur spontaneously when the jaw is opened wide (eg while yawning, yelling, eating, singing, or during prolonged dental work) or during a seizure. Some patients are susceptible because of a shallow joint.

Traumatic dislocations occur when downward force is applied to a partially opened mandible. Most dislocations are anterior.

Exclude a fracture before manipulating. It is uncomfortable for the patient but can often be reduced fairly easily by a combination of downwards and forwards traction on the mandible (place your thumbs inside the mouth and support the bone with your fingers as you pull).

Zygomatic arch fractures

Isolated fractures may be undisplaced and treated conservatively. If the fracture is displaced it may impinge on the coronoid process of the mandible and require reduction and fixation.

Maxillary fractures

Le Fort classification of maxillary fracture (Fig. 4.2h) is as follows:

- **Le Fort I:** severs the tooth-bearing portion of the maxilla from the upper maxilla. Signs include crepitus on manipulation. It causes epistaxis but rarely threatens the airway
- **Le Fort II:** the middle third of the facial skeleton is driven back and downwards. If the bite is open, the airway is at risk
- **Le Fort III:** the fracture extends into the anterior fossa via the superior orbital margins. There may be CSF rhinorrhoea

If displaced, then open reduction and intermaxillary fixation may be performed to establish correct occlusion, followed by rigid fixation.

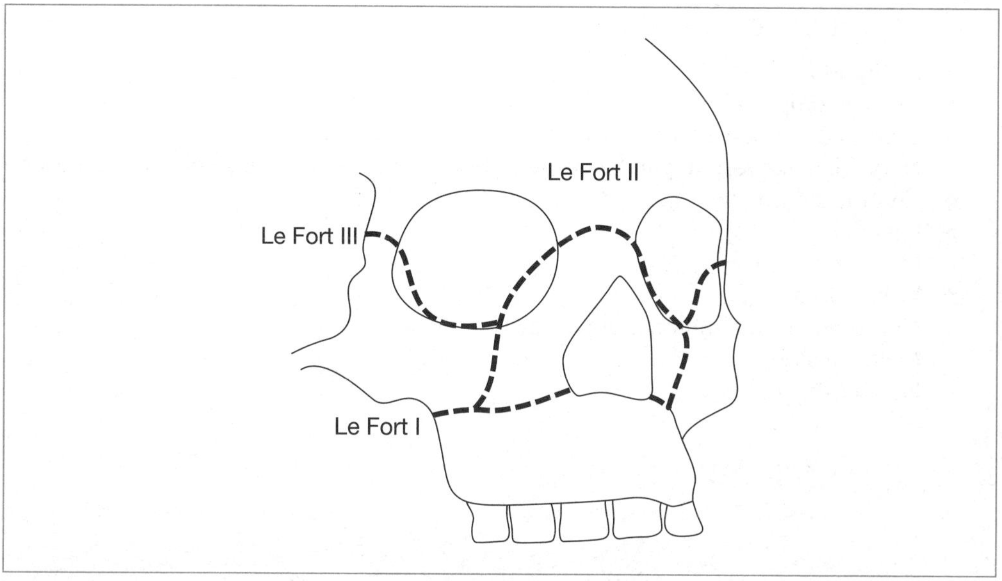

Figure 4.2h *Le Fort injury*

Mandibular fractures

These can occur in multiple locations secondary to the U-shape of the jaw and the weak condylar neck. Fractures often occur bilaterally at sites apart from the site of direct trauma. The most common sites of fracture are at the body, condyles, and angle: body 40–21%; condyle 20–15%; angle 31–20%; symphysis and parasymphysis 15–10%; ramus 9–3%; alveolar ridge 5–3%; and coronoid process 2–1%. Temporary stabilisation is performed by applying a Barton bandage (wrap the bandage around the crown of the head and jaw). A fracture of the symphysis or body of the mandible can be wired (controls haemorrhage and pain).

Soft tissue facial injury

- **Facial lacerations:** should be cleaned meticulously. Alignment of the tissues must be exact to produce a good cosmetic result. Refer complex lacerations to plastic surgery
- **Dog bites:** clean well and give appropriate antibiotic cover. Do not use primary closure
- **Rugby player's ear:** aspirate haematoma (repeat every few days) and then strap orthopaedic felt pressure pads against the head
- **Ruptured ear drum:** refer to ENT; advise against letting water into the external auditory meatus
- **Avulsed teeth:** may be replaced. If inhaled, arrange expiratory CXR
- **Bleeding socket:** bite on an adrenaline/epinephrine-soaked dressing or use sutures

Complications of facial injuries

- Aspiration
- Airway compromise
- Scars and permanent facial deformity
- Nerve damage resulting in loss of sensation, facial movement, smell, taste, or vision
- Chronic sinusitis
- Infection
- Malnutrition
- Weight loss
- Non-union or mal-union of fractures
- Malocclusion
- Haemorrhage

4.3 CHEST TRAUMA

In a nutshell ...

Life-threatening thoracic trauma

Causes 25% of trauma deaths in the UK
Fewer than 15% will require surgery
May be blunt injury, penetrating injury, or crush injury

Essential techniques for thoracic trauma

Chest drain insertion
Pericardiocentesis
Emergency thoracotomy

Likely pathologies for thoracic trauma

- Flail chest
- Pulmonary contusion
- Pneumothorax
    - Tension pneumothorax
    - Open pneumothorax
- Massive haemothorax
- Mediastinal injury
- Myocardial contusion
- Cardiac tamponade
- Aortic disruption
- Diaphragmatic rupture
- Oesophageal trauma

Types of trauma

- **Blunt** chest trauma as a result of RTAs predominates in the UK
- **Penetrating** trauma of the chest has a greater incidence in countries such as South Africa and the USA
- **Crush** trauma of the chest may be associated with cerebral oedema, congestion and petechiae due to SVC compression

Many of the conditions discussed below should be identified in the primary survey.

Procedure box: Insertion of a chest drain

Indications

Compromise in ventilation due to the presence of one of the following in the thoracic cavity:

Air
Blood
Pus
Lymph
Fluid (transudate/exudate)

Patient positioning

The site of the drain insertion depends upon the site of the fluid collection to be drained. Ultrasound may be used to locate fluid collections, and a mark placed on the skin to show an ideal site for drainage. Do not change the patient's position after marking. Alternatively a pigtail catheter inserted using a Seldinger technique may be placed for small fluid collections.

In general the drain may be inserted with the patient supine and the arm elevated. If there is grave respiratory distress and the patient is conscious the patient may be positioned sitting up and leaning forwards during the procedure.

Procedure

Perform under aseptic technique (skin preparation, gown, gloves, sterile drapes)
Identify insertion site (for large fluid collections this is usually the 5th intercostal space just anterior to the axillary line – remember the long thoracic nerve runs down the axillary line and should be avoided)
Infiltrate area with LA, taking care to site the area just above the rib – remember the intercostal neurovascular bundle runs in a groove in the underside of the lower rib border
Make a 2–3-cm transverse incision through the skin and bluntly dissect through the tissues to the parietal pleura

Puncture the parietal pleura and insert a finger into the thoracic cavity to sweep away adhesions, lung tissue and clots

Clamp the chest tube at the distal end and advance it through the incision, angled downwards towards the diaphragm for fluid collections and upwards towards the neck for collections of air

Never use the trocar as there is a high risk of damage to the lung and mediastinum

Connect the chest drain to an underwater sealed receptacle and confirm that the level swings with respiration

Suture the drain in place (you may use a purse-string to ensure that the tissues are closed tightly around the drain entry site)

Post-procedure instructions

CXR to ensure position of drain

Hazards

Never use the trocar

Never clamp a chest drain (high risk of tension pneumothorax)

Rapid drainage of fluid can result in pulmonary oedema

Complications

Damage to intrathoracic organs (lung, blood vessels, mediastinal structures)

Damage to structures of the chest wall (intercostal neurovascular bundle, long thoracic nerve)

Introduction of infection

Introduction of air to the thoracic cavity (leak around entry site; leak at site of apparatus)

Incorrect tube position

Flail chest

This is when a segment of the chest wall loses bony continuity with the rest of the thoracic cage due to multiple rib or sternal fractures. There will always be a degree of underlying lung contusion.

- Paradoxical chest wall movement means the tidal volume decreases
- Dramatic hypoxia commonly seen due to severe underlying pulmonary contusion

Signs of flail chest

Respiratory distress
Paradoxical chest wall movement
Crepitus of ribs
Hypoxia
Hypovolaemia if associated with significant blood loss

Treatment of flail chest

- Main aim of treatment is respiratory support
- IPPV is indicated if there is failure to maintain adequate oxygenation
- Drainage of any haemopneumothorax
- Adequate analgesia (epidural often helpful; intercostal block may be adequate)
- Careful fluid management essential as patients are prone to pulmonary oedema
- Operative intervention for stabilisation rarely indicated

Pulmonary contusion

Signs of pulmonary contusion

Bruising of lung tissue
Usually blunt trauma
Insidious onset of symptoms and signs
Respiratory distress
Increased airway resistance
Decreased lung compliance
Increased shunting leading to hypoxia
Atelectasis

Treatment of pulmonary contusion

- Support the respiratory system including intubation and IPPV if necessary

Tension pneumothorax

Signs of tension pneumothorax

Respiratory distress
Tracheal deviation AWAY from the side of injury
Unilaterally decreased breath sounds
Raised JVP
EMD cardiac arrest

Treatment of tension pneumothorax

- Immediate decompression
- Aspiration with a 14 G Venflon™ in the second intercostal space, clavicular line
- IV access
- Formal chest drain insertion

CXR must not delay treatment.

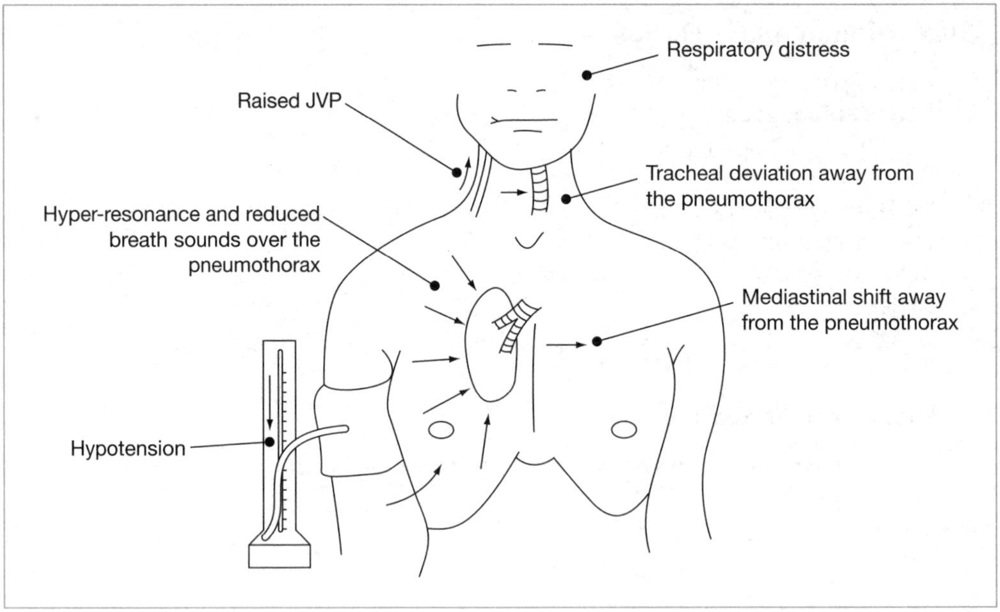

Figure 4.3a *Tension pneumothorax*

Open pneumothorax

This is a chest wound that is associated with air in the pleural space.

> **Signs of open pneumothorax**
>
> Respiratory distress
> Sucking chest wound: decreased air entry; increased percussion note over affected side

Treatment of open pneumothorax

- Occlude wound with sterile dressing; fix three sides only (flutter valve)
- Using different site, insert chest drain
- Surgical closure usually indicated

Massive haemothorax

This is 1500 mL or more blood drained from chest cavity on insertion of chest drain.

> **Signs of massive haemothorax**
>
> Hypovolaemic shock (decreased BP, tachycardia; peripheral vasoconstriction)
> Absent breath sounds
> Dull percussion note
> Signs of penetrating wound
> Increased JVP if concomitant tension pneumothorax
> Decreased JVP if hypovolaemic shock prevails

Causes of massive haemothorax

- Usually penetrating injury

Treatment of massive haemothorax

- Simultaneous drainage of haemothorax and fluid resuscitation
- Chest drain must be wide bore (> 32 Fr) AAL (anterior axillary line) 5th intercostal space
- Thoracotomy indicated if immediate loss > 2000 mL or continuing loss > 200 mL/hour

> If there are any signs of penetrating injury medial to the nipples/scapula posteriorly – assume damage to the great vessels or hilar structures.

Mediastinal injury

This is injury of any or all of the mediastinal structures:

- Heart
- Great vessels
- Tracheobronchial tree
- Oesophagus

CXR signs of mediastinal injury

Subcutaneous emphysema
Unilateral or bilateral haemothoraces
Pleural cap
Widened mediastinum
Free air in the mediastinum

Myocardial contusion

The leading cause of blunt trauma to the heart is RTAs (blunt trauma/deceleration injury).

Various injuries can occur, such as:

- Myocardial contusion (in which the myocardium is bruised and may be akinetic)
- Coronary artery dissection (which causes myocardial ischaemia, infarction, and arrhythmias)
- Cardiac rupture (usually from the atrium, which may lead to tamponade)

Cardiac blunt trauma may also be associated with other intrathoracic injuries (eg lung contusion, avulsion of vessels, aortic transection, pneumothorax).

- Myocardial contusion is the most common undiagnosed fatal injury
- Right ventricle is more often injured than the left
- Damaged heart tissue behaves similarly to infarcted myocardium

Cardiogenic shock is possible, in which case:

- Treat it early
- Treat aberrant conduction with a pacemaker if needed
- ECG changes include: premature ventricular ectopics or complexes (PVCs); sinus tachycardia; atrial fibrillation, ST changes; T-wave abnormalities; right bundle branch block (RBBB)

For a discussion of definitive treatment for blunt cardiac injury see the *Cardiothoracics* chapter in Book 2.

Cardiac tamponade

In the UK the most common penetrating cardiac traumas result from stabbing with a knife.

Cardiac chamber injury is often associated with injury to other intrathoracic regions (eg pulmonary parenchyma, hilum). The chambers most often injured are the left ventricle and the right ventricle, and injury to multiple chambers is common.

Cardiac chamber injuries proceed rapidly to pericardial tamponade. Associated chest or abdominal injuries cause hypovolaemia and pneumothorax. Failure to respond to thoracostomy tube drainage should lead to the diagnosis of pericardial tamponade being considered.

Cardinal signs of cardiac tamponade

- Raised JVP, low BP, muffled heart sounds (Beck's triad)
- Kussmaul's sign (JVP raised on inspiration)
- EMD cardiac arrest

Treatment of cardiac tamponade

Pericardiocentesis is both a diagnostic and therapeutic manoeuvre, which can decompress the pericardial space until formal cardiac surgery can be performed. A plastic cannula can be left in situ for repeated aspirations until thoracotomy is feasible. There is, however, a high false-negative diagnostic rate (50%) and a high rate of perforation of previously uninjured cardiac chambers. In one in four cases clotted blood is encountered which cannot be aspirated, though the removal of just 15–20 mL of blood can provide temporary relief.

Procedure box: Pericardiocentesis

Indications

- Cardiac tamponade
- Large pericardial effusions
- Diagnostic pericardial fluid

Contraindications

- Small, loculated or posterior effusions

Patient positioning

- Supine tilted head-up by 20°

Procedure

Performed under strict aseptic technique (gloves, gown, sterile drapes) and with full resuscitative measures in place
Infiltrate the field with 10 mL of LA
Aspirating continuously advance an 18 G needle (plastic sheathed, Seldinger catheter, or spinal needle) from the left subxiphoid approach, aiming toward the left shoulder tip
Keep an eye on the ECG as you advance the needle. An ECG lead can also be attached to the needle which will demonstrate increased T-wave voltage when the needle touches the epicardium
Blood is aspirated from the pericardial space and then a guidewire can be passed through the needle
A plastic sheath or catheter can be passed over the guidewire and left in situ (sutured in place) until urgent thoracotomy can be performed

Complications

Pneumothorax
Cardiac arrhythmia (VT)
Cardiac damage (myocardial puncture, damage to the coronary arteries)

For information on the definitive treatment for penetrating cardiac injury see the *Cardiothoracics* chapter in Book 2.

Aortic disruption

In aortic disruption:

- 90% are immediately fatal
- Deceleration injury mechanism is most common
- Site of rupture is usually ligamentum arteriosum
- Early diagnosis is essential for survival

Signs of aortic disruption

Hypovolaemia
CXR (widened mediastinum the only consistent finding)

Treatment of aortic disruption

- Involves fluid resuscitation whilst maintaining BP > 100 mmHg systolic
- Definitive treatment is surgical or stenting

Diaphragmatic rupture

Blunt trauma causes large defects in the diaphragm (allow herniation of abdominal viscera). Penetrating injuries are small and rarely life-threatening.

Signs of diaphragmatic rupture

Left side affected more than the right (right protected by liver; left more easily diagnosed)
Bilateral rupture is rare
Differential diagnoses include acute gastric dilatation, raised hemidiaphragm, loculated pneumothorax
If CXR ambiguous consider contrast radiography or CT

Treatment of diaphragmatic rupture is by surgical repair.

Oesophageal trauma

This is usually penetrating. Can follow blunt trauma to the upper abdomen (the oesophagus distends with gastric contents producing a linear tear).

Clinical signs of oesophageal trauma

Mediastinitis
Empyema

Confirmation of oesophageal trauma is by contrast studies, endoscopy, and CT.

Treatment of oesophageal trauma

- Surgical repair
- Drainage of the empyema
- Drainage of the pleural space

Emergency thoracotomy

This is commonly an **antero-lateral thoracotomy**, the procedure of choice for emergency, resuscitation room procedures, for management of cardiac or thoracic injuries, often in the context of major haemorrhage or cardiac arrest. This is discussed in the *Cardiothoracics* Chapter of Book 2.

4.4 ABDOMINAL TRAUMA

In a nutshell ...

Abdominal trauma is often missed and frequently under-estimated; therefore management should be aggressive.

Laparotomy is necessary in about 10% of blunt trauma patients, 40% of stab wound victims, and 95% of patients with gunshot wounds.

Trauma may be **blunt** or **penetrating**.

Damage may be to the:

- Abdominal viscera
- Spleen
- Liver
- Pancreas
- Intestine and mesentery
- Renal and genito-urinary systems

Blunt abdominal trauma

Blunt abdominal trauma is usually due to an RTA, a fall from a height, or a sports injury (eg rugby). The impact causes a crushing force to be applied to the organs which may result in rupture of distended hollow organs. Patients who have been involved in an RTA are also likely to have deceleration injuries.

Investigating blunt abdominal trauma

- **Baseline blood tests (including amylase):** FBC may be normal in the acute phase even with significant haemorrhage when dilution and equilibration has not yet occurred. ABG estimation may provide evidence of shock in terms of acidosis or a significant base deficit
- **Erect CXR and AXR:** these may reveal a haemothorax or pneumothorax, diaphragmatic rupture, rib fractures associated with splenic or hepatic trauma, gas under the diaphragm associated with visceral perforation, and pelvic fractures associated with massive blood loss
- **USS:** a portable scanner may provide a rapid, inexpensive way of detecting free fluid in the abdomen with a sensitivity of 86–97%

- **CT scan:** this is suitable for patients who are haemodynamically stable, but it is slow to complete. It involves moving the patient into the scanner, and relies on specialist interpretation. It provides good imaging of the retroperitoneum and is 92–98% accurate in guiding the decision to operate. It should only be used if the patient is haemodynamically stable

Diagnostic peritoneal lavage (DPL)

Diagnostic peritoneal lavage (DPL) provides a rapid way of determining whether an unstable patient with abdominal trauma requires a laparotomy. It does not reveal retroperitoneal blood loss, however, and carries a 1% complication rate, even in experienced hands. It is made more difficult by obesity, but can be up to 98% sensitive.

Indications for diagnostic peritoneal lavage

- Multiply injured patient with equivocal abdominal examination
- Suspicion of injury with difficult examination
- Refractory hypotension with no other obvious sites of haemorrhage

Contraindications to diagnostic peritoneal lavage

- Absolute (decision already made for laparotomy)
- Relative (previous abdominal surgery, obesity, advanced cirrhosis, coagulopathy, pregnancy)

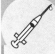

Procedure box: Technique of diagnostic peritoneal lavage

This is illustrated in Fig. 4.4a. Empty the stomach and bladder with an NG tube and a Foley catheter, respectively. Prep and drape the lower abdomen. Infiltrate LA with adrenaline/epinepehrine at the site of incision, in the line, one-third of the distance from umbilicus to pubic symphysis. Make a 2–3-cm vertical incision (long enough to expose the linea alba and peritoneum under direct vision) and dissect down in the line. Elevate the peritoneum between haemostats and carefully incise. Thread DPL catheter gently into the pelvis and aspirate gently. If blood is found, proceed to laparotomy. Otherwise, instil 1 litre of warm saline, and then allow this to drain back into the bag under gravity.

- If macroscopic blood or contamination is seen – proceed to laparotomy
- If macroscopically clear – send sample to the lab for analysis

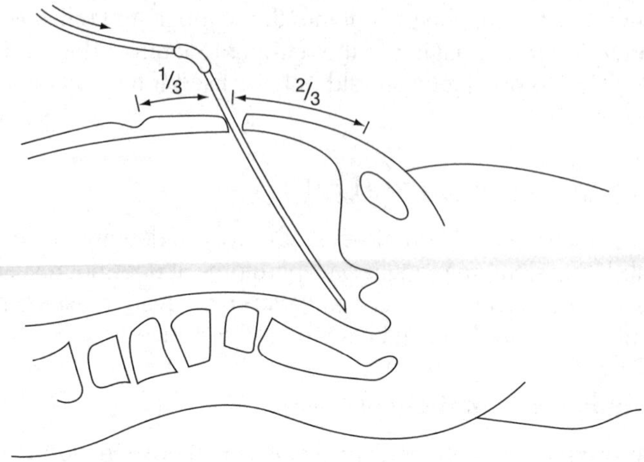

Figure 4.4a *Diagnostic peritoneal lavage*

Positive results of diagnostic peritoneal lavage

RBC > 100 000/mm^3
Gram stain showing organisms
Peritoneal lavage fluid found in urinary catheter or chest drain
WBC > 500/mm^3
GI tract contents aspirated on DPL

Penetrating abdominal trauma

- Low velocity eg knives – 3% cause visceral injury
- High velocity eg bullets – 80% cause visceral injury

These injuries commonly involve:

- Liver 40%
- Small bowel 30%
- Diaphragm 20%
- Colon 15%

Gunshot injuries are also likely to involve intra-abdominal vascular structures in 25% of cases.

Trauma to abdominal viscera

The management of trauma to individual intra-abdominal viscera is discussed in the *Abdomen* chapter of Book 2. A general outline only will be given here.

Trauma to the spleen

The spleen is one of the most commonly injured abdominal organs. Injury usually results from blunt trauma to the abdomen/lower ribs. Injury may arise from more minor trauma in children (due to the proportionally larger spleen and less robust rib cage) or in adults with splenomegaly. The injury is tolerated better in children.

- Main signs are those of haemorrhage
- Investigation depends upon whether or not the patient is haemodynamically stable
- Management depends on the degree of injury (conservative vs surgical)
- Post-splenectomy prophylaxis against infection is vital

If the patient is haemodynamically stable the possibility of splenic injury can be assessed with USS or CT (both have diagnostic accuracy of > 90%) although most trauma protocols recommend CT to exclude intra-abdominal injuries.

If the patient is unstable with obvious abdominal injuries, laparotomy is indicated after initial attempts at resuscitation. DPL is indicated only if there is doubt as to the cause of hypovolaemia (eg in unconscious multiply injured patients); some argue that it has **no role**, as less invasive investigations can be carried out if the patient is stable and immediate laparotomy is indicated if the patient is unstable.

Management is conservative unless there are signs of continuing haemorrhage, where laparotomy with splenectomy is indicated. Currently, there is a trend towards conservative management to avoid subsequent complications of overwhelming sepsis.

Long-term prophylaxis against encapsulated organisms is essential to prevent post-splenectomy sepsis syndrome. Vaccination with Pneumovax™, HIB vaccine and Meningovax™ should be administered in the post-op period. Long-term penicillin prophylaxis may also be advisable for susceptible people.

Trauma to the liver

The liver is the most frequently injured intra-abdominal organ.
Mechanisms of injury include:

- **Penetrating injuries:** knife and gunshot wounds
- **Blunt injuries:** deceleration in falls from a height or RTA

There is a hepatic injury scale which grades the liver damage from grade I (small laceration or subcapsular haematoma) to grade VI (avulsion, incompatible with survival).

Management includes simultaneous assessment and resuscitation along ATLS guidelines. If surgery is indicated, it should be performed promptly and by an appropriately experienced surgeon. Transfer to a liver unit may be necessary before or after surgery. The initial management should be along ATLS guidelines (see section 1.1).

Trauma to the pancreas

Blunt trauma to the pancreas is increasingly common and it is usually due to a compressive injury against the vertebral column from a direct blow (eg RTA, handlebar injury). It is a difficult diagnosis to make as the retroperitoneal location may mask symptoms.

- **Major injury:** proximal gland damage involving the head with duct disruption
- **Intermediate injury:** distal gland damage with duct disruption
- **Minor injury:** contusion or laceration that does not include damage to the main ducts

Amylase level may or may not be elevated; AXR may show associated duodenal injury and free gas; CT scan may be required.

Surgical intervention is reserved for major injuries. Lesser injuries can be treated with haemostasis alone. Distal injuries may require resection of the tail. Proximal injuries may require pancreaticoduodenectomy.

Trauma to the intestine and mesentery

Blunt injury leads to shearing, compression or laceration injuries. Injuries can be direct, or secondary to devitalisation when the mesenteric blood supply is compromised. Damage occurs in three ways:

- Bursting due to sudden rises in intra-abdominal pressure
- Crush injury against the vertebral column
- Deceleration injury at points where viscera are tethered (ie become intraperitoneal from retroperitoneal, or vice versa)

Penetrating injuries may cause perforation of the bowel (eg those caused by a blade) or large areas of damage (eg those from a gunshot).

Management of trauma to the intestine and mesentery

Conservative management of intestine and mesentery trauma

With repeated observation and early intervention if required (peritonism may be slow to develop)

Surgical management of intestine and mesentery trauma

Primary repair of small perforation (safer in right-sided injuries than in left-sided)
Resection with end-to-end anastomosis (if early intervention and minimal peritoneal soiling)
Defunctioning colostomy (usually due to gross contamination in a hostile abdomen)

Renal and genito-urinary injuries

Injuries to the genito-urinary tract account for 10% of all trauma.
Injury may occur to the:

- Kidney
- Ureter
- Bladder
- Urethra
- Scrotum and testes

Renal trauma is often blunt, associated with haematuria, and may be imaged using CT with IV contrast. The majority of injuries are managed conservatively (unless there is penetrating or vascular injury).

Ureteric trauma is usually penetrating or surgical and requires reconstruction.

Bladder trauma occurs when the organ is distended and is dealt a direct blow (rupture) or secondary to pelvic fracture.

Urethral injuries are usually fall-astride injuries or are associated with pelvic fracture. Beware of blood at the urethral meatus.

The scrotum and testes suffer from blunt trauma.

The management of trauma to the genito-urinary tract is discussed in Chapter 11 *Urology and Transplantation.*

4.5 TRAUMA TO THE PELVIS AND LIMBS

In a nutshell ...

The anatomy, physiology, pathology, investigation and management of individual pelvic and limb fractures are covered in detail in Chapter 2 *Orthopaedics* in Book 2. A general outline of the initial management of fractures in the trauma setting is described below, along with associated nerve and soft tissue injuries.

Trauma to the pelvis

Pelvic and acetabular fractures occur as result of high-energy trauma, so there is high incidence of associated injuries. These are severe injuries and may be associated with the loss of up to 6 litres of blood.

- **Classification:** according to mechanism of injury, or to stability of the pelvic ring
- **Investigations:** plain pelvic X-ray (ATLS), CT scan
- **Management:** initial stabilisation and later definitive fixation

The definitive management of pelvic trauma is discussed in the *Orthopaedics* chapter of Book 2.

Trauma to the limbs

Trauma to the limbs may involve damage to:
Bones
Joints
Blood vessels
Peripheral nervous system
Soft tissues and skin

In the management of limb injuries it is therefore important to examine and document the functional status of each of the components listed above. This is also important for excluding subsequent damage due to surgical management itself.

Trauma to bone

General management of fractures

- Reduce (if necessary)
- Hold
- Rehabilitate

Initial emergency measures for fractures

- Resuscitation following ATLS guidelines for all major traumas
- Temporary splint (eg sandbags, inflatable splints)
- Reposition fragment immediately if overlying skin is at risk
- For open fractures take photographs and swabs, cover with sterile dressings, give antibiotics and tetanus prophylaxis
- Assess clinically and radiologically

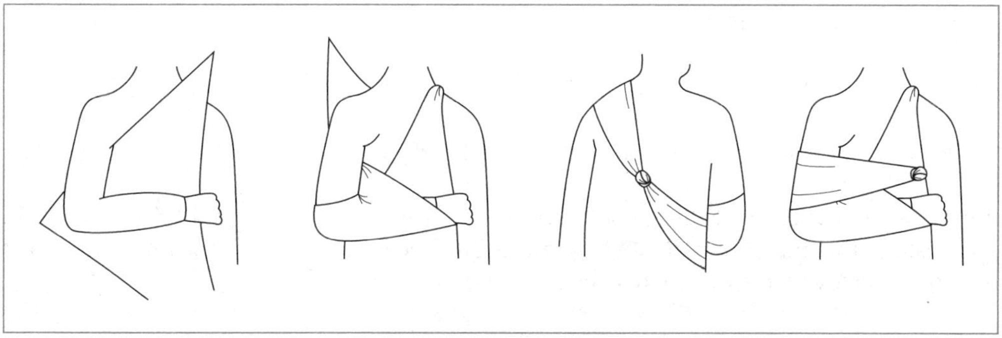

Figure 4.5a *Application of a sling*

Does the patient need to be admitted?

Admit the patient for:

- GA or other inpatient treatment required
- Observation (eg co-morbidity, multiple trauma)
- Nursing care (eg bed bound, bilateral limb fractures)
- Mobilisation with physiotherapy
- Social factors (eg elderly)
- Suspected child abuse

Local and systemic complications of fracture

Complications of fractures

Immediate complications

Internal or external bleeding
Organ injury (eg brain, lung)
Skin or soft tissues
Neurovascular damage

Late complications

General

DVT
PE
UTI
Fat embolism
Respiratory tract infection
Disuse atrophy
Osteoporosis
Psychosocial/economic factors

Local

Delayed union, non-union, mal-union
Compartment syndrome
Avascular necrosis
Infection
Joint stiffness
Secondary OA
Myositis ossificans

Finger injuries: use of a ring cutter

Presence of a ring on an injured finger may cause:

- Impedance of lymphatic drainage exacerbating swelling
- Vascular compromise in the acutely swollen digit

It may be twisted off whilst holding the proximal skin taut and using a lubricant (eg soap and water). This may be facilitated by the use of local anaesthetic in a ring block. If it cannot be removed this way then it should be cut off.

Some patients may refuse to allow a ring to be removed because of financial or sentimental value. Reassure the patient that rings can be re-formed by a good jeweller. If a patient continues to refuse to have a ring removed you must warn them about the danger of vascular compromise and then get them to sign an 'against medical advice' form which documents this warning.

Ask the patient to grasp an object, which stabilises the hand and elevates the dorsal side of the ring so it is easier to insert the ring cutter. Slide the blade of the ring cutter under the ring on the dorsal side of the hand. Once there is one cut, continue to cut completely through the ring being careful not to damage the skin. Bend the ring apart by placing pliers on either side of this break, and remove it.

For more detail about individual fractures and their management see *Orthopaedics* in Book 2. For discussion of compartment syndrome see Chapter 9 *Vascular Surgery*.

Trauma to joints

Trauma to joints may include:

Intra-articular fracture: good apposition of the fracture is important to reduce the potential for subsequent development of osetoarthritis. For further discussion see *Orthopaedics* in Book 2.

Dislocation: commonly of the digits, shoulders, and occasionally the knees. It is important to exclude associated neurovascular injury after dislocation. For further discussion see *Orthopaedics* in Book 2.

Mechanisms, complications and treatment of dislocation of individual joints is discussed in *Orthopaedics* in Book 2.

Trauma to the peripheral nerves

Acute injury to peripheral nerves is usually the result of direct mechanical trauma:

- Blunt (pressure)
- Penetrative (laceration)
- Traction (RTA and fracture)

Nerve damage is often missed, therefore assume injury present until proven otherwise. Chronic nerve injuries are more common. Leprosy is the most common cause of chronic loss of sensation worldwide, but diabetes is more common in developed countries.

Most common causes of sensation loss

In the UK	Worldwide
Diabetes mellitus (DM)	Leprosy
Peripheral vascular disease (PVD)	
Radiotherapy	

Structure of peripheral nerves

- **Endoneurium:** connective tissue around individual axons, containing collagen, capillaries and lymphatics. Protects from stretching forces
- **Perineurium:** dense connective tissue surrounding fascicle. Strong mechanical barrier. Diffusion barrier protects nerve fibres from large ionic fluxes
- **Epineurium:** outermost layer of connective tissue. Binds fascicles together and forms thick protective coat. Forms 25–75% cross-sectional area of nerve. Thicker over joints

Nerve disruption and healing

The classification of nerve lesions and process of healing is discussed in Chapter 1 *Basic Surgical Knowledge and Skills*.

Diagnosis and investigation of nerve injuries

Arterial bleeds suggest the possibility of nerve injury. Check the individual peripheral nerves, as detailed in the table.

PERIPHERAL NERVE CHECKS

	Sensory nerves	Motor nerves
Upper limb nerves		
Axillary	Regimental badge area (lateral upper arm)	Abduction of shoulder
Musculocutaneous	Lateral area of fore-arm	Flexion of elbow
Median	Palmar aspect of index finger	Abductor pollicis brevis
Radial	Dorsal web space between thumb and index finger	Wrist extension
Ulnar	Little finger	Index finger abduction
Lower limb nerves		
Femoral	Anterior aspect of knee	Knee extension
Obturator	Medial aspect of thigh	Hip adduction
Superficial peroneal	Lateral aspect of foot dorsum	Ankle eversion
Deep peroneal	Dorsal aspect of first web space	Ankle and toe dorsiflexion

Sensation can be maintained for 72 hours therefore look for sensation distortion.

Comparison of peripheral nerve function

- Hypersensitivity
- Reduced two-point discrimination
- Test with light touch
- Vasomotor function (reduced sweat production; disturbance of sympathetic function is an important early sign of nerve damage)

Electromyography

This objective investigation is time-consuming and unpleasant. It involves electrical assessment of the nerve injury and the extent of injury.

Approaches include:

- **Direct nerve stimulation:** the nerve is stimulated above and below the injury and the threshold of muscular response is compared with that of the opposite side
- **Detection of potentials within the motor unit:** surface electrodes or needle electrodes are used to establish close muscle contact; abnormal or reduced/absent action potentials indicate nerve injuries
- **Nerve conduction velocity determination:** this measures the interval between stimulation of the nerve and detection of the muscle action potential at distal sites. It is very useful for chronic lesions (eg normal velocity of the median nerve is 57 m/second, but in carpal tunnel syndrome it is 49 m/second)

None of these approaches is very effective immediately after injury as muscle stimulation continues before Wallerian degeneration is complete. When denervation is complete, fibrillation occurs.

NB: Nerve conduction is affected by age and temperature.

Treatment of nerve injuries

Aim to maximise the chance of recovery. Primary repair is always favourable as the outcome is better.

Nerve recovery

- Stump oedema occurs after 1 hour
- Axons start to sprout filopodia from the proximal to the last node of Ranvier and rely on the myelin sheath to guide them to the end organ (day 3)
- Chromatolysis (regenerative response of cell body whereby cell body enlarges) occurs in response to the increased metabolism (days 14–20)
- Distal axon undergoes Wallerian degradation (complete in 6 weeks)
- Muscle innervated by the injured nerve wastes time

During examination of the progress of a peripheral nerve injury, **Tinel's sign** represents painful paraesthesia on percussion over the area of regeneration.

Open injuries

- Always surgically explore and debride the wound thoroughly
- Clean cuts should be repaired or marked with 6.0 nylon
- Crushed/torn nerves are lightly opposed and re-operated upon at 2–3 weeks

NB: Vascular and orthopaedic injuries take priority over nerve injuries.

Closed injuries

- Mostly axonotmesis or neuropraxia
- Late surgery scar tissue should be excised; clean-cut ends should be anastomosed
- Use nerve grafts
- Use limb splints to decrease tension

Techniques for repairing nerves

Epineural
Fascicular
Grouped fascicular
Mixed repair

All wounds should be free of foreign bodies and nerves aligned with no tension.

Trauma to the soft tissues and skin

General wound management is discussed in detail in Chapter 1 *Basic Surgical Knowledge and Skills*.

In a nutshell ...

The key issues in the management of traumatic wounds are:

Assessment of devitalised tissue

Contamination

- Micro (bacteria)
- Macro (foreign bodies)

Debridement

Antibiotics and tetanus prophylaxis

Never treat a contaminated wound with primary closure.

Recognition of viable tissue

Skin viability

Look for:

- Colour and capillary return
- Bleeding from the dermal edge

Muscle viability

Accurate initial assessment of muscle viability is difficult. Debridement of dead muscle tissue is important to prevent infection. Traditionally assessment is by the **4Cs**:

C olour
C apillary bleeding
C onsistency
C ontractility

Colour is the least reliable sign – discolouration may occur due to dirt, contusion, haemorrhage, or local vasoconstriction. Transient capillary vasospasm may prevent bleeding in otherwise healthy tissue. Muscle consistency is the best predictor of viability: healthy muscle springs back into shape when compressed with forceps; non-viable muscle loses this ability and becomes gelatinous. Viable muscle fibres should twitch when squeezed with forceps.

Bone viability

Look for:

- Degree of soft tissue and periosteal stripping
- Pinpoint bleeding from debrided edges

See Chapter 1 for discussion of:

- Wound contamination
- Wound debridement
- Antibiotics and tetanus prophylaxis
- Skin loss and reconstruction

4.6 SPINAL INJURY

In a nutshell ...

The major trauma patient must be safely immobilised until the spine is cleared. At the end of the secondary survey you should have lateral C-spine X-rays and a clinical assessment of the spinal cord, which will lead you to one of the following conclusions:

1. The history, mechanism of injury and lack of clinical signs in a conscious patient who has no pain on palpation and no restriction of movement excludes a significant spinal injury
   Action: C-spine may be cleared clinically with or without adequate X-rays
2. A There is a significant mechanism of injury but the patient is conscious and has no clinical signs
   Action: C-spine may be cleared clinically but adequate imaging is advised
3. There is a significant mechanism of injury and the patient is not fully conscious or has significant distracting pain
   Action: It is difficult to clear the C-spine clinically and full imaging (which may include a CT) may be necessary
4. There are clinical signs of spinal injury, such as pain on palpation or restriction of movement or focal neurology, but no radiological signs on lateral C-spine X-rays
   Action: Full imaging is needed before clearing the C-spine (usually CT)
5. There is radiological evidence of spinal injury on C-spine X-rays
   Action: Urgent discussion with neurosurgeons, keep patient immobilised, and image the rest of the spine

The bony anatomy and neuroanatomy of the spine is covered in Book 2 in the chapter on *Elective Neurosurgery and Spinal Surgery*.

The overriding concern with spinal injuries is the risk of the trauma team either *causing* or *completing* an injury to the spinal cord, which can result in devastating and permanent neurological injury. This causes tragedy at a personal level, and has a long-term economic impact on medical resources. Utmost caution and vigilance should therefore be exercised when dealing with trauma victims at risk of having a spinal injury.

In the British Isles these injuries are most commonly seen in victims of RTAs. They are frequently associated with blunt injuries to the head, chest, and abdomen, and also with long bone fractures. If such a life-threatening injury co-exists with a suspected or proven spinal injury then it must be dealt with, whilst maintaining strict immobilisation of the spine. This is not achieved satisfactorily with a hard collar alone, but sandbags, tape, a spinal board, or in-line traction with skull tongs may be necessary until definitive treatment of the spinal injury can be safely addressed.

Trauma cases at risk of a spinal injury

- Unconscious/head injury (10% risk of associated C-spine injury)
- High-speed RTA
- Injury above the clavicle
- Sensory or motor deficit
- Brachial plexus injury
- Fall from heights more than 3 times patient's height

Injury to the spinal cord

In a nutshell ...

Assess the motor and sensory function below the level of the injury.

Complete injury: there is no motor or sensory function below the level of the injury.

Incomplete injury: there is partial motor and sensory function below the level of the injury (may also demonstrate sacral sparing with perianal sensation).

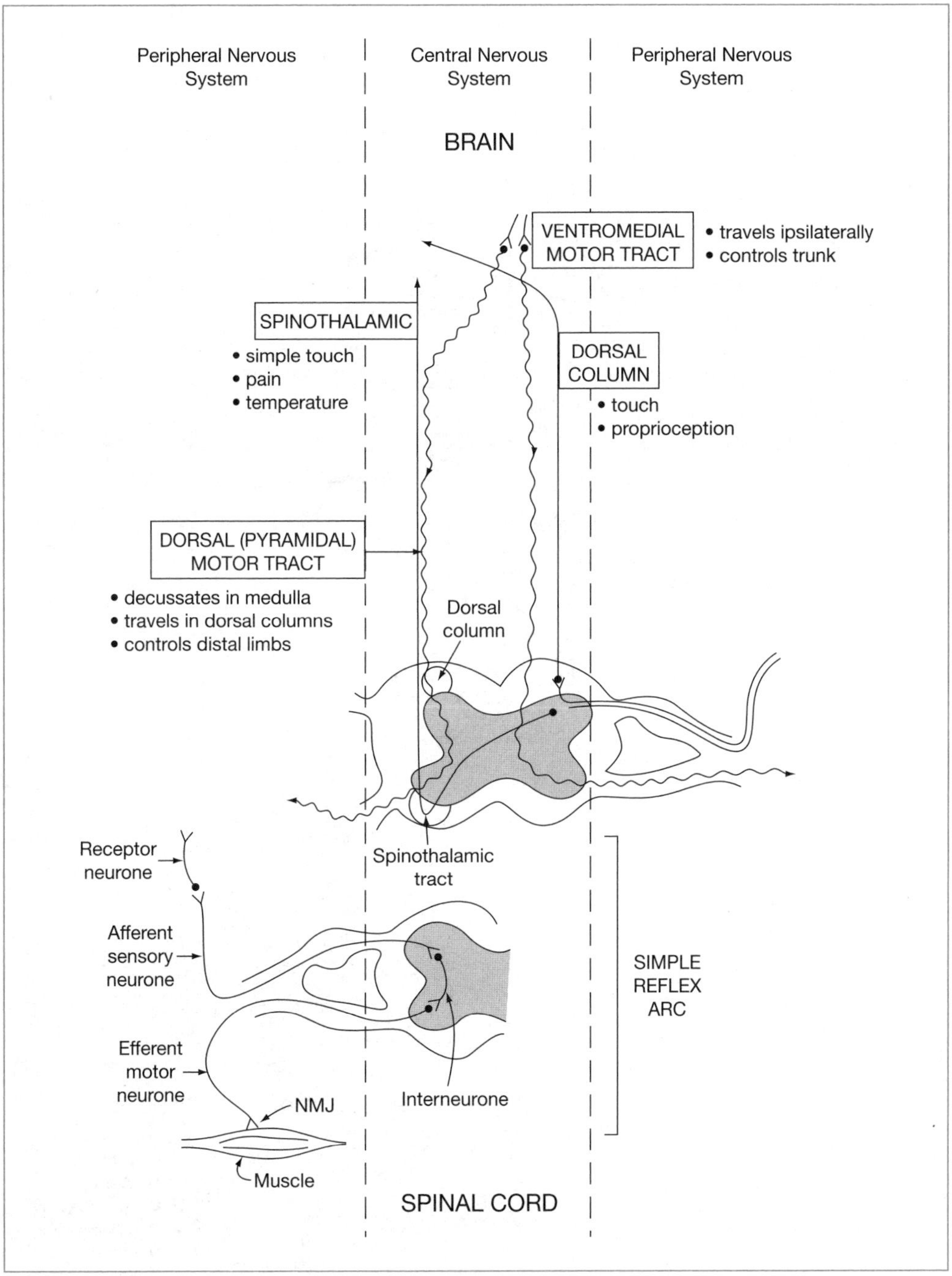

Figure 4.6a *The peripheral and central nervous systems – somatic*

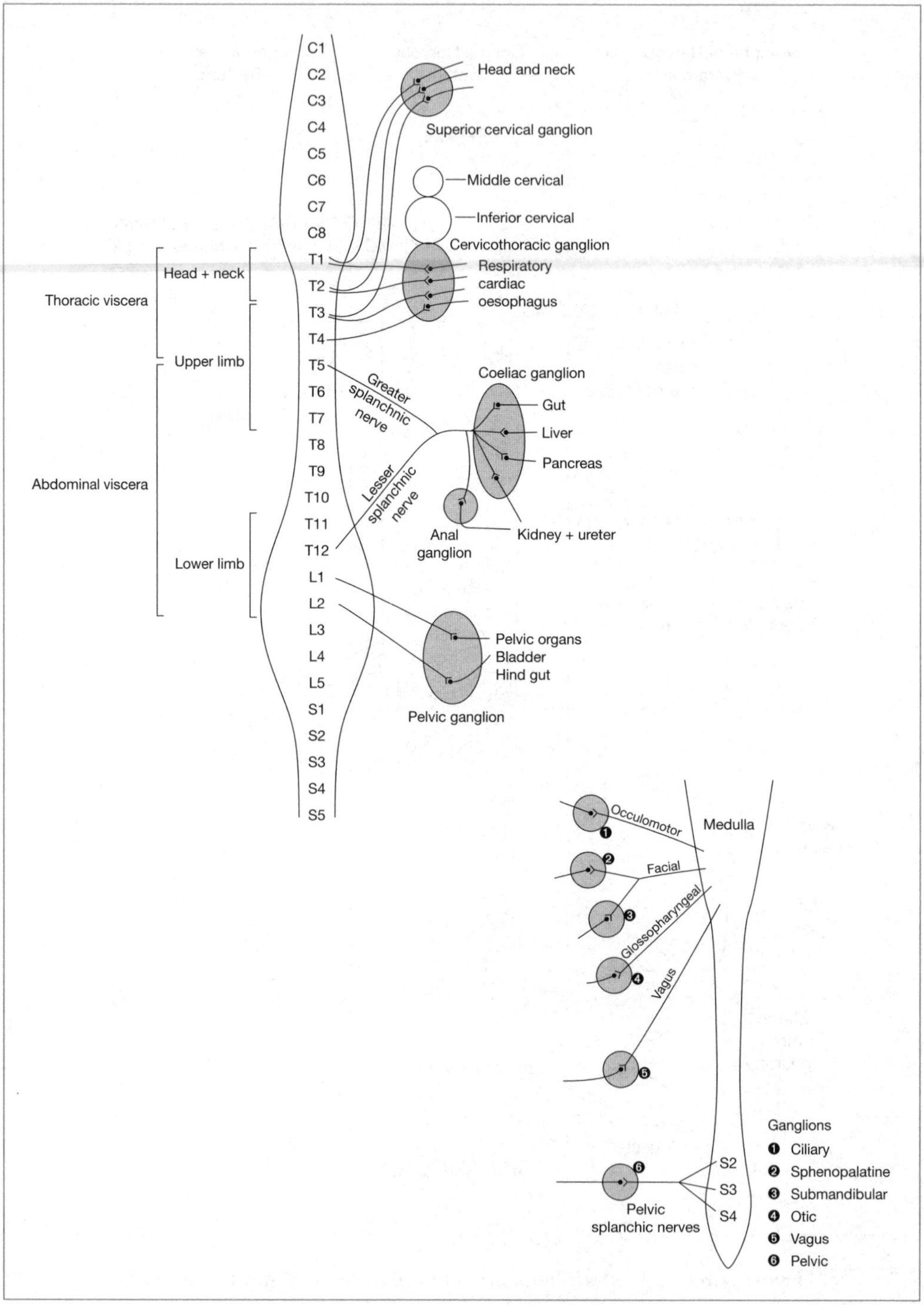

Figure 4.6b *The peripheral nervous system – autonomic*

Neurological assessment

Motor function

The assessment of motor function should reflect active movement by the patient related to each spinal level.

Movement related to spinal level

C3, C4 and C5 supply the diaphragm
C5 flexes the elbow
C6 extends the wrist
C7 extends the elbow
C8 flexes the fingers

T1 spreads the fingers
T1–T12 supply the chest wall and abdominal muscles

L2 flexes the hip
L3 extends the knee
L4 dorsiflexes the foot
L5 wiggles the toes

S1 plantar-flexes the foot
S3, S4, S5 supply the bladder, bowel, anal sphincter and other pelvic muscles

Motor function is conveyed by the ventromedial and dorsal motor tracts (see Fig. 4.6a). It is important to remember where the fibres of each tract cross in the spinal cord.

Sensory function

Pain and temperature perception are conveyed by the spinothalamic tract which supplies the contralateral side of the body (see Fig. 4.6a). Deep and superficial pain should be tested for separately (the pinch test and pricking with a broken tongue depressor, respectively). Superficial pain and light touch must be carefully distinguished as light touch is widely conveyed in the spinal cord and may be preserved when superficial pain sensation has been lost, enabling the diagnosis of a partial (as opposed to complete) spinal cord injury. Partial injuries have some potential for recovery, whereas complete injuries carry a dismal prognosis. In extreme cases the perianal and scrotal areas may be the only regions preserved (sacral sparing) and these should be carefully tested for sensation and anal contraction.

NB: loss of sensation below the level of spinal injury may obscure the diagnosis of other life-threatening injury.

The sensory levels are shown in Fig. 4.6c.

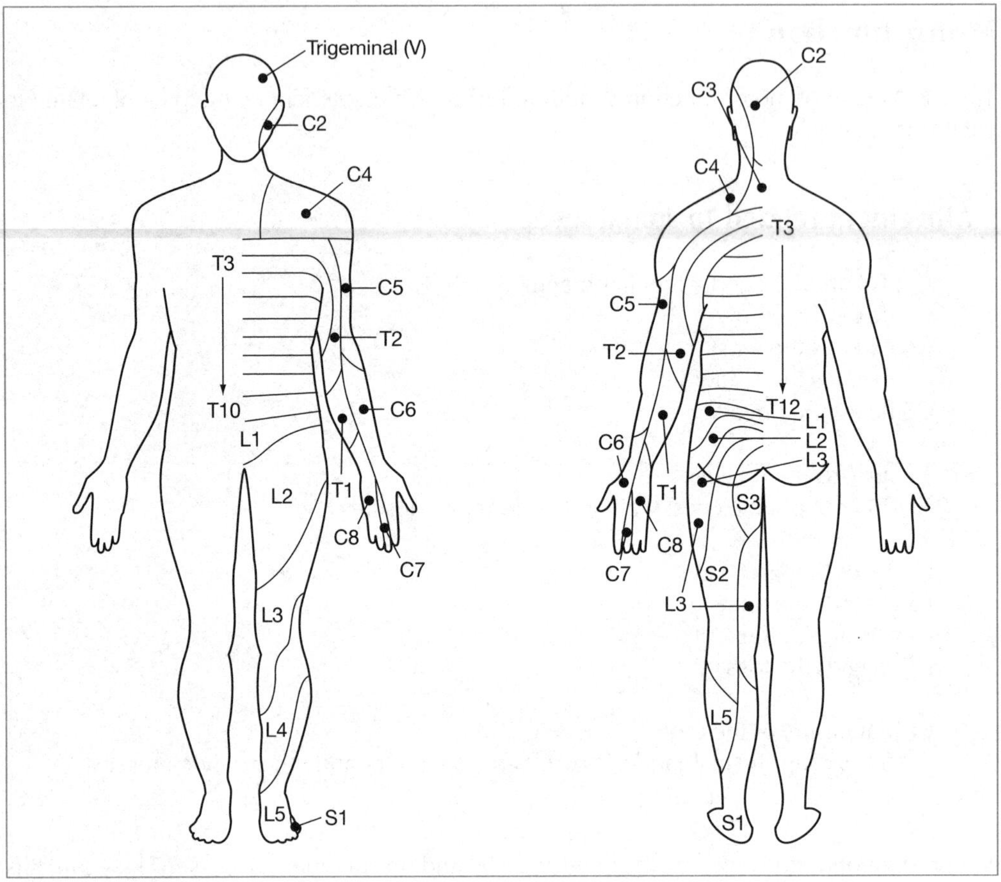

Figure 4.6c *Sensory levels*

- **Motor function:** this is transmitted via the corticospinal tracts which run on the ipsilateral side. Voluntary movement and involuntary response to painful stimuli can be assessed
- **Proprioception:** this is subserved by the posterior columns on the ipsilateral side and can be tested by joint position sense, and vibration sense using a tuning fork
- **Reflexes:** these should be assessed in the standard fashion, using a reflex hammer, and carefully documented for serial evaluation
- **Autonomic function:** evidence of damage to the autonomic nervous system can manifest as priapism and/or incontinence

Brown-Sequard syndrome

This syndrome results from hemisection of the spinal cord or disease processes affecting only one half of the cord. It results in ipsilateral motor dysfunction and contralateral sensory dysfunction below the level of the lesion. This occurs because motor fibres travel ipsilaterally in the spinal column and decussate in the brainstem. However, sensory fibres decussate in the spinal cord before ascending to the brain.

In the immediate post-injury phase, the injured spinal cord may appear completely functionless with resulting flaccidity and loss of reflexes. Several days or weeks later characteristic spasticity, hyperactive reflexes, and up-going plantar response supersede the flaccid state.

Injury to the cervical spine

In a nutshell ...

Clinical findings that suggest C-spine injury in an unconscious patient include:

- Flaccid areflexia
- Abdominal breathing (use of accessory muscles of respiration)
- Elbow flexion without extension
- Grimaces to pain above the clavicle (but not to pain below the clavicle)
- Hypotension with bradycardia (and euvolaemia)
- Priapism

NB: Accurate repeated documentation of clinical findings is essential in order to establish a baseline with which to compare trends of improvement or deterioration.

Assessment of the cervical spine

If a cervical spine injury is suspected then strict immobilisation must be maintained until accurate assessment can be performed by an adequately qualified individual. Assessment should include an accurate history, with careful consideration of the mechanism of injury and energy of impact.

Clinical symptoms in a conscious patient may include pain and neurological deficit. Clinical signs may include deformity (a palpable 'step off'), bruising, crepitus, and muscle spasm. A full radiological assessment (AP and lateral C-spine, visualisation of C7 with an effective pull-down, or a swimmer's view, and additional CT scanning if necessary).

Only when there is an absence of clinical and radiological evidence of a C-spine injury should spinal precautions be dispensed with. The cervical spine, if injured, is at particular risk during endotracheal intubation, 'log rolling', and transfer onto the operating table. During these manoeuvres, extreme caution must be exercised. For example: fibreoptic intubation avoids extending the neck from the neutral position; log rolling should be the minimum necessary to complete the secondary survey and only performed with an adequate number of trained assistants (four) in order to maintain in-line stabilisation of the C-spine.

Removing a crash helmet

The first person stands at the head of the patient. That person stabilises the patients head and neck by placing one hand on both sides of the helmet with the fingers on the patient's mandible, while someone else releases the straps.

The second person stands at the side of the patient and places their hands on either side of the patient's head with the thumb on the angle of the mandible and the fingers supporting the neck and occiput. This person is now in control of the in-line cervical stabilisation.

The first person then expands the helmet to clear the ears and slides it off (tilting it backwards to clear the nose if necessary).

Full C-spine immobilisation with collar, sandbags and tape can now be instituted.

Radiological assessment of the cervical spine

Radiographs of the C-spine are required in the following cases:

- Any injury above the clavicle
- Head injuries
- Unconscious trauma patients
- Multiply injured patients
- Brachial plexus injuries

In the first hour

Lateral C-spine radiographs are obtained as part of the standard trauma series (C-spine, chest, pelvis). Adequate views from the base of the skull to T1 must be obtained and the region of C7/T1 requires either a 'pull-down' technique, or a swimmer's view for proper assessment. The area of the atlas and axis can be rapidly assessed during CT scanning for a head injury.

It must be noted that portable films taken in the emergency setting miss up to 15% of fractures, therefore if a spinal injury is suspected on clinical grounds, then such an injury should be assumed to be present until proven otherwise. If a C-spine injury is present, then the rest of the spine needs to undergo radiological assessment.

Secondary evaluation

After the acute phase of the patient's assessment and resuscitation, if a C-spine injury is suspected or proven, then specialist evaluation by the orthopaedic or neurosurgical team will follow. This will include AP and oblique views of the C-spine, odontoid views, and CXR. Bony fragments within the spinal canal can be revealed by CT or MRI scanning. Flexion/extension views of the C-spine may also be deemed necessary and should only be performed under the strict supervision of an experienced specialist.

Specific types of cervical spine fracture

- **C1 atlas fracture:** axial loading can cause a blow-out of the ring of C1 (Jefferson fracture) best seen on the open-mouth view. A third of these are associated with a fracture of C2, but cord injuries are uncommon. These fractures are unstable and require specialist referral and management
- **C1 rotary subluxation:** usually presents in a child as torticollis. Odontoid views show the peg to be asymmetric with respect to the lateral masses of C1. No attempt should be made to overcome the rotated position of the head, and specialist referral and management is required
- **C2 odontoid dislocation:** bony injury may be absent and dislocation may be due solely to disruption of the transverse ligament on C1. Suspect this when the space between the anterior arch of C1 and the odontoid is more than 3 mm (**Steel's rule of three**: adjacent to the atlas, one third of the spinal canal is occupied by the odontoid, one third intervening space, one third spinal cord). This condition is unstable with a high risk of cord injury. Strict immobilisation and specialist management are mandatory
- **C2 odontoid fractures:** all require strict immobilisation and specialist referral:

Type 1	Above the base
Type 2	Across the base (NB: childhood epiphysis may resemble this on X-ray)
Type 3	Fracture extends onto the vertebral body

- **'Hangman's' fracture:** this results from an extension–distraction injury plus axial compression, and involves the posterior elements of C2 (in judicial hanging the slip knot was placed under the chin). This is a highly unstable injury and traction is strictly contraindicated. Strict immobilisation and specialist referral are essential
- **C3 to C7 injuries:** these can arise through a variety of mechanisms and, apart from obvious bony injury and clinical signs, they may be revealed by a haematoma reducing the space between the anterior border of C3 and the pharynx (normally < 5 mm). In children this distance is normally two thirds the width of C2 and increases on Valsalva. These require strict immobilisation, followed by specialist referral and management
- **Facet dislocations:** these may be unilateral (suspect them if the displacement between adjacent vertebral bodies is 25%) or bilateral (displacement of 50%). You may also see displacement of the spinous processes on AP views with unilateral dislocation
- **Cervical cord injuries:** at risk are injuries associated with a bone fragment from the anterior/inferior vertebral body which give the classic 'tear drop' appearance on X-ray. The posterior vertebral fragment may displace into the canal and cause cord damage

Thoracic spine injuries

These usually result in wedge fractures from hyperflexion injuries. Cord injury is uncommon but, because the canal is narrow in this region, cord injury is frequently complete when present. Thoracic spine injury more commonly occurs with a rotational injury. Wedge fractures of the thoracic vertebrae are splinted by the rib cage and only require internal fixation if the kyphosis exceeds 30° or if a neurological deficit is present.

Thoracolumbar injuries

Usually these result from hyperflexion and rotation, and they are commonly unstable. The cauda equina is at risk and will produce bladder and bowel signs, and deficits in the lower limbs. These patients are at high risk during log rolling so this may need to be minimised or deferred until X-ray studies are obtained.

Section 5
Special cases in trauma

5.1 PAEDIATRIC TRAUMA

In a nutshell ...

Accidents are the most common cause of death in children aged > 1 year. They account for 150 000 paediatric admissions and 600 deaths per year in the UK. The most common forms of accident resulting in death are RTAs, drowning, and house fires.

The assessment and resuscitation of the injured child is the same as for the adult (ABCDE) but take note of the anatomical and physiological differences.

Causes of trauma in children

The main causes of childhood deaths and accidents are shown in Fig. 5.1a.

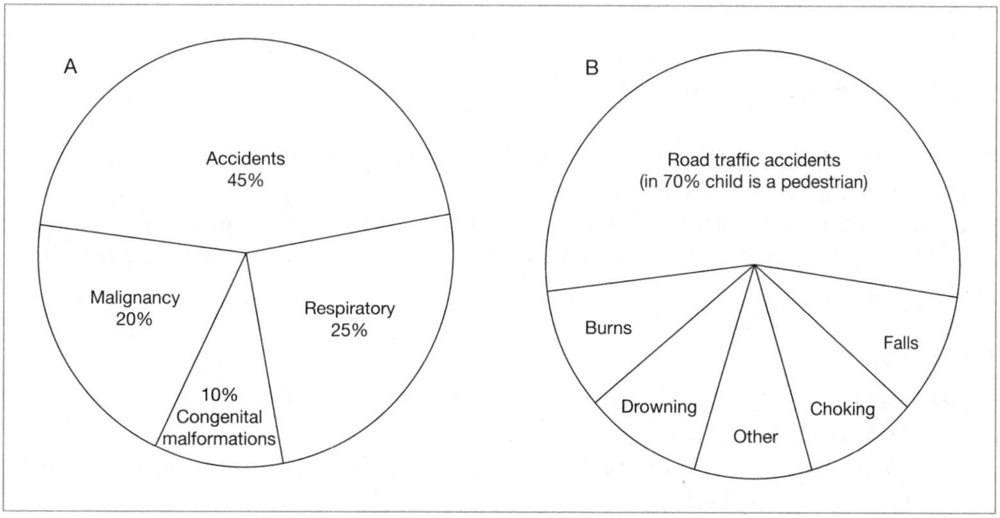

Figure 5.1a *Causes of death (A) and accidents (B) in children aged 1–14 years*

Differences between children and adults with respect to trauma

For more on paediatric physiology see the *Paediatric Surgery* chapter.

Anatomical differences in children

Children frequently have multisystem trauma because of their small size and shape.

Anatomical differences include:

- Increased force per body area
- Decreased fat layer
- Organs lie in closer proximity
- Rapid thermal losses
- Elastic skeleton often conceals underlying organ damage without fractures
- Effects of injury on growth and development

Physiological differences in children

Children tend to compensate well and therefore serious pathology goes unnoticed until decompensation occurs. Remember that pulse, respiratory rate and urine outputs vary according to the age of the child.

Psychological differences in children

Long-term effects of trauma can be social or affective resulting in learning disabilities. Communication difficulties can give rise to increased fear. Parents should always be allowed maximal contact.

Airway management

The relatively large occiput causes relatively increased flexion of the cervical spine. Soft tissues such as the tongue and tonsils are relatively large compared to the oral cavity and therefore obstruct the airway easily. A short trachea often results in right bronchus intubation. Nasal passages are narrow. Children aged < 6 months are obligate nose breathers.

Intubation

- Use straight-blade laryngoscope
- Use uncuffed ET tube to avoid subglottic oedema
- Choose a tube with a size equivalent to the girth of the child's little finger (or use the formula: (age + 4)/4)
- Use of a nasopharyngeal tube is debatable but is often safer for during transport of the child

Emergency surgical airway

- In small children (< 11 years) needle cricothyroidotomy with jet insufflation is the preferred method (surgical cricothyroidotomy is not performed because the cricoid cartilage provides the sole support for the airway in children aged < 11 years)

Breathing

Note these differences when intubating a child compared to an adult:

- Small airways are more easily obstructed (NB resistance is proportional to radius of tube)
- Muscles are more likely to fatigue
- The tracheobronchial tree is immature and is therefore more sensitive to pressure changes – be careful when using a bag and mask to minimise iatrogenic injury

Circulation

Recognition of shock may be difficult due to the great physiological reserve of children. Often the only signs are reduced peripheral perfusion and tachycardia. Greater degrees of shock may manifest as decreased consciousness and reduced responses to pain.

Remember

$CO = SV \times HR$

CO is cardiac output, SV is stroke volume, HR is heart rate.

In infants the SV is small and relatively fixed, therefore CO varies with HR. Thus the primary response to hypovolaemia is tachycardia and the response to fluid resuscitation is blunted.

Caution: increased HR is compounded by pain and fear.

NORMAL VALUES OF BP, HEART AND RESPIRATORY RATES, AND URINE OUTPUT IN CHILDREN

Age (years)	Heart rate (b.p.m.)	BP (mmHg)	Respiratory rate (breaths/min)	Urine output (mL/kg/hour)
< 1	110–160	70–90	30–40	2
2–5	95–140	80–100	25–30	1.5
5–12	80–120	90–110	20–25	1

Children aged > 12 years have values very similar to those of adults.

Chapter 5

Other useful features in assessing paediatric circulation are:

- Pulse volume
- End-organ perfusion (skin perfusion; respiratory rate; urine output; mental status)
- Temperature (toe–core gap)

PHYSIOLOGICAL RESPONSES OF CHILDREN TO HAEMORRHAGE

Organ/system	**Blood volume loss**		
	< 25%	**24–45%**	**> 45%**
Cardiovascular	Tachycardia Weak and thready	Tachycardia or bradycardia	Hypotension Pulse decreased
CNS	Lethargic Irritable Confused	Loss of consiousness Dulled response	Coma
Skin	Cool Clammy	Poor capillary refill Cold extremities Cyanotic	Pale and cold
Kidneys	Low urine output	Minimal urine output	No urine output

Intravenous (IV) access in paediatric trauma

After two attempts at percutaneous access, consider:

- In children aged < 6 years: intra-osseous needle (anterior surface of tibia 2 cm below tuberosity)
- In children aged > 6 years: venous cut-down

Fluid resuscitation in paediatric trauma

Give initial bolus of 20 mL/kg crystalloid (warmed whenever possible). Reassess, looking continually for a response to the bolus:

- Decreased HR
- Increased BP
- Increased pulse pressure
- Increased urine output
- Warm extremities
- Improved mental status

If there is no improvement with the bolus, give 20 mL/kg colloid (usually Haemaccel™). Children who do not respond to fluids may require blood (10 mL/kg).

Disability following paediatric head trauma

A child's brain is different to that of an adult. The brain grows rapidly over the first 2 years and has an increased water content. The subarachnoid space is relatively smaller and so the brain is surrounded by less CSF to cushion it in the event of impact.

The outcome of head trauma is worse in children aged < 3 and these children are particularly vulnerable to secondary brain injury. Children with an open fontanelle are more tolerant to an expanding mass because the ICP does not rise as easily (a bulging fontanelle may be palpated).

The Glasgow Coma Scale is still useful in children aged > 4. In children aged < 4 the verbal response score must be modified (eg 5 = appropriate for age, 4 = crying consolably, 3 = crying inconsolably, 2 = agitated, 1 = noiseless).

Exposure

Remember that the relatively large surface area to weight ratio of children means they lose heat quickly. Overhead heaters and blankets are essential.

NB: Remember that all drug dosages should be worked out per kg body weight.
The weight estimate in kg for those < 10 is calculated by: (age + 4) × 2.

Thoracic trauma in children

This occurs in 10% of children (and two thirds of these will have concurrent injury to the head or abdomen).

- The chest wall is more compliant, so children can have pulmonary contusions without rib fracture; therefore you should actively look for injury (rib fracture requires proportionally more force in a child than in an adult)
- Mobility of the mediastinal structures makes the child more sensitive to tension pneumothorax and flail segments
- Chest drain insertion is performed in the same way as for an adult but a smaller diameter tube is used

Abdominal trauma in children

- Decompress the stomach with an NG or orogastric tube (crying causes swallowing of air)
- Children are often managed non-operatively with repeated observation and examination (unless haemodynamically unstable)

Certain injuries are more prevalent in the child:

- Duodenal and pancreatic injuries due to handlebar trauma
- Mesenteric small bowel avulsion injuries
- Bladder rupture (shallower pelvis)
- Fall-astride injuries to the perineum

Non-accidental injury (NAI)

Always be aware of the possibility that trauma has been caused by NAI. It is estimated that up to 2% of children may suffer NAI during childhood. A number of features should raise your suspicion.

In the history:

- Late presentation
- Inconsistent story
- Injury not compatible with history (eg long bone fracture in children under walking age)
- Repeated injuries

In the examination:

- Abnormal interaction between child and parents
- Bizarre injuries (eg bites, burns, and shape of injury such as fingertip bruising)
- Peri-oral injuries
- Perianal/genital injuries
- Evidence of previous injuries (old scars, healing fracture)

If in doubt, you must refer on to the appropriate authorities (via your immediate senior and the paediatrics service – these children should be seen by a senior paediatrician). Ensure that your notes are clear and accurate. Describe what you see, not what you infer – eg say 'four circular bruises approximately 1 cm in diameter around the upper arm' rather than 'bruising from fingertips'.

The following investigations should be performed in any case of suspected physical abuse:

- Full skeletal survey – radiology of the whole skeleton to look for old or undiagnosed fractures
- Tests of clotting function, including full blood count for platelets
- Biochemistry, including bone biochemistry
- Appropriate investigations of the head if indicated
- Medical photography of any affected area

5.2 TRAUMA IN PREGNANCY

In a nutshell ...

Treatment priorities are the same as for the non-pregnant patient – treat the mother first as the fetus is reliant on her condition. Resuscitation and stabilisation need modification to account for the anatomical and physiological changes which occur in pregnancy.

The fetus may be in distress before the mother shows outward signs of shock.

Anatomical changes in pregnancy

- **1st trimester:** uterus is relatively protected by bony pelvis and thick-walled uterus
- **2nd trimester:** uterus becomes intra-abdominal and more vulnerable to injury; amniotic fluid cushions fetus
- **3rd trimester:** relative decrease in amniotic fluid and thickness of uterus, therefore fetus is more vulnerable to blunt and penetrative trauma

The placenta contains no elastic tissue and is vulnerable to shearing forces, resulting in incidences of placental abruption and damage to dilated pelvic veins.

Physiological changes in pregnancy

Oestrogen and progesterone have the following effects:

- **↓ smooth muscle tone:** decreased gastric emptying with LOS reflux, therefore risk of aspiration
- **↓ $PaCO_2$**: to 30 mmHg. This is the 'physiological hyperventilation of pregnancy' secondary to the respiratory stimulant effect of progesterone. FEV_1/FVC remains the same, but tidal volume increases by 40%
- **↑ pulse rate**
- **↑ BP:** by 10–15 mmHg in the second trimester (normalises near term)
- **↑ plasma volume:** by 50%
- **↑ cardiac output:** by 1.0–1.5 litres/minute (CVP is usually normal despite the increased total volume)

This means that pregnant women have to lose more of their total circulating volume before signs of hypovolaemia develop. Blood is shunted away from the uterofetal circulation to maintain the mother's vital signs. Therefore the fetus may be shocked before maternal tachycardia, tachypnoea, or hypotension develop. For these reasons, vigorous fluid replacement is required.

Aortocaval compression
The enlarged uterus can compress the IVC and impair venous return, reducing cardiac output by up to 40%. This can cause a drop in BP unless the pressure is minimised by placing patients in the left lateral position.

Secondary survey in pregnancy

Urgent X-rays (eg of C-spine) are still taken because the priority is to detect life-threatening injuries. The uterus can be protected with lead for all imaging except the pelvic film.

Special considerations in pregnancy

Search for conditions unique to the pregnant patient:

- Blunt/penetrating uterine trauma
- Placental abruption
- Amniotic fluid embolism
- DIC
- Eclampsia
- Uterine rupture
- Premature rupture of membranes in labour
- Isoimmunisation: prophylactic anti-D should be given to rhesus-negative mothers within 72 hours
- The Kleihauer–Betke test (maternal blood smear looking for fetal red blood cells) is specific but not very sensitive, and is therefore of little use

5.3 POST-TRAUMATIC STRESS DISORDER (PTSD)

In a nutshell ...

This occurs when a person has experienced a traumatic event involving actual or threatened death or injury to themselves or others. The individual will have felt fear, helplessness, or horror.

There are three classic symptoms which usually cluster:

- **Intrusions:** re-experiencing the event via flashbacks or nightmares
- **Avoidance:** the person attempts to reduce exposure to people, places or things that exacerbate the intrusions

- **Hyperarousal:** physiological signs of increased arousal, including hypervigilance and increased startle response

These symptoms must persist for more than 1 month after the event to qualify as PTSD, causing significant distress or impairment of social or occupational situations.

Other symptoms include:

- Insomnia
- Anorexia
- Depression with low energy
- Difficulty in focusing
- Social withdrawal

Lifetime prevalence in the USA is 5–10% (Kessler *et al.* 1995). This value increases to more than 20% in inner city populations.

Management of PTSD

If symptoms are mild and present for less than 4 weeks then a period of watchful waiting is recommended.

Psychological therapy: trauma-focused cognitive behavioural therapy should be offered to those with severe post-traumatic symptoms or with severe PTSD in the first month after the traumatic event. These treatments should be offered to everyone with PTSD over the subsequent months and should normally be provided on an individual outpatient basis.

Drug therapy: this should only be administered by a specialist and usually involves antidepressants such as paroxetine.

Chapter 6

Peri-operative Care

Sally Nicholson and Catherine Parchment Smith

Section 1

Pre-operative management of the surgical patient

In a nutshell ...

Before considering surgical intervention it is necessary to prepare the patient as fully as possible.

The extent of pre-op preparation depends on:

Classification of surgery:

- Elective
- Scheduled
- Urgent
- Emergency

Nature of the surgery (minor, major, major-plus)

Location of the surgery (A&E, endoscopy, minor theatre, main theatre)

Facilities available

The rationale for pre-op preparation is to:

Anticipate difficulties

Make advanced preparation and organise facilities, equipment and expertise

Enhance patient safety and minimise chance of errors

Alleviate any relevant fear/anxiety perceived by patient

Common factors resulting in cancellation of surgery include:

- Inadequately controlled existing medical condition
- Inadequate investigation of existing medical condition
- New acute medical condition

Classification of surgery according to the National Confidential Enquiry into Patient Outcome and Deaths (NCEPOD):

- **Elective:** mutually convenient timing
- **Scheduled:** (or semi-elective) early surgery under time limits (eg 3 weeks for malignancy)
- **Urgent:** as soon as possible after adequate resuscitation and within 24 hours
- **Emergency:** life-saving procedure with resuscitation simultaneous to surgery

Patients may be:

- Emergency: admitted from A&E; admitted from clinic
- Elective: admitted from home (usually pre-assessed)

1.1 BEFORE ADMISSION

In a nutshell ...

Pre-operative preparation of a patient before admission may include:

- History
- Physical examination
- Investigations as indicated
  - Blood tests
  - Urinalysis
  - ECG
  - Radiological investigations
  - Microbiological investigations
  - Special tests
- Consent and counselling

The pre-assessment clinic is a useful tool for performing some or all of these tasks prior to administration.

Pre-operative history

A good history is essential. Establish a good rapport with the patient. Try to ask open rather than leading questions, but direct the resulting conversation. Try to elucidate a set of differential diagnoses, and aim questions to confirm or refute your suspicions. Taking a history also gives you an opportunity to assess patient understanding and the level at which you should pitch your subsequent explanations.

A detailed chapter on taking a surgical history can be found in the new edition of the PasTest book *Short Surgical Cases for the MRCS Clinical Examination* (Chapter 7 *Information Gathering Communications Bay*). In summary, the history should cover the points in the following box.

Taking a surgical history

1. Introductory sentence
Name, age, gender, occupation.

2. Presenting complaint
In one simple phrase, the main complaint that brought the patient into hospital, and the duration of that complaint, eg 'Change in bowel habit for 6 months' or 'Right loin pain for 2 hours'.

3. History of presenting complaint
a) *The story* of the complaint as the patient describes it from when they were last well to the present
b) *Details of the presenting complaint* eg if it is a pain the site, intensity, radiation, onset, duration, character, alleviating and exacerbating factors, or symptoms associated with previous episodes
c) *Review of the relevant system/s* which may include the GI, gynaecological and urological review, but does not include the systems not affected by the presenting complaint. This involves direct questioning about every aspect of that system and recording the negatives and the positives
d) *Relevant medical history* ie any previous episodes, surgery or investigations directly relevant to this episode. Do not include irrelevant previous operations here. Ask if they have had this complaint before, when, how, and by whom
e) *Risk factors*. Ask about risk factors relating to the complaint, eg family history, smoking, high cholesterol. Ask about risk factors for having a general anaesthetic, eg previous anaesthetics, family history of problems under anaesthetic, false teeth, caps or crowns, limiting co-morbidity, exercise tolerance, or anticoagulation medications

4. Past medical and surgical history
In this section should be all the previous medical history, operations, illnesses, admissions to hospital, etc, which were not mentioned as relevant to the history of the presenting complaint.

5. Drug history and allergies
List of all drugs, dosages and times they were taken. List allergies and nature of reactions to alleged allergens. Ask directly about the oral contraceptive pill and antiplatelet medication such as aspirin and clopidogrel which may have to be stopped pre-operatively.

6. Social history
Smoking and drinking – how much and for how long. Recreational drug abuse. Who is at home with the patient? Who cares for them? Social service input? Stairs or bungalow? How much can they manage themselves?

7. Family history

Chapter 6

8. Full review of non-relevant systems
This includes all the systems not already covered in the history of the presenting complaint, eg respiratory, cardiovascular, neurological, endocrine, and orthopaedic.

Physical examination

Detailed descriptions of methods of physical examination can only really be learnt by observation and practice. Don't rely on the examination of others – surgical signs may change and others may miss important pathologies. See *Surgical Short Cases for the MRCS Clinical Examination* for details of surgical examinations for each surgical system.

Physical examination

General examination: is the patient well or in extremis? Are they in pain? Look for anaemia, cyanosis and jaundice, etc. Do they have characteristic facies or body habitus (eg thyrotoxicosis, cushingoid, marfanoid)? Are they obese or cachectic? Look at the hands for nail clubbing, palmar erythema, etc.
Cardiovascular examination: pulse, BP, JVP, heart sounds and murmurs. Vascular bruits (carotids, aortic, renal, femoral) and peripheral pulses
Respiratory examination: respiratory rate (RR), trachea, percussion, auscultation, use of accessory muscles
Abdominal examination: scars from previous surgery, tenderness, organomegaly, mass, peritonism, rectal examination
CNS examination: particularly important in vascular patients pre carotid surgery and in patients with suspected spinal compression
Musculoskeletal examination: before orthopaedic surgery

When to do an investigation:

- To confirm a diagnosis
- To exclude a differential diagnosis
- To assess appropriateness of surgical intervention
- To asses fitness for surgery

When deciding upon appropriate investigations for a patient you should consider:
- Simple investigations first
- Safety (non-invasive investigation before invasive investigation if possible)
- Cost vs benefit
- The likelihood of the investigation providing and answer (sensitivity and specificity of the investigation)

Blood tests

Full blood count (FBC)

FBC provides information on the following (normal ranges in brackets):

- Haemoglobin concentration (12–16 g/dL in males; 11–14 g/dL in females)
- WCC (5–10 × 10^9/L)
- Platelet count (150–450 × 10^9/L)

Also it may reveal details of red cell morphology (eg macrocytosis in alcoholism, microcytosis in iron deficiency anaemia) and white cell differential (eg lymphopenia, neutrophilia).

When to perform a pre-operative FBC

In practice almost all surgical patients have an FBC measured but it is particularly important in the following groups:

- All emergency pre-op cases – especially abdominal conditions, trauma, sepsis
- All elective pre-op cases aged > 60 years
- All elective pre-op cases in adult females
- If surgery is likely to result in significant blood loss
- If there is suspicion of blood loss, anaemia, haemopoietic disease, sepsis, cardiorespiratory disease, coagulation problems

Urea and electrolytes (U&Es)

U&Es provide information on the following (normal ranges in brackets):

- Sodium (133–144 mmol/L)
- Potassium (3.3–5.5 mmol/L)
- Urea (2.5–6.5 mmol/L)
- Creatinine (55–150 mmol/L)

The incidence of an unexpected abnormality in apparently fit patients aged < 40 years is < 1% but increases with age and ASA grading (American Society of Anaesthesiologists).

When to perform a pre-operative U&E

In practice almost all surgical patients get their U&Es tested but it is particularly important in the following groups:

- All pre-op cases aged > 65
- Positive result from urinalysis (eg ketonuria)
- All patients with cardiopulmonary disease, or taking diuretics, steroids or drugs active on the cardiovascular system
- All patients with a history of renal/liver disease or an abnormal nutritional state

- All patients with a history of diarrhoea/vomiting or other metabolic/endocrine disease
- All patients on an intravenous infusion for more than 24 hours

Amylase

- Normal plasma amylase range varies with different reference laboratories
- Perform in all adult emergency admissions with abdominal pain, before consideration of surgery
- Inflammation surrounding the pancreas will cause mild elevation of the amylase, dramatic elevation of the amylase results from pancreatitis

Random blood glucose (RBG)

- Normal plasma glucose range is 3–7 mmol/L

When to perform an RBG

- Emergency admissions with abdominal pain, especially if suspecting pancreatitis
- Pre-operative elective cases with diabetes mellitus, malnutrition or obesity
- All elective pre-op cases aged > 60 years
- When glycosuria or ketonuria are present on urinanalysis

Clotting tests

Prothrombin time (PT)

- 11–13 seconds
- Measures the functional components of the extrinsic pathway prolonged with warfarin therapy, in liver disease, and DIC

Activated partial thromboplastin time (APTT)

- < 35 seconds
- Measures the functional components of the intrinsic pathway and is prolonged in haemophilia A and B, with heparin therapy, and in DIC

Bleeding time

- < 10 minutes
- Prolonged with platelet dysfunction and thrombocytopenia.

Sickle cell test

Different hospitals have different protocols, but in general you would be wise to perform a sickle cell test in all patients of African or Caribbean origin in whom surgery is planned, and in anyone who has sickle cell disease in the family.

Liver function tests (LFTs)

- Perform LFTs in all patients with upper abdominal pain, jaundice, known hepatic dysfunction or history of alcohol abuse
- Remember that clotting tests are the most sensitive indicator of liver synthetic disorder and may be deranged before changes in the LFTs. Decreased albumin levels are an indicator of chronic illness and sepsis

Group and save/cross-match

When to perform a group and save:

- Emergency pre-op cases likely to result in significant operative blood loss, especially trauma, acute abdomen, vascular cases
- If there is suspicion of blood loss, anaemia, haemopoietic disease, coagulation defects
- Procedures on pregnant females

Urinalysis

When to perform pre-op urinalysis:

- All emergency cases with abdominal or pelvic pain
- All elective cases with diabetes mellitus
- All pre-op cases with thoracic, abdominal, or pelvic trauma

A **mid-stream urine** (MSU) specimen should be considered before genito-urinary operations and in pre-op patients with abdominal or loin pain.

A **urine pregnancy test** should be performed in all women of childbearing age with abdominal symptoms, or who require X-rays.

Electrocardiography (ECG)

A 12-lead ECG is capable of detecting acute or longstanding pathological conditions affecting the heart, particularly changes in rhythm, myocardial perfusion, or prior infarction.

NB: The resting ECG is not a sensitive test for coronary heart disease, being normal in up to 50%. An exercise test is preferred.

When to perform a 12-lead ECG:

- Patients with a history of heart disease, diabetes, hypertension, or vascular disease, regardless of age
- Patients aged > 60 with hypertension or other vascular disease
- Patients undergoing cardiothoracic surgery, taking cardiotoxic drugs, or with an irregular pulse
- Any suspicion of hitherto undiagnosed cardiac disease

Radiological investigations

Radiological investigations may include:

- **Plain films:** chest X-ray, plain abdominal film, lateral decubitus film, KUB film, skeletal views
- **Contrast studies and X-ray screening:** gastrograffin, IV contrast
- **Ultrasound scanning:** abdominal, thoracic, peripheral vasculature
- **Computed tomography (CT):** intra-abdominal or intrathoracic pathology
- **Magnetic resonance imaging (MRI):** particularly for orthopaedics, spinal cord compression, liver pathology

In a nutshell ...

How do X-rays work?
X-rays are electromagnetic rays that are differentially absorbed by the tissues. Plain films are the result of X-ray exposure on to photographic plates; a negative image is produced. Bone absorbs the most radiation (looks white), soft tissues of different densities and fluids absorb varying amounts (shades of grey) and gas absorbs the least (dark grey and black). A single chest X-ray is the equivalent of 3 days background radiation and an abdominal film is the equivalent of 150 days.

Chest X-ray (CXR)

When to perform a pre-op CXR

- All elective pre-op cases aged > 60 years
- All cases of cervical, thoracic, or abdominal trauma
- Acute respiratory symptoms or signs
- Previous cardiorespiratory disease and no recent CXR
- Thoracic surgery
- Patients with malignancy
- Suspicion of perforated intra-abdominal viscus

- Recent history of TB
- Recent immigrants from areas with a high prevalence of TB
- Thyroid enlargement (retrosternal extension)

Interpretation of the CXR

- **Check that the film is technically of good quality**
  - Not rotated (equal distance between the sinous processes and the end of the clavicle)
  - Adequately exposed (should see vertebrae to mid-cardiac level)
  - Lung fields expanded (should be able to count seven ribs anteriorly and nine ribs posteriorly)
- **Check name, date and orientation** (antero-posterior or postero-anterior?)
- **Follow a systematic approach:** look at the heart, mediastinum, lung fields, diaphragm, other soft-tissues and bones
  - **Heart:** should be less than half the width of the thorax
  - **Mediastinum:** may be widened in trauma or aortic dissection, trachea should be central
  - **Lung fields:** left hilum should be slightly higher than right; look for hyperexpansion (COAD); look for masses (eg tumour or old TB), shadowing (eg consolidation or fluid), collapse (eg pneumothorax)
  - **Diaphragm:** right side is usually higher; look for free gas (NB easier on the right as the stomach bubble is on the left); look for abnormally high diaphragm (eg lobar collapse or traumatic rupture)
  - **Soft tissues:** surgical emphysema (eg from IV line insertion or chest trauma)
  - **Bones:** rib fractures (eg single or flail chest segment)

Plain abdominal film (AXR)

When to perform an AXR

Plain abdominal films should be performed when there is:

- Suspicion of obstruction
- Suspicion of perforated intra-abdominal viscus
- Suspicion of peritonitis

Interpreting an AXR

- **Check name and date**
- **Identify bowel regions:** small bowel tends to lie centrally and has valvulae conniventes (lines cross from one wall to the other); large bowel lies peripherally with haustrae (only partially cross the diameter of the bowel)

Look at the **gas pattern**:

- **Localised ileus:** due to peritonitis in that region and sometimes called a sentinel loop (eg right upper quadrant in cholecystitis, centrally or left upper quadrant loop in pancreatitis, right lower quadrant loop in appendicitis and left lower quadrant in diverticulitis)

- **Central gas pattern:** ascites
- **Dilated bowel:** distal obstruction or pseudo-obstruction
- **Extraluminal gas:** produces a double contrast pattern in which the bowel wall is seen clearly as it is highlighted by gas on either side (Rigler's sign)

Look for calcification:

- Renal or ureteric (best seen on KUB), vascular calcification, faecoliths

Contrast studies

Contrast studies are performed by instilling a radio-opaque compound into a hollow viscus or the blood stream. Occasionally patients may have true allergies to intravenous contrast (approx 1:1000) and intravenous contrast should be used cautiously in patients with renal impairment.

- **Upper GI tract contrast studies:** oral contrast agents such as barium and gastrograffin may be used as a 'swallow' to demonstrate tumours, anastomotic leaks or obstruction in the oesophagus, stomach and small bowel
- **Bowel contrast studies:** barium and gastrograffin may also be used for enema studies to identify tumours, anastomotic leaks or obstruction
- **Cholangiography:** Contrast is used during ERCP to demonstrate stones, strictures and tumours of the bile ducts and head of pancreas
- **Renal contrast studies:** Intravenous contrast is excreted by the kidneys and thus used to highlight the anatomy of the collecting ducts, ureters and bladder as an intravenous urogram (IVU). Contrast may also be instilled in a retrograde manner into the bladder to demonstrate urethral rupture after trauma
- **Angiography:** Intravenous contrast may be used to image the major vessels and demonstrate vascular occlusive disease, malformations, emboli and thrombosis. Digital subtraction angiography (DSA) is a technique providing reverse negative views and requires less contrast to be administered. Many vascular patients are arteriopaths with poor renal function and so contrast must be used judiciously. Alternative contrast agents that are not nephrotoxic include a stream of small CO_2 bubbles which eventually dissolve in the blood and are excreted through the respiratory system

Screening studies

X-ray screening involves the production of a continuous image by an image intensifier. Bombardment with X-rays causes fluorescence of phosphor crystals within the machine translated into an image on screen. This allows a procedure to be guided by visualising the needle tip or contrast flow in real time.

Rather than a transient exposure to X-rays, screening therefore delivers a higher radiation dose to the patient and surrounding personnel must wear shielding.

Ultrasound scanning (USS)

In a nutshell ...

How does ultrasound work?
Ultrasound is the use of pulsed high frequency sound waves that are differentially reflected by tissues of different densities.

Uses of ultrasound
Ultrasound can be combined with Doppler as Duplex scanning (to assess blood flow) or with computer technology to form a 3-D image. Ultrasound is commonly used for imaging of the abdomen, pelvis, cardiac anatomy and thorax and vasculature. It is used for:

- **Diagnosis** eg liver metastasis, renal pathology, fluid collections
- **Monitoring** eg obstetrics, vascular graft patency
- **Treatment** eg guiding percutaneous procedures such as drain insertion, radiofrequency ablation

Ultrasound does not involve exposure to radiation. It works by using pulsed high-frequency sound waves (1–5 megaHz) emitted from the ultrasound probe. The sound is generated by vibration of a piezoelectric crystal when a transient electrical field is applied to it. These pulses of sound are differentially reflected by the planes between different tissues (eg tissue and fluid or fluid and air). The higher the density of the object, the more sound is reflected. If all the sound is reflected (eg off a calcified object) then an acoustic shadow appears beyond that object. Reflected waves are identified by the same probe and are analysed by the machine into distance and intensity. This is then displayed as a two-dimensional image on a screen.

The incorporation of the Doppler effect to ultrasound (called Duplex scanning) has allowed assessment of blood flow in peripheral and visceral vessels. The moving blood changes the frequency of the echo reflected to the probe – creating a higher frequency if it is moving towards the probe and a lower frequency if it is moving away from the probe. How much the frequency is changed depends upon how fast the object is moving.

Recent developments to ultrasound include three-dimensional imaging. Several two-dimensional images are acquired by moving the probes across the body surface or rotating inserted probes. The 2-D scans are then combined by computer software to form 3-D images.

Advantages of ultrasound

- No radiation
- Good visualisation of soft tissues, fluids and calculi
- Duplex can be used to assess blood flow
- Can be used to guide percutaneous techniques

Disadvantages of ultrasound

- Limited by dense structures that deflect sound waves (eg bone)
- Limited by body habitus (obesity)
- Difficult to accurately visualise the retroperitoneum
- Operator dependant

Computed tomography (CT scanning)

In a nutshell ...

How does CT work?

CT images are created from the integration of X-ray images as the X-ray tube travels in a circle around the patient. The density of different tissues causes differential X-ray attenuation which is recorded as an image with different levels of grey.

- **Image enhancement:** scanning may be performed with or without IV contrast to demonstrate vessels and enhance vascular lesions
- **Radiation dose:** CT scans represent multiple X-rays, so the cumulative radiation dose is high

CT images are created from the integration of X-ray images. Images are displayed as stacked slices of the whole (like slices in a loaf of bread). The X-rays are directed through the slice from multiple orientations as the X-ray tube and detectors travel in a circle around the patient. X-rays are differentially scattered or absorbed due to the density of the different tissues. This X-ray attenuation is recorded by the X-ray detector. A specialised algorithm is then used by the computer to display the X-ray attenuation levels on the screen as different levels of grey. These densities are different for gas, fluid and tissues and can be measured in Houndsfield units. The patient platform then moves an automated distance ready for the next image or slice.

To maximise their effectiveness in differentiating tissues while minimising patient exposure, CT scanners use a limited dose of relatively low-energy X-rays. They acquire data rapidly to minimise artefact created by movement of the patient during scanning (eg breathing, voluntary movement). In order to do this they use high-output X-ray sources and large, sensitive detectors.

Magnetic resonance imaging (MRI)

In a nutshell ...

How does MRI work?
MRI uses a magnetic field to image tissues based on movement of their hydrogen atoms in response to a radiofrequency pulse.

Pros and cons of MRI
Main advantages are the lack of radiation and clarity of soft tissue imaging. However, it is expensive and unsuitable for patients with claustrophobia or metal implants.

MRI uses powerful magnets to detect the movement of hydrogen atomic nuclei. The main magnet creates a stable magnetic field with the patient at the epicentre. This causes the atomic nuclei of hydrogen atoms in the tissues to align in the same direction. A radiofrequency (RF) pulse is then generated by the coil and passed through the tissues, causing the hydrogen atoms to resonate or vibrate. When the RF pulse is turned off, the hydrogen protons slowly return to their natural alignment within the magnetic field and release their excess stored energy. This movement is identified by the coil and sent to the computer system. Different tissues have characteristic readings. Additionally, the RF pulse can be altered to produce different responses from normal and abnormal tissues. This 'weights' the images, improving visualisation of different aspects.

- **T1 weighted images:** There is a wide variance of T1 values in normal tissue and so these images show good separation of solid structures and anatomy. Fat has the highest signal intensity (white) and other tissues have varying signal intensities (shades of grey) with fluids giving the lowest intensity (black). These images may be used in conjunction with IV contrast such as gadolinium to look at enhancing lesions
- **T2 weighted images:** T2 weighting doesn't give as much anatomical detail. It may be better for imaging some pathology. In T2-weighted images fluids give the brightest signal

Advantages of MRI

No radiation
Can identify vasculature without the use of contrast
Can produce images in any plane (eg sagittal and coronal)
Less bony artefact than CT

Disadvantages of MRI

- Expense
- Claustrophobia
- Contraindicated in patients with metal implants
- Longer imaging time than CT
- Not good for bony resolution

Microbiological investigations

The use and collection of microbiological specimens is discussed in Chapter 2 *Infection and Inflammation*.

Investigating special cases

Co-existing disease

- CXR for patients with severe rheumatoid arthritis (they are at risk of disease of the odontoid peg causing subluxation and danger to the cervical spinal cord under anaesthesia)

Major-plus cases

- Specialised cardiac investigations (eg echocardiography, cardiac stress testing, MUGA scan) used to assess pre-op cardiac reserve
- Specialised respiratory investigations (eg spirometry) to assess pulmonary function and reserve

Investigations relating to the organ in question

- Angiography or Duplex scanning in arterial disease before bypass
- Renal perfusion or renal isotope imaging or liver biopsy before transplant
- Colonoscopy, barium enema or CTC before bowel resection for cancer

Consent and counselling

Informing the patient of the decision to operate

It is often said that the best surgeon knows when *not* to operate.

The decision to undertake surgery must be based on all available information from thorough history, examination and investigative tests.

In the case of elective surgery, the operating surgeon has usually seen the patient in the outpatient clinic and has gone through the options for treatment. The patient and surgeon then decide upon the treatment option and the decision to operate; principles, consequences and practicalities of the surgery are usually explained in general terms at this point. This is not the same as gaining consent but is an important stage of the process of informing the patient. In some specialities, clinical nurse practitioners or other support staff may be accessed to support the patient (eg breast care nurse prior to mastectomy, colorectal nurse specialist prior to an operation resulting in a stoma). This helps to prepare the patient for the surgery and its consequences and facilitates the consent at a later date.

Counselling

Medical staff spend most of their working life in and around hospitals, so it is easy to forget how the public view hospital admission, operative procedures, and the post-op stay on the ward. These stays can, as we know, be more lengthy for some than others and it's important that we remember to be understanding about our patients' needs.

It is important for you to recognise that all patients are different – in their ages, in their beliefs, and in their worries.

General concerns of the surgical patient

Is this the first time the patient has stayed in hospital?

Never forget that *all* operative procedures are significant to the patient, no matter how simple we believe the case to be.

Good communication is essential so that the patient knows what to expect beforehand and can make an informed decision:

- Check you know the patient well enough and understand their problem enough to explain it to them!
- Choose the setting
- Explain the diagnosis in terms they will understand
- Explain the possible options
- Explain between conservative and operative managements of the condition
- Ask if they have any thoughts about their options
- Explain what option you think is best and why
- Ask if they have any questions
- Give them the option to ask you questions later

Think about potential questions from the patient and address them in your explanation:

- What are the risks of anaesthetic and surgery?
- Will I wake up?
- What will I wake up with?
    - Lines
    - Tubes and catheters

    - Colostomy
    - Transplant
    - Amputated limbs
- What if things go wrong?
- How long will I stay in hospital?
- Will I die?

Specific considerations of the individual

Knowledge

- Information available on the internet, books, patient information leaflets, friends and relatives
- Is their understanding correct?

Employment

- Physical vs desk work

Social network

- Support if breaking bad news
- Isolated living conditions
- Family nearby
- Young children

Physical issues/deformity

- Amputation
- Mastectomy
- Burns and skin grafts
- Colostomy/ileostomy bags
- Scars
- Multiple trauma

Psychological issues

- Sexual function after mastectomy or orchidectomy
- Having another person's organ inside them after transplant (often associated with 'survivor guilt')
- Brain damage after head injury
- Loss of control (their life in our hands)
- Potential death

Recovery and what to expect

- Blood tests
- Potential for further operations

- Fatigue
- Loss of function
  - Incontinence
  - Poor mobility
- Infection

Re-admission

- Wound dehiscence
- Infection
- Failure of operation
  - Was it their fault?
  - Depression

Recurrent admission/prolonged hospital stay

- Institutionalisation
- Safer in hospital than at home?
- Social support at home?

Additional requirements for different patient groups

Young adults

- Physical changes from procedure
- Scars
- Acne from drugs
- Body image and psychosexual effects (eg stoma)

Adults

- Functional changes
- Will I still be able to play with my kids?

Elderly people

- Do the benefits outweigh the risks?

Presenting information to patients

- Discuss diagnoses and treatment options at a time when the patient is best able to understand and retain the information
- Use up-to-date written material, visual and other aids to explain complex aspects of the diagnosis or treatment where appropriate
- Make arrangements to meet particular communication needs (eg with translators or deaf signers)
- Discuss the possibility of the patient bringing a friend or relative or making a tape-recording of the consultation

- Use accurate data to explain the prognosis of a condition and probabilities of treatment success or the risks of failure
- Ensure distressing information is given in a considerate way, and offer access to counselling services and patient support groups
- Allow the patient time to absorb the material, perhaps with repeated consultations or written back-up material
- Involve nursing or other members of the healthcare team
- Ensure voluntary decision making: you may recommend a course of action but you must not put pressure on the patient to accept your advice. Ensure that the patient has an opportunity to review their decision nearer the time

Responding to questions: you must respond honestly to any questions the patient raises, and, as far as possible, answer as fully as the patient wishes.

Withholding information: you should not withhold information necessary for decision making unless you judge that disclosure of some relevant information would cause the patient serious harm (not including becoming upset or refusing treatment). You may not withhold information from a patient at the request of any other person including a relative.

If a patient insists they do not want to know the details of a condition or a treatment, you should explain the importance of knowing the options and should still provide basic information about the condition or treatment unless you think this would cause the patient some harm.

Records: You should record in the medical records what you have discussed with the patient and who was present. This helps to establish a timeline and keeps other members of staff informed as to what the patient knows. You must record in the medical records if you have withheld treatment and your reasons for doing so.

The consent procedure is vital and may be commenced pre-operatively. For more information on consent see Chapter 8.

Pre-assessment

The pre-assessment clinic aims to assess surgical patients 2–4 weeks pre-admission for elective surgery.

Pre-assessment is timed so that the gap between assessment and surgery is:

- Long enough so that a suitable response can be made to any problem highlighted
- Short enough so that many new problems are unlikely to arise in the interim

The timing of the assessment also means that:

- Surgical team can identify current pre-op problems
- High-risk patients can undergo early anaesthetic review

- Peri-operative problems can be anticipated and suitable arrangements made (eg book ITU/HDU bed for the high-risk patient)
- There is a chance for assessment by allied specialties (eg dietician, stoma nurse, occupational therapist, social worker)
- The patient can be admitted to hospital closer to the time of surgery, thereby reducing hospital stay

The patient should be reviewed again on admission for factors likely to influence prognosis (eg new chest infection, further weight loss).

Pre-assessment is run most efficiently by following a set protocol for the pre-operative management of each patient group. The protocol-led system has several advantages:

- The proforma is an aide memoire in clinic
- Gaps in pre-op work up are easily visible
- Reduces variability between clerking by juniors

However, be wary of pre-ordered situations as they can be dangerous and every instruction must be reviewed on an individual patient basis. For example, the patient may be allergic to the antibiotics which are prescribed as part of the pre-assessment work up and alternatives should be given.

1.2 AFTER ADMISSION

In a nutshell ...

Once the patient is admitted for surgery, there are several important pre-operative processes:

- Identification
- Documentation
- Optimisation
  - Resuscitation
  - Controlling co-morbidity (see section 2 Pre-operative management of co-existing disease)
  - Nutrition
- Prophylaxis
- Consent and marking

Identification

Patient identification is essential. All patients should be given an identity wristband on admission to hospital. This should state clearly and legibly their name, date of birth, ward and consultant. They should also be given a separate red wrist band documenting allergies. Patient identification is checked by the nursing team on admission to theatre.

Documentation

Medical documents (medical notes, drug and fluid charts, consent forms and operation notes) are legal documents. All entries to the notes should be written clearly and legibly. Always write the date, time and your name and position at the beginning of each entry.

Documentation often starts with clerking. Record as much information as possible in the format described above for history and examination. The source of information should also be stated (eg from patient, from relative, from old notes, from clinic letter, from GP).

Accurate documentation should continue for each episode of patient contact including investigations, procedures, ward rounds and conversations with the patient about diagnosis or treatment.

File documents in the notes yourself otherwise they will get lost. This is important to protect both the patient and yourself. From a medicolegal point of view, if it is not documented then it didn't happen.

Optimisation

In a nutshell ...

Morbidity and mortality increase in patients with co-morbidity.

Optimising the patient's condition gives them the best possible chance at a good surgical outcome.

In patients with severe co-morbidity the CEPOD recommend the following:

- Discussion between surgeon and anaesthetist before theatre
- Adequate pre-operative investigation
- Optimisation of surgery by ensuring:
  - An appropriate grade of surgeon (to minimise operative time and blood loss)
  - Adequate resuscitation
  - Critical care is available

It is essential that the acutely ill surgical patient is adequately resuscitated and stabilised before theatre. In extreme and life-threatening conditions this may not be possible (eg ruptured AAA, trauma).

Additionally, in order to achieve the maximal benefit and minimise the risks of elective surgery it is necessary to optimise the patient's medical condition before theatre.

Resuscitation of patients for emergency surgery

Treat pain: pain results in the release of adrenaline and can cause tachycardia and hypertension. Pain control before anaesthesia reduces cardiac workload.

Correct dehydration: many acute surgical patients require IV fluids to correct dehydration and restore electrolyte balance. Insertion of a urinary catheter is vital to monitor fluid balance carefully with hourly measurements. Severe renal impairment may require dialysis before theatre.

Correct anaemia: anaemia compromises cardiac and respiratory function and is not well tolerated in patients with poor cardiac reserve. The anaemia may be acute (acute bleed) or chronic (underlying pathology). If anaemia is acute, transfuse to reasonable Hb and correct clotting.

Decompress the stomach: insert an NG tube to decompress the stomach as this reduces the risk of aspiration on anaesthetic induction.

Optimisation of patients for elective surgery

Control underlying co-morbidity: specialist advice on the management of underlying co-morbidities (cardiovascular, respiratory, renal, endocrinological) should be sought. For example, optimisation of cardiac medication for a patient with angina pre-operatively will reduce the risk of peri-operative myocardial infarction. This may be done as an outpatient in the case of elective surgery or occasionally requires inpatient care. This is covered in more detail in section 2 *Pre-operative management of co-existing disease*.

Nutrition: good nutrition is essential for good wound healing. Malnourished patients do badly and a period of pre-operative dietary improvement (eg build-up drinks, enteral feeding, TPN) improves outcome. See section 2.9.

Prophylaxis

Pre-operatively prophylaxis includes:

- Starting beneficial interventions:
- Minimising known associated risks
  - DVT prophylaxis with LMW heparin and TED stockings
  - Antibiotic prophylaxis in cases of infection and sepsis (often given by the anaesthetist in theatre)

- Prescribing drugs known to improve outcome eg pre-operative β-blockers in vascular surgery (to improve cardiovascular outcomes)
- Stopping potentially harmful factors:
  - Stopping medications (eg the oral contraceptive pill for a month, aspirin or clopidogrel for a week before surgery)
  - Stopping smoking: improves respiratory function even if the patient can only stop for 24 hours

Consent and marking

Obtaining consent

The GMC gives the following guidelines (General Medical Council 1998).

Obtaining consent

Provide sufficient information which includes:

- Details of diagnosis
- Prognosis if the condition is left untreated and if the condition is treated
- Options for further investigations if diagnosis is uncertain
- Options for treatment or management of the condition
- The option not to treat
- The purpose of the proposed investigation or treatment
- Details of the procedure including subsidiary treatment such as pain relief
- How the patient should prepare for the procedure
- Common and serious side effects
- Likely benefits and probabilities of success
- Discussion of any serious or frequently occuring risks
- Lifestyle changes which may be caused by the treatment
- Advice on whether any part of the proposed treatment is experimental
- How and when the patient's condition will be monitored and reassessed
- The name of the doctor who has overall responsibility for the treatment
- Whether doctors in training or students will be involved
- A reminder that patients can change their minds about a decision at any time
- A reminder that patients have a right to seek a second opinion
- Explain how decisions are made about whether to move from one stage of treatment to another (eg chemotherapy)
- Explain that there may be different teams of doctors involved (eg anaesthetists)
- Seek consent to treat any problems which might arise and need dealing with while the patient is unconscious or otherwise unable to make a decision
- Ascertain whether there are any procedures to which a patient would object (eg blood transfusions)

Ask patients whether they have understood the information and whether they would like more before making a decision. Sometimes asking the patient to explain back to you, in their own words, what you have just said clarifies areas that they do not really understand and may need more explanation.

The legal right to consent

The ability to give informed consent for different patient ages and groups is discussed fully in Chapter 8 *Surgical Outcomes, Research, Ethics and the Law.*

Who obtains consent

The responsibility is that of the doctor providing the treatment or undertaking the investigation. If obtaining consent is delegated to someone other than the doctor providing the treatment the person to whom the task is delegated should be:

- Suitably trained and qualified
- Have sufficient knowledge of the treatment and understand the risks
- Act in accordance with the above GMC guidelines

The doctor providing the treatment remains responsible for ensuring the patient has been given sufficient time and information to make a decision.

Pre-operative marking

This should be performed after consent and before the patient has received pre-medication. Marking is essential to help avoid mistakes in theatre. Marking whilst the patient is conscious is important to minimise error. Pre-operative marking is especially important if the patient is having:

- a unilateral procedure (eg on a limb or the groin)
- a lesion excised
- a tender or symptomatic area operated on (eg an epigastric hernia)
- a stoma created

Marking for surgery

Explain to the patient that you are going to mark the site for surgery
Confirm the procedure and the site (including left or right) with the notes, the patient and the consent form
Position the patient appropriately (eg standing for marking varicose veins, supine for abdominal surgery)
Use a surgical marker that will not come off during skin preparation
Clearly identify the surgical site using a large arrow

1.3 DAY-CASE SURGERY

In a nutshell ...

In day-case surgery a patient is admitted for investigation or operation on a planned non-resident basis, but they nonetheless require facilities for recovery. Day-case surgery may be performed under GA, regional, or LA. Many different procedures are now suitable for day-case surgery. There are advantages and disadvantages when considering a patient for day-case surgery.

Patients should have full verbal and printed instructions including:

- A brief description of the surgical problem
- An outline of the nature of the surgery to be undertaken
- Pre-operative instructions
- Post-operative instructions as well as details about the nature of possible complications, what to do about them, and when and who to contact for advice
- Advice on when to return to work and other activities
- Instructions about any appropriate appointments for follow-up or suture removal

Advantages of day surgery

A firm date and time for operation with less risk of cancellation
Minimum time away from home (especially in paediatric surgery)
Greater efficiency of operating list scheduling
Release of inpatient beds
Cost effective

Disadvantages of day surgery

Requirement of adequate aftercare at home
Restriction of surgery and anaesthesia to experienced staff
Requirement for inpatient admission or readmission in cases of unexpected, complications, inadequate analgesia, etc

Contraindications to day-case surgery

Medical contraindications

- Unfit (ASA class >II)
- Obese (BMI > 35)
- Specific problems (eg bowel resections)
- Extent of pathology (eg large scrotal hernia)
- Operation longer than 1 hour
- Psychologically unsuitable
- Concept of day surgery unacceptable to patient

Social contraindications

- Lives further than a 1-hour drive from the unit
- No competent relative or friend to accompany or drive patient home after surgery and/or to look after the patient at home for the first 24–48 hours post-operatively
- At home there is no access to a lift (for an upper floor flat), telephone, or indoor toilet and bathroom

Some common procedures suitable for day-case surgery

General surgery

- OGD
- Varicose vein surgery
- Colonoscopy
- Excision of breast lumps
- Hernia repair – inguinal, femoral, umbilical, para-umbilical and epigastric
- Pilonidal sinus

Urological surgery

- Circumcision
- Excision of epididymal cyst
- Cystoscopy +/– biopsy
- Reversal of vasectomy
- Hydrocoele surgery

ENT surgery

- Myringotomy and insertion of grommets
- Submucous resection
- Submucosal diathermy of turbinates
- Direct laryngoscopy and pharyngoscopy

Orthopaedic surgery

- Carpal tunnel release
- Arthroscopy
- Release of trigger finger
- Amputation of finger or toe
- Dupuytren's contracture surgery
- Ingrowing toenails

Paediatric surgery

- Circumcision
- Repair umbilical hernia
- Inguinal herniotomy
- Orchidopexy
- Hydrocoele surgery

Ophthalmic surgery

- Cataract surgery
- Correction of squint

Plastic surgery

- Correction of 'bat' ears
- Insertion of tissue expanders
- Blepharoplasty
- Nipple and areola reconstruction
- Breast augmentation

Gynaecological surgery

- D&C
- Laparoscopy
- Termination of pregnancy
- Laparoscopic sterilisation

Other considerations

Day surgery should ideally be performed in dedicated day-case units, controlling their own waiting lists and scheduling. They should ideally be on the ground floor, with their own entrance, wards, theatres, and staff. Patient satisfaction, adequacy of post-operative analgesia, complications and admission rates should be regularly audited.

Section 2

Pre-operative management of co-existing disease

2.1 PRE-OPERATIVE MANAGEMENT OF MEDICATIONS

In a nutshell ...

If a patient is having surgery:

- Review pre-existing medication
  - Document pre-operative medications
  - Decide which drugs need to be stopped pre-operatively
  - Decide on alternative formulations
- Prescribe pre-operative medication
  - Prescribe prophylactic medication
  - Prescribe medication related to the surgery
  - Prescribe pre-med if needed
- Be aware of problems with specific drugs
  - Steroids and immunosuppressants
  - Anticoagulants and fibrinolytics

Review pre-existing medication

Peri-operative management of pre-existing medication

Document pre-operative medications

Decide whether any drugs need to be stopped before surgery

- Stop oral contraceptive (OCP) 4 weeks before major or limb surgery – risk of thrombosis
- Stop MAOI antidepressants – they interact with anaesthetic drugs, with cardiac risk
- Stop antiplatelet drugs 7–14 days pre-operatively – risks of haemorrhage

Decide on alternative formulations for the peri-operative period

- eg IV rather than oral; heparin rather than warfarin

Regular medications should generally be given – even on the day of surgery (with a sip of clear fluid only). If in doubt ask the anaesthetist. This is important especially for cardiac medication. There are some essential medications (eg anti-rejection therapy in transplant patients) that may be withheld for 24 hours in the surgical period but this should only be under the direction of a specialist in the field.

Prescribe pre-operative medication

Medication for the pre-operative period

Pre-existing medication (see above for those drugs that should be excluded)
Prophylactic medication
- eg DVT prophylaxis
- eg antibiotic prophylaxis

Medication related to the surgery
- eg laxatives to clear the bowel before resection
- eg methylene blue to aid surgical identification of the parathyroids

Anaesthetic premedication (to reduce anxiety, reduce secretions etc)

Be aware of problems with specific drugs

Steroids and immunosuppression

Indications for peri-operative corticosteroid cover
This includes patients:

- With pituitary–adrenal insufficiency on steroids
- Undergoing pituitary or adrenal surgery
- On systemic steroid therapy of > 7.5 mg for > 1 week before surgery
- Who received a course of steroids for > 1 month in the previous 6 months

Complications of steroid therapy in the peri-operative period

- Poor wound healing
- Increased risk of infection
- Side effects of steroid therapy (eg impaired glucose tolerance, osteoporosis, muscle wasting, fragile skin and veins, peptic ulceration)
- Mineralocorticoid effect (sodium and water retention, potassium loss and metabolic alkalosis)
- Masking of sepsis/peritonism
- Glucocorticoid deficiency in the peri-operative period (may present as increasing cardiac failure which is unresponsive to catecholamines, or addisonian crisis with vomiting and cardiovascular collapse)

Management of patients on pre-op steroid therapy

This depends on the nature of the surgery to be performed and the level of previous steroid use.

- **Minor use:** 50 mg hydrocortisone IM/IV pre-operatively
- **Intermediate use:** 50 mg hydrocortisone IM/IV with pre-med and 50 mg hydrocortisone every 6 hours for 24 hours
- **Major use:** 100 mg hydrocortisone IM/IV with pre-med and 100 mg hydrocortisone every 6 hours for at least 72 hours after surgery

Equivalent doses of steroid therapy: hydrocortisone 100 mg, prednisolone 25 mg, dexamethasone 4 mg.

Anticoagulants and fibrinolytics

Consider the risk of thrombosis (augmented by post-surgical state itself) vs risk of haemorrhage.

Warfarin

- Inhibits vitamin K-dependant coagulation factors (II, VII, IX and X) as well as protein C and its co-factor, protein S
- Illness and drug interactions may have unpredictable effects on the level of anticoagulation
- Anticoagulative effects can be reversed by vitamin K (10 mg IV; takes 24 hours for adequate synthesis of inhibited factors) and fresh frozen plasma (15 mL/kg; immediate replacement of missing factors)
- Stop 3–5 days before surgery and replace with heparin; depends upon indication for anticoagulation (eg metal heart valve is absolute indication, but AF is relative)
- INR should be < 1.2 for open surgery and < 1.5 for invasive procedures

Heparin

- Mucopolysaccharide purified from intestine
- Binds to antithrombin III and thus inhibits factors IIa, IXa, Xa and XIIa
- May be unfractionated or fractionated (LMWH)

Uses of heparin include:

- General anticoagulant (should be stopped 6 hours before surgery)
- Treatment of unstable angina
- Maintenance of extracorporeal circuits (eg dialysis, bypass)
- Flush for IV lines to maintain patency
- In vascular surgery before temporary occlusion of a vessel to prevent distal thrombosis

Unfractionated heparin

Given by continuous infusion (short half-life)
Check APTT every 6 hours and adjust rate until steady state (ratio of 2 to 3) achieved

Fractionated heparin (low-molecular-weight heparin, LMWH)

Inhibits only factor Xa
Increased half-life and more predictable bioavailability (compared to unfractionated form)
Can be given once daily (eg tinzaparin) or twice a day (eg enoxaparin)
Can cause an immune reaction (heparin-induced thrombocytopenia, HIT); LMWH is less likely to do so
Effects can be reversed by use of protamine 1 mg per 100 units of heparin (may cause hypotension and in high doses, paradoxically, may cause anticoagulation)
Can be used during pregnancy (non-teratogenic)

Antiplatelet agents

- Increasingly used (eg aspirin, dipyridamole, clopidogrel, abciximab)
- Decrease platelet aggregation and reduce thrombus formation
- May be used in combination
- Should be stopped 7–14 days before major surgery otherwise there is a risk of uncontrollable bleeding

Fibrinolytics

- Examples include streptokinase and alteplase
- Act by activating plasminogen to plasmin which undertakes clot fibrinolysis
- Used in acute MI, extensive DVT, and PE
- Contraindicated if the patient has undergone recent surgery, trauma, recent haemorrhage, pancreatitis, aortic dissection, etc

For discussions of the management of immunosuppression in the peri-operative period see *Urology and Transplantation* in Book 2. DVT prophylaxis in the peri-operative period is covered in Chapter 4 *Haematology*.

2.2 PRE-OPERATIVE MANAGEMENT OF CARDIOVASCULAR DISEASE

In a nutshell ...

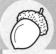

Cardiac comorbidity increases surgical mortality (includes ischaemic heart disease, hypertension, valvular disease, arrhythmias and cardiac failure).

Special care must be taken with pacemakers and implantable defibrillators.

In general it is necessary to:

- Avoid changes in heart rate (especially tachycardia)
- Avoid changes in BP
- Avoid pain
- Avoid anaemia
- Avoid hypoxia (give supplemental oxygen)

Additionally, the details of pre-operative assessment prior to cardiac surgery is covered in Book 2 *Cardiothoracics*.

Ischaemic heart disease

Pre-operative considerations

Known risk factors must be identified in the history (eg smoking, hypertension, hyperlipidaemia, diabetes, including a positive family history). A careful examination of the heart and lungs must be performed. Remember that ischaemia **may be silent**.

New York Heart Association (NYHA) classification

Grade 1 No limitation on ordinary physical activity

Grade 2 Slight limitation on physical activity; ordinary activity results in palpitations, dyspnoea or angina

Grade 3 Marked limitation of physical activity; less than ordinary activity results in palpitations, dyspnoea or angina

Grade 4 Inability to carry out any physical activity without discomfort; symptoms may be present at rest

Recent MI dramatically increases the risk of re-infarction in the peri-operative period, ie 80% in the first 3 weeks, 25–40% in the first 3 months, and 10–15% in 3–6 months. After 6 months the risk drops to 5% and is normally the minimum time period that is an acceptable risk for an elective procedure. Obviously the risk must be balanced against any potential benefit of a surgical procedure.

Investigation of patients with cardiac disease

Investigation of **all** patients with previous cardiac disease includes:

Electrocardiogram (ECG)

- Look for previous infarct, ischaemia at rest, BBB or LVH (these are evidence of strain)
- Acts as a baseline for comparison in the future enabling new changes to be distinguished from pre-existing abnormalities

CXR

- Look at heart size, evidence of failure, fluid, evidence of infection, and suspicious shadows if smoking history

FBC

- Correction of anaemia is essential as it compromises cardiac and respiratory function and is not well tolerated in patients with ischaemic disease
- May require iron supplements or even staged transfusion

Electrolytes

- Potassium and magnesium levels may affect cardiac functioning and should be optimised
- Bear in mind that electrolyte disturbances occur in patients treated with diuretics

Some patients require more sensitive tests of cardiac function:

- Exercise ECG
- Echocardiogram with left ventricular ejection fraction (LVEF)
- Dobutamine stress test
- Coronary angiogram if lesion suspected

Always bear in mind that a patient may need their cardiac condition optimised by a cardiologist. It may be necessary to arrange angioplasty or CABG before other elective procedures are attempted).

Intra-operative considerations for patients with cardiac disease

Cardiac effects of GA include:

- Systemic vascular resistance decreases (induction decreases arterial pressure by 20–30%)
- Tracheal intubation decreases BP by 20–30 mmHg
- Causes myocardial depression (IV agents less than inhaled agents)
- Cardiac irritability increases (increased sensitivity to the catecholamines released in response to surgery predisposes to arrhythmia)

Cardiac effects of regional anaesthesia include:

- Vasodilation (blocks sympathetic outflow)
- May be combined with GA for pain control

Hypertension

Causes of hypertension

Essential hypertension
Pain
Anxiety (eg white-coat hypertension)
Fluid overload
Hypoxia and hypercapnia

If the diastolic blood pressure is > 110 mmHg then elective procedures should be discussed with the anaesthetist and possibly postponed until better control can be achieved. After appropriate pain relief take three separate BP readings, separated by a period of at least 1 hour, to help exclude anxiety or discomfort as a cause.

Newly diagnosed hypertension must be assessed for possible reversible aetiological factors (eg renal disease, endocrine diseases such as phaeochromocytoma, pregnancy, the OCP, and coarctation of the aorta).

Chronic (longstanding) hypertension puts the patient at increased risk of cardiovascular disease, cerebrovascular events, and renal impairment. These patients are also at higher risk of hypertensive crises. These conditions need to be excluded or optimised, if possible, before an elective surgical procedure. Left ventricular hypertrophy (whether clinically, radiologically, or electrocardiographically detected) is directly related to myocardial ischaemia. Poorly controlled hypertension in the immediate pre-op period predisposes the patient to peri-operative cardiac morbidity and must be avoided.

Post-operative hypertension is common and is most often due to pain. It may be due to omission of usual cardiac drugs immediately before surgery (in general these drugs should always be given pre-operatively; if in doubt, speak to your anaesthetist).

Valvular disease

Patients with valvular disease are susceptible to endocarditis if they become septic. Prophylactic antibiotics are important. They may also be on long-term anticoagulation.

Aortic stenosis

Associated with a 13% risk of peri-operative death (risk increases with increasing stenosis to 50% for patients with critical aortic stenosis). Symptomatic AS produces syncope, dyspnoea and angina. On examination there may be an ejection systolic murmur (radiates to the carotids), a soft or absent second heart sound and pulsus parvus. The valve needs assessing with echocardiography (valve area $< 1\ cm^2$ or gradient of > 50 mmHg indicates critical AS).

Mitral stenosis

May predispose to pulmonary hypertension and right cardiac failure. Clinically look for mitral facies, diastolic murmur and AF (increased pressure chronically enlarges the left atrium). Must be given prophylactic antibiotics for invasive procedures. Minimise fluid overload and changes in cardiac rate.

Arrhythmias

Atrial fibrillation (AF)

Common arrhythmia giving an irregularly irregular beat. Due to short circuiting of the electrical impulses of the atria resulting in disorganised muscle contraction. Causes reduced efficiency of the atria to pump prime the ventricles.

Common causes of atrial fibrillation

Acute causes

- Fluid overload
- Sepsis (especially chest)
- Ischaemic event
- Alcohol
- PE
- Dehydration
- Thyrotoxicosis

Chronic causes

- Ischaemic or valvular disease

Questions to ask yourself about each case of AF

Is it reversible?

- Acute: may be reversible (consider ways to reduce or remove causes listed above)
- Chronic: rarely reversible (eg irreversibly dilated atria, ischaemic disease)

Is the rate compromising cardiac output?

- Indication of the need for and the speed of intervention; consider oral medication (eg digoxin) versus IV medication (eg amiodarone) vs DC cardioversion

Does the patient need anticoagulating?

- AF predisposes to thrombotic events (blood in the auricles of the atria moves sluggishly and forms clots which are then expelled into the systemic circulation – commonly causing CVA)

Pacemakers and implanted ventricular defibrillators

Problems during the surgical period include:

- Interactions with diathermy current: electrical interference with device (eg causing resetting, rate increases or inhibition); current travelling down wires and causing myocardial burn
- Effect of anaesthetic agents on pacing and sensing thresholds
- Problems with rate control devices; may not allow physiological responses (eg tachycardia)

Ask yourself the following questions

- Reason for insertion?
- Continuous or demand model?
- If continuous, is it working optimally? (ie is the ECG showing captured beats – large electrical spike seen before each ventricular contraction?)

Patients should have the pacemaker evaluated by cardiology before and after surgery as they will be able to assess and advise on any changes required to the settings.

Always use bipolar diathermy if possible and check for deleterious effects. Unipolar diathermy current may pass down pacing wires causing cardiac burns so advice should be sought from the cardiologist if unipolar diathermy is thought to be necessary.

Cardiac failure

- Due to acute or chronic ischaemic or valvular disease
- Exercise tolerance is a good indictor of cardiac reserve; ask:
  - How far can you walk?
  - Can you manage a flight of stairs without getting short of breath?
- Morbidity and mortality increase proportionally to severity of CCF
- Ask for a cardiology review in order to optimise fully (eg ACE inhibitors, diuretics) before surgery

Care with fluid management in the peri-operative period is essential – remember that these patients may require their regular diuretics.

2.3 PRE-OPERATIVE MANAGEMENT OF RESPIRATORY DISEASE

In a nutshell ...

Respiratory disease commonly includes COPD, asthma, cystic fibrosis, bronchiectasis and infections

Optimise any reversible component of the condition and avoid surgery during infective exacerbations of the disease

Encourage smoking cessation (even if just for 24 hours pre-operatively)

NB: Patients with respiratory disease may be on regular long-term steroids.

Chronic obstructive pulmonary disease (COPD) and asthma

COPD is pathologically distinct, but frequently co-exists with bronchospasm. It may be difficult to determine the importance of each condition in an individual. Generalised air flow obstruction is the dominant feature of both diseases.

History and examination of patients with COAD/asthma

Questions should be directed at:

- Patient's exercise tolerance (eg walking distance on the flat)
- Any recent deterioration resulting in hospital admission
- Previous admission to ITU for ventilation

- Need for home oxygen, and present medical therapy (eg need for steroids)
- Current smoking habit, or when smoking was stopped
- Changes on examination (eg are they consistent with chronic lung disease/focal infective exacerbations)

Investigation of COPD and asthma

Assess baseline levels with lung function tests:

- FEV_1/FVC ratio (if < 50% the risk of post-op respiratory failure is increased)
- ABGs confirming CO_2 retention in pure chronic bronchitis
- Sputum cultures and sensitivity in the presence of a productive cough
- CXR

Management of COPD and asthma

- Give pre-operative salbutamol (nebulisers)
- Must treat any reversible component (eg infective exacerbations)
- Consider regional anaesthesia for body surface/lower extremity surgery
- Intra-operative nitrous oxide can rupture bullae leading to a tension pneumothorax, so use opioids in doses that are not associated with pronounced respiratory depression
- Ensure humidification of inspired gases
- Post-operatively, offer advice regarding smoking; provide chest physiotherapy; administer CPAP in an HDU setting; provide adequate pain relief allowing deep breathing and early mobilisation; nurse in an upright position in bed, monitoring oxygen saturation

Hypoxia in the peri-operative setting is most commonly due to inadequate ventilation or respiratory depression with opiates rather than loss of hypoxic drive due to prolonged high-concentration oxygen therapy. However, the latter should always be borne in mind when dealing with patients with chronic respiratory disease.

Tuberculosis (TB)

Many patients have evidence of old TB disease or previous anti-TB surgery on CXR. This is not usually a problem, but the resulting lung change and reduced respiratory capacity may need consideration.

Active TB should be considered in recent immigrants from areas where TB is endemic, and in immunosuppressed and HIV patients. They may require pre-operative CXR, sputum culture, Mantoux testing (if they haven't had previous BCG) and treatment if appropriate.

Bronchiectasis and cystic fibrosis

Both conditions cause chronic productive cough with airway inflammation and recurrent infective exacerbations. Assess pre-operative respiratory function carefully and send a pre-operative sputum culture and ABG to act as baseline information. Input from respiratory physicians is advisable.

Active physiotherapy, bronchodilators and treatment of residual infections are required before elective surgery. Post-operative physiotherapy at least three times per day is essential.

Smoking

Short-term effects of smoking

- Nicotine increases myocardial oxygen demand
- Carbon monoxide reduces oxygen delivery by binding to haemoglobin
- Carboxyhaemoglobin levels fall if stopped prior to 12 hours pre-surgery
- High carboxyhaemoglobin can give false pulse oximetry readings
- Airway irritability and secretions are increased

Long-term effects of smoking

- Reduces immune function, increases mucous secretion
- Reduces clearance and causes chronic airway disease (cessation needs to be longer than 6–8 weeks to bring about an improvement)
- Increased risk of ischaemic heart disease

Intra-operative considerations in patients with respiratory disease

Site and size of incision

Upper abdominal incisions result in an inability to breathe deeply (basal atelectasis) or to cough (retained secretions), and have a higher incidence of respiratory complications compared to lower abdominal incisions (30% vs 3%, respectively). In patients with known respiratory disease, think about the optimal incision site (eg transverse rather than midline).

Analgesia

Optimise analgesia using a combination of local and regional techniques to allow deep breaths and coughing as required. Remember local infiltration intra-operatively. Infiltration of LA eg Chirocaine™ into the rectus sheath is helpful in upper midline incisions in those with compromised respiratory function.

Anaesthetic agents

Anaesthetic agents have the following effects:

- Reduce muscle tone and thus functional residual capacity
- Increase airway resistance and reduce lung compliance
- Cause atelectasis in dependant zones of the lung causing pulmonary vascular shunting
- Increase ventilatory dead space

2.4 PRE-OPERATIVE MANAGEMENT OF ENDOCRINE DISEASE

In a nutshell ...

- Diabetes mellitus
- Thyroid problems
- Parathyroid problems

Pre-operative management of diabetes mellitus

Peri-operative management of diabetes mellitus

- Avoid hypoglycaemia (especially under anaesthesia – risk of cerebral damage)
- Avoid hyperglycaemia (osmotic diuresis and dehydration)
- Supply enough insulin (prevent ketoacidosis)
- Be aware of increased risks of post-operative complications (infective, arteriopathic, etc)

Reasons for good glycaemic control

- Prevention of ketosis and acidaemia
- Prevention of electrolyte abnormalities and volume depletion secondary to osmotic diuresis
- Impaired wound strength and wound healing when plasma glucose concentration is > 11 mmol/L
- Hyperglycaemia interferes with leucocyte chemotaxis, opsonisation and phagocytosis and thus leads to an impaired immune response
- Avoidance of hypoglycaemia in an anaesthetised patient

Pre-operative precautions in diabetics

- Full pre-op history and examination (diabetes is associated with increased risk of ischaemic heart disease, hypertension, PVD, autonomic and peripheral neuropathy, renovascular disease and renal failure, impaired vision, susceptibility to gastric reflux and delayed gastric emptying)
- Check U&Es
- Urinalysis for proteinuria

- ECG
- Confirm adequate glycaemic control (see below)

Peri-operative precautions in diabetics

- Place first on operating list (reduces period of starvation and risk of hypoglycaemia)
- Protect pressure areas (especially with PVD and neuropathy)
- At risk from increased infection and arteriopathic disease (renal, cardiac, neurological, peripheral) post-operatively
- Involve diabetologists in peri-operative management of patients with brittle bone disease
- Involve patients themselves in the management of their diabetes during this period; they are usually very knowledgeable and have managed their disease for a long time

Assessment of pre-op control of diabetes

- Daily glucose measurements from the patient's diary
- HbA1c measurement (assesses glycaemic control over the last 8 weeks by levels of glycosylation of haemoglobin)
  - Good control < 6.5
  - Adequate control 6.5–8.0
  - Poor control > 8.0

Management of diabetes

Management of NIDDM (non-insulin dependent diabetes mellitus)

Optimise control pre-operatively and continue normal oral hypoglycaemic control until the morning of surgery (except chlorpropamide and metformin which may need to be reduced or stopped 48 hours in advance – can predispose to lactic acidosis). Post-operatively monitor BM regularly and institute a sliding scale of intravenous insulin if the patient is unable to tolerate oral diet immediately. Restart patients back on their normal oral hypoglycaemic regimen as soon as enteral diet is recommenced.

Management of IDDM (insulin dependent diabetes mellitus)

Achieve good pre-op control and admit the patient the night before surgery. Monitor the patient's BM from admission, and commence the patient on a sliding scale of insulin on the morning of surgery. Restart regular insulin once the patient is eating and drinking normally and observe closely for sepsis. Only discharge the patient once their control is within recognised limits as their insulin requirements may well increase transiently after a stressful stimulus such as surgery.

Pre-operative management of thyroid problems

For more details of thyroid physiology, pathology and management, see Chapter 5 *Endocrine Surgery* in Book 2. Problems associated with thyroid disease include:

- **Local effects:** for example, large thyroid goitre can cause vocal cord palsy (recurrent laryngeal nerve damage) airway compromise (dyspnoea and stridor), laryngeal deviation and difficult intubation
- **Hormonal effects:** problems arise in patients with poorly controlled hypothyroidism or hyperthyroidism undergoing major emergency procedures (see *Endocrine Surgery* in Book 2)

Hyperthyroidism

This should be controlled before surgery:

- Propylthiouracil decreases hormone synthesis (but increases vascularity)
- Potassium iodide reduces gland vascularity
- Propanolol reduces systemic side effects of thyroxine

Increased risks associated with lack of pre-op preparation:

- Cardiac: tachycardia, labile BP, arrhythmia
- 'Thyroid crisis' can be precipitated by surgery. This is a syndrome of excessive and uncontrolled thyroxine release which may result in hyperthermia, life-threatening cardiac arrhythmia, metabolic acidosis, nausea, vomiting and diarrhoea, mania and coma

Hypothyroidism

Hypothyroidism reduces physiological responses:

- Low cardiac output and increased incidence of coronary artery disease (hyperlipidaemia)
- Blood loss poorly tolerated
- Respiratory centre less responsive to changes in partial pressure of O_2 and CO_2
- Sensitive to opiate analgesia

Hypothyroidism carries increased risks of:

- Myocardial ischaemia
- Hypotension
- Hypothermia
- Hypoventilation
- Hypoglycaemia
- Hyponatraemia
- Acidosis

Pre-operative management of parathyroid problems

For more details of parathyroid physiology, pathology and management, see Chapter 5 in Book 2 *Endocrine Surgery*.

Hyperparathyroidism

- **Primary** hyperparathyroidism is due to a secretory parathyroid adenoma
- **Secondary** hyperparathyroidism is parathyroid hyperplasia due to chronic hyper-stimulation
- **Tertiary** hyperparathyroidism is autonomous hypersecretion

Problems in hyperparathyroidism:

Increased calcium levels; decreased phosphate levels
Increased risks of:
Renal impairment (needs careful rehydration and fluid balance, monitoring of catheter and CVP line)
Urinary calcium excretion (which may be enhanced by judicious use of diuretics)
Hypertension
Hypercalcaemic crisis (may occur in the elderly or in those with malignant disease)

Hypoparathyroidism

Problems in hypoparathyroidism

Decreased calcium levels; increased phosphate levels
Increased risks of:
- Stridor
- Convulsions
- Decreased cardiac output

Manage with careful IV calcium replacement

2.5 PRE-OPERATIVE MANAGEMENT OF NEUROLOGICAL DISEASE

In a nutshell ...

- Epilepsy
- Cerebrovascular disease
- Parkinson's disease

Pre-operative management of epilepsy

Aim to avoid seizures in the peri-operative period by minimising disruption to the maintenance regimen of medication:

- Avoid disturbances of GI function (affects medication absorbance) and electrolyte balance
- Give usual medications up to the point of surgery
- Replace oral medications with parenteral formulations if required
- Neurology advice may be required for patients whose epilepsy is hard to control

Pre-operative management of cerebrovascular disease

- Avoid changes in BP (hypo/hypertension) and manage fluids carefully as arteriopaths have a relatively rigid vascular system
- Continue anticoagulants in the form of heparin unless contraindicated
- Position neck so as to avoid syncope
- Examine and carefully document pre-operative and early post-operative neurological status
- Delay elective surgery if there has been a recent CVA (risk of subsequent CVA increased 20-fold if surgery is performed in < 6 weeks; aim to wait for 6 months)
- Indications for carotid endarterectomy (see Chapter 10 *Vascular Surgery*)

Pre-operative management of Parkinson's disease

Parkinson's disease is due to reduced dopaminergic activity in the substantia nigra (may be degenerative, drug-induced, post-traumatic). Typical symptoms include tremor, postural instability, rigidity and dyskinesia. Peri-operative issues include:

- Postural hypotension
- Dysphagia and aspiration

- Compromised respiratory function
- Urinary retention
- Confusion, depression, hallucination
- Difficulties with speech and communication

Pre-operative medications and Parkinson's disease

Patients with Parkinson's disease are often on multiple medications and this must be managed carefully. They are at risk of drug interactions. Timing of medications must be optimised to allow the best control of the condition during waking hours ('on' and 'off' periods) as symptoms occur rapidly if doses of regular medications are missed. Consider individual special needs when arranging analgesia (may not cope with PCAS, for instance). Domperidone is a good anti-emetic as it does not have significant antipyramidal effects.

2.6 PRE-OPERATIVE MANAGEMENT OF LIVER DISEASE

In a nutshell ...

Patients with cirrhosis and liver disease do badly and have a high mortality rate with elective surgery.

Problems to anticipate include:
- Bleeding due to coagulopathy
- Encephalopathy
- Increased risk of infection
- Increased risk of renal failure
- Hypoglycaemia
- Acid–base and electrolyte imbalances
- Underlying cause (eg malignancy, EtOH abuse and withdrawal)

Distinguish between biliary obstruction (cholestatic jaundice) and chronic decompensated liver failure (hepatocellular jaundice) and manage the patient accordingly.

Pre-operative management of patients with jaundice

Fluid balance

Hypoalbuminaemia and fluid overload are common in jaundiced patients and lead to pulmonary/peripheral oedema as well as ascites. There may be sodium retention and hypokalaemia due to secondary hyperaldosteronism, which may be further complicated by the use of spironolactone or other diuretics.

Acid–base balance

A combined metabolic and respiratory alkalosis may occur. This will cause the oxygen dissociation curve to shift to the left and decrease oxygen delivery to the tissues.

Clotting

Due to a decrease in vitamin K absorption in cholestatic jaundice there is reduced synthesis of factors II, VII, IX and X and there may also be a thrombocytopenia if there is portal hypertension (due to hypersplenism).

Hepatorenal syndrome

Renal failure may be precipitated by hypovolaemia. Hepatorenal syndrome has a very poor prognosis.

Drug metabolism

Many drugs, including anaesthetic agents, undergo metabolism by the liver and may therefore have a prolonged duration of action. Hypoalbuminaemia impairs drug binding and metabolism and may lead to elevated serum levels.

Other complications

- Hypoglycaemia may occur due to depleted glycogen stores
- Wound failure and infection are increased in the jaundiced patient
- Risk of infectivity to surgeon and hospital personnel if infective hepatitis (patients require hepatitis screen if considered high-risk)

CHILD'S CLASSIFICATION OF THE SEVERITY OF CHRONIC LIVER DISEASE

	A	B	C
Bilirubin	< 35	35–50	> 50
Albumin	> 35	30–35	< 30
Ascites	None	Mild to moderate	Severe
Encephalopathy	None	Mild	Advanced
Nutrition*	Good	Moderate	Poor
Risk of surgery	Good	Fair	Poor

*Pugh's modification replaces nutrition with prothrombin time.

Pre-operative management of cholestatic jaundice

- If possible relieve jaundice before surgery (eg an endoscopically performed sphincterotomy to drain common bile duct stones)
- Keep the patient well hydrated in an attempt to avoid hepatorenal syndrome
- Check the prothrombin time and administer vitamin K 10 mg IV daily (maximum effect after three doses) or fresh frozen plasma within 2 hours of a surgical procedure
- In the presence of biliary obstruction/anticipated manipulation of the biliary tree administer prophylactic antibiotics to avoid cholangitis

Pre-operative management of chronic liver failure

- Fluid and electrolyte management (**NB:** even if there is a low serum sodium these patients have a high total sodium due to secondary aldosteronism and so additional sodium load in fluids should be avoided)
- Management of ascites (drain if tense, spontaneous bacterial peritonitis)
- Prevention of encephalopathy (restricted nitrogen, regular lactulose, sedative avoidance, prophylactic antibiotics such as metronidazole)
- Management of coagulopathy (vitamin K and fresh frozen plasma)
- Nutritional support (plus vitamin supplementation)

Pre-operative management of alcohol withdrawal

- Dangerous
- May cause confusion and aggression
- Symptoms often occur at night

Predicting patients who will suffer from withdrawal allows prescription of a sensible prophylactic regimen (eg reducing dose of chlordiazepoxide from four times per day down to zero over 7–10 days) rather than acute management with large doses of sedatives which can be dangerous.

2.7 PRE-OPERATIVE MANAGEMENT OF RENAL FAILURE

Renal failure may be acute or chronic. Details of the causes, physiology and management of renal failure can be found in Chapter 4 *Critical Care*.

Patients in established renal failure pose specific problems in peri-operative care. Fluid and electrolyte balance may be deranged and drug/metabolite excretion disturbed. Severe uraemia can directly affect the cardiovascular, pulmonary, haematological, immunological and CNS. Avoid nephrotoxic drugs in those with borderline or impaired renal function.

Classification of renal failure

- **Pre-renal** eg haemorrhage (blood); burns (plasma); vomiting (crystalloid)
- **Renal** eg diabetes; glomerulonephritis
- **Post-renal** eg retroperitoneal fibrosis (medially deviated ureters); benign prostatic hyperplasia (with chronic retention); pelvic malignancies

Pre-operative problems in patients with renal failure

Complications encountered pre-operatively in patients with established renal failure may include:

- Fluid overload, oedema
- Hypoalbuminaemia (nephrotic syndrome)
- Electrolyte abnormalities (hyperkalaemia, hyponatraemia)
- Metabolic acidosis
- Higher incidence of arterial disease (ischaemic heart disease and PVD), diabetes and hypertension
- Susceptibility to infection (uraemia suppresses the immune system)

Pre-operative management of established renal failure involves:

- Dialysis before surgery with regular monitoring of fluid/electrolyte balance
- Reduce doses of drugs excreted by kidney (eg morphine)
- Involvement of the renal team

NB: When establishing IV access in a patient with severe end-stage renal failure avoid potential arteriovenous fistula sites (eg cephalic vein). Veins on the hands can be used.

2.8 PRE-OPERATIVE MANAGEMENT OF RHEUMATOID DISEASE

Rheumatoid disease encompasses a range of disorders from joints and arthritis to connective tissue diseases and vasculitis.

Rheumatoid arthritis (RA) is a common relapsing and remitting autoimmune condition resulting in progressive joint swelling and deformity (see *Orthopaedics* in Book 2). Prevalance is about 3% in females and 1% in males.

Increased risks at time of surgery for RA patients

Cardiac: increased risk of valve disease (valvular inflammation occurs as part of the disease and can damage mitral and tricuspid valves)
Anaemia: of chronic disease
Respiratory disease: patients often have pleural nodules, pulmonary fibrosis and effusions which may compromise reserve
Peripheral neuropathy: be careful of pressure areas
Renal impairment: may be due to nephritis or medication
Skin: poor wound healing due to underlying disease and steroid use
C-spine: 15% of RA patients have atlantoaxial instability of the C-spine that may be associated with pathological fracture of the odontoid peg, and which predisposes them to atlantoaxial subluxation (horizontal/vertical) and this risk is increased during anaesthesia; subluxation can result in:

- Medullary compression and sudden death
- Spinal cord compression (acute/chronic); causes difficulty with clumsy hands, stiff legs, gait, balance
- Occipitocervical pain

Patients with neurological symptoms and signs (including tingling of hands or feet) or those with persistent neck pain should have a pre-operative C-spine X-ray.

2.9 PRE-OPERATIVE MANAGEMENT OF NUTRITIONAL STATUS

In a nutshell ...

Nutritional depletion pre- and post-surgery increases morbidity and mortality.

Malnutrition may be due to:

- Decreased intake
- Increasingly catabolic states
- Impaired digestion or absorption of nutrients

Nutritional support improves outcome and follows a hierarchy:

- Oral supplementation
- Enteral tube feeding
- Parenteral nutrition

Body mass index (BMI)

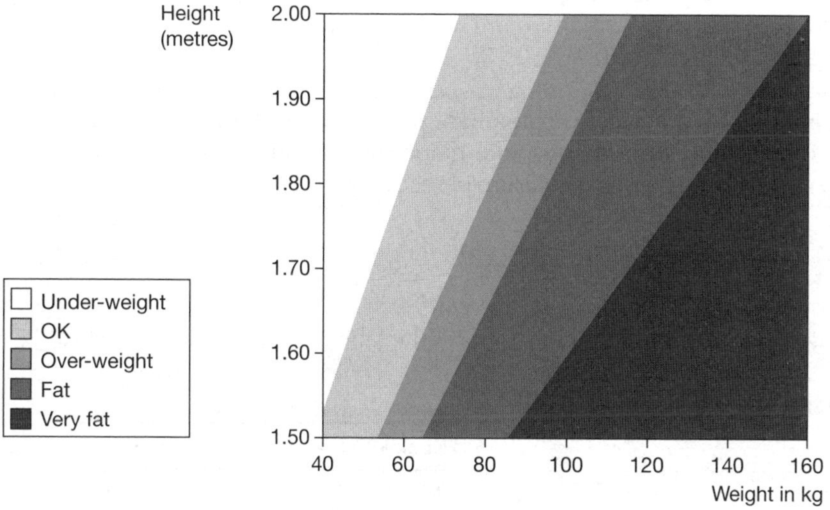

Figure 2.9a *Body mass index*

BMI is calculated with the formula below (NB: dry weight should be calculated, so exclude extra fluid weight due to ascites, renal failure, etc).

$$BMI = weight\ (kg)/height^2\ (m)$$

Body habitus is classified on the basis of BMI as follows:

< 16	Severely malnourished	
< 19	Malnourished	
20–27	Normal	
27–30	Overweight	
30–35	Obese	
35–40	Morbidly obese (if also demonstrates co-morbidities)	
> 40–50	Morbidly obese	
50–60	Super obese	These are predominantly American definitions
60–70	Super super obese	
70>	Ultra obese	

Chapter 6

Information about nutritional status may also be determined by:

- Degree of recent weight loss (> 5% mild; 10% moderate; > 15% severe)
- Percentage of expected body weight (< 85% moderate; < 75% severe)
- Physical measurements: mid-arm muscle or triceps skinfold thickness
- Serum albumin levels

NB: albumin is also a negative acute-phase protein whose levels fall in sepsis and inflammation. Therefore it is not an absolute marker for nutritional status – however, a rising albumin is the most useful as a measure of recovery.

Nutritional requirements

Daily nutritional requirements are shown in the table.

DAILY NUTRITIONAL REQUIREMENTS

	Kcal/kg/day	Protein g/kg/day
Baseline	25	0.8
Catabolic states	30–35	1.3–2.0
Hypercatabolic states	40–45	1.5–2.5

Also required are the following micronutrients:

- Electrolytes: sodium, potassium, calcium, chloride, magnesium, phosphate, fluoride
- Vitamins: A, B series, C, D, E, K
- Trace minerals: copper, iodine, iron, manganese, selenium, zinc

Malnutrition

Malnutrition is starvation that induces a low-grade inflammatory state, which causes tissue wasting and impaired organ function. Many patients (especially those with chronic disorders, malignancy and dementia) may be suffering from malnutrition. Surgery may induce anorexia and temporary intestinal failure, exacerbating the problem. The post-operative catabolic state and the stress (inhibition of the normal ketotic response) can cause muscle metabolism and weaken the patient.

Malnutrition in hospital patients is common:

- Up to 40% of surgical patients are nutritionally depleted on admission
- Up to 60% may become nutritionally depleted during admission

Malnutrition has prognostic implications for increased post-op complications:

- Poor wound healing and dehiscence
- Immunocompromise leading to infection (chest and wound)
- Organ failure

Causes of malnutrition in the surgical patient

Decreased intake

Symptoms such as loss of appetite, nausea, vomiting
Conditions such as alcoholism
Inability to feed oneself (trauma, stroke, dementia)
Disease of the mouth, pharynx, or oesophagus
Primary pathology (eg dysphagia due to tumour)
Opportunistic infection (eg *Candida*)

Increasingly catabolic state

Due to disease process eg sepsis, infection and pyrexia (especially chronicity)
Cachexia due to malignancy (some tumours cause muscle wasting and weight loss out of proportion to their size eg oesophageal cancers)
Organ failure (eg renal or hepatic failure)
Major surgery itself (trauma)

Impaired digestion or absorption

Primary disease of GI tract (eg inflammation, obstruction, fistulae)
Visceral oedema in patients with protein malnutrition
Ileus

- Post abdominal surgery
- Intra-abdominal sepsis
- Electrolyte imbalance (eg hypokalaemia, hyponatraemia)

Assessment of malnourished patients

History

- Duration of illness
- Weight loss
- Reduced appetite
- Risk factors (eg alcohol, malignancy)

Examination

- Sunken eyes
- Loose skin

- Reduced tissue turgor
- Apathy
- Weight loss

Investigation

- Arm circumference/triceps skinfold thickness
- Serum albumin
- FBC
- Transferritin
- Retinol binding protein

Malnourished patients requiring elective surgery should be considered for pre-operative and peri-operative feeding.

Obesity

Obese patients are at increased risk of surgical complications for many reasons.

Respiratory

- Decreased chest wall compliance, inefficient respiratory muscles, and shallow breathing prolong atelectasis and increase the risk of pulmonary infections
- Oxygen consumption is increased due to metabolic demand from adipose tissue and increased muscular work of breathing
- Increasing obesity causes respiratory impairment and chronic hypoxia, tolerance to hypercapnia and polycythaemia
- Sleep apnoea can result in cardiac failure

Aspiration

- Increased gastric volume and high intra-abdominal pressure predispose to gastric aspiration

Wound healing

- Poor quality abdominal musculature predisposes to dehiscence
- Increased adipose tissue predisposes to haematoma formation and subsequent wound infection

Technical problems

- Surgery takes longer and is more difficult due to problems of access and obscuring of vital structures by intra-abdominal fat deposits
- Technical problems arise with IV cannulation and subsequent phlebitis

Assessment of obese patients

Obesity increases risks of:

Hyperglycaemia (insulin resistance)
Hypertension and ischaemic heart disease
Gallstones
Osteoarthritis

For elective surgery in obese patients, the pre-op assessment should include:

- Measurement of the patient's BMI
- Discuss with anaesthetist (may require specialist)
- Referral to a dietician
- Blood glucose estimation and restoration of glycaemic control
- Measurement of blood gases (hypoxia and hypercarbia reflect respiratory impairment), and respiratory function tests (FEV_1/FVC) of < 75% in patients with obstructive pulmonary disease

Consideration of treatment for obesity before major surgery (eg weight loss regimen, procedure such as gastric bypass in the morbidly obese)

Nutritional support

These are tailored to the protein, calorific, and micronutrient needs of the patient. It follows a hierarchy, using oral supplementation if possible, enteral tube feeding if oral feeding cannot supply the required nutrients, and parenteral feeding only if enteral feeding is not possible.

Oral supplementation

- Can be used between or instead of meals
- Variety available (milk or fruit-juice based)
- High in protein and calories
- Not all contain micronutrients
- Examples include Complan™

Enteral tube feeding

Enteral feeding is the best route because it preserves GI mucosal integrity. If the patient cannot take enough nutrients in orally, tube feeding is the next step.

Enteral tube options include:

- Nasogastric (NG) tube or nasojejunal (NJ) tube (may be fine bore)
- Percutaneous endoscopic gastrostomy (PEG) or jejunostomy (PEJ). This may be useful in patients who have had facial, laryngeal or oesophageal surgery and cannot have a nasogastric tube
- Feeding gastrostomies or jejunostomies may be inserted on the ward, under radiological control endoscopically or at open surgery

Feeds include:

- Polymeric (whole protein, carbohydrate, and fat)
- Small molecule (short peptides, free amino acids and elemental fats)
- Specific feeds (eg low sodium diets in liver failure)
- Feed is delivered at pre-set speed by a pump, and gastric residual volume is checked to assess absorption
- A feed-free period allows gastric pH to fall and is important to control bacterial colonisation (see also *Bacterial Translocation* in Chapter 7 *Critical Care*)

Complications of enteral feeding tubes

- Feeding tube displaced or blocked
- Metabolic (hyperglycaemia, micronutrient deficiencies)
- Diarrhoea
- Aspiration

Parenteral nutrition

This is used only if enteral feeding is not possible or is contraindicated.

Feeding is via venous access which may be:

- Peripheral vein (long line, PICC line)
- Central access (jugular or subclavian line)
- May be tunnelled, cuffed or have a subcutaneous port

Sterile feeds are made up either to standard or to individual prescription. Feeding may be cyclical or continuous.

Catheter complications

- Risks of insertion
- Thrombosis
- Infection

Metabolic complications

- Hyperglycaemia
- Electrolyte and fluid imbalance
- Hepatic dysfunction
- Immune compromise
- Metabolic bone disease

Nutritional planning in surgical patients

Pre-operative considerations

- Dietician pre-op assessment of high-risk patients
- Encourage increased oral intake
- Oral supplementation (high protein and high calorie drinks, NG/PEG feeding)

Operative considerations

- Think about placement of tubes for enteral feeding (especially PEJ)

Post-operative considerations

Colorectal surgery

Traditionally the post-operative feeding regimen for bowel surgery was a stepwise progression guided by improving clinical signs (eg passing of flatus) thus: NBM, sips and small volumes of clear fluids, soft diet, normal diet. This has changed in recent years, with many surgeons allowing free fluids on day 1 and diet as tolerated.

- Early feeding has been shown to improve early outcome measures even in the presence of a bowel anastomosis
- Chart food intake and monitor daily on ward rounds
- Weigh patients regularly
- Patients who have had laparoscopic bowel resections are typically eating and drinking on day 2, and fit for discharge on day 4 or 5.

Upper GI surgery

Oesophageal and gastric resections are typically combined with a feeding jejunostomy placed intra-operatively so the patient can resume enteral feeding very soon after surgery. Many surgeons will then do a water contrast swallow on day 10 of high-risk anastomoses before allowing oral feeding.

Maxillofacial and pharyngeal surgery

These patients will typically have a gastrostomy feeding tube. Depending on the surgery, this may be permanent.

Section 3
The operating theatre

3.1 THEATRE DESIGN

Position

- Theatres ideally should be close to the surgical wards, ITU, sterile supplies unit, A&E and radiology/CT

Layout

- Clean areas and corridors should be separate from dirty areas and sluices, for instance
- Anaesthetic rooms should be adjacent to the theatre
- Adequate space is required for such things as storage and staff recreation

Environment

- Ideal temperature of 20–22° C to maintain patient and staff comfort
- Humidity control
- Clean filtered air enters via ceiling, leaves via door flaps (higher pressure in ultra-clean/clean areas; lower in dirty areas)
- Power, piped gas, anaesthetic gas scavenging system, suction
- Adequate lighting

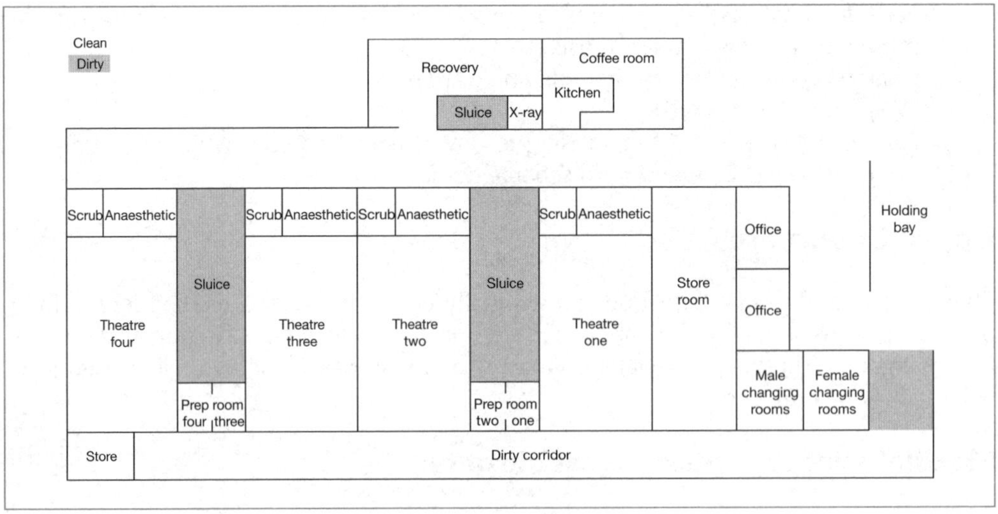

Figure 3.1a *Theatre design*

3.2 CARE OF THE PATIENT IN THEATRE

In a nutshell ...

The three Ps of patient care in theatre are:

- Pre-induction checks
- Preventing injury to the anaesthetised patient
- Preserving patient dignity

Pre-induction checks

Care of the patient in theatre starts on entering the theatre complex with **pre-induction** – which involves correct identification of patient and name band, operation, site, operation side, information about starving (if for GA), allergies, blood available (if required), and that consent form is signed.

Preventing injury to the anaesthetised patient

Causes of injury to the anaesthetised patient

General

- Transferring anaesthetised patients on and off the operating table
- Positioning of patients for the duration of surgery

Specific

- Injury to oral cavity during intubation (see section 4.6)
- Use of diathermy/laser/tourniquet (see section 3.3)
- Use of laser (see section 3.4)
- Use of torniquet (see section 3.5)
- Pressure areas not protected
- Joint injury
- Nerve injuries
- Eye injuries
- Skin injuries
- Muscle injuries

Pressure-area injury

- Risk factors: elderly, immobile, steroids, PVD
- Risk areas: sacrum, heels, back of the head
- Prevention: padding, heel protectors

Joint injury

- Risk factors: lithotomy position, 'breaking' the table
- Risk areas: prosthetic hip joints, cervical spine, limbs
- Prevention: co-ordinated lifting, head support, care with transfers

Eye injury

- Eyes should be closed and taped

Nerve injury

- Risk factor: excessive arm abduction

Prevention of injuries:

- Brachial plexus: for abduction of < 80° pronate hand and turn head
- Ulnar nerve causing claw hand: excessive flexion, avoid full flexion trauma with poles from stretchers
- Lateral popliteal causing foot drop: padding nerve of fibula in lithotomy position
- Femoral nerve causing loss of knee extension: avoid extension of hip

Skin injury

- Burns (may be due to diathermy earth, by patient touching metal on operating table or by use of flammable skin preparation, which may be ignited by diathermy, so put tape over rings or body piercings to protect site)
- Allergies (to dressings or skin preparations)
- Explosions (may be caused by flammable skin preparations, or ignition of anaesthetic or colonic gases)

Muscle injury

- Compartment syndromes may occur after prolonged surgery eg in lithotomy position

Preserving patient dignity

The operating surgeon and all the staff in contact with the anaesthetised patient have a responsibility to ensure that the patient is cared for in a way which preserves their dignity. Try to imagine that the patient is your relative and deal with them in a way that you feel is acceptable.

In particular:

- Avoid unnecessary exposure of the patient
- Avoid inappropriate comments or personal observations
- Respect clinical confidentiality
- Discourage disrespectful behaviour and report it if it persists

Remember that you are the patient's advocate. A good surgeon is one whom one would wish to operate on a member of one's own family. The patient should have good treatment, but should also be treated well, whether awake or asleep.

3.3 DIATHERMY

How diathermy works

Diathermy is used for cutting tissues and haemostasis. Heat is generated by the passage of high-frequency alternating current through body tissues. Locally concentrated high-density currents generate local temperatures of up to 1000 °C. Currents of up to 500 mA are safe at frequencies of 400 kHz to 10 MHz. There is no stimulation of neuromuscular tissue at frequencies above 50 kHz.

Diathermy settings

Cutting

- Continuous output
- High local temperature causes tissue disruption, some vessel coagulation and vaporisation of water

Coagulation

- Pulsed output of high-frequency current at short intervals
- Tissue water vaporisation and vessel coagulation

Blend

- Continuous sine-wave current with superimposed bursts of higher intensity

Monopolar

- High power unit (400 W) generates high-frequency current
- Current passes from active electrode (HIGH current density) which is the tip of the pencil held by the surgeon through the body, returning via patient plate electrode (LOW current density) to generator
- Forceps point, spatula, or diathermy scissors commonly used
- Alternate return pathway if patient touching earthed metal objects (may cause burns in older machines); most modern diathermy machines do not have earth-referenced generators

Placement of the patient plate electrode

- Good contact on dry, shaved skin; kinking must be avoided
- Contact surface area at least 70 cm^2 (minimal heating)
- Away from bony prominences and scar tissue (poor blood supply means poor heat distribution)
- Normally on patient's thigh or back
- Avoid metal prostheses (eg hip)

NB: Incorrect placement is the most common cause of accidental diathermy burns. Most systems have an alarm system if there is a fault.

Bipolar

- Lower power unit (50 W)
- Current passes between two limbs of diathermy forceps only
- No need for patient plate electrode
- Inherently safer BUT no use for cutting or touching other instruments to transfer current (buzzing)
- Useful for surgery to extremities: scrotum, penis or on digits

Diathermy safety

Safe use of diathermy

Ensure patient is not touching earthed metal (older machines)
Avoid pooling of inflammable agents (alcohol, inflammable gases)
Use a pedal
Use lowest practicable power setting
Keep active electrode in contact with target tissue and in view
Do not use too close to important structures (skin, blood vessels, nerves)
Don't use monopolar on narrow pedicles (penis, digits, dissected tissue block, spermatic cord)
Place plate away from metallic implants (eg prosthetic hips)

Causes of diathermy burns

- Incorrect plate electrode placement
- Careless technique (eg using spirit-based skin preparation fluid, not replacing electrode in a quiver after use)
- Use of diathermy on appendages (eg penis) where a high current can persist beyond the operative site
- Use of diathermy on large bowel should be avoided as explosions have been reported

3.4 LASER

LASER is an acronym for **L**ight **A**mplification by the **S**timulated **E**mission of **R**adiation.

Mechanism of action of lasers

Lasers produce light by high voltage stimulation of a medium, causing it to emit photons which are then reflected around the medium exciting other particles, which release further photons in phase with the initial photons. This process is repeated until a very high density of in-phase photons is achieved (coherent light), some of which is allowed to escape through a partially reflected mirror (the beam).

At a cellular level they vaporise tissue by evaporating water (for cutting or ablation) and coagulate proteins (for haemostasis)

Examples of uses

- Argon-beam laser: eye surgery, endoscopic ablations
- CO_2 laser: ENT ablation surgery, cervical ablation surgery
- Nd–YAG laser: endoscopic debulking surgery or GI bleeder coagulation; laparoscopic surgery

Advantages of lasers

Access: can reach difficult areas as the beam can be projected through narrow spaces, or down endoscopes
Selective effects: eg argon lasers selectively absorb red pigments (eg in blood vessels)
Precision: very fine beams can be used for cutting and/or coagulation
Minimal damage to surrounding tissues

Dangers of lasers

Retinal or corneal damage
Fire risk
Damage to structures beyond the target if burns through target
Burns (patient or operator)
Beam may be invisible

3.5 TOURNIQUETS

A tourniquet is an occlusive band applied temporarily to a limb to reduce blood flow.

Uses of tourniquets

- Prevent excessive bleeding in limb surgery allowing a clear operative field (eg for vascular anastomosis or orthopaedic surgery)
- Isolation of a limb for perfusion (eg Bier's block)
- Should not be used as a first-aid measure to arrest bleeding

Application of tourniquets

Simple tourniquets:

- Elastic tourniquets for phlebotomy
- Rubber tourniquet for digital surgery (eg ingrowing toenail)

Limb tourniquets:

- Check monitor or cuff before application
- Ensure application to correct limb and adequate breadth tourniquet (too thin may cause pressure necrosis)
- Apply tourniquet before skin preparation, avoiding vital structures (eg testicles)
- Place plenty of padding beneath tourniquet
- Inflate appropriately to 50 mmHg over systolic BP in upper limb, 100 mmHg over systolic BP in lower limb for adults; note the time of application
- The cuff should be deflated to allow reperfusion every 90 minutes (upper limbs) or 120 minutes (lower limb)

Complications of tourniquets

- Damage to skin, soft tissues or joints during application
- Chemical burns due to skin preparation getting under tourniquet
- Pressure necrosis from over-tight tourniquet, insufficient padding on prolonged application
- Distal ischaemia, venous or arterial thrombosis
- Haemorrhage following release

3.6 OPERATING THEATRE ETIQUETTE

Before arriving

- Look at the list (preferably the day before)
- Look at the notes for each patient
- Visit and examine patients that you are going to operate on
- Familiarise yourself with the procedures to be performed

On arrival

- Be prompt
- Wear appropriate scrubs, shoes and hat
- Display your ID badge so that people know who you are
- Introduce yourself to the surgeon, sister and anaesthetist
- Be helpful: with gowning and gloving, with patient transfers, etc

During procedure

- Be courteous to all members of the team
- Concentrate on what the surgeon is doing
- Keep your hands still (movement is distracting) and in plain view on the table
- Take opportunities to learn (ask about the case, its management, the surgical techniques used)
- Speak when it is appropriate to do so. Some surgeons hate to be distracted by chatter; others enjoy companiable conversation. It is best to keep quiet and concentrate during challenging moments of the operation.

After the procedure

- Clean the patient properly before dressing the wound (Betadine™ is sticky – it is uncomfortable to lie in and painful to clean off when the patient is awake)
- Help with patient transfers
- Write microbiology and histopathology request cards as fully as possible
- Keep your log book up to date
- Read the operation note and discuss or read up on any aspects of the surgery you do not understand

Section 4

Anaesthetics

Anaesthesia is the rendering of part (local anaesthesia) or all (general anaesthesia) of the body insensitive to pain or noxious stimuli.

For the purposes of the MRCS examination, a surgical SHO would be expected to know about:

- Local and regional anaesthesia
- Sedation
- General anaesthesia
- Pain control

4.1 LOCAL ANAESTHESIA

In a nutshell ...

- Local anaesthetic agents work by altering membrane permeability and preventing the passage of nerve impulses
- They can be used in a variety of ways to effect local or regional anaesthesia
    - Topical
    - Direct infiltration
    - Field block
    - Ring block
    - Individual nerve block
    - Plexus block
    - Intravenous regional anaesthesia
    - Spinal anaesthesia
    - Epidural anaesthesia
- Use of local anaesthetic agents thus has the advantage of avoiding the risks of general anaesthetic

Mode of action of local anaesthetics

- Work by altering membrane permeability to prevent passage of nerve impulses
- Stored as acidic salt solutions (following infiltration the base is released by the relative alkalinity of the tissue – hence LA is ineffective in acidic conditions such as in infected wounds)
- Often used in combination with GA to reduce opiate analgesic and GA requirements
- Ideal LA has low toxicity, high potency, rapid onset, and long duration

Local anaesthetic agents

Dosage of local anaesthetic agents:

0.5% = 5 mg/mL
1% = 10 mg/mL
2% = 20 mg/mL, etc

LAs should be used at their lowest concentration and warmed to body temperature to decrease pain on injection. Adrenaline/epinephrine may be used with LAs to slow systemic absorption and prolong duration of action.

NB: Never use local anaesthetic agents containing adrenaline (epinephrine) near end-arteries (eg digits, penis) as this may result in ischaemic necrosis.

DOSAGES AND USES OF LOCAL ANAESTHETIC AGENTS

	Maximum dose	Plus adrenaline/ epinephrine	Uses
Lidocaine	3 mg/kg	5 mg/kg	Infiltration Nerve blocks Epidurals
Bupivacaine (Marcain™)	2 mg/kg	3 mg/kg	Infiltration Nerve blocks Epidurals Spinals – high cardiotoxicity
Prilocaine	6 mg/kg	6 mg/kg	Regional nerve blocks, Bier's block – high cardiotoxicity
Cocaine	–	–	ENT
Ropivacaine	–	–	Like bupivacaine but less cardiotoxic

Chapter 6

Advantages of local and regional anaesthesia

- No systemic use of drugs (reduced side effects compared to a GA)
- Good depth of analgesia in local area only
- No requirement for mechanical ventilation
  - Better for patients with chronic respiratory disease
  - No atelectasis and infection risk
  - Less risk of gastric aspiration
- May be used in conjunction with reduced level of GA (evidence for reduced morbidity and mortality)
- May be continued for post-operative reasons:
  - Analgesia (eg epidural for laparotomy)
  - Respiratory function (allows deep inspiration and pain-free chest physiotherapy)
- Less cardiac stress during surgery (reduced ST changes seen)
- Reduced post-operative ileus
- Reduced incidence of DVT

Complications of local anaesthetics

Drug toxicity can be local or systemic.

Local toxicity

- Inflammatory response
- Nerve damage from needle or intraneural injection

Systemic toxicity

- Allergy
- May occur from over-dosage, inadvertent IV administration, absorption from highly vascular areas or cuff failure in Bier's block
- Causes perioral tingling and paraesthesia, anxiety, tinnitus, drowsiness, unconsciousness, seizures, coma, apnoea, paralysis and cardiovascular collapse (negatively inotropic and vasodilation)

Management of toxicity: stop administration of LA, then perform ABC resuscitation – protect airway, intubate and ventilate if necessary. Give IV fluids, and consider inotropic support.

Topical local anaesthetic

This is in the form of a cream or a spray and is used for routine procedures where only superficial anaesthesia is required, for example:

- EMLA cream before cannulation in children
- Lidocaine (lignocaine) gel before urethral catheterisation
- Xylocaine™ spray before gastroscopy

Infiltration of local anaesthesia

This is used typically for removal of small skin lesions.

Procedure box: Infiltration of local anaesthetic

- Check there are no allergies and there is no contraindication for using a local anaesthetic agent with adrenaline (epinephrine)
- Check the maximum safe dose for the patient and draw up only that amount, checking the vial yourself
- Use a fast-acting agent such as lidocaine
- Using an orange or blue needle, first raise a subcutaneous wheal along the line of the proposed skin incision (this will be an ellipse around a skin lesion, for example)
- Keeping the needle in the same site as much as possible, inject deeper into the subcutaneous tissue to the level of the estimated dissection, aspirating before you inject in any area where there may be vessels
- If you draw blood, do not inject, as intravenous lidocaine can cause arrhythmias
- Wait a few moments and test the area for sensation with forceps before incision. Remember that even lidocaine takes 10–20 minutes to take full effect
- Use leftover local to infiltrate if the patient reports sensation

Field block and ring block

A field block is infiltration of a local anaesthetic agent in such a way as to effect anaesthesia in the entire operating field. This may involve blocking a nerve that supplies the area. For example, when performing an inguinal hernia repair under local anaesthetic, a surgeon may combine a direct infiltration of local anaesthesia with an injection of local anaesthetic into the ileoinguinal nerve above the anterior superior ileac spine.

A ring block is a type of field block where the area to be blocked is a digit or the penis. An entire finger or toe can be made completely numb by injecting a millilitre or two of local anaesthetic just to either side of the proximal phalynx at the level of the web space. The nerve runs here with the digital artery and vein, so adrenaline (epinephrine)-containing local anaesthetic agents should never be used for a ring block, as they might render the digit ischaemic by putting the end arteries into spasm . A ring block can be used for manipulation of dislocated fingers, ingrowing toenail procedures and for post-operative analgesia after circumcision.

Brachial plexus block

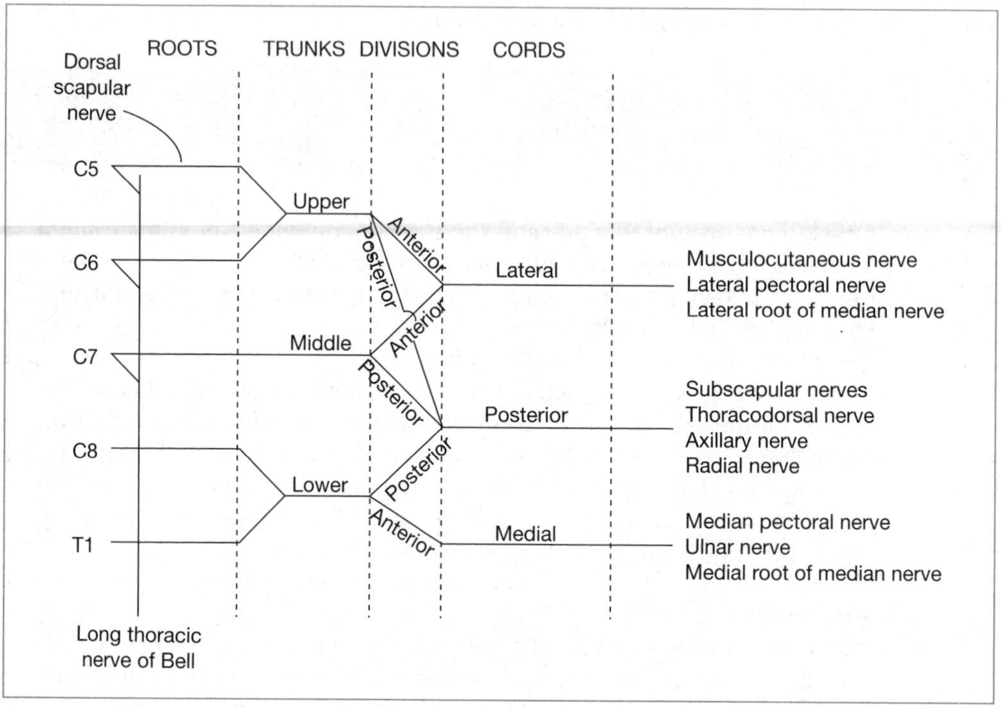

Figure 4.1a *The brachial plexus*

The brachial plexus is formed from the nerve roots C5–T1 which unite to form the main trunks (upper, middle and lower) which divide into anterior and posterior nerve divisions at the level of the clavicle. These subdivide into cords as they enter the axilla and the cords are named according to their position relative to the second part of the axillary artery (medial, lateral and posterior). The cords subdivide as the plexus passes through the axilla.

Brachial plexus blocks may be performed at different levels:

- Interscalene block (trunks)
- Supra/infraclavicular block (divisions)
- Axillary block (cords)

If injected into the fascial covering of the plexus the anaesthetic will track up and down providing a good block. These blocks are good for post-op pain relief as they last for several hours.

Femoral block

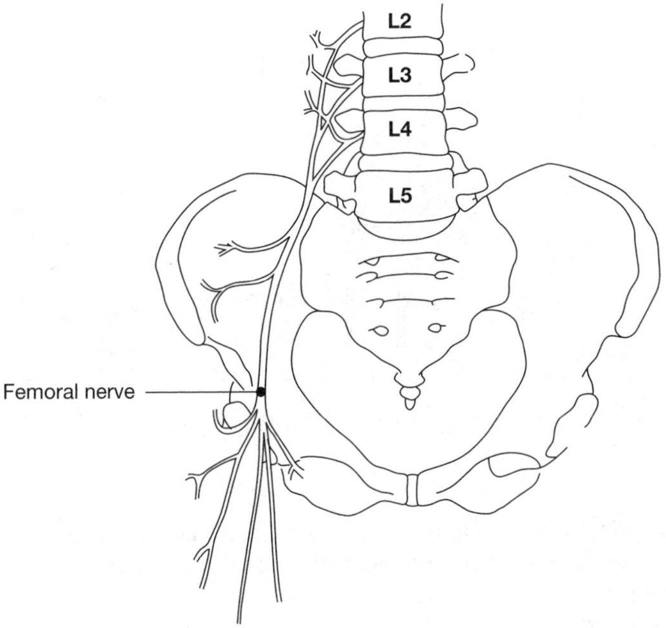

Figure 4.1b *The femoral nerve*

The femoral nerve arises from L2–4 and passes downwards on the posterior wall in the groove between the psoas and iliacus muscles. It lies on the ileopsoas as it passes under the inguinal ligament to enter the thigh, laterally to the vascular bundle and femoral sheath. The femoral nerve then divides in the femoral triangle and supplies the muscles of the anterior thigh, cutaneous nerves of the anterior thigh and the saphenous nerve.

The femoral nerve lies at a point which is 1 cm lateral to the pulsation of the femoral artery as it exits from under the inguinal ligament and 2 cm distal to the ligament. Deep infiltration of local anaesthetic at this point will produce a femoral block (NB avoid injecting into the femoral vessels). This is suitable for analgesia covering the anterior thigh, knee and femur.

Sciatic block

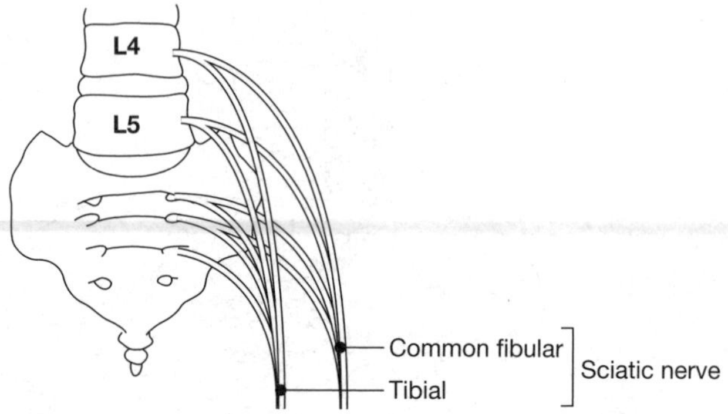

Figure 4.1c *The sciatic nerve*

The sciatic nerve arises from the lumbosacral nerve roots L4–S3 and exits under the biceps femoris muscle. It undergoes early organisation into common peroneal and tibial portions which run together centrally down the back of the thigh under adductor magnus. They usually divide in the distal third of the thigh, although this may occur at a higher level in some individuals.

The sciatic nerve block can be performed by a lateral, anterior or posterior approach and is suitable for ankle and foot surgery. The sciatic nerve lies 2 cm lateral to the ischial tuberosity at the level of the greater trochanter. Sciatic nerve blocks may be of slow onset (up to 60 minutes) so be patient with your anaesthetist.

Bier's block

This is IV regional anaesthesia, usually into the upper limb.

Technique for Bier's block

- IV access – both arms!
- Exsanguinate limb (eg Eschmark bandage)
- Apply double cuff tourniquet (with padding)
- Inflate upper cuff to approximately 300 mmHg
- Inject approximately 40 mL 0.5% prilocaine IV into isolated arm
- Inflate lower cuff (over anaesthetised segment)
- Release upper cuff (reduces cuff pain and acts as safeguard)

Intercostal nerve blocks

Useful for invasive procedures (eg chest drain insertion) and analgesia (eg flail chest or fractured ribs, breast surgery). The intercostal nerve runs with the vascular bundle under the overhanging edge of the rib. Feel for the posterior angle of the rib at the posterior axillary line and insert the needle just below the edge of the rib ('walk' the needle off the rib if necessary). Inject local anaesthetic (NB risk of pneumothorax).

Spinal anaesthesia

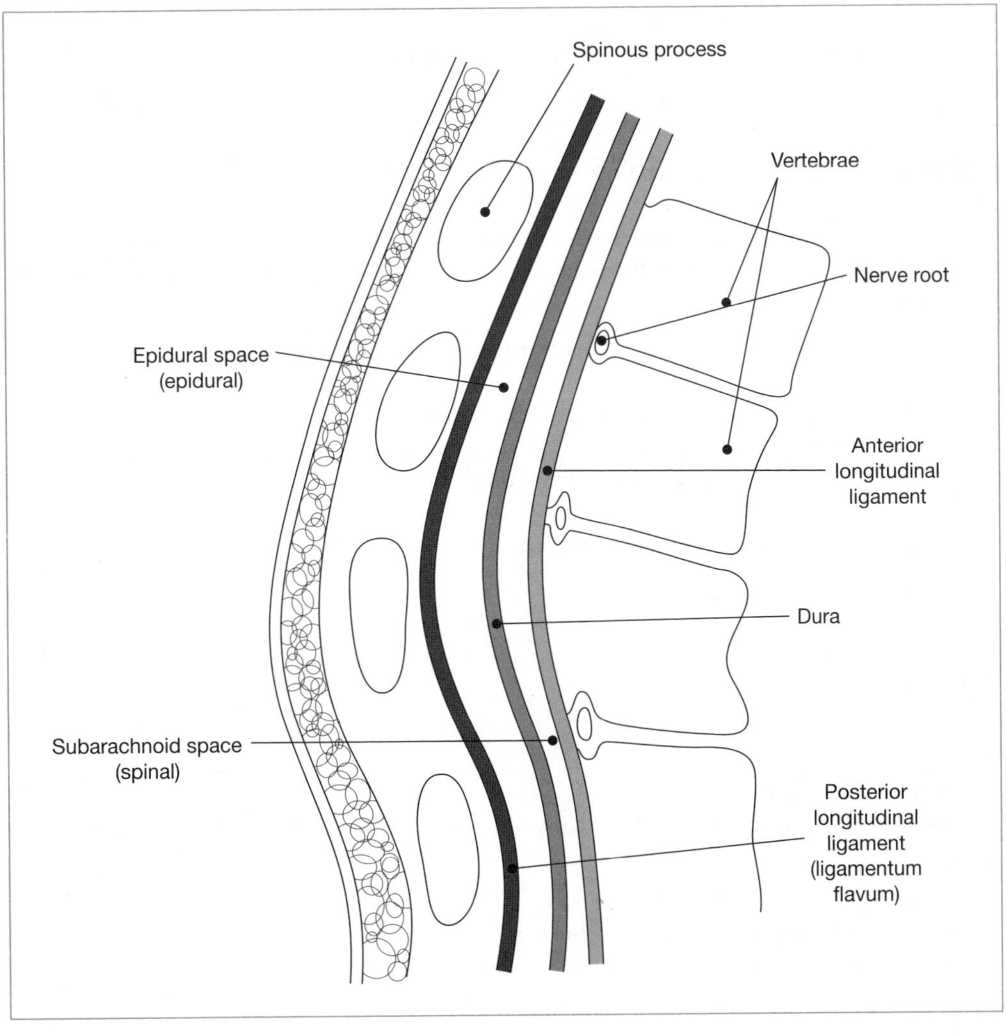

Figure 4.1d *Spinal anatomy*

Useful for lower abdominal, perineal and lower limb surgery. It is contraindicated in patients who are anticoagulated, are septic, have had previous back surgery or aortic stenosis.

- Introduce via fine-bore needle into spinal (subarachnoid space) at L1–L2 level (by the cauda equina)
- Low dose, low volume, rapid (< 5 minutes) onset
- Duration 3–4 hours
- Mainly used for peri-operative pain relief

Complications of spinal anaesthesia

- Toxicity
- Hypotension (avoid in severe cardiac disease)
- Headache, meningism, neurological disturbance
- Urinary retention

Epidural anaesthesia

This is introduced via large-bore needle to feed the catheter into the extradural space (as the needle passes through the ligamentum flavum there is a change in resistance signifying placement in the correct location).

- Situated at level of nerve roots supplying surgical site (lumbar for pelvic surgery; thoracic for upper abdominal)
- High dose, high volume, delayed (> 5 minutes) onset
- Duration of continuous infusion: up to a few days
- Can be used for peri- and post-op pain relief

Complications of epidural anaesthesia

- Dural tap
- Backache
- Infection
- Haematoma
- Urinary retention

Monitoring the level

Anaesthetic spreads caudally and cranially in both spinals and epidurals.

- Level is controlled by:
  - Initial level of placement
  - Patient positioning (eg head-down tilt)
  - Volume and concentration of anaesthetic
- Level is described by the dermatome affected:
  - Nipples T5
  - Umbilicus T10
  - Inguinal ligament T12

- High block may cause respiratory depression, and impair cough and deep inspiration (respiratory arrest at C4 level)

Spinal haematoma and abscess

- Haematoma may occur on needle insertion and epidural catheter removal
- Catheters should not be removed when the patient is anticoagulated (can be removed 12 hours post low-dose heparin followed by 2 hours delay before any further doses)
- Risk of epidural abscess increases if left in situ for > 72 hours

4.2 SEDATION

In a nutshell ...

Sedation is the administration of drug(s) to alleviate discomfort and distress during diagnostic and therapeutic interventions, with maintenance of patient responsiveness and protective reflexes. Allows for rapid recovery and avoids GA.

Sedation can be used:

- As a premedication anxiolytic
- As an amnesiac (eg relocation of dislocated shoulder)
- As an adjunct to regional anaesthesia
- During invasive interventions such as endoscopy
- In critical care (eg to tolerate endotracheal intubation)

Patients must be monitored carefully.

- Supplemental oxygen (mask or nasal cannulae)
- Cardiovascular: ECG leads and monitor
- Respiratory: pulse oximetry
- CNS: responsive and obeying commands

Avoid sedating high-risk patients (eg elderly, obese, cardiorespiratory disease).

Be prepared for adverse reactions by ensuring the following:

- Presence of an assistant
- Resuscitation equipment ready and nearby
- IV cannula left in for emergencies (**NEVER** use a butterfly needle to administer sedation)

- Drug is titrated slowly against response (especially if combined with opiate as increased risks of cardiorespiratory depression)
- Monitor until full consciousness is regained and discharge home with a responsible adult

For a discussion of common drugs used see section 4.4 of this chapter on premedication.

4.3 GENERAL ANAESTHESIA

In a nutshell ...

General anaesthesia induces

Narcosis (unconsciousness)
Analgesia
Muscle relaxation

It does this in a controlled and reversible manner, so the patient suffers no pain and has no recollection of the experience, and the surgeon has ideal operating conditions.

Stages of general anaesthesia

Pre-op assessment and preparation
Induction and muscle relaxation
Maintenance and monitoring
Recovery
Post-op monitoring and transfer

Pre-operative anaesthetic assessment

The anaesthetist will assess the patient fully pre-operatively, ideally to assess and try to minimise risks of general anaesthesia, to counsel the patient, and may prescribe premedication.

ASA grading (estimation of risk for anaesthesia and surgery)

Class 1 Normal healthy individual
Class 2 Patient with mild systemic disease
Class 3 Patient with severe systemic disease that limits activity but is not incapacitating
Class 4 Patient with incapacitating disease that is a constant threat to life
Class 5 Moribund patient not expected to survive with or without an operation

Premedication

Objectives and functions of premedication:

- Anxiolytic effect
- Causes sedation and enhancement of hypnotic effect of GA
- Causes amnesia
- Dries secretions
- Anti-emetic effect
- Increases vagal tone
- Modification of gastric contents

Benzodiazepines

These are sedative, anxiolytic and amnesic.

- **Midazolam**
  - Induction of anaesthesia
  - Sedation during endoscopy and procedures performed under LA
  - Hypnotic effect
  - Used for premed
  - Used for treatment of chronic pain
  - Is water soluble, has short duration, gives rapid clear-headed recovery
  - Dose is 0.05–0.1 mg/kg by slow IV injection
  - May cause over-sedation or respiratory depression
  - Can be reversed with flumazenil (which may itself cause seizures)
  - All patients having midazolam sedation should have IV access, pulse oximetry, ECG monitoring, resuscitation facilities available and should not drive or operate machinery for 24 hours afterwards
- **Temazepam:** 10–20 mg orally 1 hour pre-surgery
- **Diazepam:** oral or IV; longer duration than other benzodiazepines and more difficult to reverse

Droperidol

- A butyrophenone
- Anti-emetic, neuroleptic, α-blocker
- Prolonged duration action and 'locked in' syndrome may cause problems
- Rarely used

Opioids

- Analgesic and sedative
- Examples are papaveretum (Omnopon™) 20 mg IM, morphine 10 mg IM
- Can be reversed with naloxone (Narcan™)

Anticholinergics

- Competitive acetylcholine antagonists at muscarinic receptors
- Dry secretions; prevent reflex bradycardia
- Example: atropine 300–600 μg IV pre-induction

- **Glycopyrronium**
    - Less chronotropic effect than atropine
    - Doesn't cross the BBB
    - 200–400 μg IV/IM pre-induction
- **Hyoscine** (scopolamine)
    - As for atropine but more sedative and anti-emetic
    - May cause bradycardia, confusion, ataxia in elderly
    - 200–600 μg SC/IM 60 minutes pre-induction

Antacids

These are used to prevent aspiration of gastric contents (causing Mendelson syndrome) in patients at risk (eg pregnancy, trauma patients (not starved), obese, hiatus hernia). For example:

- Cimetidine 400 mg PO 1–2 hours pre-surgery
- Ranitidine 50 mg IV or 150 mg PO 1–2 hours pre-surgery
- Omeprazole 20 mg PO 12 hours pre-surgery

Additional medication

Patients may also be given (according to case):

- Steroids
- Prophylactic antibiotics
- Anticoagulants
- Immunosuppressants (eg if undergoing transplant)

Induction of general anaesthesia

This is the administration of drug(s) to render patient unconscious before commencing surgery. May be intravenous or inhalational. The IV route is quicker, but requires IV access, so inhalation induction may be the method of choice in children, in people who are needle phobics, or who are difficult to cannulate. IV induction agents are liquid soluble, and thus hydrophobic. IV induction agents are also used for maintenance of anaesthesia, by slow IV infusion.

- **Thiopentone sodium** is a commonly used induction agent. It is a barbiturate which appears as a pale yellow powder with a bitter taste and a faint smell of garlic. It is given in an alkaline solution (pH 10.8) and thus is irritant if injection occurs outside the vein. It causes a smooth and rapid induction but has a narrow therapeutic window and overdose may cause cardiorespiratory depression. It is a negative inotrope and can result in a drop in BP. There is often associated respiratory depression. It sensitises the pharynx and cannot be used with laryngeal airways

- **Propofol** is more expensive than thiopentone but has the advantage of a slight anti-emetic effect. It is a phenol derivative which appears as a white aqueous emulsion, and may cause pain on injection. It gives a rapid recovery without a 'hangover' and has a lower incidence of laryngospasm which makes it the agent of choice if using a laryngeal mask. It causes vasodilatation and is a negative inotrope resulting in a drop in BP, and therefore it is not recommended for hypovolaemic patients
- **Etomidate** is less myocardial depressive, so is better used in cardiovascularly unstable patients

Inhalational anaesthetics may also be used for induction and are discussed later in this chapter.

Complications of induction agents

Complications include:

- Hypotension
- Respiratory depression
- Laryngeal spasm
- Allergic reactions
- Tissue necrosis from perivenous injection

The effects are especially pronounced in hypovolaemic patients.

Contraindications include previous allergy and porphyria. For a discussion of intubation see Chapter 7 *Critical Care*.

Muscle relaxants

Depolarising muscle relaxants

Depolarising muscle relaxants work by maintaining muscle in depolarised (or relaxed) state.

The main example is **suxamethonium.** This has a structure similar to two acetylcholine molecules and acts in the same way as acetylcholine at the neuromuscular junction. The rate of hydrolysis, by plasma cholinesterase, is however much slower, thus depolarisation is prolonged, resulting in blockade. Its action therefore cannot be reversed. Because it acts on the acetylcholine receptor there is an initial period of muscle fasciculation which may be painful and distressing to the patient.

It is the most rapid-acting of all the muscle relaxants and is therefore useful when rapid tracheal intubation is required (crash induction). It has a duration of 2–6 minutes in normal individuals, but some people have a deficiency of plasma cholinesterase and thus have prolonged response (scoline apnoea).

Complications of depolarising muscle relaxants

- Muscle pain
- Hyperkalaemia
- Myoglobinaemia
- Bradycardia
- Hyper- or hypotension
- Malignant hyperpyrexia

Contraindications of depolarising muscle relaxants

- Patients prone to hyperkalaemia, especially burns victims
- History or family history of malignant hyperpyrexia
- History or family history of bronchospasm

Non-depolarising muscle relaxants

All have a slower onset than suxamethonium, but longer duration. Atracurium or benzylisoquinolinium have intermediate duration.

- **Atracurium** undergoes non-enzymatic metabolism independent of hepatic or renal function and thus has a safety-net advantage for critically ill patients. It does, however, cause significant histamine release in some people, which can cause cardiovascular problems or redness at the site of injection. Other benzylisoquinoliniums include cisatracurium and gallamine
- **Vecuronium** is an aminosteroid of intermediate duration. Other aminosteroids include pancuronium
- **Reversal agents:** neostigmine is used to reverse non-depolarising neuromuscular blockade, but the resulting muscarinic action may induce a profound bradycardia and is therefore given with atropine or glycopyrronium

Factors causing prolonged neuromuscular blockade

- Hypothermia
- Acidosis
- Hyperkalaemia
- Increasing age
- Concurrent use of suxamethonium
- Inhalational anaesthetics

People with myasthenia gravis have a lower number of post-synaptic receptors due to autoantibodies against them; this makes these patients more sensitive to non-depolarising muscle relaxants, but resistant to suxamethonium.

Maintenance of general anaesthesia

Inhalational anaesthetics are usually used for maintenance of anaesthesia, after IV induction, but can be used for induction eg in children.

- **Halothane** is a volatile liquid anaesthetic of the halogenated hydrocarbon class. Inhalation is well tolerated and non-irritant, which means that it rarely causes patients to cough or hold their breath. It is a very potent anaesthetic. Halothane causes respiratory depression resulting in the retention of CO_2. In addition, it is a negative inotrope, resulting in a decrease in heart rate and BP. It is also a mild general muscle relaxant
- **Enflurane** is a halogenated ether volatile liquid anaesthetic. It causes respiratory and myocardial depression resulting in a decrease in cardiac output and a rise in $paCO_2$. It is best avoided in epilepsy as it has been shown to cause EEG changes. It may cause hepatotoxicity and hyperthermia but less commonly than halothane. Free fluoride ions are a product of metabolism and may result in the very rare complication of fluoride-induced nephrotoxicity
- **Isoflurane** is the inhaled anaesthetic of choice for most surgical procedures and is also a halogenated ether. It is an isomer of enflurane but only an insignificant amount is metabolised by the patient. Hepatotoxicity is rare and malignant hyperthermia is as common as with other agents. Respiration is depressed and respiratory tract irritation may occur. There is a decrease in systemic vascular resistance due to vasodilatation and BP falls. This may result in an increase in heart rate and rarely in 'coronary steal' syndrome
- **Sevoflurane** is a recently introduced volatile liquid anaesthetic. It produces a rapid induction and recovery which means that post-op pain relief must be planned well
- **Nitrous oxide** is a potent analgesic but only a weak anaesthetic. This would therefore require greater than atmospheric pressure to produce effective anaesthesia. It does, however, potentiate the effect of other inhalational anaesthetic agents allowing a reduction in the dose required. A mixture of 50% nitrous oxide and oxygen (Entonox™) is used for analgesia, especially in obstetrics and emergency departments. Nitrous oxide will diffuse into any air-containing space. It diffuses more rapidly than nitrogen, and can lead to distension of the bowel. It must not be used in those who have recently been diving, exposed to high atmospheric pressures, or who are suspected of having a gas-filled space (eg pneumothorax or pneumocephalus). Exposure to nitrous oxide for prolonged periods of time causes suppression of methionine synthetase which leads to myelosuppression and a megaloblastic anaemia. Prolonged exposure should therefore be avoided

Contraindications of inhalational anaesthetics

Pyrexia following administration of halothane or a history of jaundice is an absolute contraindication to its use.

The major disadvantage of halothane is its association with severe hepatotoxicity (1 in 30 000) with a 50% mortality. The risk is increased with repeated exposures over a short period of time and is known to occur in theatre personnel where there have been inadequate or faulty gas exhaust systems

Like all inhalational anaesthetics, apart from nitrous oxide, it is also associated with malignant hyperthermia.

Patient monitoring during anaesthesia

These are the recommendations for standards of monitoring of the Association of Anaesthetists of Great Britain and Ireland.

Patient monitoring during anaesthesia

- Continuous presence of an adequately trained anaesthetist and clinical observation
- Regular arterial pressure and heart rate measurements (recorded)
- Continuous display ECG throughout anaesthesia
- Continuous analysis of gas mixture oxygen content (with audible alarm)
- Oxygen supply failure alarm
- Tidal/minute volume measurement
- Ventilator disconnection alarm
- Pulse oximeter
- Capnography with moving trace
- Temperature measurement available

Complications of general anaesthesia

In a nutshell ...

- Allergies
- Age
- Anaesthetic agents used (short-acting vs long-acting)
- Accidents
- Problems with intubation
  - Sore throat
  - Damage to structures in the mouth
  - Difficult airways and failed intubation
- Problems with anaesthetic drugs
  - Anaphylaxis
  - Malignant hyperpyrexia
  - Post-op nausea and vomiting (PONV)
  - Drowsiness

- Trauma to the unconscious patient
- Cardiovascular complications
  - Myocardial ischaemia
  - Hypo/hypertension
  - Arrhythmias
- Respiratory complications
  - Airway obstruction
  - Hypoventilation and hypoxia
  - Residual neuromuscular blockade
  - Gastric aspiration

Problems with intubation

Post-intubation patients may complain of a sore throat due to the endotracheal tube. This usually settles spontaneously but a search for other causes (eg *Candida* in immunocompromised people) should be undertaken if it does not.

Trauma to structures in the mouth, predominantly the soft palate and teeth, may occur. Dislodged teeth may be aspirated.

Airway management and intubation may be difficult because of:

- Abnormal anatomy (eg small mouth, large tongue)
- Atlantoaxial instability (eg Down syndrome, rheumatoid arthritis)
- Endocrine disorders causing glycosylation or enlargement of tissues (diabetes, acromegaly)
- Morbid obesity and obstructive sleep apnoea
- Pathology causing tracheal deviation

Options for managing difficult airways include:

- Optimal head position
- Pressure on the larynx
- Bougie
- Fibre-optic intubation (may be performed awake)
- Alternatives such as laryngeal mask

Failed intubation may require the procedure to be abandoned. Failed intubation with inability to ventilate necessitates an alternative airway (eg surgical or needle cricothyroidotomy).

Anaphylaxis

This is a severe allergic reaction to an epitope which is characterised by massive release of histamine and serotonin.

- Commonly occurs as a reaction to muscle relaxants, antibiotics and NSAIDs
- Clinical features include bronchospasm, angioedema and laryngeal oedema, urticaria and cardiovascular collapse
- Management involves stopping administration of the causative agent, preservation of the airway, IV administration of chlorpheniramine 10–20 mg, hydrocortisone 100–300 mg, and sometimes IM or IV adrenaline/epinephrine is required

Complications of general anaesthesia

In a nutshell ...

Minor complications include:
Damage to oral cavity and contents (intubation)
Sore throat (intubation)
Headache
Post-op nausea and vomiting
Urinary retention

Major complications include:
Death (1 in 160 000)
Gastric content aspiration
Hypoxic brain injury
MI
Respiratory infection

Gastric content aspiration

Induction is the riskiest time for gastric aspiration. Even patients undergoing a regional block should be starved pre-operatively in case there are complications and the anaesthetic has to be converted to a full GA.

Risk factors include:

- Raised intra-abdominal pressure (obese, pregnant, intra-abdominal catastrophe)
- Known GORD or hiatus hernia
- Trauma

- Drugs (eg opiates)
- Children
- Delayed gastric emptying due to disease
  - Metabolic (diabetes, renal failure)
  - Gastric motility (head injury)
  - Obstruction (at pylorus, due to ileus, mechanical bowel obstruction)

Risks reduced by:

- No solids for preceding 6 hours, clear fluids only (no milk)
- NBM for 4 hours pre-operatively
- Regular medications taken with sip of clear fluids only
- Decompress the stomach with NG tube if ileus present

Malignant hyperpyrexia

Pathology of malignant hyperpyrexia
This condition may be triggered by all inhalational anaesthetics, except nitrous oxide, and also by suxamethonium. It is a rare life-threatening condition (1 in 150 000) which requires recognition and treatment.

It is a familial disorder thought to be of autosomal dominant inheritance in which there appears to be a rapid influx of Ca^{2+} into muscle cells resulting in actin/myosin activation and muscle rigidity.

Signs include hyperthermia, muscle rigidity, tachycardia, tachypnoea and DIC. There is an increase in oxygen demand and CO_2 production leading to a metabolic acidosis, as well as hyperkalaemia.

Treatment of malignant hyperpyrexia
Dantrolene sodium 1 mg/kg by rapid IV injection, repeated to a maximum dose of 10 mg/kg. Surface cooling and cool IV fluids may be administered. Hyperventilation will help reduce $paCO_2$. The patient will need to be nursed on ITU and carefully monitored for signs of renal failure. The patient and family must be counselled as to further risks and the possibility of genetic inheritance.

Post-operative nausea and vomiting (PONV)

Occurs in about 20% patients if no prophylaxis is used.

Aetiology of PONV

- Patient factors
  - Previous history of PONV
  - Children > adults
  - Women > men
  - Obesity

- Drugs
  - Anaesthetic agents (eg nitrous oxide, etomidate, ketamine)
  - Opioid analgesics
- Certain procedure groups
  - Gynaecology (especially ovarian)
  - Head and neck, ophthalmic, ENT
  - Bowel and gallbladder surgery
- Early oral intake
- High spinal anaesthesia
- Movement causing disorientation

Management of PONV

- Prophylactic anti-emetics
- Follow the analgesic ladder
- Metoclopramide is ineffective – use cyclizine 50 mg three times daily
- Can combine anti-emetics (research shows that this is more effective than monotherapy) eg ondansetron and droperidol

Trauma to the unconscious patient

Injury can occur whilst the patient is unconscious.

- Nasal injury from NG tubes
- Corneal injury to eyes if left untaped
- Nerve injury
- Joint injury (eg hyper-extension)
- Pressure injury

Cardiovascular complications

- Myocardial ischaemia
- Cardiac failure
- Hypotension/hypertension
- Arrhythmias

These are covered in more detail in Chapter 7 *Critical Care*.

Respiratory complications

Airway obstruction

May be due to:

- Reduced pharyngeal muscular tone
- Laryngeal oedema
- Laryngeal spasm
- Bronchospasm after extubation

Hypoventilation

- Reduced respiratory drive
  - Sedative drugs and opioid analgesics
  - Anaesthetic agents
- Elevated abdominal pressures due to distension, obesity, abdominal compartment syndrome
- Abdominal pain
- Pre-existing respiratory disease
- Residual neuromuscular blockade occurs due to inadequate reversal at the end of the operation (neostigmine)

Hypoxia

- Hypoventilation
- Pathology causing VQ mismatch
- Increased oxygen requirements

Gastric aspiration

Induction is the riskiest time for gastric aspiration. Even patients undergoing a regional block should be starved pre-operatively in case there are complications and the anaesthetic has to be converted to a full GA.

- **Risk factors**
  - Raised intra-abdominal pressure (obese, pregnant, intra-abdominal catastrophe)
  - Known GORD or hiatus hernia
  - Trauma
  - Drugs (eg opiates)
  - Children
  - Delayed gastric emptying due to disease
    - Metabolic (diabetes, renal failure)
    - Gastric motility (head injury)
    - Obstruction (at pylorus, due to ileus, mechanical bowel obstruction)
- **Risk reduction**
  - No solids for preceding 6 hours; clear fluids only (no milk)
  - NBM for 4 hours pre-operatively
  - Regular medications taken with sips of clear fluids only
  - Decompress the stomach with NG tube if ileus present

4.4 PAIN AND ITS MANAGEMENT

In a nutshell ...

Pain is an unpleasant sensory and emotional experience associated with actual or potential tissue damage. It is a protective mechanism.

The physiological experience of pain is called **nociception.** It comprises four processes:

- Transduction (anti-inflammatories act here)
- Transmission (local anaesthetics act here)
- Modulation (TENS machine exploits pain gating)
- Perception (opiates act here)

The physiological aspects of pain may be modified by pharmacological means.

Transduction of pain stimuli

This is the translation of a noxious stimulus into electrical activity at the sensory endings of nerves. A noxious stimulus can be mechanical, chemical or thermal. The pain receptors in the skin and other tissues are all free nerve endings. The noxious stimulus results in tissue damage and inflammation. Non-steroidal analgesics reduce pain by inhibiting prostaglandins, which sensitise pain receptors to noxious stimuli.

Nociceptive neurones can change in their responsiveness to stimuli, especially in the presence of inflammation.

- In areas of damaged tissue the nociceptive threshold is decreased; normally noxious stimuli result in an exaggerated response (**primary hyperalgesia**) as in the extreme sensitivity of sunburned skin
- In damaged tissue there can be a lower pain threshold in areas beyond the site of injury (**secondary hyperalgesia**)
- In damaged tissue normally innocuous stimuli (eg light touch) can cause pain (**allodynia**); for example, a light touch in peritonitis can cause severe pain
- In damaged tissue pain is prolonged beyond the application of the stimuli (**hyperpathia**)

Transmission of pain impulses

Impulses travel in A fibres (fast) and C fibres (slow). A fibres transmit acute sharp pain. C fibres transmit slow chronic pain. This 'dual system' of pain transmission means that a painful stimulus results in a 'double' pain sensation, a fast sharp pain followed by slow burning pain. 'Fast' pain involves a localised reflex flexion response, removing that part of the body from the injurious stimulus, therefore limiting tissue damage. Although C fibre pain is not well localised it results in immobility, which enforces rest and therefore promotes healing of the injured part.

- A fibres terminate at two places in the dorsal horn; lamina 1 and lamina 5
- C fibres terminate in lamina 2 and lamina 3 of the dorsal horn (an area called the **substantia gelatinosa**)
- These primary afferent fibres synapse onto 2nd-order neurones in the dorsal horn (the neurotransmitter here is **substance P**)
- The majority of these 2nd-order neurones cross over in the **anterior white commissure** about one segment rostrally and ascend as the **lateral spinothalamic tract**; in the brainstem this is called the **spinal lemniscus**
- The 2nd-order neurones eventually synapse in the thalamus (**ventral posterolateral nucleus**)
- From here the 3rd-order neurones pass through the **internal capsule** to the **somaesthetic area** in the **post-central gyrus** of the cerebral cortex, for conscious perception and localisation of the pain. This projection is **somatotopic**
- Although A fibres project to the cortex, the C fibres nearly all terminate in the reticular formation, which is responsible for the general arousal of the CNS

Modulation of pain

Central mechanisms

Sometimes these central mechanisms are called the descending antinociceptive tract. The tract originates in the peri-aqueductal grey and peri-ventricular area of the mid-brain, and descends to the dorsal horn of the spinal cord; here enkephalins are released which cause pre-synaptic inhibition of incoming pain fibres.

Throughout the descending antinociceptive tract there are receptors which respond to morphine; the brain has its own natural opiates known as endorphins and enkephalins which act along this pathway (opiate analgesics act via these opioid receptors).

Spinal mechanisms

Opioids act directly at the spinal laminae inhibiting the release of substance P (the neurotransmitter involved between the primary and secondary afferent fibres). This is the mechanism exploited by epidural injection, for example.

Mechanical inhibition of pain

Stimulation of mechanoreceptors in the area of the body where the pain originates can inhibit pain by stimulation of large A fibres. (This is why analgesia is induced by rubbing the affected part or by applying TENS.) TENS (transcutaneous electrical nerve stimulation) involves applying a small electrical current over the nerve distribution of the pain, which activates the large sensory fibres and inhibits pain transmission through the dorsal horn. This is known as 'pain gating'.

Perception of pain

This occurs in the thalamus and sensory cortex.

Referred pain

This is when pain is perceived to occur in a part of the body topographically distinct from the source of the pain. Branches of visceral pain fibres synapse in the spinal cord with some of the same 2nd-order neurones that receive pain fibres from the skin. Therefore when the visceral pain fibres are stimulated, pain signals from the viscera can be conducted through 2nd-order neurones which normally conduct pain signals from the skin. The person then perceives the pain as originating in the skin itself.

Visceral pain

Viscera have sensory receptors for no other modality of sensation except pain. Localised damage to viscera rarely causes severe pain. Stimuli that cause diffuse stimulation of nerve endings in a viscus can cause pain which is very severe (eg ischaemia, smooth muscle spasm, distension of a hollow viscus, chemical damage to visceral surfaces).

- Visceral pain from the thoracic and abdominal cavities is transmitted through sensory nerve fibres which run in the sympathetic nerves – these fibres are C fibres (transmit burning/aching type pain)
- Some visceral pain fibres enter the spinal cord through the sacral parasympathetic nerves, including those from distal colon, rectum and bladder
- Note that visceral pain fibres may enter the cord via the cranial nerves (eg the glossopharyngeal and vagus nerves) which transmit pain from the pharynx, trachea and upper oesophagus

If a disease affecting a viscus spreads to the parietal wall surrounding the viscera, the pain perceived will be sharp and intense. The parietal wall is innervated from spinal nerves, including the fast A fibres.

Localisation of pain

Visceral pain is referred to various dermatomes on the body surface. The position on the surface of the body to which pain is referred depends on the segment of the body from which the organ developed embryologically. For example, the heart originated in the neck and upper thorax, therefore the visceral pain fibres from the surface of the heart enter the cord from C3 to T5. These are the dermatome segments in which cardiac pain may be perceived. Pain from organs derived from the fore-gut is felt in the upper abdomen. Pain from organs derived from the mid-gut is felt in the mid-abdomen, and pain from organs derived from the hind-gut is felt in the lower abdomen.

Parietal pain (eg from parietal peritoneum) is transmitted via spinal nerves which supply the external body surface. A good example is acute appendicitis.

- A colicky umbilical pain appears to 'move' to the RIF and becomes constant
- Visceral pain is transmitted via the sympathetic chain at the level of T10; this pain is referred to the dermatome corresponding to this area, ie around the umbilicus; this is colicky pain associated with obstruction of a hollow viscus (the appendix)

Where the inflamed appendix touches the parietal peritoneum, these impulses pass via spinal nerves to level L1–L2. This constant pain will be localised in the RIF (at McBurney's point, a third of the distance from anterior superior iliac spine to the umbilicus).

Pharmacology of pain

The analgesic ladder

Step 1 Simple analgesics (paracetamol, NSAIDs)
Step 2 Compound analgesics (co-proxamol, co-codamol, etc)
Step 3 Opiate (oral morphine remains drug of choice)

Routes for administration of analgesics

Oral	Sublingual
Intramuscular	Rectal
Intravenous	Inhalational
Subcutaneous	Epidural
Transdermal	Spinal

Paracetamol

- Mildly analgesic and antipyretic
- No significant anti-inflammatory activity

Side effects of paracetamol

- Overdosage can cause liver damage

Non-steroidal anti-inflammatory drugs (NSAIDs)

- Examples: diclofenac, ibuprofen
- Anti-inflammatory, analgesic and antipyretic actions
- Mainly act peripherally but have some central action
- Mechanism of action is by inhibition of the enzyme cyclo-oxygenase (this therefore inhibits synthesis of prostaglandins, and prostaglandins normally sensitise pain receptors to noxious stimuli)

Side effects of NSAIDs

- Prostaglandins are important in gastric mucus and bicarbonate production, so gastric irritation and peptic ulceration may result if production of them is inhibited (especially in elderly patients)
- Nephrotoxicity: chronic use can cause interstitial nephritis, papillary necrosis and urothelial tumours
- Increased bleeding results from decreased platelet adhesiveness because of inhibition of thromboxane production
- Bronchospasm in asthmatics (use should be avoided)
- May cause gout (especially indomethacin)
- May displace warfarin or other drugs from plasma proteins
- Aspirin overdosage causes metabolic acidosis and respiratory alkalosis

Opioid analgesics

- Examples: morphine, diamorphine, fentanyl
- Cause analgesia, euphoria and anxiolysis
- Act centrally and peripherally at opiate receptors
- Three main types of receptor: mu (μ), kappa (κ), delta (δ)

Side effects of opiates

- Central side effects of opiates
  - Respiratory depression (by acting on respiratory centre)
  - Nausea and vomiting (by acting on chemoreceptor trigger zone)
  - Hypotension, especially if hypovolaemic or if taking vasodilating drugs (common cause of post-operative hypotension)
  - Meiosis
  - Tolerance and addiction

- Peripheral side effects of opiates
  - Constipation
  - Delayed gastric emptying
  - Urinary retention
  - Spasm of the sphincter of Oddi
  - Pruritis

Routes of administration of opiates

- **Oral opioids**
  - Codeine phosphate, dihydrocodeine, co-dydramol, co-proxamol
  - Not useful immediately after major surgery, because of nausea and vomiting and delayed gastric emptying
  - Very useful after day-case surgery and 3–4 days after major surgery
- **Intramuscular opioids**
  - Commonest form of post-op analgesia, even though they are ineffective in providing effective analgesia in up to 40% of patients
  - There is a five-fold difference in peak plasma concentrations among different patients following administration of a standard dose of morphine, with the time taken to reach these levels varying by as much as seven-fold
  - The minimum effective analgesic concentration (MEAC) may vary by up to four-fold between patients
  - The 'standard' dose is likely to be optimal for a minority of patients
- **Intravenous opioids**
  - Continuous infusion leads to effective analgesia, but with significant risk of respiratory depression
  - Patient-controlled analgesia is the safest form
  - Epidural opioid analgesia (see below)
- **Slow-release opioids**
  - Morphine sulfate tablets (MST) have modified release over 12 hours (therefore give twice daily)
  - To calculate dose: titrate oral dose required to provide relief, then divide total daily oral dose into two daily MST doses
  - Always provide additional Oramorph™ when required for breakthrough pain

Patient-controlled analgesia (PCA)

- Now widely used for post-operative analgesia
- Administered via a special microprocessor-controlled pump, connected to the patient via an intravenous line, and which is triggered by pressing a button in patient's hand
- A pre-set bolus of drug is delivered, and a timer prevents administration of another bolus for a specified period (lock-out interval)
- A loading dose of opioid must be given at the start to achieve adequate analgesia

- The patient titrates the level of analgesia
  - eg morphine 50 mg in 50 mL saline (1 mg morphine per mL)
  - Bolus = 1 mL (1 mg morphine)
  - Lock-out time = 5 minutes
  - 4 hour limit = 30 mg morphine

Advantages of patient-controlled analgesia

- Dose matches patient requirements
- Decreased nurse workload
- Painless (no IM injections)
- Placebo effect from patient autonomy

Disadvantages of patient-controlled analgesia

- Technical error can be fatal (be very wary of background infusions)
- Expense of equipment

Cautions in the use of patient-controlled analgesia

- A dedicated IV cannula should be used to ensure the drug from the PCA does not accumulate retrogradely
- Monitor respiratory rate and level of sedation
- Patient must be orientated and fully understand how to use the system for it to be effective; use may be difficult for some patients (eg those with rheumatoid arthritis)

Management of analgesia

Remember to work up the ladder towards opiates. There are often substitutions that can be made:

- Co-codamol 2 tablets four times daily is equivalent to morphine 6–8 mg 4-hourly
- Paracetamol should be given **regularly** as a starting point
- **Non-opioids** (eg aspirin, NSAIDs, paracetamol) can control bone pain

The starting dose of morphine should be titrated to pain (eg 10 mg 4-hourly) unless the patient is elderly or has hepatorenal impairment.

With opiates, always prescribe:

- Anti-emetic for first 2 or 3 days
- Aperient to prevent constipation
- Transdermal fentanyl or alternative oral drugs (eg OxyNorm™) are useful if tolerance is poor

Acute pain

Methods of assessing acute pain

Subjective measures of acute pain

- Verbal scale
  - None
  - Mild
  - Moderate
  - Severe
- Visual analogue score
  - Ranging from worst pain ever (10) to no pain at all (0)
  - Smiley faces, sad faces (for children)

Objective measures of acute pain

- Most are indirect (eg blood pressure variations, vital capacity)

Post-operative pain relief

Inadequate analgesia

Inadequate post-op pain relief may be due to:

- Expectation (of the patient, nursing staff, or medical team)
- Prescription method: prescribe prophylactically and regularly rather than on-demand
- Inability to use or intolerance of the pain relief method (eg if the patient is immobile, arthritic, or confused and so unable to use a PCAS)

Harmful effects of undertreated acute pain

Cardiovascular effects

- Tachycardia
- Hypertension
- Increased myocardial oxygen consumption

Respiratory effects

- Splinting of the chest wall and therefore decreased lung volumes
- Atelectasis
- Inability to cough adequately, therefore sputum retention
- Infection

Gastrointestinal effects

- Reduced gastric emptying and bowel movement

Genito-urinary effects

- Urinary retention

Musculoskeletal effects

- Muscle spasm
- Immobility (therefore increased risk of DVT)

Psychological effects

- Anxiety
- Fear
- Sleeplessness

Neuroendocrine effects

- Secretion of catecholamines and catabolic hormones, leading to increased metabolism and oxygen consumption, which promotes sodium and water retention and hyperglycaemia

Management of post-operative pain

The realistic aim of pain relief is not to abolish pain completely, but to ensure the patients are comfortable and have return of function with a more rapid recovery and rehabilitation. Two fundamental concepts prevail:

- Preventing the development of pain is more effective than treating established pain – give pre-emptive analgesia, prior to surgical trauma, with parenteral opioids, regional blocks, or NSAIDS
- It is difficult to produce safe, effective analgesia for major surgery with a single group of drugs (monomodal therapy). Better analgesia is achieved with combinations of drugs that affect different parts of the pain pathway (multimodal therapy) – usually a combination of local anaesthetics, opioids and NSAIDs

NB: If possible choose the least painful incisions (eg lower abdominal or transverse incisions).

Strategies for effective post-operative analgesia

'Balanced analgesia' is the best method. This involves combining several therapeutic modalities to optimise pain relief and minimise unwanted adverse effects.

Pre-emptive analgesia

- Multimodal therapy
- Use regular non-opioid analgesic initially (eg paracetamol or NSAID, if not contraindicated) for minor surgery
- Use regional or local analgesia techniques (eg epidural or peripheral nerve blocks); they are especially effective in the immediate post-anaesthetic period
- In major surgery, opioids will be needed as an addition to the above to enhance analgesia; they are especially useful in the immediate post-op period and are still the mainstay for routine post-op pain relief. IV opioids are preferred as dose-delivery of IM injections is erratic and has greater complications
- IV opioids are best administered in the form of PCAS

The acute pain service (APS)

Each hospital should have an acute pain service team who should be responsible for the day-to-day management of patients with post-op pain. This is a multidisciplinary team using medical, nursing and pharmaceutical expertise. Anaesthetists have a major role to play, since they not only initiate post-operative analgesic regimens such as PCA and epidural infusions, but also are very familiar with the drugs and equipment. Protocols for the strict management of PCA and epidural regimens are essential.

Chronic pain

In a nutshell ...

Chronic pain is pain that persists after a time period when it would be expected that healing is complete.

The aetiology involves physical neural system rewiring and behavioural and psychosocial factors. It is very difficult to manage and requires specialist knowledge (often an anaesthetic subspecialty).

Management strategies include:

Assessment of chronic pain states
Multimodal therapy
Pain clinics

Aetiology of chronic pain

Neural system rewiring

In chronic pain states there are microscopic neural changes in the dorsal horn, spinal cord, and brain. Neural connections are altered, resulting in central plasticity. These changes result in a reduced pain threshold (hyperalgesia, in which there is exaggerated local response to non-painful stimulus), connection of mechanoreceptive neurons to pain pathways (allodynia, in which non-painful stimuli are perceived as painful), and increased receptive field size for pain neurons (equivalent to the spread of pain to nearby areas). Examples of this plasticity of the CNS are phantom limb pain and the pain of peripheral neuropathy.

Behavioural and psychosocial issues

Depression or anxiety occurs in 58% of chronic pain patients and there is a higher than normal incidence of personality disorder. Psychological issues may represent aetiological factors or occur as the sequelae to an unpleasant condition.

Types of chronic pain

- May be skeletal, spinal, joint, muscle or neuropathic (eg burning)
- Commonly back pain and headaches

Assessment of chronic pain

- History of injury, medication use and co-morbid illness (physical and psychological)
- Pain history (amount, duration, constant vs intermittent, description eg shooting vs burning)
- Identify effects of condition on physical, psychological, social and financial aspects of the patient's life to establish functional status
- Exclude a treatable underlying medical condition
- Identify behaviour patterns that may respond to behaviour modification techniques
- Identify realistic treatment goals and time course

Multimodal therapy for chronic pain

- Functional rehabilitation (MDT approach – nurses, psychologists, physiotherapists and occupational therapists) co-ordinated in pain clinic
- Medication:
  - NSAIDs and tramadol for flare-ups
  - Long-acting opioids (eg MST, transdermal fentanyl) for analgesia maintenance
  - Anti-epileptics (gabapentin, lamotrigene) and antidepressants (TCAs or SSRIs) for neuropathic pain

Pain in malignancy

Pain from malignancy is a combination of:

- Neuropathic pain (due to invasion of nerves)
- Nociception (due to tissue damage)

Management of malignant pain:

- Follow the analgesic ladder (may require opioid analgesia)
- Aim for regular, oral medication
- Regional blocks (eg coeliac plexus block)
- Radiotherapy can provide pain relief
- CT-guided stereotactic percutaneous destructive procedures

Palliative care

In a nutshell ...

Palliation is the care of patients who are not responsive to curative treatment and have a terminal condition.

It aims to address physical, mental and spiritual needs and achieve the highest quality of life possible (with the emphasis on quality rather than quantity).

Patients may be nursed at home, in a hospice, or as a hospital inpatient.

Common symptoms in palliative care

- Pain
- Shortness of breath
- Fatigue
- Dry mouth
- Appetite loss, nausea, vomiting, diarrhoea and cachexia
- Anxiety, depression and confusion

Analgesics in palliative care

- By mouth (where possible)
- By the clock (prescribe regularly as 'p.r.n.' = **p**ain **r**elief **n**egligible!)
- By the analgesic ladder

Parenteral analgesia

- For patients who cannot take things by mouth
- SC administration has been shown to be as effective as IM in terminal care
- Diamorphine is the drug of choice
  - May need anti-emetic in pump if not previously on opiate
  - Diamorphine SC dose is equivalent to a quarter to a third of the oral dose of morphine
  - SC infusion preferable to IV infusion
- Less potentiation
- Easier management
- Can discharge to home/hospice with SC pump

Potential problems with pumps

- Miscalculations with rate and delivery of setting of pump
- Mechanical failure of pump
- Reaction at injection site (IV/SC)

Treatment of pain and distressing symptoms in palliative care

Pain	
Colic	Loperamide 2–4 mg q.d.s. hyoscine
Gastric distension	Domperidone
Muscle spasm	Relaxant (eg diazepam, baclofen)
Nerve pain-compression	Dexamethasone
Nerve irritation	Amitriptyline, carbamazepine, TENS, nerve blocks
Liver pain (capsular stretching)	Dexamethasone
Respiratory	
Dyspnoea	Morphine, diazepam, dexamethasone
Excess respiratory secretions	Hyoscine
Cough	Morphine (short-acting better than MST)
GI	
Hiccoughs	Antacid, metoclopramide, chlorpromazine
Anorexia	Prednisolone, dexamethasone, Megace™
Constipation	Lactulose, co-danthrusate
Nausea and vomiting	Haloperidol (due to morphine)
Skin/mucous membranes	
Pruritus	Antihistamine
Dry mouth	Artificial saliva, oral candidiasis treatments

Neurological	
Headache	Dexamethasone if raised ICP
Hypoxia	Oxygen
Confusion/sedation	Consider drugs/hypercalcaemia/brain mets
Confusion/agitation	Haloperidol, chlorpromazine
Convulsions	Phenytoin, carbamezapine, rectal diazepam

Section 5

Post-operative care of the surgical patient

5.1 WARD ROUNDS

In a nutshell ...

Surgical ward rounds should:

- Be fast and effective
- Ideally be performed AM and PM
- Be accompanied by a nurse who knows the patients
- Provide comprehensive patient review
- Deal with ward requests at the time (ie early)
- Be associated with effective communication between MDTs:
  - Verbally
  - Via request cards written with accurate information required for investigations to be performed by other specialities
  - Via written patient notes

Aims of the ward round

- **Identify problems** arising overnight or during the day
- **Check observations**
  - Pulse, BP, respiratory rate, oxygen saturations
  - Blood glucose
  - Fluid balance (input vs output)
  - Nutritional status and intake
- **Check for pain**
  - Score
  - New/old
  - Appropriateness of current analgesic regimen:
    - PCAS
    - Epidural

    - Analgesic ladder on drug chart
    - Neuropathic (especially in amputees)
    - Pain team referral
- **Ask for and look at sputum production**
- **Perform a targeted examination** of patient
  - Cardiorespiratory (including calves for DVT)
  - Abdomen
  - Wound
    - Erythema
    - Slough
    - Dehiscence
    - Collection
- **Observe wound and drains**
  - Wound status and sutures
  - Output and content of drain
  - Removal of drains, NG tubes, catheters, cannulas
- **Check blood results, requests and patterns of change**
  - Haemoglobin
  - WCC
  - LFTs
  - Renal function
- **Check imaging results and requests**
  - US +/– Dopplers
  - CXR
  - AXR
  - CT scans
- **Approve/arrange for transfer of patients to and from critical care services**
- **Maintain communication with:**
  - Ward sister and nurses
  - Your seniors
  - Other medical teams (eg warn the on-call team of specific problems needing review)
  - MDTs for review of specific problems (eg physiotherapy, specialist nurses, dietician)
  - Discharge planning
- **Update documentation in notes:**
  - Legible, clear, correct, **useful** notes
  - Write date, time and your full name and position in capitals at the start of **every entry**. Get into this habit tomorrow!
  - Write every time the patient is reviewed
  - Remember that it is a legal requirement to include this information
  - Documentation should include information about:
    - Patient's current status
    - Patient's progress (eg results of scans)
    - Try the mnemonic SOAP (symptoms, observations, action, plan)

- The information should allow the on-call team to accurately assess the patient (regularly updated summary sheets at the front of the notes are extremely useful if called to see someone in the middle of the night or in emergencies)

5.2 POST-OPERATIVE MONITORING

In a nutshell ...

Basic non-invasive monitoring comprises:
Pulse
Blood pressure
Respiratory rate
Oxygen saturations
Temperature
Urine output
Cardiac monitoring

Additional invasive monitoring (often in a critical care setting):
CVP (central venous pressure)
ABG (arterial blood gas)
PAWP (pulmonary artery wedge pressure)

Pulse, BP and ECG monitoring

This is mandatory throughout induction of anaesthesia, maintenance and recovery. Heart rate can be obtained from ECG monitoring, pulse oximetry or intra-arterial BP monitoring.

BP can be estimated by manual sphygmomanometry, automatic sphygmomanometry measurement or directly by intra-arterial pressure monitoring via a catheter placed into a peripheral artery, usually the radial.

Cardiac monitoring

Post-operatively patients may be monitored by cardiac monitor, especially in a critical care setting. This provides a continuous cardiac rhythm trace and measurement of the pulse rate.

Pulse oximetry

Pulse oximeters measure the arterial oxygen saturation (SaO_2) – not the partial pressure of oxygen (paO_2). Probes are attached to either the fingers or ear lobes and contain two light emitting diodes (one red, one infrared) and one detector.

The instrument pulses infrared light of wavelengths 660 nm to 940 nm through the tissues. A constant 'background' amount is absorbed by skin, venous blood and fat, but a changing amount is absorbed by the pulsatile arterial blood. The constant amount is subtracted from the total absorbed to give the amount absorbed by arterial blood. Because oxygenated and deoxygenated Hb absorb differing amounts at the two wavelengths, the instrument is able to calculate a percentage of saturated Hb from the ratio of the two. Skin pigmentation does not affect the readings.

However, observation of the haemoglobin dissociation curve may show that a significant fall in the paO_2 occurs before the SaO_2 decreases (15–20-second delay).

Problems with pulse oximetry

Delay: calculations are made from a number of pulses hence there is a delay of about 20 seconds between the actual and displayed values
Abnormal pulses: atrial fibrillation, hypotension/vasoconstriction, tricuspid incompetence (pulsatile venous component)
Abnormal Hb or pigments: carbon monoxide poisoning (eg smokers), methaemoglobinaemia, bilirubin
Interference: movement/shivering, electrical equipment (eg diathermy), bright ambient light (eg in theatre)
Poor tissue perfusion
Nail varnish (coloured or not)
NB: Pulse oximetry only measures oxygenation, not ventilation. CO_2 content of blood is a reflection of ventilation (measured using a capnograph or ABGs).

Intra-arterial BP monitoring

Indications for intra-arterial monitoring

- Critically ill or shocked patients
- Major surgery (general, vascular, cardiothoracic, orthopaedic or neurosurgery)
- Surgery for phaeochromocytomas
- Induced hypotension
- Those requiring frequent blood gas analysis (ie severe pre-existing lung disease undergoing any major operation)

Complications of intra-arterial monitoring

- Embolisation
- Haemorrhage
- Arterial damage and thrombosis
- Sepsis
- Tissue necrosis
- Radial nerve damage

Urine output

Renal perfusion is closely linked to cerebral perfusion. Urine output is a good indicator of renal perfusion and thus of overall fluid balance and adequate resuscitation in a sick patient.

Catheterisation and hourly urine measurement is mandatory in:

Massive fluid or blood loss
Shocked patients – whatever the cause
Major cardiac, vascular, or general surgery
Surgery in jaundiced patients (hepatorenal syndrome)
Pathology associated with major fluid sequestration 'third space loss' (eg bowel obstruction, pancreatitis)

Invasive monitoring

Central venous pressure (CVP) monitoring

CVP is a guide to circulating volume status and myocardial contractility. CVP lines are normally placed with the tip in the superior vena cava from either an internal jugular or subclavian venous approach using the Seldinger method.

The normal CVP range for adults is 8–12 cmH_20.

The CVP can be read intermittently with a manometer, or continuously using a transducer connected to an oscilloscope. It is essential when the measurement is taken for the transducer to be at the level of the right atrium, and for the reading to be taken during respiratory end-expiration.

CVP lines can also be used for administering total parenteral nutrition (TPN) or toxic drugs (eg vancomycin).

They are indicated in critically ill patients and in major surgery if there is likely to be a complicated post-operative course, or in patients with a poor cardiac reserve where fluid balance may prove difficult to assess correctly.

The most common approaches are via the internal jugular or subclavian vein, the latter being more hazardous in a patient with chronic lung pathology where the risk of pneumothorax may have potentially more dangerous consequences. An aseptic Seldinger technique is employed using a metal guide wire.

Complications of central venous lines

Complications of CVP lines

Common complications
- Sepsis
- Pneumothorax
- Incorrect placement (position should be confirmed with a CXR)

Less common complications
- Brachial plexus injury
- Phrenic nerve injury
- Carotid or subclavian artery puncture
- Thoracic duct injury

Uncommon but potentially fatal complications
- Tension pneumothorax
- Air embolism (head-down position in ventilated patient) employed during insertion, (aspirate blood prior to flushing lines)
- Haemothorax
- Lost guidewire

For further discussion see section on *Venous Access* in the *Critical Care* chapter.

Pulmonary artery wedge pressure (PAWP)

Pulmonary artery pressure catheters (Swan–Ganz catheters) may be required when the central venous pressure (CVP) does not correlate with pressure in the left atrium as in the following conditions:

- Left ventricular failure
- Interstitial pulmonary oedema
- Valvular heart disease
- Chronic severe lung disease

They are also of value for the calculation of cardiac output and systemic vascular resistance (eg use of inotropes following cardiac surgery).

Most catheters have at least four lumens:

- Distal lumen (at the tip) which should lie in a peripheral pulmonary artery
- Proximal lumen ~ 25 cm from the tip, which should lie in the right atrium
- Balloon lumen
- Thermistor lumen, which is used to measure temperatures

The catheter is inserted into a central vein, connected to an oscilloscope, and advanced into the right atrium (shown by the venous waveform). The balloon is then inflated with air and floated into the right ventricle and then into the pulmonary artery. Further advancement will occlude a branch of the pulmonary artery and show a typical 'wedging' waveform. When occluded there is a column of fluid from the end of the catheter to the left atrium and left arterial pressure can be measured. The balloon is then deflated to prevent pulmonary infarction.

Cardiac output can be measured indirectly by infusing a small amount of cold glucose solution through the proximal lumen and measuring the temperature with the thermistor. If the volume and temperature are known the degree of dilution can be determined and thus the cardiac output can be calculated.

5.3 POST-OPERATIVE COMPLICATIONS: GENERAL

In a nutshell ...

Post-operative complications may be categorised by **time of occurance** ie:

Immediate
Early
Late

They may also be classified according to their **underlying cause:**

General complications of surgery

Haemorrhage
Pyrexia
Venous thromboembolism
Wound complications and surgical site infection

Complications specific to the operation, such as:
Anastomotic leak
Infection of prosthetic material
Hypocalcaemia after parathyroid surgery

Complications related to patient co-morbidity
Can affect any system: cardiac, respiratory, GU, GI, neurological

Risk factors for post-operative complications

- Extremes of age
- Obesity
- Cardiovascular disease
- Respiratory disease
- Diabetes mellitus
- Liver disease
- Renal disorders
- Steroids and immunosuppressant drugs

Complications may be **immediate**, **early** or **late** and may *also* be **specific** to the operation or **general** to any operation.

- **Immediate complications** occur within 24 hours of surgery
- **Early complications** occur within the 30-day period after the operation or during the period of hospital stay
- **Late complications** occur after the patient has been discharged from hospital or more than 30 days after the operation

Remember:

Prophylaxis
Early recognition
Early management

Haemorrhage

- **Primary haemorrhage** occurs during the operation; it should be controlled before the end of the operation
- **Reactionary haemorrhage** occurs usually in the first few hours after surgery, as a result of the patient warming up (vasodilating) and the blood pressure coming up after anaesthesia

- **Secondary haemorrhage** occurs a number of days after the operation; the cause is usually infection-related, but can also be related to sloughing of a clot, or erosion of a ligature

Predisposing factors for haemorrhage

- Obesity
- Steroid therapy
- Jaundice
- Recent transfusion of stored blood
- Disorders of coagulation
- Platelet deficiencies
- Anticoagulation therapy
- Old age
- Severe sepsis with DIC

Prevention of haemorrhage

- Recognise patients at risk
- Reverse risk factors if possible
- Liaise with haematologist about managing disorders of coagulation
- Control of infection
- Meticulous surgical technique

Management of haemorrhage

- Resuscitate
- Correct coagulopathy
- Surgical haemostasis if necessary
- Packing may be necessary

Post-operative pyrexia

Pyrexia is a common complication. Consider:

Is it a correct measurement?

- How was the temperature measured?

What is the trend?

- New onset
- Persistent elevation
- 'Swinging'

Is it due to an infection?

- DVT and PE can present with low-grade pyrexia
- Compartment syndrome may cause pyrexia
- Early pyrexia may be a response to surgical trauma or blood transfusion

Is there evidence of systemic involvement?

- Rigors
- Shivering
- Sweating

Is it related to drugs or infusions?

- Allergy
- Blood transfusion reaction
- Gelofusin can cause reactions

Recent culture results?

- Tailor the correct antibiotic specific to the bacteria grown

Different causes tend to manifest at different time points in the post-operative period, as shown in the box. However, these are not absolute and you should consider all causes.

Post-operative pyrexia

Day 1–3

Atelectasis
Metabolic response to trauma
Drug reactions (including to IV fluids)
SIRS (systemic inflammatory response syndrome)
Line infection
Instrumentation of a viscus or tract causing transient bacteraemia

Day 4–6

Chest infection
Superficial wound infection
Urinary infection
Line infection

Day 7 onwards

Chest infection
Suppurative wound infection
Anastomotic leak
Deep abscess
DVT

Investigation of a post-op pyrexia

- Bloods for FBC including white cell count (WCC) and neutrophil count
- Septic screen
  - Blood for culture (take from peripheral site and a separate sample through any potentially infected line; send line tips for culture)
  - Urinalysis
  - Wound swab
  - Sputum culture
  - Stool culture (eg antibiotic associated colitis)
- Tailor special investigations to examination findings (eg CXR for respiratory symptoms or signs; abdominal CT to look for deep abscess)

Note: in the 24 hours after surgery, CRP will almost always be raised due to trauma and so should not be measured routinely; an upwards trend in CRP measurements is a sensitive marker of infection (CRP increases within 24 hours of an insult).

Post-operative pyrexia is covered in detail in Chapter 2 *Infection and Inflammation*.

Venous thromboembolism

DVT and PE are discussed in Chapter 4 *Haematology*.

Post-operative wound and surgical site infections

Wound infections are discussed in detail in Chapter 2 *Infection and Inflammation*.

Risk factors for wound complications

- Type of operation
  - Potentially contaminated operations (eg elective operations on GI tract)
  - Contaminated operations (eg perforated duodenal ulcer)
  - Dirty operations (eg faecal peritonitis)
- Obesity
- Haematoma
- Diabetes
- Steroids
- Immunosuppression
- Malnutrition
- Obstructive jaundice

- Foreign material
  - Vascular grafts
  - Joint replacements
  - Heart valves
  - Mesh for hernia

NB: Effects of infection in cases with implanted prosthetic material can be devastating.

Prophylaxis for wound infections

- Identify patients at risk
- Reduce/control risk factors
- Meticulous surgical technique
- Antibiotic prophylaxis
- Bowel preparation

Treatment of wound complications

Wound infections

- Ensure adequate drainage
- Send pus for culture and sensitivity
- Debride if necessary
- Appropriate dressings
- Antibiotics only if acute infection (cellulitis, septic)
- Dehiscence requires urgent surgical repair

Abscesses

- Drain – radiological, surgical
- Treat underlying cause (eg anastomotic leak)

Septicaemia/septic shock

- Early recognition
- Treat source of sepsis
- Organ support as required on ITU

Complications of specific surgery

Complications of GI surgery

- Anastomotic haemorrhage or leak (+/– peritonitis or abscess)
- Visceral injury (due to adhesions)
- Ileus
- Oesophageal surgery: reflux, fungal infections, strictures
- Gastric surgery: 'dumping syndrome', nausea, pancreatitis
- Biliary surgery: leaks, bile duct injuries, strictures
- Small bowel surgery: short gut syndrome, malabsorption
- Colorectal surgery: stoma formation, anastomotic leaks, wound infection

Complications of vascular surgery

Carotid surgery

- TIA/CVA
- Hyperperfusion syndrome
- Patch dehiscence and secondary haemorrhage
- Cranial nerve injuries

AAA repair

- Damage to adjacent structures (eg left renal vein)
- Prosthetic infection
- Acute ischaemic colitis
- Retroperitoneal haematoma

Bypass grafting

- Anastomotic leaks or rupture
- Graft thrombosis and failure (+/– amputation)
- False aneurysm formation
- Compartment syndrome
- Disease progression

Venous surgery

- Damage to nerves (saphenous and sural)
- DVT
- Major venous injury (to femoral vein)

Complications of cardiothoracic surgery

Cardiac surgery

- Arrhythmia
- Low cardiac output
- MI

Pulmonary surgery

- Persistent air leak
- Atelectasis
- Bronchopleural fistula
- Empyema

Complications of orthopaedic surgery

- Prosthetic infection
- Joint dislocation
- Peri-prosthetic fracture
- DVT

Complications of urological surgery

Renal surgery

- Haemorrhage
- AV fistula
- Urinary leaks

Ureteric surgery

- Stenosis
- Obstruction
- Hydronephrosis

Bladder surgery

- Ileus
- Rectal injury
- Sexual dysfunction

Prostate surgery

- Urinary retention
- Retrograde ejaculation

Complications of plastic surgery

- Unsightly scarring
- Flap failure and necrosis

Complications of breast surgery

- Damage to axillary structures
- Seroma, haematoma and wound infection
- Lymphoedema and limited movement of arm
- Recurrence and breast deformity

5.4 POST-OPERATIVE COMPLICATIONS: CARDIOVASCULAR

In a nutshell ...

More than 50% of post-operative anaesthetic complications are cardiovascular, including:

- Problems with pulse rate
- Problems with blood pressure
- Myocardial infarction/ischaemia
- Congestive cardiac failure
- Tachyarrhythmias
- Sudden death

Cardiovascular disease is the most common medical problem in pre-operative patients in the developed world; and one which is associated with considerably increased morbidity and mortality during the surgical period.

Cardiology consultations and review prior to surgery is essential in patients with pre-existing cardiac disease to optimise their outcome. Consideration of the potential risks and benefits is essential pre-operatively.

In all patients at risk of cardiac complications consider:

- **Oxygen**
- **Physiotherapy:** to prevent basal atelectasis
- **Haemoglobin:** levels should be at least 10g/dL
- **ECG**
- **Invasive monitoring:** CVP and PAWP (in critical core setting only)
- **Avoidance of tachycardia and hypertension:** by increasing myocardial oxygen consumption, and lowering BP (afterload) with vasodilators
- **Good diastolic BP:** promotes coronary blood flow
- **Adequate analgesia:** reduces circulating catecholamines and stress response, thereby decreasing myocardial oxygen consumption
- **Prevention of hypothermia:** increases systemic oxygen consumption, especially below 35 °C
- **Elective ventilation:** reduces the work of breathing and prevents respiratory acidosis
- **Adequate fluid balance:** euvolaemia to reduce risk of pulmonary oedema

Problems with pulse rate

Tachycardia

Causes of post-operative tachycardia:

- Pain
- Anxiety
- Shock/hypovolaemia (+ weak thready pulse)
- Infection and sepsis (+ pyrexia + bounding pulse)
- PE
- Dysrhythmias
- SVT (eg atrial fibrillation)
- VT (with or without cardiac output)
- Ventricular ectopic beats

Bradycardia

Causes of post-operative bradycardia

- Heart block (eg inferior MI)
- Sedative drugs
- Hypothermia
- Hypothyroidism

Initial management of tachycardia or bradycardia

Consider:

- Analgesia
- Anxiolytics
- MI
- Fluid balance
- Cardiac failure
- Pulmonary oedema

Useful adjuncts

- Full cardiorespiratory examination
- 12-lead ECG
- Cardiac monitor
- Cardiac drugs/temporary pacing wires/permanent pacemakers

Cautions

- Elderly or patients on β-blockers/calcium-channel blockers may not become tachycardic
- Elderly easily pushed into pulmonary oedema
- Arteriopaths have less cardiac reserve
- Athletes have a resting bradycardia
- Children may maintain a normal pulse rate with sudden decompensation

Problems with blood pressure

The systemic BP is produced by the transmission of left ventricular systolic pressure, while the diastolic pressure is maintained by vascular tone, and an intact aortic valve. The diurnal variation of BP describes how pressures are higher during the day than at night.

Despite some degree of variability, in a resting adult the systolic pressure should not exceed 150 mmHg, and the diastolic pressure should be less than 90 mmHg.

Remember:

Is this new? Check BP on admission/pre-assessment, and intra-operative and immediately post-operative recordings. Look at the trend.

Is there evidence of haemodynamic compromise with hypotension?

Dizzy/collapse
Poor urine output
Pale
Tachycardic

What is the risk to the patient of persistent hypertension?

Think about the degree of elevation of BP
Timescale
Causation (eg Have recent antihypertensive drugs been omitted? Recent CVA causes hypertension to optimise cerebral circulation)
Effects of treatment (eg sudden fall in BP has deleterious effects)

Hypotension

Common causes of post-operative hypotension include:

- Hypovolaemia
  - Insufficient IV fluid (increased insensible losses)
  - Haemorrhage
  - Third-space loss
- Cardiogenic
  - Cardiac failure
  - Pulmonary oedema
  - Anaemia
- Thrombosis and embolism
  - PE
  - MI
- Hypersensitivity reaction
  - Allergy and anaphylaxis
  - Transplanted organ rejection

Hypertension

Common causes of post-operative hypertension include:

- Omission of usual regular antihypertensives
- Pain
- Anxiety
- Essential hypertension
- Fluid overload
- Intracranial event
- Underlying pathology (eg phaeochromocytoma)

Initial management of hypotension or hypertension

Consider

- Further investigation and monitoring (eg CVP)
- Co-morbidities and past medical history
- Nature of operation
- Fluid challenges
- Transfusion requirement
- Drugs

Useful adjuncts

- Analgesia
- Prolonged observation
- Anxiolytics
- Antihypertensives (eg titrated IV labetolol)
- ECG

Cautions

- Do not change antihypertensive medication (or add new) if the BP readings are a one-off. Remember that observation of the trend is the key
- Systolic pressures are higher in the elderly due to atherosclerosis

Myocardial infarction (MI)

Risk factors associated with increased incidence of post-op myocardial infarction

- Recent infarction (surgery within 3 months of previous MI increases risk of further MI to 25%; elective operations should be delayed by a minimum of 6 months)
- Coronary artery stenosis
- Prolonged surgery
- Surgery type
  - Vascular
  - Major abdominal
  - Cardiothoracic
- Poor left ventricular function (LVF)
- Pre-existing cardiac disease
- Angina
  - Chronic stable vs unstable
  - Pre-operative angioplasty for left main stem or triple vessel disease
- Hypertension
  - Doubles the risk of peri-operative MI
  - Should be treated pre-operatively or postponement of elective surgery until controlled
- Arrhythmias
  - Rates > 100 b.p.m

Reducing the risk of myocardial infarction peri-operatively

- Pre-operative optimisation of BP and anti-anginals
- Stop smoking!
- Local/regional anaesthesia vs general
- Shorten procedure
- Invasive monitoring
- High dependency/intensive care available

Clinical features of myocardial infarction

- Central, crushing chest pain
- May radiate to jaw, back or down left arm (common innervation)
- May also be silent
- Look for associated cardiac compromise and hypotension
- Peak occurrence on post-op day 3–4

Investigating myocardial infarction

ECG changes (affected leads identify territory of infarct):

- ST segment elevation (> 1 mm) and reciprocal depression in other leads
- Inverted T waves (sub-endocardial MI)
- Q wave development (full wall thickness MI)
- Enzyme changes post MI
  - CK-MB (creatinine kinase-myocardial bound) peaks at 12–24 hours
  - ALT peaks at 20–30 hours
  - LDH peaks at 30–48 hours
  - Troponin T rises after 12 hours and is a useful diagnostic tool
- Echocardiogram
  - Looks for areas of dyskinetic cardiac muscle
  - Assesses left ventricular function
  - Assesses damage to valves

Management of myocardial infarction

- Remember that myocardial ischaemia occurs when need exceeds supply
  - Maximise oxygen delivery to the myocardium
  - Minimise myocardial oxygen consumption by controlling rate
  - Optimise haemoglobin level
- Relieve pain with nitrates (eg GTN or IV) and diamorphine (NB titrate to BP)
- Aspirin 300 mg orally reduces mortality by 27%
- May require IV β-blockers
- May require management with ACE inhibitors for cardiac failure

Potential sequelae of myocardial infarction

- Hypotension
- Ventricular failure and cardiogenic shock
- Arrhythmias
- Conduction defects
- Rupture of septum, chamber or valve
- Ventricular aneurysm
- Cardiac arrest

Congestive cardiac failure (CCF)

May be due to:

- Pump dysfunction
- Fluid overload
- High output states (eg sepsis, hyperthyroidism)

May be acute or chronic.

Clinical features of CCF

Right ventricular failure

- Peripheral oedema (lower limbs and sacrum)
- Raised jugular venous pressure (JVP)

Left ventricular failure

- Shortness of breath
- Orthopnoea, paroxysmal nocturnal dyspnoea (PND)
- Third heart sound
- Bi-basal inspiratory crepitations

Cardiogenic shock

- Raised JVP
- Hypotension
- Loss of cardiac pump function due to:
  - MI
  - Acute valvular regurgitation
  - Pericardial tamponade
  - PE
  - Advanced heart failure

Causes of exacerbation of CCF

- Arrhythmias
- Fluid retaining drugs (eg NSAIDs)
- Anaemia
- Infection
- Thyroid disease
- Fluid overload

Investigating CCF

- ECG: shows ischaemia, arrhythmia
- CXR: shows bi-basal shadowing and bats wing oedema, fluid in the horizontal fissure, upper lobe diversion, pleural effusion, and cardiomegaly

Management of CCF

- Give oxygen
- Treat underlying cause (ischaemia or arrhythmia)
- Diuretics
- Vasodilators (eg IV nitrates) to reduce the afterload on the heart
- May require inotropes

Cardiac arrhythmias

Causes of arrhythmias

- Cardiac ischaemia
- Conduction defects
- Acidosis
- Hypercapnoea
- Hypoxaemia
- Electrolyte imbalance
  - Potassium > 6 mmol/L
  - Hypo- and hypercalcaemia
  - Hypomagnesaemia
- Hypovolaemia
- Infection (usually causes atrial fibrillation)
- Pain and anxiety
- Drugs
  - Inotropes
  - Anaesthetic

Clinical features of cardiac arrhythmias

Symptoms and signs of cardiac arrhythmias

- May be ventricular or supraventricular in nature
- May be asymptomatic
- Palpitations
- Haemodynamic instability and cardiac compromise (hypotension, dizziness, sweating)
- VT may be pulseless (see cardiac arrest pathway)

Investigating cardiac arrhythmias
Elucidate the underlying cause (see above).

Management of cardiac arrhythmias

- Give oxygen
- Assess degree of haemodynamic compromise (may require sedation and DC cardioversion urgently)
- Correct underlying contributory causes (eg hypercapnoea, electrolyte disturbance)
- Anti-arrhythmic drugs (eg digoxin, amiodarone, esmolol)

5.5 POST-OPERATIVE COMPLICATIONS: RESPIRATORY

In a nutshell ...

Respiratory problems are very common following surgery. Risk factors include:

- Patient factors
- Anaesthetic factors
- Post-operative factors
- Trauma

The management of respiratory problems is covered in detail in Chapter 7 *Critical Care*.

Risk factors for respiratory problems

Patient factors

- Age
- Pre-existing respiratory disease
- Smoking
- Obesity
- Pre-existing cardiac disease
- Excessive sedation
- Immobility
- Post-operative pain
- Upper abdominal/thoracic wounds
- One-lung ventilation

Anaesthetic factors

- Reduced residual capacity resulting from supine position and raising of diaphragm
- V/Q mismatching: increased **shunt** – perfused but not ventilated; increased **dead space** – ventilated but not perfused
- Impaired host defences: impaired protective reflexes (eg gag and cough); dry anaesthetic gases hinder ciliary function

Post-operative factors

- Residual anaesthetic agents (muscle relaxants)
- Analgesia/sedatives (eg opiates)
- Pain restricting respiratory effort and adequate cough
- Lying supine

Trauma factors

- Cord lesions
- Analgesia
- Pain
- Pneumothorax
- Lung contusion

Common respiratory post-operative pathology

- Basal atelectasis (commonest)
- Bronchopneumonia
- PE
- Pleural effusion
- Pneumothorax
- Respiratory failure
- ARDS/acute lung injury

Investigating post-op respiratory problems

- CXR
- ABGs (see Chapter 7 *Critical Care* on interpretation)
- ECG to exclude cardiac cause

Management of post-op respiratory problems

- Risk factors corrected before surgery
- Adequate post-operative analgesia (epidural is ideal for major abdominal surgery)
- Minimal sedation
- Regular physiotherapy
- Antibiotics if evidence of infection
- Drainage of effusion/pneumothorax
- Ventilatory support if necessary

Post-operative respiratory management is discussed in Chapter 7 *Critical Care*.

5.6 POST-OPERATIVE COMPLICATIONS: RENAL

In a nutshell ...

Post-operative genito-urinary problems can be subdivided into:
- Acute renal failure
  - Causes
  - Prophylaxis
  - Treatment
- Urinary tract infection

Acute renal failure

The physiology of the kidney, renal failure definition, classification, causes and management are discussed in detail in Chapter 7 *Critical Care*. A summary of the management of post-operative renal failure is given below.

Management of acute renal failure

Acute renal failure in the post-operative period may be due to pre-renal, renal or post-renal causes.

First review the patient's history, surgical notes, medications and fluid-balance chart since surgery. Check the catheter is not blocked.

Pre-renal causes: post-operative oliguria and subsequent renal impairment is most often due to dehydration. Give a fluid challenge of 500 mL and repeat until you are sure that the patient is well filled. (NB beware pulmonary oedema in the elderly.) A CVP line may be needed to monitor response to fluid

Renal causes: stop all nephrotoxic drugs (such as NSAIDs or gentamicin). Replace with non-nephrotoxic alternatives

Post-renal causes: investigate potential bladder outflow obstruction. Exclude prostatic hypertrophy or blocked urinary catheter. An USS of the renal tract will exclude most post-renal causes of ARF

All patients with oliguria or renal impairment post-operatively should be managed with a urinary catheter and hourly urine volume measurements.

Additionally, consider in all cases of renal impairment:

- Oxygenation
- Adequate circulation
- Avoidance of fluid overload (indication for dialysis)
- Routine bloods
  - Hyperkalaemia (a life-threatening complication that needs treating if K+ is > 6.0 mmol/L). Check ECG (peaked T waves). Treat with IV calcium, insulin and glucose and oral calcium resonium
  - Hyponatraemia
- Arterial blood gas: metabolic acidosis is an indication for dialysis
- Imaging
  - US
  - Antegrade or retrograde pyleography
- Renal replacement therapy (see Chapter 11 *Urology and Transplantation*)

The golden rule is: DON'T IGNORE OLIGURIA! Some patients will respond to a simple fluid challenge, and some will need full intervention. If the patient remains oliguric, do not delay treatment; more intervention is needed. As a rule, for every 2 hours that a post-operative patient is oliguric he should be reviewed by a more senior doctor. Hence no registrar should ever be unaware that one of her patients has not passed urine for 6 hours!!

Consider the following scenario:

- **2 AM:** The nurse informs the house officer that a patient has had a urine output of 5 mL per hour for the last 2 hours. The house officer manages the patient as above, reviewing notes, history, medications, surgery and fluid charts, flushes the catheter and gives several boluses of 500 mL fluid
- **4 AM:** The SHO is called. Despite 2 litres fluid bolus, the output is still only 3–5 mL per hour. The SHO repeats blood gases, U&Es, inserts a CVP line, gives fluid until the CVP is > 10 and then gives a bolus of 40 mL furosemide (frusemide)
- **6 AM:** The registrar is called. The CVP is 16, urea and creatinine have doubled, there is a compensated acidosis on the blood gases, and only 10 mL of urine was produced after the bolus of furosemide. The patient is otherwise well with no abdominal signs and a stable Hb. The patient is transferred to the HDU, discussed with the on-call intensivist and renal physicians, bloods and gases are repeated, and an USS of the renal tract is arranged. A further bolus of furosemide is given with no result, so a diuretic infusion is commenced
- **8 AM:** The consultant is informed. The patient has a worsening acidosis and hypercalcaemia and his urea and creatinine have deteriorated further. He is on HDU with a CVP line in, has a CVP of 16–20 and is on an insulin, dextrose and calcium gluconate infusion. The intensive care physicians are monitoring the situation with you and the renal physicians will be reviewing the patient on their round at 9 AM. He is on a diuretic infusion with a plan for haemofiltration if he fails to respond, and a renal ultrasound is booked for 8.30 AM. The consultant is impressed by his team's management

It would have been unacceptable to leave this man oliguric from midnight until morning without increasing his care. Prompt management of oliguria is vital, and every member of the team has a role to play.

Urinary tract infections (UTIs)

Remember:

- Most infections arise from the introduction of bowel flora via the urethra into the bladder
- Increased risk in catheterised patients (duration of catheterisation is important, around 90% develop infection if indwelling > 2 weeks)
- Causative organisms are usually coliforms

Symptoms of urinary tract infections

- Dysuria
- Frequency
- Urgency
- Loin pain
- Fever
- Haematuria

Investigating urinary tract infections (UTIs): Urinalysis

- **Nitrites:** suggesting Gram-negative bacteria (common culprits!) which convert nitrates to nitrites
- **Leucocytes:** raised levels suggest inflammatory process in renal tract; no leucocytes suggests sterile pyuria. Causes include:
  - TB of renal tract
  - Neoplasia
  - Calculi

Urinary tract infection is discussed in Chapter 11 *Urology and Transplantation*. Empirical treatment is discussed in Chapter 2 *Infection and Inflammation*.

5.7 POST-OPERATIVEL COMPLICATIONS: GASTROINTESTINAL

In a nutshell ...

- Paralytic ileus
- Antibiotic-associated colitis
- Decompensation of liver disease

Paralytic ileus

Paralytic ileus is a type of functional bowel obstruction. It may be caused or exacerbated by the conditions below.

Common causes of paralytic ileus

- Open abdominal and pelvic surgery (handling and air drying of the bowel)
- Metabolic and electrolyte disturbances
  - Hypokalaemia
  - Hypothermia
  - Diabetic ketoacidosis
  - Uraemia
- Reflex inhibition of motor activity
  - Spinal injury
  - Retroperitoneal haemorrhage
  - Head injury
  - Chest infection
- Drug-induced
  - Tricyclic antidepressants
  - GA
- Peritoneal sepsis

Clinical aspects of paralytic ileus

- Presents as prolonged bowel inactivity
- Recent history of abdominal surgery or cause as above
- Typically effortless vomiting and abdominal distension on post-op day 2 or 3
- No flatus or faeces passed
- Painless
- Absent bowel sounds
- Plain AXR shows loops of small intestine distended with gas and an empty colon

- Must be differentiated from a mechanical obstruction
- Fluid sequesters in the inactive bowel contributing to third-space loss

Management of paralytic ileus

- Prevent excessive bowel handling and cover with moist swabs in theatre
- Correct electrolyte imbalances
- Promptly treat infections
- Sometimes neostigmine is used to stimulate bowel activity (NB should not be used in those with cardiac history)

Antibiotic-associated colitis

Prolonged antibiotic usage may result in alteration of the bowel flora and an antibiotic associated colitis. Pseudomembranous colitis is caused by toxin-producing *Clostridium difficile*, which undergoes overgrowth in the gut as normal gut flora are reduced by antibiotic usage. Focal necrosis of the surface mucosa is followed by inflammation and fibrin exudation, which produce the 'pseudomembrane' and diarrhoea. See *Abdomen* in Book 2.

Decompensation of liver disease

Patients with chronic liver disease are at risk of decompensation during the operative period. For further discussion see Chapter 7 *Critical Care*.

5.8 REHABILITATION

For surgeons the ultimate goal is success of surgery. However, this does not just mean getting patients off the operating table; it includes post-operative care and rehabilitation during that time, and eventually getting the patient successfully back into the community with any adjustments and help that are necessary.

- What is the physical injury or operation?
- What is the likely outcome and effect on physical status?
- What is the existing home situation?

Things to consider include:

- Multidisciplinary team input
- Communication with:
  - Patient
  - Relatives
  - Nurses
  - Social services

- Transfer possibilities:
  - Home (+/– increased level of care)
  - Increased level of care (residential home or nursing home)
  - Hospice
  - Rehabilitation unit

Specific rehabilitation needs

Some injuries or procedures have specific rehabilitation needs, for example:

- Multiple trauma
- Head injuries
- Stoma patients
- Amputation
- Mastectomy
- Transplant

Rehabilitation of multiple trauma victims

Consider the following:

- Age and pre-hospital function
- Understanding and acceptance of injuries
- Long-term analgesia requirements
- Goal setting (ideal vs realistic)
- Early physiotherapy
- Occupational therapy (time-frame)
- Employment and income issues
- Employment and income issues if self-employed:
  - More likely to want to re-start work early whether their rehab is complete or not
  - Family need money
- Employment and income issues if company-employed:
  - Sick pay
  - Stigma of 'being on the sick'
- Psychological issues
  - Psychiatric review
  - Social worker
  - Support groups

Rehabilitation of patients with head injuries

This will largely depend on the extent of the original head injury and the sequelae of that injury.

- **Skull fractures**
  - Vault
  - Basal skull

- **Intracranial injuries**
  - Extradural
  - Subdural
  - Diffuse: concussion/diffuse axonal injury
- **Facial injuries**

Consider the following:

- **Scar tissue and plastic surgery** (revision and follow-up)
- **Post-concussion syndrome**
  - Amnesia
  - Prolonged nausea and vomiting
  - Dizziness
  - Anosmia
- **Autonomic dysfunction**
- **Cerebral cortex damage**
  - Emotional outbursts
  - Cognitive changes
- **Depression**
- **Post-traumatic epilepsy**
  - 5% closed head injuries
  - 15% severe head injuries
- **Speech therapy**
- **Occupational therapy**
- **Physiotherapy**

Rehabilitation of patients with a stoma

After stoma formation, consider:

- **Patient's pre-operative understanding and acceptance**
  - Explanation
  - Stoma nurse discussion
  - Discussion with patients with existing stoma
- **Ileostomy** bearing in mind:
  - Younger patients
  - Concerns about odour
  - Patients can contact The Ileostomy Association to discuss problems (http://www.the-ia.org.uk/)
- **Colostomy** bearing in mind:
  - Older patients
  - Acceptance is harder in later years, because of physical, psychosexual and psychosocial issues
  - Concerns about odour
  - Co-morbidities
  - Neoplasia
  - Arthritis (and changing bags)

- **Bag problems** eg high output and leakage
- **Skin problems** eg irritation and infection
- **Future operations** ie reversal or refashioning

Rehabilitation after amputation

Special considerations include:

- **Post-op infection:** high risk
- **Commonly revised** if not healing
    - Digital
    - Transmetatarsal
    - Below knee
    - Above knee
    - Hindquarter
- **Phantom limb pain**
- **Chronic pain team referral**
- **Prosthetic referral**
    - Correct fitting
    - Skin rubbing
- **Physiotherapy** and appliances
- **Psychotherapy**
    - Acceptance of limb loss
    - Acceptance of mobility changes (prosthesis, wheelchair, dominant arm)
- **Co-morbidities**
    - Continuation of smoking
    - Diabetes mellitus
    - Atherosclerosis
    - Renal impairment

Rehabilitation after mastectomy

After mastectomy, consider:

- **Age**
- **What it means to the patient**
    - Many assume the impact of mastectomy on the elderly will be smaller than in young patients
    - Many assume elderly patients will not want a reconstruction
- **Cosmetic results** (were yours and the patients expectations the same?)
- **Psychosexual problems**
    - Body image pre-op
    - Body image post-op

- **Counselling**
  - Breast nurses
  - Well patients
- **Lymphoedema**
- **Shoulder exercises**
- **Venesection** not from the axillary clearance arm
- **Long-term pain**

Rehabilitation after transplantation

Consider the following in transplant patients:

- **Compliance**
  - Regular blood tests
  - Regular clinics
  - Medications
- **Aetiology**
  - Fulminant hepatic failure can present suddenly at an early age
  - Life-long abstinence from alcohol for alcoholics
- **Immunosuppression:** life-long
  - Tablets every day
  - Side effects
  - Secondary organ damage
  - Renal impairment
- **Rejection**
  - Can be acute or early in the recovery phase
  - Early recognition
- **Psychological problems:** recognise early
  - Acceptance of organ
  - Depression
  - Inability to cope
  - Knowledge about the donor can sometimes help
  - Guilt
- **Community support**
  - Transplant games
  - Fellow patients

5.9 PSYCHOLOGICAL INFLUENCES ON RECOVERY

In a nutshell ...

Psychological effects of surgery should be considered in all patients. All require a degree of counselling and rehabilitation.

Psychological problems after surgery include:

- Confusion
- Depression
- The effects of chronic pain
- Long post-operative recovery

Post-operative confusion

Acute confusional states are common after surgery, although reports of incidence vary.

Risk factors for post-op confusion

- Male > female
- Elderly > young
- Alcohol abuse
- Pre-operative dementia or cognitive impairment
- Electrolyte imbalance

Exacerbating factors for post-op confusion

- Hypotension and poor cerebral perfusion
- Sepsis
- Hypoxia
- Electrolyte imbalances
- Drug effects, interactions and withdrawal
- Pain and anxiety
- Cerebral events (eg CVA, TIA)

Management of post-op confusion

- Assess and correct underlying causes if possible
- Be careful with prescription of sedatives in the elderly; small doses of medication can be given pre-emptively rather than large doses in the middle of the night
- See section on management of delirium tremens

Post-operative depression

This affects 4.5% of surgical patients. Pre-operative psychiatric illness, complications of surgery and long-stay patients are at high risk of developing depression. Certain procedures are more strongly associated with its development:

- Cancer surgery
- Cardiothoracic surgery
- Transplantation
- Breast surgery

Clinical features include low mood, tearfulness, insomnia, apathy and anorexia. Management should be in conjunction with psychiatric referral and includes supportive measures and medication.

Chronic pain may contribute to depression.

Long stay patients also have high levels of depression. Factors affecting the long-stay patient include:

- Immobility (eg complications, bed sores, DVT)
- Colonisation (eg MRSA)
- Institutionalisation
- Depression

Response to surgery and disease

Factors influencing the response to surgery and disease are:

- Pre-operative emotional state
- Accuracy of expectations
- Ability to choose and feelings of control over the outcome
- Personality traits (eg type A personality is associated with catecholamine release; optimists have better outcomes than pessimists)
- Coping and relaxation strategies
- Social support

Additional sources of psychological support

Nurses
Social services (eg ward-based social workers)
Physiotherapists (encouragement and aims)
Counsellors and psychotherapists
Chronic pain team
Drugs (eg antidepressants)

Breaking bad news

This is discussed in more detail in *Surgical Short Cases for the MRCS Clinical Examination*.

Compassion and honesty is required.

This should **not** be done on the ward round in front of large groups of people and remember that the curtains around the bed are **not** soundproof.

If possible take the patient to an office or private space or return at the end of the round in order to speak to them personally. Many patients already expect the worst and you should sound out their expectations. They may not wish to have full knowledge of their diagnosis and prognosis and you should identify how much they want to be told by giving information in small amounts and assessing their reaction. Patients may need information to be repeated several times in different ways at a later date.

The six steps to breaking bad news

Getting started

- **Get the physical context right.** In person, not by phone or letter
- **Where?** In a private room. Curtains drawn around the bed. Both sitting down
- **Who should be there?** A relative, friend, or nurse, as the patient wishes
- **Starting off.** Normal courtesies apply: say hello, use the patient's name, introduce yourself. Start with a general question to get a two-way conversation going, assess the patient's mental state and make the patient feel that you care: How are you today? Are you up to having a chat for a few minutes?

Find out how much the patient knows

- **How much has the patient been told?** How much have they understood?
- **What is the style of the patient's statements?** This will guide you to the level at which you have to pitch your information. Do they talk in simple terms? Or are they very well educated with good medical knowledge and wide vocabulary?
- **What is the emotional content of the patient's statements?** Distressed, anxious, brave but trembly, off-hand and defensive, hostile, or in denial?

Find out how much the patient wants to know

You could ask the patient:

- Would you like me to give you the full details of the diagnosis?
- Are you the type of person who wants to know all the details of what's wrong, or would you prefer if I just tell you what's going to happen next?

- If your condition is serious, how much would you like to know about it?
- That's fine. If you change your mind or want any questions answered at future visits, just ask me at any time. I won't push information at you if you don't want it

Share information

- **Decide on your agenda** (Diagnosis, Treatment plan, Prognosis, Support)
- **Start from the patient's starting point** (Aligning)
  - Repeat to the patient what they have said to you and reinforce those things they have said that are correct. This shows them that you take their point of view seriously and respect them
  - Give them the information that you need to, clearly, to educate them
  - Give information in small chunks with warning shots: Well, the situation does appear to be more serious than that
  - Do not use jargon: say tumour AND THEN cancer, not space-occupying lesion or malignancy
  - Check how they receive this and clarify: Am I making sense? Do you follow what I'm saying?
  - Make sure you both mean the same thing: Do you understand what I mean when I say it's incurable?
  - Repeat the important points
  - Use diagrams and written messages
  - Use any printed or recorded information available
  - Check your level: Is it too complicated or too patronising?
  - Listen for the patient's agenda: Is there anything you particularly want to talk through or are worried about?
  - Try to blend your patient's agenda with the patient's
  - Be prepared for a 'last minute' query, a hidden question, or the patient trying to 'lead' the interview

Respond to the patient's feelings

- Identify and acknowledge the patient's reaction
- Allow silence if needed
- Denial is perfectly natural and should be challenged only if causing serious problems for the patient
- Anger and blame need to be acknowledged; exploring the causes can follow later
- Despair and depression must be acknowledged. Allow the patient to express his feelings and offer support
- Awkward questions such as 'How long have I got?' may have no honest answer and you may have to reply with an open question, an empathic response, or silence in some situations
- Collusion, where relatives ask the doctor not to tell the patient, is a common request. It must be made clear that the duty of the doctor lies first to the patient, but the reasons for collusion need to be explored

Planning and follow-up

Planning for the future is a good way to alleviate the bewildered, dispirited, disorganised thoughts of a patient who has just received bad news.

- Demonstrate an understanding of the patient's problem list
- Identify problems that are 'fixable' and those that are not
- Make a plan: put 'fixable' problems in order of priority and explain what you are going to do about each one
- Prepare the patient for the worst and give them some hope for the best
- Identify coping strategies for the patient and reinforce them
- Identify other sources of support for the patient and incorporate them
- Make a contract and follow it through
- Summarise the plan you have formulated
- Check there are no outstanding issues
- Outline what will happen next and what the patient is expected to do
- Make sure you leave an avenue open for further communication (eg follow-up appointment with doctor or associated medical professional, such as a breast-care nurse)

Grief

Be aware of the normal stages of grief as shown in the box.

Response to bad news or grief

- Denial
- Anger
- Bargaining
- Depression
- Acceptance

These responses to bad news may not occur in a pre-defined order and there is no predictive timeline for how long these feelings will last. The intensity of the reaction depends upon the intensity of the feeling of loss on hearing the bad news.

Chapter 7

Critical Care

Sam Andrews and Claire Ritchie Chalmers

Section 1
The structure of critical care

1.1 LEVELS OF CARE

In a nutshell ...

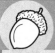

Critical care provision is classified into four levels:

Level 0	Normal ward
Level 1	Enhanced care. Nurse ratio of about 3 to 1. Monitored
Level 2	High dependency. Nurse ratio of 2 to 1. Single organ failure (not ventilated)
Level 3	Intensive care. Recovery units. Nurse ratio of 1 to 1. Multiorgan failure. Ventilation

Recovery units

After a general anaesthetic, patients are routinely transferred to a recovery unit that provides level 3 critical care before transfer to the ward. The recovery unit provides continued invasive monitoring for:

- Detection of continuing effects of anaesthetics (see *Post-Anaesthetic Complications* in Chapter 6)
- Detection of early complications of surgery (eg haemorrhage, severe pain)

Criteria for discharge to ward:

- Spontaneous airway maintenance
- Awake and non-drowsy
- Comfortable and pain-free
- Haemodynamically stable and well perfused
- No evidence of haemorrhage

The high-dependency unit (HDU)

The HDU provides level 2 critical care. It is appropriate for patients who require more input than a general ward can give, or have single organ failure but do not require ITU care or ventilation. These patients benefit from a higher ratio of nurses to each patient, allowing for increased levels of monitoring and therapy.

Outreach services may provide early access to skilled advice and allow earlier initiation of critical care. Referral should be from specialty consultant to ITU consultant.

The intensive treatment unit (ITU)

The ITU provides level 3 critical care. ITU beds in the UK account for 1% of the total beds. An ITU should have a minimum of 4 beds to be efficient and they often have 8 to 12 beds. Bed occupancy should be around 70% but is often much higher due to insufficient capacity.

The ITU should ideally be near and on the same floor as:

- A&E
- Theatres
- Radiology
- Blood bank

Admission to ITU

- For elective, emergency, or prophylactic treatment
- For potentially reversible conditions (not if outlook is futile)
- For specialised or high level of monitoring
- For mechanical support of organs (eg ventilation, dialysis)
- For failure of more than one system

Discharge from ITU

- Discharge to HDU can occur sooner than to a general ward
- Decided by senior ITU staff
- Care is handed over to specialty team

Staffing in critical care

Medical staff

- **ITU director:** should have specialty training in intensive care medicine (CCST in intensive care medicine will be required in the future), and base specialty from Anaesthetics, Medicine, Surgery, or A&E. More than 80% consultants are from Anaesthetics
- **ITU consultants:** covering all daytime sessions and on-call rota

- **Trainee:** 24-hour dedicated cover by, SHOs, SpRs, or Fellows from the above specialities

It is recommended that trainees in acute specialties should have at least 3 months training in ITU.

Nursing staff
There should be about seven whole-time equivalents per ITU bed. Nurses have an increasing degree of autonomy with roles in fluid therapy, weaning and ventilation, and inotrope titration.

Costs of critical care

- Approximately £1000–£1800 per bed per day
- Non-survivors consume greater costs

Rationale for critical care

Reasons for poor outcome in the critically ill

- Inadequate ward care
- Late referral to ITU
- Cardiac arrest (it is estimated that up to 80% are predictable prior to arrest)

Improvement in survival
This is possible because of:

- Earlier critical care intervention
- Better critical care training of medical and nursing staff in critical care principles
- Systems to identify physiological deterioration earlier
- ITU staff are expanding their roles into the wards and emergency rooms

1.2 SCORING SYSTEMS IN CRITICAL CARE

Early warning systems

These are needed to recognise ill patients on the ward early and institute critical care. They can be based on a physiological score including parameters like:

- Airway compromise
- Respiratory rate and effort
- Heart rate
- BP
- Urine output
- GCS
- *Anything* that makes ward staff suspicious

Examples of early warning systems

Many hospitals use a medical early warning system (MEWS) in order to identify the critically ill patient and highlight deterioration of a previously stable patient. The MEWS system converts vital signs into a numerical score. Nursing staff have a set threshold at which a doctor must be called to assess the patient.

The MEWS score takes into consideration:

- Haemodynamic parameters (pulse and BP)
- Temperature
- Urine output
- Respiratory rate
- Level of consciousness

Scoring systems

Scoring systems enable comparison between units and evaluation of new/existing treatments by case-mix adjustment for differences in the severity of illness of patients. Average mortality in ITUs is 25–30%.

- **Standardised mortality ratio (SMR):** calculated on the unit for diagnostic groups and can be compared with national standards (eg ICNARC)
- **Acute physiology, age and chronic health evaluation (APACHE I, II and III).** This has three point-scoring components:
  - Acute physiology based on GCS, blood results, haemodynamic and urine output variables
  - Age
  - Chronic health
- **Simplified acute physiology score (SAPS):** reduces the APACHE scoring system to 14 variables

Other scoring systems

- **Injury severity score (ISS)** correlates severity of injury in three anatomical areas, scoring up to 5 and squaring the result. Maximum score is 75. Used for audit
- **Revised trauma score (RTS)** where TRISS = ratio of RTS and ISS
- **Mortality prediction model** or mortality probability model (MPM)
- **Standardised mortality ratio (SMR)** is the ratio of estimated deaths (MPM) and actual deaths
- **Therapeutic intervention scoring system (TISS)** is used to measure nursing workload; points are attributed to different therapeutic interventions received by patients
- **Quality of life data** eg QALYs

NB: No scoring system can predict with certainty outcomes in individual patients and should not be used to influence clinical decision making.

1.3 CARE OF THE CRITICALLY ILL

Transportation of critically ill patients

In a nutshell ...

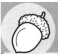

Provision of care to the critically ill patient requires:

- An understanding of the levels of care provision available and the rationale for critical care (see section 1.1)
- An understanding of the physiology of homeostasis (see section 2 of this chapter)
- An appreciation of the anatomy and physiology of each of the organ systems, how they fail, and how we support them (see section 3–8 of this chapter)
- Consideration of other aspects, ie transfer issues, sedation and analgesia (see below)

The standard of care provided during inter-hospital transfer must be the same as that provided on the ITU.

Patients should be transported:

- When adequately resuscitated
- When as stable as possible
- With a secure airway (ie endotracheal intubation)
- With adequate IV access (at least two large-bore cannulas)
- With full monitoring capability (pulse, BP, oxygen sats, end-tidal CO_2)
- With appropriately qualified staff in attendance (doctor and ITU nurse or ODP). Some units, especially paediatrics, have specialist patient retrieval teams
- With all the equipment and drugs that may be needed for resuscitation

Communication between sending and receiving centres must be exemplary. All the involved medical and surgical teams should have a written and verbal doctor-to-doctor handover, and all relevant radiology, lab results and notes should be sent with the patient.

Documentation of the transfer period must be completed.

1.4 SEDATION AND ANALGESIA IN CRITICAL CARE

Sedation in critical care

Aims of sedation

- Relieve anxiety
- Help synchronisation with the ventilator
- Encourage natural sleep
- Permit unpleasant procedures

Drugs for sedation

- **Bolus dosing:** prevents over-sedation but is inconvenient
- **Infusion:** risk of over-sedation. Can be discontinued each day until rousable then re-started as necessary
- **Benzodiazepines (eg midazolam):** reduce anxiety and are amnesic. Can accumulate with infusions, and are inexpensive
- **Propofol:** rapid elimination. Does not accumulate but is expensive (however avoiding increased length of stay due to over-sedation may offset cost). May cause hypotension

Analgesia in critical care

Aims of analgesia

- Reduce stress response due to pain
- Respiratory depression helps ventilator synchronisation
- Epidural analgesia post-surgery gives excellent analgesia avoiding IV administration

Drugs for analgesia

- **Opioids** are the mainstay administered by infusion.
- **Morphine:** for analgesia and anxiolysis. Apnoea may occur, and gastrointestinal stasis. It's inexpensive, but may accumulate. Its metabolite, morphine-6 glucuronide, accumulates in renal failure and is more potent than morphine
- **Alfentanil:** cleared by hepatic clearance. Accumulation less likely but variable metabolism in the critically ill. Expensive

Regulation of analgesic effect

- Ramsay score of 1–6: 1 is anxious, 6 is unresponsive, 2–4 is appropriate normally
- Sedation may not be required if a tracheostomy is used
- To assess pain, visual analogue scales or pain scores can be used

Section 2
The physiology of homeostasis

In a nutshell ...

Homeostasis is the maintenance of a stable internal environment. This occurs on two levels:

Normal cellular physiology relies on controlled conditions, including temperature, pH, ionic concentrations and O_2/CO_2 levels

System physiology within the body requires control of blood pressure and blood composition via the cardiovascular, respiratory, GI, renal and endocrine systems of the body

These variables oscillate around a set point, with each system drawn back to the normal condition via the homeostatic mechanisms of the body.

Homeostatic feedback works on the principles of:

- Detection via sensors
- Afferent signalling
- Comparison to the 'set point'
- Efferent signalling
- Effector action

2.1 THE BASIC PHYSIOLOGY OF THE CELL

Structure of the cell

In a nutshell ...

Cells are the building blocks of the body. They consist of elements common to all cells and additional structures that allow the cell to perform specialised functions.

Elements common to all cells include:

- Cell membrane
- Cytoplasm

- Nucleus
- Organelles
  - Mitochondria
  - Endoplasmic reticulum
  - Golgi apparatus
- Lysosomes

Cell membrane

The cell membrane is a phospholipid bilayer formed by the hydrophobic interactions of the lipid tails with the hydrophilic phosphate groups on the outside. Cholesterol molecules are also polarised with a hydrophilic and hydrophobic portion. This forms a major barrier that is impermeable to water and water-soluble substances, allowing the cell to control its internal environment. The membrane is a fluid structure (like oil floating on water) allowing its components to move easily from one area of the cell to another.

There are a number of proteins that are inserted into or that span the cell membrane and act as ion channels, transporter molecules, or receptors. These trans-membrane proteins may be common to all cells (eg ion channels) or reflect the specialised function of the cell (eg hormone receptors).

Cytoplasm

The cytoplasm is composed of:

- **Water:** 70–85% of the cell mass. Ions and chemicals exist in dissolved form or suspended on membranes
- **Electrolytes:** predominantly potassium, magnesium, sulfate and bicarbonate, and small quantities of sodium and chloride
- **Proteins:** the two types are structural proteins and globular proteins (predominantly enzymes)
- **Lipids:** phospholipids and cholesterol are used for cell membranes. Some cells store large quantities of triglycerides (as an energy source)
- **Carbohydrates:** may be combined with proteins in structural roles but are predominantly a source of energy

Under the cell membrane a network of actin filaments provides support to the cytoplasm, essentially rendering it the consistency of jelly. In the centre of the cell around the nucleus, the cytoplasm is essentially liquid. There is also a cytoskeleton consisting of tubulin microtubules that enables the cell to maintain its shape and to move by extension of cellular processes called pseudopodia.

Dispersed in the cytoplasm are the intracellular organelles such as the nucleus, mitochondria, golgi apparatus and endoplasmic reticulum. There are also fat globules, granules of glycogen, and ribosomes.

The cytoplasm is a complex and busy region of transport between the cell membrane and the intracellular organelles. Binding of molecules to cell-surface receptors activates secondary messenger systems such as cyclic adenosine monophosphate (cAMP) and inositol triphosphate (IP_3).

The nucleus

A double phospholipid membrane surrounds the nucleus and this is penetrated by nuclear pores which allow access to small molecules. The nucleus contains the DNA and is the primary site of gene regulation.

The bases of DNA comprise two purines, adenine (A) and guanine (G) and two pyrimidines, thymidine (T) and cytosine (C) – A forms a bond with T, and G forms a bond with C. DNA is a double helix with a backbone of deoxyribose sugars either side of the paired nitrogenous bases that act as the code.

DNA is stored in the nucleus in a condensed form, wrapped around proteins called histones. When condensed the genes are inactive. The DNA unwinds from the histone protein when the gene becomes activated. The two strands separate to allow transcription factors access to the DNA code. The transcription factor binds to the gene promoter region and allows an enzyme called RNA polymerase to produce complementary copies of the gene in a form known as messenger RNA (mRNA). Messenger RNA is then transported to the ribosomes for translation into protein.

Mitochondria

These structures generate > 95% of the energy required by the cell. Different cells have variable numbers. They are bean-shaped with a double membrane – the internal membrane is folded into shelves where the enzymes for the production of energy are attached. Mitochondria can self-replicate and contain a small amount of DNA.

Endoplasmic reticulum (ER)

This is a network of tubular structures with the lumen of the tube connected to the nuclear membrane. These branching networks provide a huge surface area of membrane and are the site of the major metabolic functions of the cell. They are responsible for the majority of synthetic processes producing lipids and proteins in conjunction with the attached ribosomes.

The ribosome is responsible for translating the mRNA into protein. The mRNA travels along the ribosome (and may pass through several ribosomes simultaneously, like beads on a string). Each amino acid binds to a small molecule of transfer RNA (tRNA) which has a triplet of bases that correspond to the amino acid that it is carrying. These bases are complementary to the bases on the mRNA strand. ATP is required to activate each amino acid. The ribosome then catalyses peptide bonds between activated amino acids.

Golgi apparatus

The Golgi apparatus is structurally similar to the ER and lies as stacked layers of tubes close to the cell membrane. Its function is secretion. Substances to be secreted leave the ER by becoming enclosed in a pinched off piece of membrane (a vesicle) and travel through the cytoplasm to fuse with the membrane of the Golgi body. They are then processed inside the Golgi to form secretory vesicles (or lysosomes) which bud off the Golgi and fuse with the cell membrane, disgorging their contents.

Basic cellular functions

In a nutshell ...

Basic cellular functions are common to all cells. They include:

- Transport across membranes
- Generation of energy from carbohydrates and lipids
- Protein turnover

Transport across membranes

Molecules may be moved across cell membranes by:

- **Simple diffusion:** this occurs down a concentration gradient or down an ionic gradient. It depends on the permeability of the membrane to the molecule. There is no energy requirement for this process
- **Simple facilitated diffusion:** this also occurs down a concentration gradient, but the molecule becomes attached to a protein molecule that facilitates its passage (for example, a water-soluble molecule that would be repelled by a cell membrane attached to a carrier molecule that can pass easily through a cell membrane). There is no energy requirement for this process
- **Primary active transport:** in which energy from ATP is used to move the molecule against a concentration or ionic gradient. This is also called a 'pump'
- **Secondary active transport:** in which energy is used to move a molecule against a concentration or ionic gradient. This energy comes from the associated movement of a second molecule down a concentration gradient. If both these molecules are moving in the same direction this is called 'co-transport'. If they are moving in opposite directions this is called 'counter-transport'

- **Endocytosis and exocytosis:** these processes involve a piece of membrane budding off from the cell membrane to envelop a substance which is then internalised by the cell (endocytosis). Conversely, secretory vesicles from the Golgi apparatus may fuse with the cell membrane releasing their contents outside the cell (exocytosis)

The sodium–potassium pump

This pump (also called the Na^+/K^+ ATPase) is used by cells to move potassium ions into the cell and sodium ions out of the cell. It is present in all cells of the body and maintains a negative electrical potential inside the cell. It is also the basis of the action potential.

The Na^+/K^+ ATPase consists of two globular protein subunits. There are two receptor sites for binding K^+ ions on the outside of the cell and three receptor sites for binding Na^+ on the inside of the cell. When three Na^+ ions bind to the receptors on the inside of the cell, ATP is cleaved to ADP, releasing energy from the phosphate bond. This energy is used to induce a conformational change in the protein which extrudes the Na^+ ions from the cell and brings the K^+ ions inside the cell. As the cell membrane is relatively impermeable to Na^+ ions this sets up a concentration and therefore an ionic gradient (called the electrochemical gradient). Water molecules tend to follow the Na^+ ions, protecting the cell from increases in volume that would lead to cell lysis. Additionally K^+ ions tend to leak back out of the cell more easily than Na^+ ions enter.

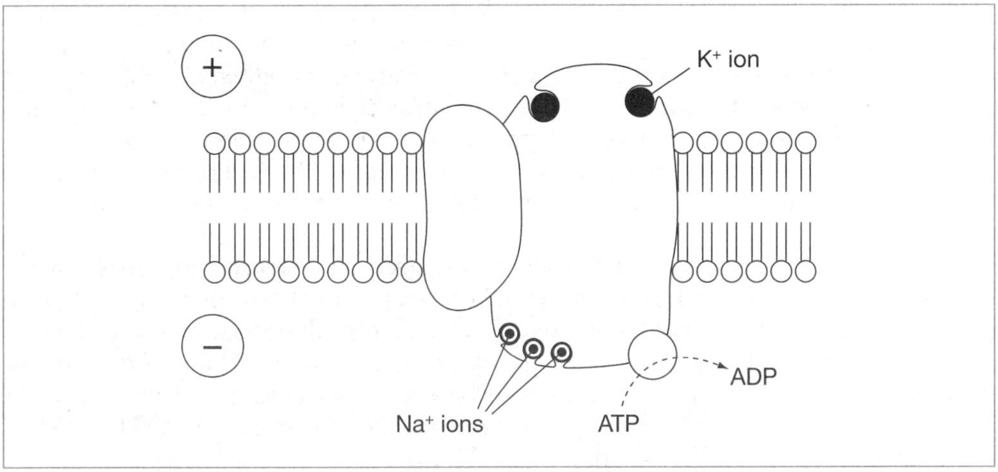

Figure 2.1a *The sodium–potassium pump*

Generating energy

Cells generate energy by combining oxygen with carbohydrate, fat, or protein under the influence of various enzymes. This is called **oxidation** and results in the production of a molecule called adenosine triphosphate (ATP) which is used to provide the energy for all cellular processes. The energy is stored in the ATP molecule by two high-energy phosphate bonds and is released when these bonds are broken.

Energy is used for:

- **Synthesis** – Synthesis of any chemical compound requires energy. All cells synthesise proteins, phospholipids, cholesterol, and the purine/pyrimidine building blocks of DNA. In addition, some cells have specialised secretory roles (eg hormone production)
- **Membrane transport** – Active transport of ions and other substances requires energy
- **Mechanical work** – Specialised cells (eg muscle cells) require energy for mechanical work. Other cells also require energy for amoeboid and ciliary movement

Energy from carbohydrate

The smallest component of the carbohydrate molecule is its monomer, glucose. Glucose enters the cell via facilitated diffusion using a glucose transporter molecule in the phospholipid membrane. This process is increased by the hormone insulin. Inside the cell, glucose is phosphorylated to form glucose-6 phosphate. Phosphorylated glucose is either stored as a polymer (via glycogenesis to form glycogen) or utilised immediately for energy. Energy is produced from glucose by glycolysis and then oxidation of the end products of glycolysis (via Krebs cycle).

In glycolysis the glucose molecule is broken down in a stepwise fashion releasing enough energy to produce one molecule of ATP at each step. This results in 2 molecules of pyruvic acid, 2 molecules of ATP and 4 hydrogen atoms. Pyruvic acid is combined with co-enzyme A in the mitochondria to form acetyl-co-enzyme A (acetyl-coA) and ATP. This combines with water in the Krebs cycle, releasing 2 molecules of ATP, 4 molecules of carbon dioxide, 16 hydrogen atoms and the co-enzyme A to be used again. The hydrogen ions combine with NAD^+ and undergo oxidative phosphorylation to produce the majority of the ATP.

Energy can also be released in the absence of oxygen by **anaerobic glycolysis**. When oxygen is not available then oxidative phosphorylation cannot take place. Glycolysis to produce pyruvic acid does not require oxygen and so this still occurs, producing a small amount of energy. In the absence of oxygen the pyruvic acid, NAD^+ and hydrogen ions combine to form lactic acid. When oxygen becomes available again the lactic acid breaks down releasing the pyruvic acid, NAD^+ and hydrogen ions and these can then be used for energy by oxidative phosphorylation.

Energy from lipids

The basic component of a lipid is the fatty acid. Lipids are transported from intestine to the liver in the blood as small aggregates, called chylomicrons, along the portal vein to the liver. The liver processes lipids to basic fatty acids. It also synthesises triglycerides from carbohydrates and produces cholesterol and phospholipids. Spare fat is stored in adipose tissue (modified fibroblasts that contain up to 95% of their volume as triglycerides).

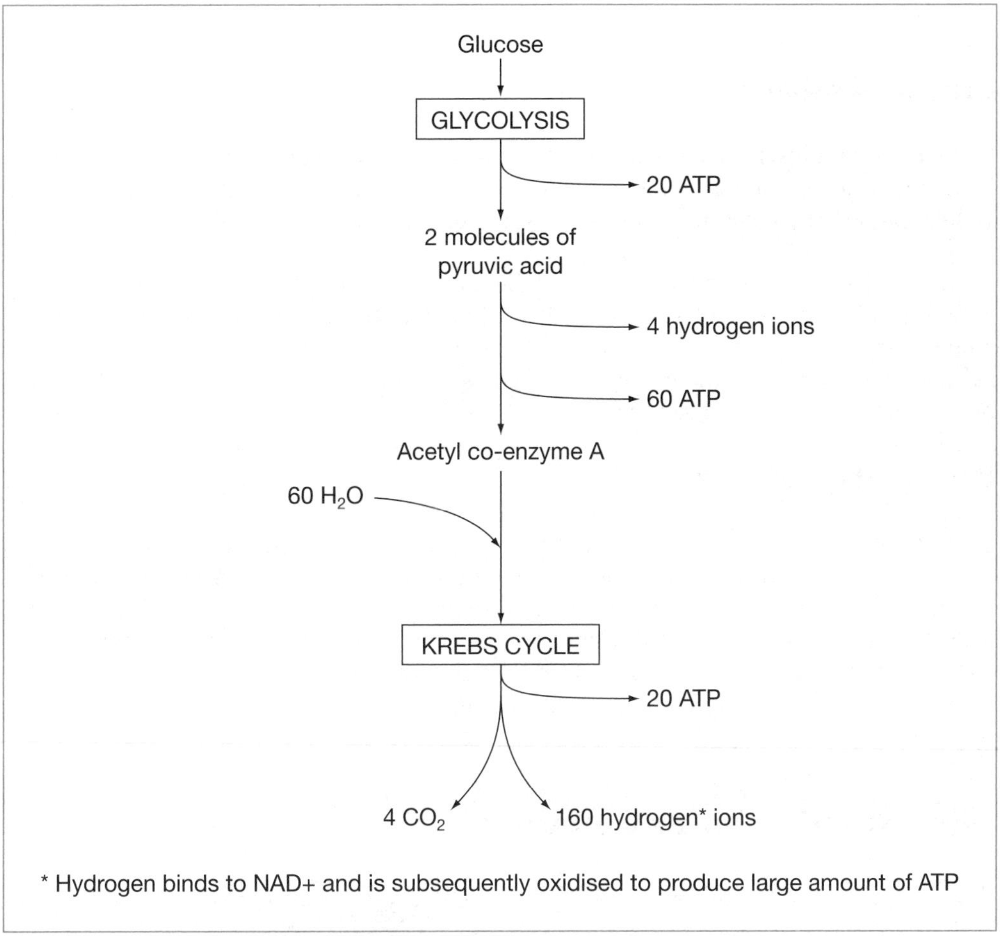

Figure 2.1b *Energy production from glucose*

Lipids can be used as fuel. Triglycerides are hydrolysed to free fatty acids and glycerol in the liver (which enters the carbohydrate pathway described above). Fatty acids are transported into the hepatocyte mitochondria where molecules of acetyl-coA are sequentially released from the fatty acid chains. Each time a molecule of acetyl-coA is released, 4 hydrogen atoms are also produced and these undergo oxidative phosphorylation, releasing large amounts of ATP. The acetyl-coA condenses to form acetoacetic acid and other ketones and this is released from the liver into the bloodstream to supply other tissues with energy. Cells take up the acetoacetic acid and turn it back into acetyl-coA which is transported to the mitochondria. The acetyl-coA then enters the Krebs cycle as described above. Usually levels of ketones in the blood are low. If the predominant source of energy is coming from fat then these levels rise. This may occur in starvation (when the body is metabolising its own fat stores), diabetes (when a lack of circulating insulin prevents glucose transport into the cells) or in very high fat diets.

Protein turnover

Protein synthesis

Proteins are absorbed from the GI tract and transported in the blood as their basic component, amino acids. Amino acids are taken up by the cells and almost immediately form cellular proteins by creation of peptide linkages directed by the ribosomes.

There are 20 different amino acids – 10 of the amino acids can be synthesised by the body ('non-essential' amino acids) and the other 10 have to be supplied in the diet ('essential' amino acids). The non-essential amino acids are synthesised from ketones. Glutamine acts as an intracellular store which can then be converted into other amino acids by the action of enzymes such as the transaminases.

Protein degradation

Only if cells have achieved maximal protein storage are amino acids 'deaminated' and used as energy or stored as fat. Ammonia is produced during deamination and converted into urea in the liver. This is then excreted from the bloodstream via the kidney. In severe liver disease this process is insufficient and may lead to the accumulation of ammonia in the blood (resulting in encephalopathy and eventually coma). During starvation, when the body has exhausted its stores of glycogen and fat, amino acids begin to be liberated and oxidised for energy.

Specialised cellular functions

In a nutshell ...

Some cells have specialised functions. They include:
- The action potential
- Synapses
- The neuromuscular junction
- Muscle contraction

The action potential

The transmission of signals along an excitable cell (ie nerve or muscle) is achieved by a self-propagating electrical current known as an action potential.

Generation of an action potential

All cells have an electrochemical gradient maintained by Na^+/K^+ ATPase. This results in a net internal negative charge and a net external positive charge. The difference between the two is called the **resting potential** of the cell membrane and is approximately –70 mV.

The action potential is initiated by a stimulus which alters the resting potential of the membrane. If the stimulus is big enough (usually about 15–35 mV and referred to as the **threshold level**) it increases the resting potential enough to start a chain of events resulting in a dramatic change in potential (called **depolarisation** or the **action potential**).

Changes in the resting potential of the membrane alter its permeability to sodium ions. This is thought to be because the resting potential determines whether certain ion channels (called voltage-gated sodium channels) are open or not. When the resting potential increases as a result of a stimulus, the gated sodium channels open and sodium ions flood into the cell down their electrochemical gradient. The membrane potential continues to increase as these positively charged ions enter the negatively charged cell. The gated sodium channels open wider as the membrane potential increases resulting in a positive feedback loop. At the peak of depolarisation (about 50 mV) the gated sodium channels start to close.

Depolarisation opens voltage-gated potassium channels and potassium moves out of the cell to try and restore the resting potential. This is called **repolarisation**. Depolarisation can not occur again until the resting potential has been restored and this is called the **refractory period**.

Differences in the action potential between nerve and muscle

In cardiac and smooth muscle cells there are also calcium channels. In the resting state calcium is pumped out of the cell and so there is a higher concentration in the extracellular fluid than inside the cell. Increases in the membrane potential open voltage-gated calcium channels. These increase depolarisation but work more slowly than the sodium channels. The action potential in these cells therefore has a plateau which delays the recovery of the resting potential. This allows for prolonged and complete contraction of the muscle cell compared to the action potential in neurons which re-sets itself quickly to transmit the repetitive impulses of coded messages. Skeletal muscle has an action potential similar to nerve. Repetitive firing can result in tetany with multiple sustained contraction and no effective relaxation.

Rhythmical spontaneous depolarisation occurs in some tissues, such as the sinoatrial node of the heart and the smooth muscle cells of the GI tract that are responsible for peristalsis. No stimulus is necessary to cause depolarisation in these cells. This is because the cell membrane is relatively leaky to sodium ions. As sodium ions leak into the cell, the resting potential rises and depolarisation occurs spontaneously. The influx of sodium is seen in the slow up-sweep of the action potential in these cells.

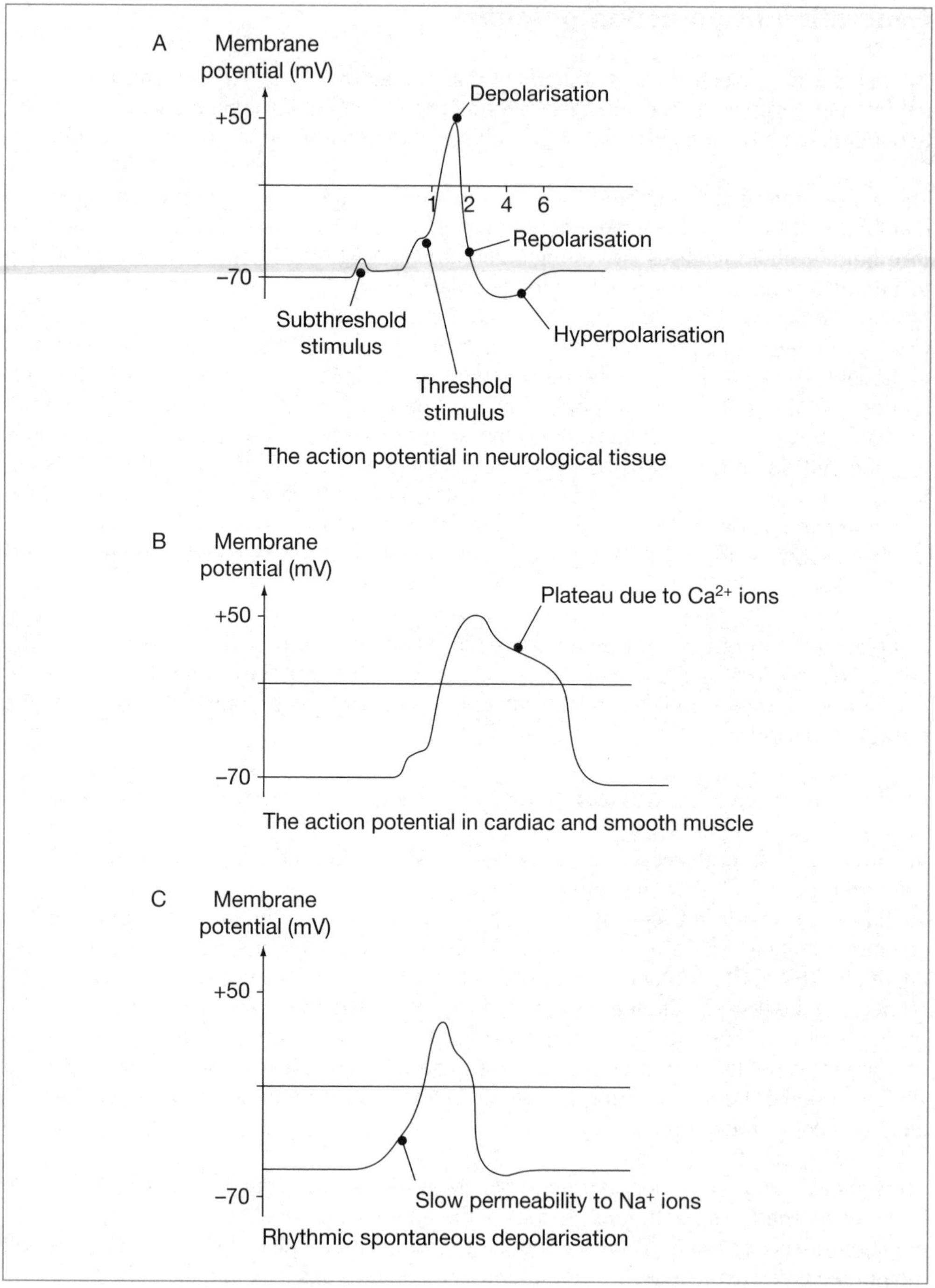

Figure 2.1c *The action potential*

Transmission of the action potential

The action potential can be propagated along the membrane by setting up small local circuits. The stimulus depolarises a small area of the membrane which reverses its polarity. As sodium ions flow into the cell through the depolarised part of the membrane they diffuse locally in either direction. This alters the resting potential of the neighbouring parts of the membrane and acts as a stimulus for depolarisation.

The action potential travels in an 'all or nothing' manner, whereby if a stimulus is sufficient to cause depolarisation then the impulse generated has a fixed amplitude regardless of the strength of the stimulus. The strength of the stimulus is reflected in the frequency of the impulse.

Conduction of the action potential

Depolarisation travels smoothly along the membrane in unmyelinated nerve fibres. Myelinated fibres have Schwann cell wrapped around them (like Swiss rolls). These cells insulate the membrane and force the depolarisation to jump rapidly from bare area to bare area. These bare areas are called the **nodes of Ranvier** and this form of conduction is much faster than straightforward transmission; it is called **saltatory conduction**.

Synapses

The **synapse** is the connection between one neuron and the next. The end terminal of the axon is called the **synaptic bulb** and this is separated from the **post-synaptic membrane** by the **synaptic cleft**. In the end terminal of the axon are many mitochondria and Golgi apparatus, which are responsible for the synthesis of a chemical **neurotransmitter**. The neurotransmitter is stored in secretory vesicles in the synaptic bulb.

When an action potential reaches a synapse it stimulates the opening of calcium ion channels. The influx of calcium draws the secretory vesicles to the pre-synaptic membrane and causes them to exocytose their contents. The neurotransmitter diffuses across the synaptic cleft and stimulates receptors on the post-synaptic membrane. These receptors alter the permeability of the post-synaptic membrane to sodium ions and this change in the resting potential acts as a stimulus to depolarise the membrane of the target neuron.

Often a single action potential is insufficient to accomplish depolarisation of the neuron, and many action potentials arriving in rapid succession are required. This is called **temporal summation**. Alternatively, near-simultaneous firing of many synapses onto a single target cell may also be sufficient to result in depolarisation of the target neuron. This is called **spatial summation**.

A single neuron may have as many as 100 000 synaptic inputs. These may be excitatory or inhibitory. The balance between excitatory input (the excitatory post-synaptic potential or EPSP) and inhibitory input (the inhibitory post-synaptic potential or IPSP) from other neurons will determine whether the neuron will fire. This integrates information allowing negative feedback and modifications to be made to the original impulses.

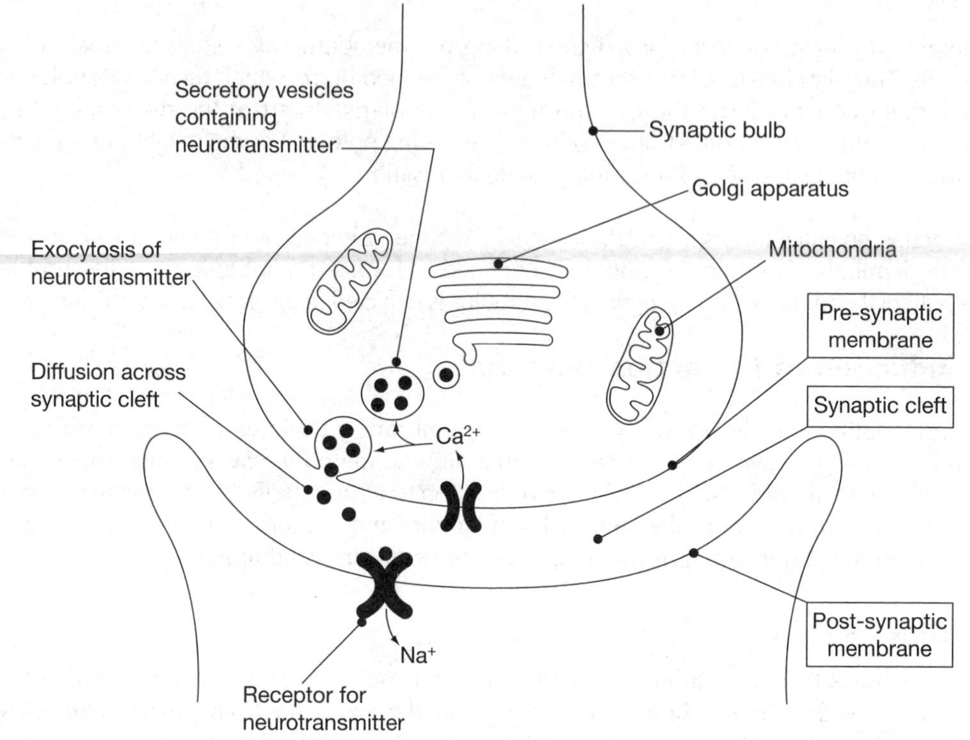

Figure 2.1d *The synapse*

Excitatory neurotransmitters include:
- Acetylcholine
- Noradrenaline (norepinephrine)
- Glutamate

Inhibitory neurotransmitters include:
- Dopamine
- Gamma-aminobutyric acid (GABA)
- Glycine
- Serotonin (5-HT)

The neuromuscular junction (NMJ)

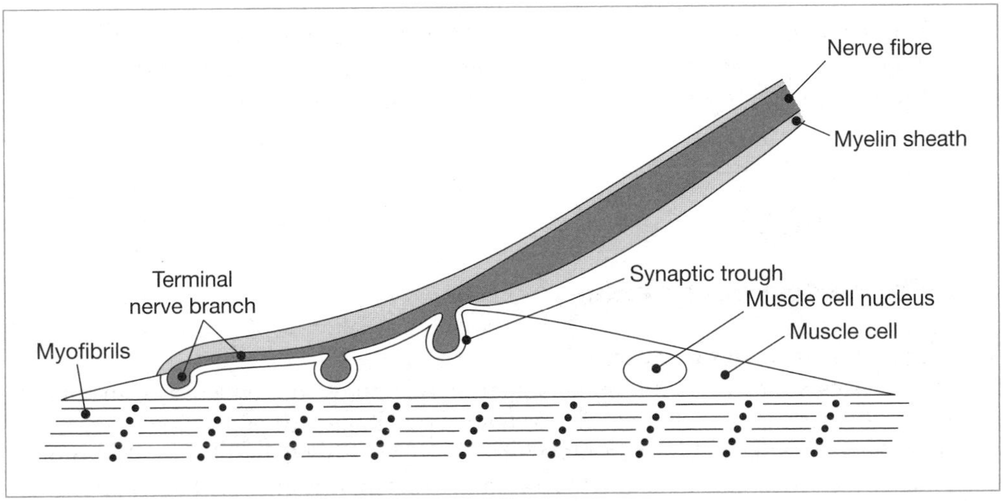

Figure 2.1e *The neuromuscular junction*

The nerve fibre forms a junction with the muscle fibre at its mid-point. Action potentials transmitted to the muscle therefore travel in both directions to the either end of the muscle fibre. This is called the motor end-plate and it is insulated with Schwann cells. When the action potential reaches the terminal of the nerve it triggers the release of hundreds of secretory vesicles of acetylcholine into the synaptic trough. The muscle membrane of the synaptic trough has multiple acetylcholine receptors which act as gated ion channels. On binding acetylcholine these channels open allowing sodium ions to flood into the cell, depolarising the membrane and generating an action potential. The acetylcholine in the synaptic trough is rapidly inactivated by the acetylcholinesterase enzyme in the synaptic trough.

Disease and drugs acting on the NMJ

Myasthenia gravis: this is an autoimmune condition that involves development of antibodies against the acetylcholine receptor. The end-plate potentials are therefore too weak to adequately stimulate the muscle fibres. The hallmark of myasthenia gravis is muscle weakness that increases during periods of activity and improves after periods of rest. Certain muscles, such as those that control eye and eyelid movement, facial expression, chewing, talking, and swallowing, are often involved. The muscles that control breathing and neck and limb movements may also be affected

Acetylcholine mimetic drugs: act in the same manner as acetylcholine but are not sensitive to acetylcholinesterase and so have a longer duration of action. They include methacholine and nicotine

NMJ blockers: act competitively with acetylcholine for the receptor and are known as the curariform drugs
NMJ activators: inactivate acetylcholinesterase (eg neostigmine, physostigmine) and result in persistence of the acetylcholine in the synaptic trough, with resulting persistence of muscle contraction

Muscle contraction

Skeletal muscle contraction

The structure of skeletal muscle

Skeletal muscles are composed of longitudinal muscle fibres surrounded by a membrane called the sarcolemma. Each muscle fibre is made up of thousands of myofibrils. Myofibrils are composed of actin and myosin filaments. These are essentially polymerised protein molecules which lie in a parallel orientation in the sarcoplasm. They partially interdigitate and so under the microscope the myofibrils appear to have alternating dark and light bands. Between the myofibrils lie large numbers of mitochondria. Wrapped around the myofibrils is a large quantity of modified endoplasmic reticulum called the sarcoplasmic reticulum.

The ends of the actin filaments are attached to a Z disc. The Z disc passes through neighbouring myofibrils attaching them together into a muscle fibre. This gives the fibres a striped or 'striated' appearance. The area between the Z discs is called the sarcomere. In the relaxed state the actin molecules overlap very slightly at the ends. In the myofibril, the I band represents areas where the actin molecule does not overlap the myosin, and the A band represents areas where both actin and myosin overlap. So (as shown in Fig. 2.1f) when the muscle contracts the A band stays the same length but the I bands become much smaller.

The mechanism of contraction of skeletal muscle

The action potential is transmitted through the muscle fibre by invaginations of the membrane deep into the centre of the fibre (called transverse or T-tubules). Depolarisation of the T-tubule membrane stimulates the release of calcium ions from the sarcoplasmic reticulum in the muscle fibre. These calcium ions cause the actin and myosin molecules to slide along one another resulting in contraction of the myofibrils. This process is called **excitation–contraction coupling**.

This sliding mechanism works by interaction between the myosin heads and the active site on the actin molecule. The actin fibres are made up of actin, tropomyosin, and troponin molecules. The tropomyosin and troponin form a complex that covers and inhibits the actin active site until it binds with four calcium ions. This induces a conformational change in the molecule which uncovers the actin active site. The myosin molecule has cross bridges on which there are ATPase heads. These heads bind to the actin active site and ATP is used to enable the myosin molecule to 'walk along' the actin molecules. The calcium ions are then pumped back into the sarcoplasmic reticulum.

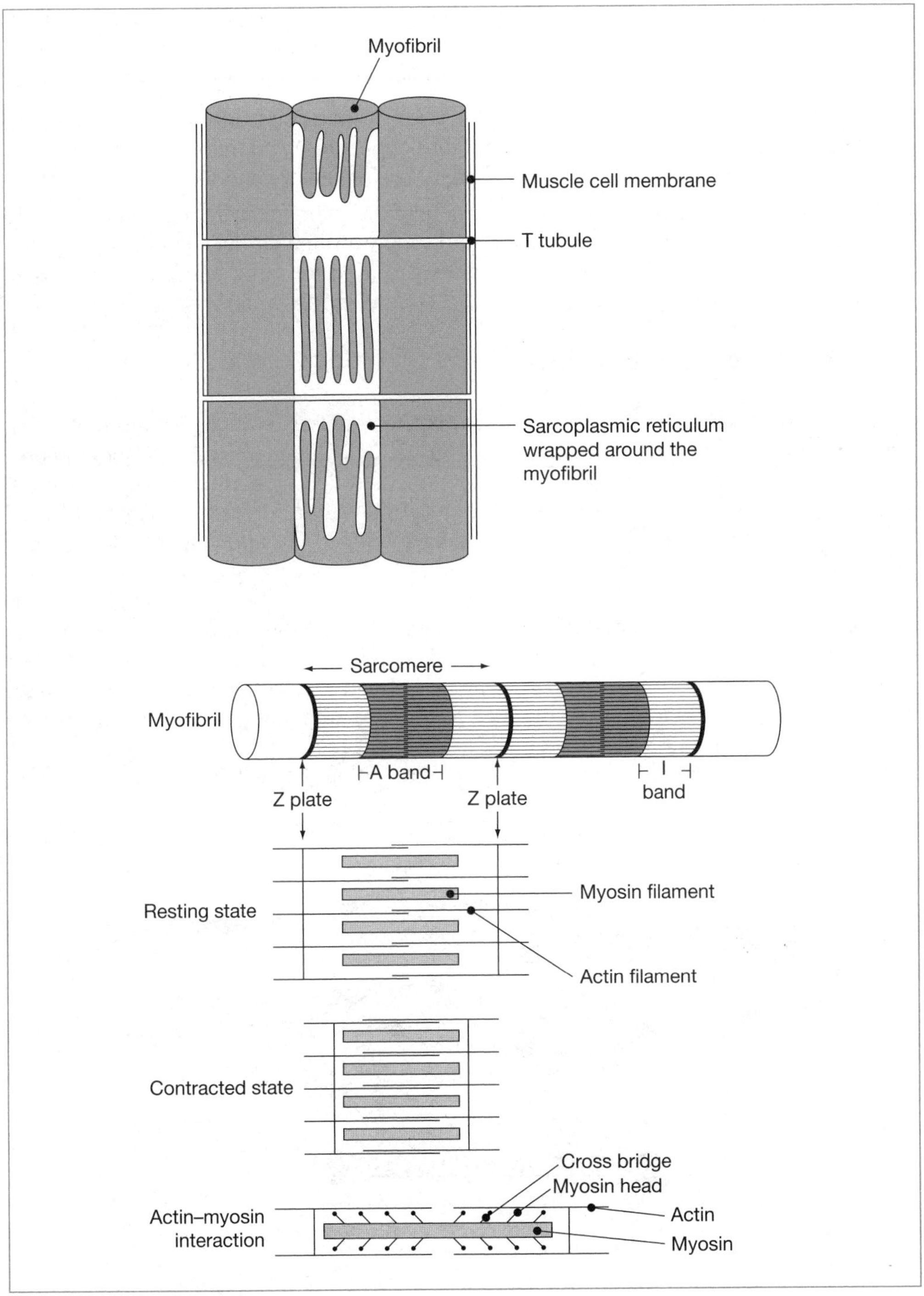

Figure 2.1f *The structure of the myofibril*

Muscles are composed of 'fast-twitch' and 'slow-twitch' fibres and there are other fibres which lie between these two extremes. Depending on their function, an entire muscle is made up of a variable mixture of these two types of fibre.

- **Slow-twitch fibres (type I)** are smaller with an extensive blood supply, contain myoglobin to act as an oxygen store (and thus appear red) and mitochondria for oxidative phosphorylation. These fibres are used for prolonged or continuous muscle activity
- **Fast-twitch fibres (type II)** are larger, have extensive sarcoplasmic reticulum for rapid release of calcium ions, and minimal blood supply as they produce energy by glycolysis and not oxidative phosphorylation. They are used for rapid and powerful muscle contraction. They have no myoglobin and therefore appear white

Smooth muscle contraction

Smooth muscle cells contain muscle fibres that may act as a single or multiple units. Smooth muscle composed of multiple units is usually richly innervated and under neurological control, compared to single units that are controlled by non-neurological stimuli. Single unit smooth muscle is found in the gut, biliary tree, ureters, uterus and blood vessels. These smooth muscle cells are joined by gap junctions, allowing free flow of ions from one cell to the next (known as a syncytium).

Smooth muscle contains bundles of actin filaments attached at either end to a dense body (which serve the same role as the Z disc) and are arranged surrounding a myosin filament. The dense bodies of neighbouring cells may be bonded together to form protein bridges that transmit contractile force from one cell to the next. The actin and myosin in smooth muscle interact as described for skeletal muscle, but there is no troponin molecule – instead they contain a molecule called calmodulin. On binding calcium ions, calmodulin

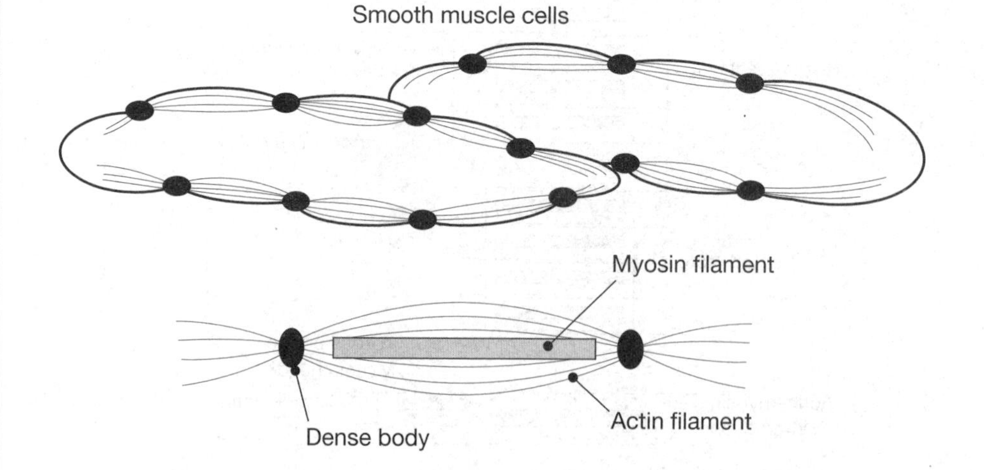

Figure 2.1g *The smooth muscle cell*

activates myosin kinase, which phosphorylates and activates the myosin cross-bridges. Contraction occurs in a far more prolonged fashion and is halted only when the myosin head is de-phosphorylated by another enzyme called myosin phosphatase.

Smooth muscle contraction may be induced by nervous impulses as discussed previously. Additionally, smooth muscle may be induced to contract or relax by local tissue factors and hormones. For example, local hypoxia, carbon dioxide and increased hydrogen ion concentration all cause smooth muscle relaxation in the blood vessels, which results in vasodilation. Hormones cause smooth muscle contraction when the smooth muscle contains hormone-specific receptors; these often act as ion gates which open when stimulated by the relevant hormone.

Cardiac muscle contraction

Cardiac muscle is striated and contains actin and myosin filaments which contract in the same manner as described for skeletal muscle.

2.2 METABOLISM AND THE CATABOLIC STATE

The metabolic response to surgery

In a nutshell ...

Trauma can be defined as any stress on the body (including surgery itself). This provokes a metabolic and physiological response. This response occurs:

- Locally (inflammation and wound repair)
- Generally with systemic involvement (ebb and flow pattern)

It involves an initial **catabolic** phase followed by a rebuilding **anabolic** phase.

Stress provokes a metabolic response. Stress may include:

- Injury
- Surgery
- Sepsis
- Dehydration
- Starvation
- Hypothermia
- Anaesthesia
- Severe psychological stress

The nature, severity, and duration of the metabolic response are variable and depend on:

- Nature and degree of trauma
- Presence of sepsis
- Co-existing systemic disease
- Drugs
- Age (reduced in children and the elderly)
- Gender (reduced in young women)
- Nutritional state (malnutrition reduces metabolic response)

The response to injury can be considered to occur as both local and general phenomena:

- Local response: management of wounds (inflammation and subsequent wound healing)
- General response: acts to conserve fluid and provide energy for repair processes

It is described as an ebb and flow pattern by Cuthbertson (1932).

The ebb and flow phases of the metabolic response to trauma

The ebb phase

- Occurs in the first few hours (< 24 hours)
- Acts as a protective mechanism, conserving circulating volume and minimising demands on the body
- Effects include:
  - ↓ oxygen consumption
  - ↓ enzymatic activity
  - ↓ cardiac output
  - ↓ basal metabolic rate
  - ↓ body temperature
  - ↑ production of acute-phase proteins
- Modulated by catecholamines, cortisol and aldosterone

The flow phase

- Occurs later (> 24 hours)
- Describes a hypermetabolic state
- Effects include:
  - ↑ oxygen consumption
  - ↑ glucose production
  - ↑ cardiac output
  - ↑ basal metabolic rate
  - ↑ body temperature
  - ↓ weight loss

- Initially this phase is **catabolic** (3–10 days), which allows mobilisation of the building blocks of repair; it is controlled by glucagons, insulin, cortisol, and catecholamines
- Subsequently the process becomes **anabolic** (10–60 days) with repair of tissue, repletion of stores of fat and protein and weight gain; it is controlled by growth hormones, androgens and ketosteroids (growth hormone and insulin-like growth factor are dependant on calorie intake)

The catabolic state

In a nutshell ...

Catabolism is a destructive mechanism in which large organic molecules are broken down into their constituent parts providing building blocks for synthesis and releasing ATP.

Anabolism is a constructive mechanism in which small precursor molecules are assembled into larger organic molecules with utilisation of an energy source, ATP.

- **Glucose:** glucose is released from the liver by glycolysis and seriously ill patients may develop a state of glucose intolerance. Serum glucose is high and the turnover rapid. The liver produces glucose from the catabolism of proteins and fats to maintain the high serum levels
- **Fat:** this is initially released from adipose tissue under control of interleukins and TNF. Lipases release glycerol and fatty acids from triglycerides. Glycerol is used for gluconeogenesis and fatty acids are oxidised for energy
- **Protein:** skeletal muscle breakdown occurs at an increased rate due to a proteolysis-inducing factor (PIF) secreted after trauma. Muscle loss results in a supply of alanine and glutamine. Amino acids are used for gluconeogenesis and synthesis of acute-phase proteins. This results in a negative nitrogen balance as up to 20 g/day of nitrogen is excreted in the urine and it peaks after several days

Severe loss of muscle mass causes a reduction and eventually failure in immunocompetence predisposing to overwhelming infection. Gut mucosal integrity also relies on a supply of amino acids and a reduction in this supply (especially of glutamine) predisposes to bacterial translocation.

Glucose is incredibly important in the response to trauma and the metabolic response is geared to providing as much as possible. Nutritional support for patients in shock is therefore composed of 65–70% glucose with the rest of the calories supplied by means of emulsified fat.

Management of the metabolic response

- Minimise the initial insult if possible (eg minimal access surgery)
- Give aggressive fluid and electrolyte management to prevent a decrease in tissue perfusion and fluid shifts
- Provide sufficient oxygen (by respiratory support and ventilation if necessary)
- Control glucose levels
- Control pain (pain and anxiety cause hormonal release and potentiate an increase in the metabolic response)
- Manage body temperature (warming/cooling, medication)
- Prevent and control associated sepsis
- Optimise nutrition to provide energy for repair
- Support failing organ systems (renal replacement therapy, respiratory support, cardiac support)

Production and utilisation of energy in the body

In a nutshell ...

Metabolism = anabolism + catabolism

Energy produced from catabolism of food is utilised in:

- Energy for necessary synthesis and anabolism
- Energy for heat
- Energy storage
- Energy for external work

Energy is measured in joules or calories. These are essentially measures of heat (1 K calorie is the amount of heat needed to produce a rise of 1 °C in 1 kg of water.

Energy supplied by different foodstuffs:

- 1 g carbohydrate = 4.1 Kcal
- 1 g protein = 5.3 Kcal
- 1 g fat = 9.3 Kcal

Energy production by the body can be measured by direct or indirect calorimetry.

- **Direct calorimetry** relies on measurement of the heat released by the body; this is difficult to do and so remains experimental (eg Atwater–Benedict chamber)

- **Indirect calorimetry** measures bodily processes associated with the consumption and production of energy (eg oxygen consumption and CO_2 production with Benedict apparatus)

The respiratory quotient (RQ) is the ratio of O_2 consumption to volume of CO_2 produced per unit of time. It reflects the fuel used to produce the energy (a diet of pure carbohydrate produces an RQ of 1.0, of pure protein 0.8, and of pure fat 0.7.

Metabolic rate

> ***In a nutshell ...***
>
> The basal metabolic rate (BMR) is the minimal calorific requirement to sustain life.
> It can be measured in $Kcal/m^2/hour$.
> It is affected by a number of different factors (eg age, sex, and temperature, and catabolic states like burns).

Measurement of BMR

BMR is measured in $kcal/m^2/hour$ (about 35–40 $Kcal/m^2/hour$ per adult male). Calorific requirement can also be estimated by the equation:

$$BMR = \text{body mass (kg)} \times 20 \text{ kcal}$$

Thus, for example, a 70 kg man will have a baseline daily requirement of 1400 kcal if he sleeps all day.

20 Kcal are required to maintain 1 kg of body mass. This does not take energy required for external work into account and so additional calories are required for movement.

BMR increases in injury states when the body is catabolic (eg burns where the BMR doubles to about 45 kcal per kg of body mass).

Factors affecting BMR

- Age (higher in the young due to higher lean body mass)
- Height (taller people have higher BMRs)
- Surface area
- Sex (lower by 10% in women)
- Race (higher in Caucasians than in Asians)

- Growth states (higher in children and pregnancy/lactation)
- Body composition (higher BMR with more lean tissue)
- Pyrexia (↑ BMR)
- Environmental temperature (both heat and cold ↑ BMR)
- Malnutrition and starvation (↓ BMR)
- Food (protein ↑ BMR)
- Hormones (catecholamines and thyroxine ↑ BMR)
- Stress and mental status (stress ↑ BMR; depression ↓ BMR)
- Physical exercise (can ↑ BMR 10–20-fold)
- Sleep (↓ BMR)

2.3 FLUID BALANCE

In a nutshell ...

Body fluids are predominantly composed of:

- Water
- Ions
- Proteins

The movement of fluids within the body and across capillary membranes depends on the relative concentration of these three components in each compartment.

Different concentrations of these components exert forces across cell membranes. The net movement of fluid depends on the balance of these forces. These forces include:

- Osmotic pressure
- Hydrostatic pressure

Body fluid composition

Water distribution within the body

Water makes up about 60% of a man and 50% of a woman (due to higher body fat) and 75% of a child. The majority of water in the body is from oral intake. In addition, a small volume (150–250 mL/day) is produced as the result of oxidation of hydrogen during the oxidative phosphorylation phase of metabolism.

- Total body water (TBW) is the total volume of water in the body
- Extracellular fluid (ECF) is the fluid outside the cells

- Intracellular fluid (ICF) is the fluid inside the cells (given by TBW – ECF)
- Plasma is blood without cells, containing proteins, water and electrolytes

Transcellular fluid is defined as being separated by a layer of epithelium; it includes CSF, intra-ocular, pleural, synovial, and digestive secretions and gut luminal fluid. Volume is relatively small. If the transcellular compartment is very large, it may be called the 'third space' because fluid in this compartment is not readily exchangeable with the rest of the ECF.

- Intravascular volume is the fluid within the vascular compartment
- Interstitial fluid is the fluid within tissues (given by ECF – intravascular volume)

Distribution of water in a 70 kg man

Total body water is 45 litres (57%).

One-third is extracellular fluid (15 litres)

Plasma (3.5 litres)
Interstitial/tissue fluid (8.5 litres)
Lymph (1.5 litres)
Transcellular fluid (1.5 litres)

Two-thirds is intracellular fluid (30 litres) found in the cell cytoplasm

Distribution of ions in the body

ION COMPOSITION OF BODY FLUIDS

Ions	Extracellular fluid (mmol/L)	Intracellular fluid (mmol/L)
Cations		
Na+	135–145	4–10
K^+	3.5–5.0	150
Ca^{2+} ionised	1.0–1.25	0.001
Ca^{2+} total	2.12–2.65	–
Mg^{2+}	1.0	40
Anions		
Bicarbonate	25	10
Chloride	95–105	15
Phosphate	1.1	100
Organic anions	3.0	0
Protein	1.1	8

In intracellular fluid (ICF)

- K^+ and Mg^{2+} are the main **cations**
- Phosphate, proteins and organic ions are the main **anions**

In extracellular fluid (ECF)

- Na^+ is the main **cation**
- Chloride (Cl^-) and bicarbonate (HCO_3^-)are the major **anions**

Regulation of potassium (K^+)

Potassium is the main intracellular cation and its levels inside the cell are maintained by the Na^+/K^+ ATPase pump that was discussed earlier in this chapter. Plasma levels of potassium are tightly regulated as hypokalaemia and hyperkalaemia may manifest in abnormalities of cardiac function.

Control of potassium levels in the plasma

Potassium levels in the plasma are controlled by:

- Dietary Intake
- Renal excretion
- Plasma pH
- Hormones (insulin, adrenaline/epinephrine and aldosterone)

- **Dietary intake:** foods that are high in potassium include bananas, chocolate, avocado, baked beans, lentils, tomatoes and milk
- **Renal excretion:** filtration of potassium in the renal tubule depends on the plasma concentration. However, the resorption of sodium in the collecting ducts is dependant on exchange for potassium. This is controlled by aldosterone which is produced in response to low plasma sodium and low blood pressure. Aldosterone may also be produced in response to high plasma potassium levels
- **Plasma pH:** hydrogen ions move in and out of cells in exchange for potassium ions. When hydrogen levels in the plasma rise, hydrogen enters the cell in exchange for potassium, thus raising the plasma potassium levels. When hydrogen levels in the plasma fall, hydrogen leaves the cell in exchange for potassium thus lowering the plasma potassium levels. Additionally, in an attempt to retain hydrogen ions in alkalotic states the kidney preferentially secretes potassium
- **Hormones:** insulin, adrenaline (epinephrine) and aldosterone stimulate cellular uptake of potassium. Hyperaldosteronism (in renal artery stenosis, cirrhosis, nephrotic syndrome and severe heart failure) is associated with hypokalaemia

Drugs that affect potassium levels in the body

Drugs that increase potassium levels
- Angiotensin-converting enzyme (ACE) inhibitors
- Angiotensin II receptor antagonists
- Cyclosporin
- Potassium salts

Drugs that decrease potassium levels
- Loop and thiazide diuretics
- Corticosteroids
- Beta-2 agonists
- Amphotericin
- Theophylline

Regulation of sodium (Na^+)

Sodium is the most common extracellular cation and it is important in regulating the amount and distribution of water in the body. Excess sodium results in water retention and too little sodium may result in neuromuscular dysfunction. Total body sodium levels depend on amounts ingested and the amount of renal excretion. The concentration of sodium in the body depends on the amount of total body water. Non-renal excretion (eg sweat, faeces) is commonly small but may be significant if there is prolonged diarrhoea or large surface area burns.

- **Sodium intake:** high sodium levels stimulate the hypothalamus and generate thirst. The addition of salt to food and consumption of high sodium foodstuffs depends on dietary habits
- **Sodium excretion:** sodium is filtered freely through the glomerular membrane of the kidney and so the sodium concentration in the filtrate depends on the plasma sodium. 65% of the sodium filtered is passively reabsorbed in the proximal convoluted tubule and the remainder is actively reabsorbed by the Na^+/K^+ pump in the ascending limb of the loop of Henle. Atrial natrurietic factor (ANF) is produced in response to fluid overload and promotes sodium excretion by decreasing resorption. Antidiuretic hormone (ADH) is produced in response to increased plasma osmolality and acts to increase water resorption and restore sodium concentration

Plasma proteins

Because the capillary barrier is readily permeable to ions but impermeable to proteins, plasma proteins principally determine the osmotic pressure within the capillary. Albumin accounts for 75% of this osmotic pressure within the capillary lumen.

Fluid movement across the capillary membrane

The capillary

The capillary is the site of fluid and solute exchange between the interstitium of the tissues and the bloodstream. Arterioles become meta-arterioles and then capillary beds. The flow through each capillary is regulated by a pre-capillary sphincter which controls flow through the capillary bed. A capillary is a single layer of endothelial cells surrounded by a basement membrane. There are potential spaces between adjacent cells and their size regulates permeability to solutes.

Osmotic pressure

Osmosis is a form of diffusion of water molecules across a semipermeable membrane when there is a different concentration (**osmolality**) of solutes on either side. This is because the number or concentration of particles in solution on either side of the membrane generates **osmotic pressure**. Water is drawn by osmotic pressure, moving from regions of low osmotic pressure to regions of higher osmotic pressure. Osmotic pressure can be generated by ions (eg Na^+ or Cl^-) or by proteins.

- **Capillary osmotic pressure** refers to the pressure generated by the plasma proteins inside the capillary. It is sometimes called colloid osmotic pressure, or even oncotic pressure
- **Tissue osmotic pressure** refers to the pressure generated by the interstitial fluid. The oncotic pressure of the interstitial fluid depends on the interstitial protein concentration and the permeability of the capillary wall to proteins. The more permeable the capillary barrier is to proteins, the higher the tissue osmotic pressure

Hydrostatic pressure

Hydrostatic pressure is the difference between the capillary pressure (ie perfusion pressure generated by the blood pressure) and the pressure of interstitial fluid within the tissues.

- **Capillary hydrostatic pressure** is determined by the blood pressure and the differential between arterial and venous pressures
- **Tissue hydrostatic pressure** is determined by the interstitial fluid volume and by the compliance of the tissue, which is related to the ability of the tissue volume to increase and accommodate more fluid

Movement of fluid across capillary membranes: The Starling hypothesis

The distribution of ECF between plasma and the interstitial space is regulated at the membrane of the capillaries and lymphatics.

The movement of fluid at the capillary membrane is shown in Fig. 2.3a. In normal tissue there are few proteins in the interstitial fluid and the capillary is impermeable to plasma proteins and so the osmotic pressure across the membrane is considered to be constant (about 25 mmHg).

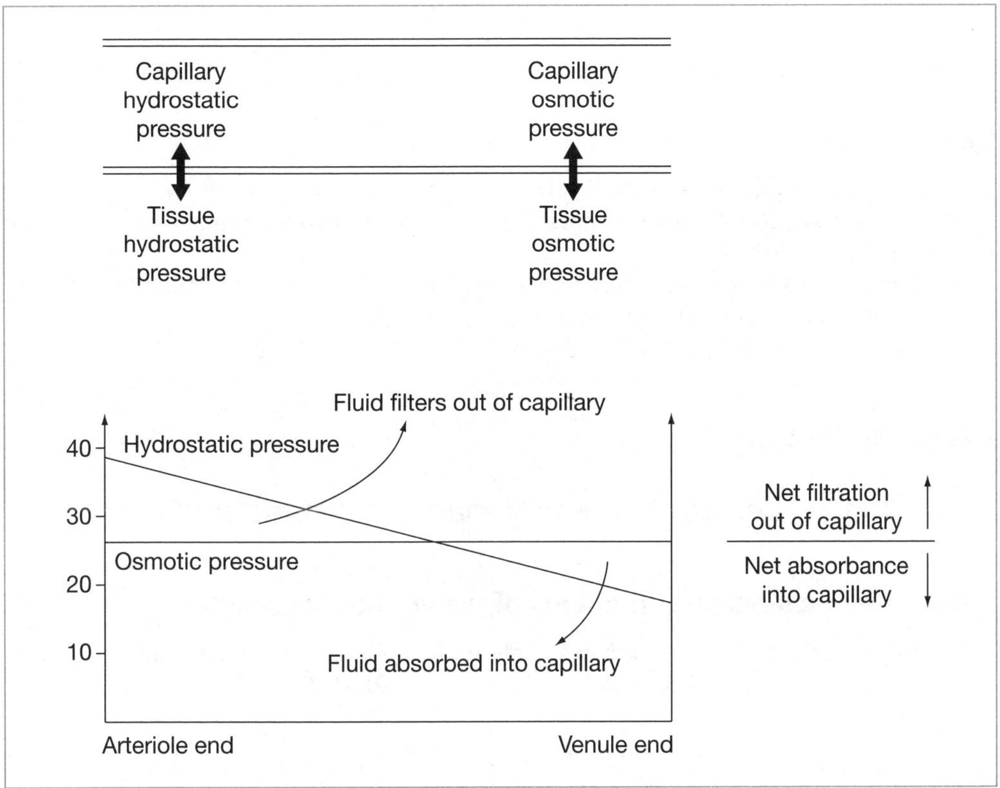

Figure 2.3a *The movement of fluids across the capillary membrance*

Additionally the tissue hydrostatic pressure is relatively constant. The capillary hydrostatic pressure is high at the arterial end of the capillary, favouring net filtration of fluid into the interstitium. As fluid moves along the capillary towards the venous end, the hydrostatic pressure falls.

There tends to be a net flow of water out of the capillary into the interstitium at the arteriolar end of the capillary, and a net flow back into the capillary at the venular end of the capillary.

Starling equation

Movement of fluid = K = filtration constant for the capillary membrane

K = outward pressure – inward pressure

Where:
Outward pressure = capillary hydrostatic pressure + tissue osmotic pressure
Inward pressure = tissue hydrostatic pressure + capillary osmotic pressure

Oedema

This describes the clinical observation of excess tissue fluid (ie interstitial fluid).

Causes of oedema

- Increased capillary hydrostatic pressure (eg venous obstruction, fluid overload)
- Decreased capillary oncotic pressure (eg causes of hypoproteinaemia – nephrotic syndrome, cirrhosis)
- Increased tissue oncotic pressure (eg resulting from increased capillary permeability due to burns or inflammation)
- Decreased tissue hydrostatic pressure

Fluid management

Daily fluid and electrolyte maintenance requirements

Daily maintenance requirements of water and electrolytes

Electrolyte/water	Per kg body weight (mmol)	Total average male adult (mmol)
Na^+	1–1.5	70–100
K^+	1.0	70
Cl^-	1.0	70
PO_4^{3-}	0.2	14
Ca^{2+}	0.1	7.0
Mg^{2+}	0.1	7.0
Water	35 mL	2500 mL

AVERAGE DAILY WATER BALANCE FOR SEDENTARY ADULT IN TEMPERATE CONDITIONS

Intake (mL)		**Output (mL)**	
Drink	1500	Urine	1500
Food	750	Faeces	100
Metabolic	350	Lungs	400
		Skin	600
Total	2600	Total	2600

Fever increases maintenance fluid requirement by 20% of the daily insensible loss for each 1 °C rise. Most clinicians give an extra 1 litre per 24 hours for each 1 °C rise.

In general, fluid maintenance needs can be gauged by maintaining an adequate urine output (> 0.5 mL/kg/hour). The patient's daily weight is also essential for adequate assessment.

(NB: Mechanical ventilation also increases insensible fluid loss).

DAILY GI SECRETIONS AND ELECTROLYTE COMPOSITION

	Volume (mL/24 hour) (range in brackets)	Na^+ (mmol/L)	K^+ (mmol/L)	Cl^- (mmol/L)	HCO_3^- (mmol/L)
Saliva	1500 (1000–15 000)	10	26	10	30
Stomach	1500 (1000–2500)	60	10	130	-
Duodenum	Variable (100–2000)	140	5	80	-
Ileum	3000 (100–9000)	140	5	104	-
Colon	Minimal	60	30	40	-
Pancreas	500 (100–800)	140	5	75	115
Bile	800 (50–800)	145	5	100	35

Summary of fluid balance considerations

Patient size and age
Abnormal ongoing losses, pre-existing deficits or excesses, fluid shifts
Renal and cardiovascular function
Look at fluid balance charts over preceding 24 hours
Check serum electrolytes

Fluid loss and surgical trauma

Fluid loss and surgical trauma

Surgical trauma
↓
ADH release and aldosterone from adrenal glands
↓
Water conservation, Na^+ retention, K^+ excretion

Therefore peri-operative fluid balance must be carefully monitored in relation to electrolytes and volume.

Sources of excess fluid loss in surgical patients

- Blood loss (eg trauma, surgery)
- Plasma loss (eg burns)
- GI fluid loss (eg vomiting, diarrhoea, ileostomy, bowel obstruction)
- Intra-abdominal inflammatory fluid loss (eg pancreatitis)
- Sepsis
- Abnormal insensible loss (eg fever, mechanical ventilation with no humidification)

It is essential for an accurate fluid chart to be kept. This records all fluid intake (oral and IV) and all output (urine, drain fluid, GI contents, etc), and provides a balance for each 24 hours, once insensible loss has been estimated.

Assessing fluid depletion

Patient evaluation

History

Thirst, obvious fluid loss
Fluid intake, fluid output
If patient on ward or ITU check charts for fluid balance

Examination

Dry mucous membranes
Sunken eyes
Low skin elasticity
Low urine output
Increase in heart rate
Low pulse pressure, low BP
Confusion
Low capillary refilling

Investigations in dehydration

Simple indicators of dehydration are a rising haematocrit and albumin, and a raised urea, particularly in the presence of low-volume concentrated urine.

Central venous pressure (CVP)

- Normal range 3–8 cmH_2O
- Single values are not as useful as looking at the trend
- CVP measurement is best used as a guide to adequacy of treatment (ie it can be used to monitor response to a fluid challenge)

Consider a fluid challenge of 200 mL of colloid.

- In a dehydrated patient the CVP will rise in response to the challenge and then fall to the original value
- In a well-filled patient there will be a substantial rise (2–4 cmH_2O for 5 minutes) in the CVP
- If there is no over-filling, the CVP will rise by > 4 cmH_2O and will not fall again

NB: CVP may be artificially elevated if rapid filling has occurred prior to measurement (due to venoconstriction), as occurs following rapid filling in 'shocked' patients.

Pulmonary arterial occlusion pressure (PAOP)

CVP reflects the function of the right ventricle which usually parallels left ventricular function. In cardiac disease, however, there may be a disparity between the function of the two ventricles. The Swan–Ganz catheter has a balloon on the tip with a pressure transducer beyond the balloon. The catheter is placed so that the balloon lies in a branch of the pulmonary artery, and when the balloon is inflated, the pressure beyond the balloon gives a good guide to the left atrial pressure – the pulmonary arterial occlusion pressure, or PAOP. This gives a better indication of the state of filling of the systemic circulation than the CVP, although usually measurement of CVP will suffice.

Routes of fluid replacement

Enteral fluids

Oral fluid replacement is suitable if the GI tract is functioning and the deficiency is not excessive (ie post-obstructive diuresis). However, this is not always possible (eg paralytic ileus following surgery).

Parenteral fluids

IV fluid replacement is needed if the GI tract is not functioning properly or if rapid fluid replacement is required. Parenteral fluids can broadly be divided into crystalloid, colloid, and blood.

- **Crystalloids:** electrolyte solution in water. They form a true solution and can pass through a semipermeable membrane. They diffuse out quickly into the interstitial space
- **Colloids:** regarded as plasma substitutes. Do not dissolve into a true solution and cannot pass through a semipermeable membrane. Contain high-molecular weight molecules and remain in the intravascular compartment longer than crystalloids. They provide oncotic pressure
- **Blood:** see Chapter 4 *Haematology*

Fluid administration

Types of fluid replacement

Water

This is given as a 5% dextrose solution. Dextrose is a carbohydrate monomer and is metabolised leaving net pure water.

Crystalloid solutions

All are isotonic with body fluid.

- **Normal saline** (0.9%) Contains 154 mmol/L Na^+, 154 mmol/L Cl^-
- **5% dextrose** Contains 278 mmol/L dextrose (calorific content is negligible)
- **Dextrose saline** (0.18% saline; 4% dextrose) Contains 30 mmol/L Na^+, 30 mmol/L Cl^-, 222 mmol/L dextrose
- **Hartmann's solution** Contains 131 mmol/L Na^+, 5 mmol/L K^+, 29 mmol/L HCO_3^-, 111 mmol/L Cl^-, 2 mmol/L Ca_2^+
- **Ringer's solution** Contains 147 mmol/L Na^+, 4 mmol/L K^+, 156 mmol/L Cl^-, 2.2 mmol/L Ca^{2+}

Colloid solutions

- Albumin (4.5%)
  - Natural blood product
  - MR 45–70 000 (natural, therefore broad range MR)
  - No clotting factors
  - Small risk of anaphylaxis
  - Limited availability/expensive
- Gelatins (Haemaccel™/gelofusine/Volplex™)
  - Modified gelatins (from hydrolysis of bovine collagen)
  - Half-life 8–10 hours
  - Low incidence allergic reaction

NB: Haemaccel contains K^+ and Ca^{2+} therefore if mixed with citrated blood in a giving set, leads to coagulation of the residual blood.

Dextrans

- Glucose polymers
  - Dextran 40: average MR is 40 000
  - Dextran 70: average MR is 70 000
- Half-life 16 hours
- Dextran 40 is filtered by the kidney but Dextran 70 is not, therefore Dextran 70 stays in circulation for longer
- Dextran interferes with cross-matching blood and coagulation (forms red blood cell rouleaux) – it is also nephrotoxic and can cause allergic reactions

Hetastarch

- 6% hetastarch in saline
- Half-life 16–24 hours
- MR 120 000
- Must limit dose to 1500 mL/kg (excess leads to coagulation problems)
- Low incidence anaphylaxis/and no interference with cross-matching
- Expensive

If water is given to a patient, it will rapidly distribute throughout the ECF with a resultant fall in ECF osmolality. Since osmolality must be the same inside and outside the cell, water will move from ECF to ICF until the osmolalities are the same. Thus water distributes throughout the whole body water. Since the intravascular space only comprises about 7.5% of the total body space, only 7.5% of infused water will stay in the intravascular compartment, and a large amount of fluid will need to be given to increase significantly the plasma volume.

If isotonic crystalloids are infused, the fluid will stay in the ECF. There is no change in osmolality inside or outside the cells, and so there is no net flow of water into the cells. The saline will distribute throughout the extracellular space. The ECF makes up about 35% of the body water, and less saline will need to be given than water to lead to a corresponding increase in plasma volume.

Colloid solutions (albumin, starch solutions, gelatins) stay in the plasma compartment since the capillary membrane is impermeable to colloid. Consequently less colloid will need to be given than both water and saline to lead to a corresponding increase in plasma volume.

Use of common fluids

When prescribing fluid regimens for patients, we need to take three things into account:

- Basal requirements
- Continuing abnormal losses over and above basal requirements
- Pre-existing dehydration and electrolyte loss

Basal fluid requirements

Common daily maintenance regimens for a 70 kg adult in a temperate environment

Regimen A

1 litre normal saline + 20 mmol KCl over 8 hours
1 litre 5% dextrose + 20 mmol KCl over 8 hours
1 litre 5% dextrose + 20 mmol KCl over 8 hours

This provides: 3 litres water, 60 mmol K^+, 150 mmol Na^+

Regimen B
1 litre dextrose saline + 20 mmol KCl over 8 hours
1 litre dextrose saline + 20 mmol KCl over 8 hours
1 litre dextrose saline + 20 mmol KCl over 8 hours

This provides: 3 litres water, 60 mmol K^+, 90 mmol Na^+.

NB: Metabolism of dextrose may lead to effectively administering hypotonic saline. Therefore, regimen B is only suitable in the short-term.

Correction of pre-existing dehydration

Patients who are dehydrated will need to be resuscitated with fluid over and above their basal requirements. The important issues are:

- To identify which compartment or compartments the fluid has been lost from
- To assess the extent of the dehydration

The fluid used to resuscitate the patient should be similar to that which has been lost. It is usually easy to decide where the losses are coming from. Bowel losses come from the ECF, pure water losses come from the total body water, and protein-containing fluid is lost from the plasma. There is frequently a combination of these.

Fluid regimens and potassium (K^+)

In the first 24 hours after non-cardiac surgery, potassium is often omitted from the IV fluid regimen. There is a tendency for potassium to rise during and after surgery because of:

- Cell injury (high intracellular potassium concentration released into plasma)
- Blood transfusions
- Decreased renal potassium clearance due to transient renal impairment in the immediate post-op period
- Opposed action of insulin by 'stress hormones' tend to cause potassium release from the cells
- However, potassium should be replaced in patients who are on intravenous fluids for prolonged periods of time

Therefore peri-operative fluid balance must be carefully monitored in relation to electrolytes and volume.

It is essential for an accurate fluid chart to be kept. This records all fluid intake (oral and IV) and all output (urine, drain fluid, GI contents, etc), and provides a balance for each 24 hours, once insensible loss has been estimated.

2.4 ACID–BASE BALANCE

In a nutshell ...

The products of metabolism are predominantly acids (CO_2 and organic acids). Maintenance of a stable pH is initially achieved by buffer systems. The excess acid is then excreted via the lungs and kidneys.

An **acid** is a proton or hydrogen ion donor
A **base** is a proton or hydrogen ion acceptor

Acidaemia is arterial blood pH of < 7.35
Alkalaemia is arterial blood pH of > 7.45

Acidosis is an abnormal condition demonstrated by a decrease in arterial pH
Alkalosis is an abnormal condition demonstrated by an increase in arterial pH

pH is the logarithm (to the base 10) of the reciprocal of the hydrogen ion concentration, thus: $pH = \log_{10} 1/[H^+] = -\log_{10} [H^+]$
pKa is the pH of a buffer at which half the acid molecules are undissociated and half are associated

Acids, bases and buffers

Normal physiological function depends on a narrow range of pH (centred around pH 7.4). The major products of metabolism are acids (CO_2 and organic acids). The body prevents the pH level straying too far from the ideal with the use of buffering systems and by excretion of the excess acid via the lungs and the renal system.

A buffering system usually consists of a weak acid and its conjugate base.

$$HB \Longleftrightarrow H^+ + B^-$$

Where HB is a weak acid, H^+ is the hydrogen ion, and B^- is the conjugate base.

This resists changes in pH as the addition of any acid reacts with the free base ions (and the reaction moves to the left to provide replacement B^- ions for those in solution that have just been used to neutralise the acid). Conversely, the addition of alkali reacts with the free H^+ ions (and the reaction moves to the right to provide replacement H^+ ions for those in solution that have just been used to neutralise the base).

Intracellularly, proteins and phosphates act as buffers. Extracellularly, the bicarbonate buffer system is of major importance. This can be illustrated by the Henderson–Hasselbach equation.

The Henderson–Hasselbach equation

The Henderson–Hasselbach equation is based on the relationship between CO_2 and bicarbonate (HOC_3^-) in the blood. In the bicarbonate buffer system, the weak acid and base are carbonic acid and bicarbonate:

$$H_2CO_3 \Leftrightarrow H^+ + HCO_3^-$$

The carbonic acid (H_2CO_3) dissociates in the blood to form $CO_2 + H_2O$:

$$CO_2 + H_2O \Leftrightarrow H_2CO_3$$

Therefore:

$$CO_2 + H_2O \Leftrightarrow H_2CO_3 \Leftrightarrow H^+ + HCO_3^-$$

The addition of acid will shift this equation to the left to provide replacement HCO_3^- ions for those in solution that have just been used to neutralise the acid. The addition of alkali will shift the equation to the right to provide replacement H^+ ions for those in solution that have just been used to neutralise the alkali.

The Henderson–Hasselbach equation

The equation is given by:

$$pH = pKa + \log \frac{[base]}{[acid]}$$

That is:

$$pH = pKa + \log \frac{[HCO_3]}{[H_2CO_3]}$$

This equation describes the relationship of arterial pH to bicarbonate and $PaCO_2$.

It is derived from the reaction of CO_2 with water, thus:

$$CO_2 + H_2O \Leftrightarrow H_2CO_3 \Leftrightarrow H^+ + HCO_3^-$$

The carbonic acid can be expressed as CO_2, thus:

$$pH = pKa + \log \frac{[HCO_3^-]}{pKaCO_2}$$

Where pKa is a constant, and K is a constant.

This buffer system aims to minimise pH change, so if $PaCO_2$ goes up then HCO_3^- goes up; and if $PaCO_2$ goes down then HCO_3^- goes down.

Excretion of excess acid and alkali

The bicarbonate buffering system will not restore large changes in pH. Excess H^+ and HCO_3^- ions are excreted via the lungs and the kidneys.

Excretion via the lungs

The respiratory mechanism is a rapid-response system that allows CO_2 to be transferred from pulmonary venous blood to alveolar gas and excreted in expired gas. Brainstem respiratory centres respond directly to the levels of CO_2 by detecting H^+ in the blood. High levels cause an increase in the rate of respiration, blowing off CO_2 and decrease acidity. Dysfunction of the mechanics or control of ventilation can lead to retention of CO_2 and a rise in H^+ (respiratory acidosis) or over-excretion of CO_2 and a fall in H^+ (respiratory alkalosis).

Excretion via the kidneys

Excretion of excess acid and alkali occurs more slowly by renal compensation. The body produces more acid than base each day and so the urine is usually slightly acidic (pH 6.0). It relies upon the excretion of hydrogen ions in the urine by secretion of H^+ ions in the distal nephron. Additionally, HCO_3^- ions are generated in the renal tubules. Renal dysfunction (whether pre-renal, renal, or post-renal) will prevent hydrogen ion excretion, resulting in a metabolic acidosis.

The excretion of excess acid requires buffer systems in the urine. These are phosphate and ammonia:

$$H^+ + HPO_4^- \Longleftrightarrow H_2PO_4$$

$$H^+ + NH_3 \Longleftrightarrow NH_4^+$$

Respiratory acidosis

Respiratory acidosis results in a primary disturbance of increased pCO_2 leading to a decrease in pH and a compensatory increase in HCO_3^-.

Causes of respiratory acidosis

Depression of the respiratory centre

- CVA
- Cerebral tumour
- Drugs (narcotics/sedatives)
- Encephalitis

Decreased chest wall movement
Neuromuscular disorder (eg myasthenia gravis)
Trauma/surgery
Ankylosing spondylitis

Pulmonary disease (known as type II respiratory failure)
COPD
Pneumonia

Respiratory alkalosis

Respiratory alkalosis results from the primary disturbance of a decreased $PaCO_2$ leading to an increase in pH and a compensatory decrease in HCO_3^-.

Causes of respiratory alkalosis

Stimulation of the respiratory centre
CNS disease (eg CVA, encephalitis)
Hypermetabolic state (eg fever, hyperthyroidism, sepsis)
Exercise
Hypoxia (eg pneumonia, pulmonary oedema, pulmonary collapse or fibrosis)

Excess mechanical ventilation (by patient or ventilator)
Anxiety
Certain drugs (eg aspirin)

Metabolic acidosis

Metabolic acidosis results from the primary disturbance of a decreased HCO_3^- or increased H^+ leading to a decrease in pH and a compensatory decrease in $PaCO_2$.

Causes of metabolic acidosis

Increased anion gap
Renal glomerular failure
Overdose (eg salicylate – also causes respiratory alkalosis; see above)
Lactic acidosis – inadequate tissue perfusion (hypovolaemia, ischaemic gut)

Ketoacidosis – diabetic or alcoholic
Renal tubular acidosis
Acetazolamide therapy
Ureterosigmoidostomy

Normal anion gap
Excess acid intake (eg parenteral nutrition)

Metabolic alkalosis

This occurs in diarrhoea, fistulas, and proximal renal tubular acidosis. It results from the primary disturbance of an increase in HCO_3^- or a decrease in H^+ leading to an increase in pH and a compensatory increase in $PaCO_2$ (although clinically this effect is small).

Causes of metabolic alkalosis

Excess alkali intake
Alkali abuse
Over-treatment of acidosis

Excess loss of acid
Vomiting

Increased urinary acidification
Diuretics
Excess aldosterone
Hypokalaemia

Compensation in acid–base balance

During a disturbance in the acid–base status there is an attempt by the body to try to correct the disturbance. There are two main mechanisms:

- Manipulation of $PaCO_2$ by the respiratory system: this is rapid but not as effective as renal compensation
- Manipulation of HCO_3^- by the kidneys: this is slow but more effective than respiratory compensation

NB: Compensatory changes do not bring the pH to normal; they simply change the pH towards the normal range.

Interpretation of acid–base balance

From the Henderson–Hasselbach equation it can be seen that if a patient has a change in acid–base status, three parameters also change:

- pH
- HCO_3^- concentration
- $PaCO_2$

Blood gas machines measure pO_2, pH and pCO_2 directly. Bicarbonate is calculated from the Henderson–Hasselbach equation.

Other important variables given by the blood gas machine include:

- **Actual bicarbonate**: the concentration of bicarbonate measured in the blood sample at the $PaCO_2$ of the patient
- **Standard bicarbonate:** the concentration of bicarbonate in the blood sample when the $PaCO_2$ is normal (ie if there was no respiratory disturbance). Therefore this gives information about metabolic changes

Normal standard bicarbonate is 22–26 mmol.

- Greater than this → **metabolic alkalosis**
- Less than this → **metabolic acidosis**

Standard base excess is the amount of acid/base needed to be added to the sample to return the pH to the normal range.

Normal ranges of arterial blood gases

pH	7.35–7.45
H^+	36–44 mmol/L
pO_2	10–14 kPa (75–100 mmHg)
pCO_2	4–6 kPa (35–42 mmHg)
HCO_3^-	22–26 mmol/L

Interpretation of the ABG

When interpreting the arterial blood gas it helps to follow a logical schematic such as the one below:

1. Is the patient hypoxic?

pO2 < 10 kPa

How much inspired O_2 are they on?

2. Is the patient acidotic or alkalotic?

Look at the pH:

Normal arterial blood pH = 7.40 ± 0.02
Acidotic pH < 7.38
Alkalotic pH > 7.42

3. Is the primary disturbance respiratory or metabolic?

Look at the pCO_2 and the serum HCO_3^-.

A respiratory disturbance primarily alters the arterial pCO_2
A metabolic disturbance primarily alters the serum HCO_3^-

RESPIRATORY acidosis	RESPIRATORY alkalosis
↑ pCO_2 ↔ or ↑ HCO_3^- HCO_3^- remains normal unless there is metabolic compensation when HCO_3^- increases as it is retained by the kidney	**↓ pCO_2 ↔ or ↓ HCO_3^-** HCO_3^- remains normal unless there is metabolic compensation when HCO_3^- decreases as it is excreted by the kidney
METABOLIC acidosis	**METABOLIC alkalosis**
↓ HCO_3^- ↔ or ↓ pCO_2 (pCO_2 remains normal unless there is respiratory compensation when pCO_2 decreases due to hyperventilation)	**↑ HCO_3^- ↔ or ↑ pCO_2** pCO_2 remains normal unless there is respiratory compensation when pCO_2 increases due to hypoventilation

Compensation occurs within the two systems when the pH becomes disturbed. This occurs rapidly in the case of the respiratory system by changing the rate of respiration to 'blow off' or conserve CO_2. The kidney is responsible for metabolic compensation and this responds more slowly (approximately 4 hours with maximal compensation at 4 days) with the net gain or loss of HCO_3^- ions.

4. In metabolic acidosis is there a difference in the anion gap?

The anion gap is the calculated difference between negatively charged (anion) and positively charged (cation) electrolytes. It provides diagnostic information in cases of metabolic acidosis.

The anion gap

Normally this is 10–16 mmol/L.

In the body, to maintain electrical chemical neutrality, the number of cations equals the number of anions. The main cations in the body are sodium and potassium. The main anions in the body are chloride, bicarbonate, proteins, phosphates, sulfates and organic acids. Usually the ions which are measured are sodium, potassium, bicarbonate and chloride.

CALCULATING THE ANION GAP

Cations		**Anions**	
Na^+	140 mmol/L	Cl^-	105 mmol/L
K^+	5 mmol/L	HCO_3^-	30 mmol/L
Total	145 mmol/L	Total	135 mmol/L

In the example shown in the table the difference is 10 mmol/L and therefore the anion gap is 10 mmol/L.

This anion gap is made up of anions which are not usually measured.

Why is this important?

- An increased anion gap = **metabolic acidosis**
- The cause of this metabolic acidosis will be due to retention of acid other than HCl (eg lactic acid)

Section 3
The cardiovascular system in critical care

3.1 ANATOMY OF THE HEART AND MEDIASTINUM

The anatomy of the mediastinum

The mediastinum (the space between the pleural cavities) contains the heart and great vessels, the oesophagus, the trachea and bifurcation, the thoracic duct, and the phrenic and vagus nerves. An anatomical plane passing through the sternal angle and the lower border T4 divides it.

Divisions of the mediastinum

Superior	Above this plane
Anterior	In front of fibrous pericardium
Middle	Containing fibrous pericardium and heart
Posterior	Behind fibrous pericardium

The pre-vertebral and pre-tracheal fascia from the neck extends into the superior mediastinum. Neck infection will therefore:

- Pass into the anterior mediastinum if in front of pre-tracheal fascia in the neck
- Be confined to the superior mediastinum in front of the vertebral bodies if behind the pre-vertebral fascia in the neck

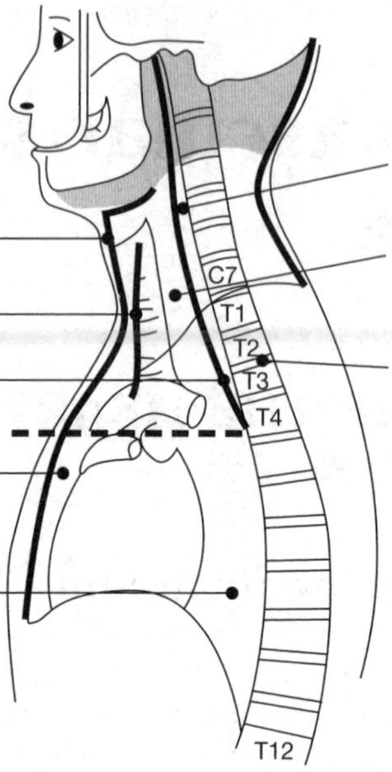

Figure 3.1a *Divisions of the mediastinum demonstrating continuity with the tissue spaces of the neck*

The superior mediastinum

Boundaries of the superior mediastinum

Anterior	Manubrium
Superior	Thoracic inlet (often clinically referred to as thoracic outlet)
Inferior	Plane through T4
Posterior	Bodies of T1 to T4

Contents of the superior mediastinum

The great vessels are contained within the superior mediastinum (veins on right, arteries on left). There is more 'dead space' on the right side (to accommodate venous distension) therefore fluid in the mediastinum may collect there.

Arteries in the superior mediastinum

The arch of the aorta lies wholly in the superior mediastinum, behind the manubrium.

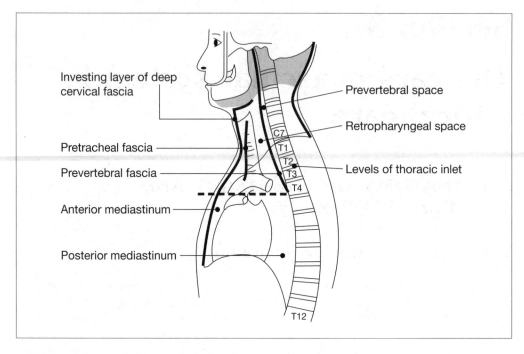

Important arterial branches in the superior mediastinum

Brachiocephalic trunk: arises behind the manubrium; termination of the left brachiocephalic vein lies in front of the artery; it divides behind the right sterno-clavicular joint into the right subclavian artery and the right common carotid artery

Left common carotid artery: passes up next to the trachea into the neck; there are no branches in the mediastinum

Left subclavian artery: supplies the head and neck, the upper limb and some thoracic wall structures; there are no branches in the mediastinum

Ligamentum arteriosum

The fibrous remnant of fetal ductus arteriosum (between the pulmonary artery and aortic arch). The left recurrent laryngeal nerve (from the vagus) hooks around it.

Veins in the superior mediastinum

- **Brachiocephalic veins** are formed behind the sternoclavicular joints, from internal jugular and subclavian veins: the **right** passes vertically downwards; the **left** passes nearly horizontally through the superior mediastinum behind the manubrium, and meets the right brachiocephalic vein at the lower border of the first costal cartilage on the right
- **Superior vena cava** (SVC) is formed by the two brachiocephalic veins and passes vertically downwards behind the right sternal border, through the pericardium and joins the right atrium at the lower border of the third right costal cartilage; the azygos vein drains into the SVC behind the sternal angle, opposite the second right costal cartilage

Nerves in the superior mediastinum

Phrenic nerves

- Supplied by C3 to C5 (mainly C4) – 'keeps diaphragm alive'
- Passes in front of the lung root on each side
- Adjacent to the mediastinal pleura throughout its mediastinal course (ie lies as far medial as possible in the thorax)
- Medial relations are different on each side (see box)

Medial relations of the phrenic nerve

Right phrenic nerve medial relations (venous structures throughout its course)

Right brachiocephalic vein
Superior vena cava
Right atrium
Inferior vena cava

Passes through the vena caval foramen in central tendon of diaphragm.

Left phrenic nerve medial relations

Left common carotid artery
Left subclavian artery
Arch of aorta (lateral to superior intercostal vein)
Pericardium over left ventricle

Passes through muscular part of diaphragm to left of pericardium.

Vagus nerves

These lie as medial in their course as structures permit.

- Right vagus nerve
  - Lateral to trachea
  - Passes behind lung root
  - Enters oesophageal plexus in mid-line (with left vagus)
  - Right recurrent laryngeal branch given off in root of neck
  - Hooks around the right subclavian artery (non-recurrent in 1–2% of cases)
- Left vagus nerve
  - Separated from trachea by left common carotid and subclavian arteries and passes over the aortic arch
  - Passes behind lung root
  - Enters oesophageal plexus

Left recurrent laryngeal branch

- Given off on the aortic arch
- Hooks around the ligamentum arteriosum and passes up on the right side of the aortic arch

Recurrent laryngeal nerves

- Supply trachea and adjacent oesophagus

The laryngeal nerves are extremely important due to their innervation of the muscles of the larynx and their potential for injury in thyroid surgery.

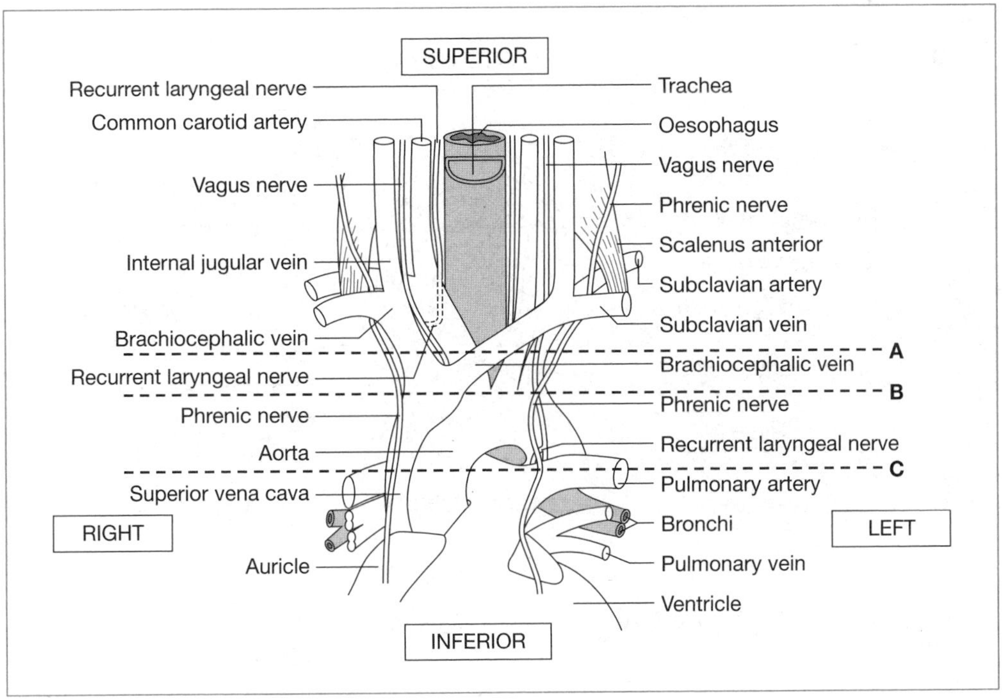

Figure 3.1b *Lines A, B and C on this figure correspond to horizontal sections A, B, and C in Figs 3.1c, 3.1d and 3.1e respectively*

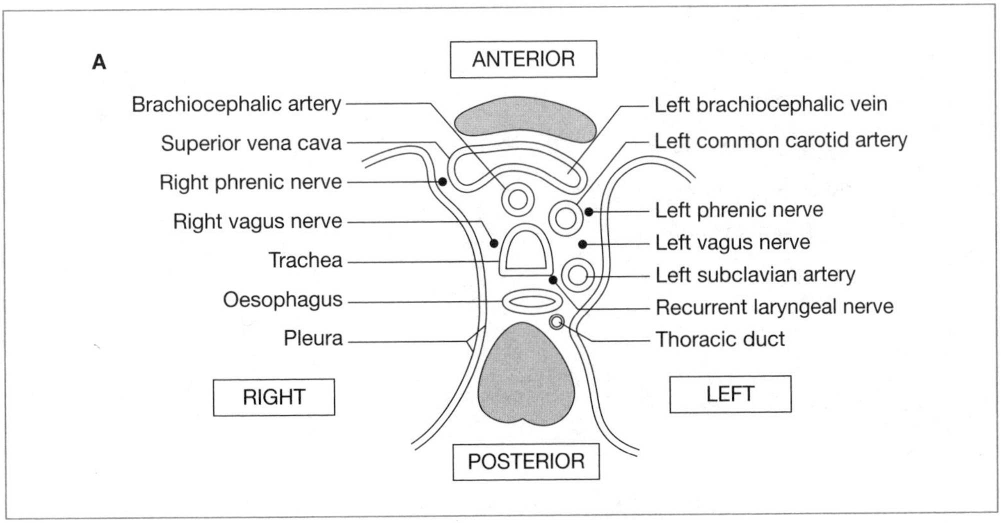

Figure 3.1c *Transverse section through T3*

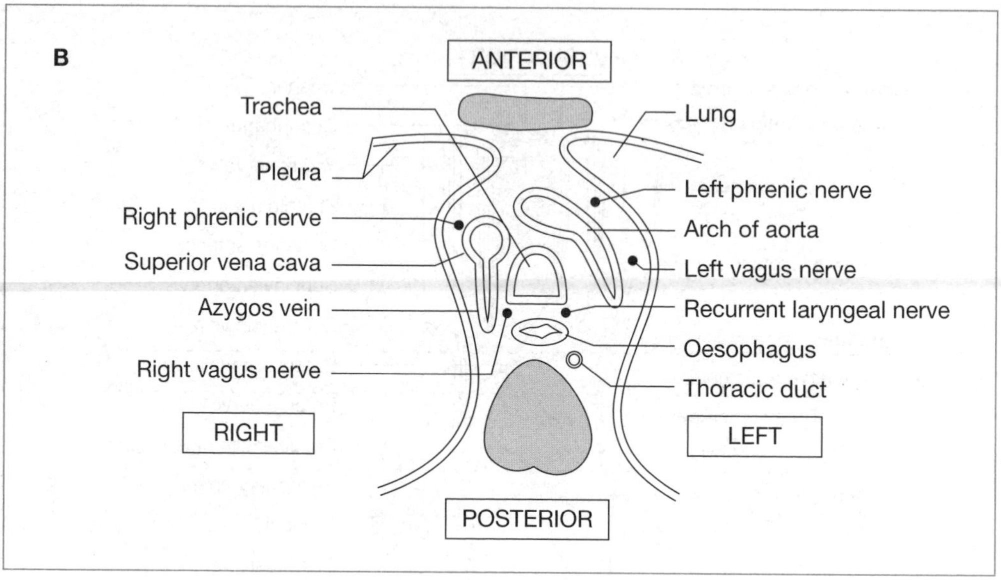

Figure 3.1d *Transverse section through T4*

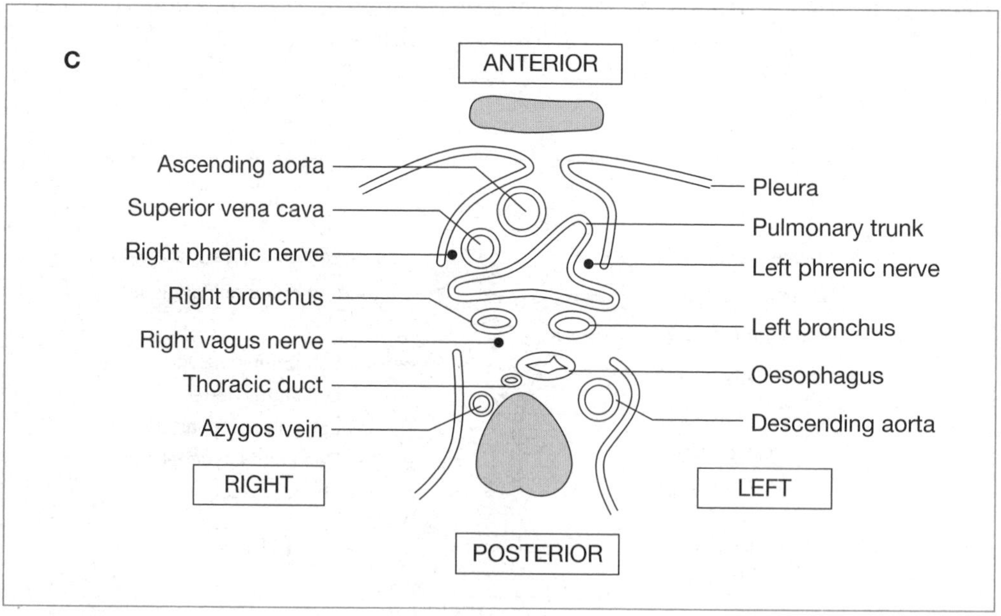

Figure 3.1e *Transverse section through T5*

Cardiac plexus

- Sympathetic and parasympathetic afferent fibres
- Supply SA node, AV node and bundle, ventricular myocardium
- Also contain afferent pain fibres

Other structures in the superior mediastinum

Trachea

- Continuation of larynx
- Commences in neck at level of C6
- Bifurcates just below manubrium
- Thoracic part descends in superior mediastinum in front of oesophagus to upper part of posterior mediastinum

Oesophagus

- Crossed by arch of the aorta on the left and azygos vein on the right

The anterior mediastinum

Contains the thymus (although the thymus may only be present in the anterior part of the superior mediastinum).

- Surgical approach is via median sternotomy
- Continuous through superior mediastinum with pre-tracheal space of the neck

The middle mediastinum

- Pericardium and heart
- Adjoining parts of the great vessels
- Lung roots
- Phrenic nerves

Pericardium

- Fibrous (outer part):
  - Fuses with all vessels except IVC
  - Blends with central tendon of the diaphragm
  - Also attached to the sternum (sterno-pericardial ligaments)
  - Supplied by the phrenic nerve
- Serous (inner part):
  - Parietal (outer layer) has phrenic nerve supply
  - Visceral (inner layer) has no sensation
  - Transverse and oblique sinuses = folds of pericardium between parietal and visceral layers

NB: Pericardiocentesis = needle aspiration of fluid (eg blood) in pericardial cavity.

The posterior mediastinum

Boundaries of the posterior mediastinum

Anteriorly: pericardium (upper part), posterior part of the diaphragm (lower part)
Posteriorly: T4 to T12

Contents of the posterior mediastinum

- Descending aorta (commences at lower border of T4; exits posterior mediastinum at mid-line at level of T12 by passing behind the crura of the diaphragm)
- Oesophagus (commences at C6 and ends at cardia of the stomach at level of T10; exits posterior mediastinum at level of T10)
- Thoracic lymph nodes
- Thoracic duct
- Azygos veins
- Thoracic sympathetic trunk

The anatomy of the heart

Borders of the heart

Left border
Mostly left ventricle
Auricle of left atrium (upper part)
Surface marking: apex to lower border left 2nd costal cartilage, 2 cm lateral to the sternum

Right border
Right atrium
Surface marking: level of 3rd–6th right costal cartilage, right margin of the sternum

Inferior border
Mostly right ventricle
Small amount of left ventricle (which forms the apex)
Surface marking: right 6th costal cartilage to apex (usually left 5th intercostal space, in mid-clavicular line)

Surfaces of the heart

- Anterior/sternocostal surface
  - Right atrium and ventricle, small amount of left ventricle, forming left border
- Diaphragmatic surface
  - Right atrium, receiving IVC; antero-posterior AV groove
  - Part of both ventricles (1/3 right, 2/3 left)
- Posterior surface/base of heart
  - Left atrium, receiving pulmonary veins

Tissues of the heart

- Epicardium (outer part)
- Myocardium (muscle layer; makes up the bulk of the heart)
- Endocardium (inner part of the chambers of the heart)

Valves of the heart

Tricuspid valve

- Three cusps (anterior, posterior and septal)
- Surface marking: behind sternum, level of 5th and 6th costal cartilages
- Auscultation area: 5th intercostal space, right sternal edge

Pulmonary valve

- Three semilunar cusps (anterior, left and right)
- Surface marking: left of mid-line behind sternum, level of 3rd costal cartilage
- Auscultation area: 3rd costal cartilage, left sternal edge

Mitral valve

- Cusps (large anterior and small posterior)
- Surface marking: left of mid-line behind sternum, level of 4th intercostal space
- Auscultation area: at the apex beat

Aortic valve

- Three cusps (right, left and posterior)
- Surface marking: left of mid-line behind sternum, level of 3rd intercostal space
- Auscultation area: 2nd intercostal space, right sternal edge

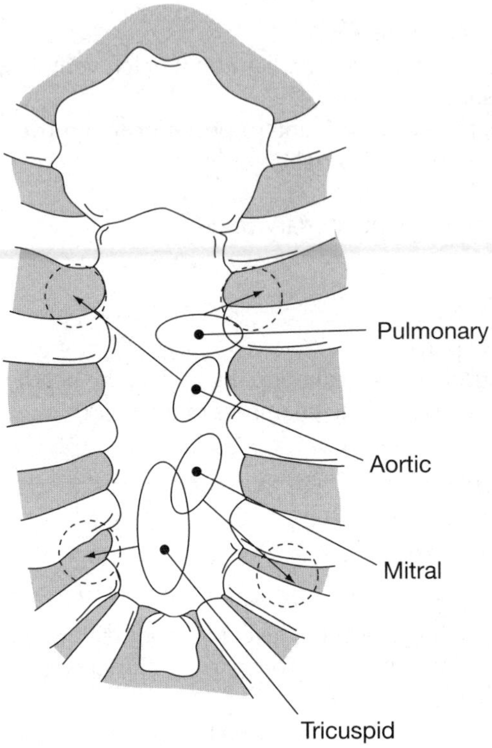

Figure 3.1f *Surface markings of the heart valves. The arrows indicate the directions in which sounds of the closing valves are propagated and the dashed circles indicate the generally preferred sites for auscultation*

Conducting system of the heart

This is formed by specialised cardiac muscle cells and initiates, co-ordinates and controls the rhythm of cardiac muscle contraction.

Main elements of the conducting system of the heart:

- **Sino-atrial node (SA node):** acts as a pacemaker for the heart; situated in the wall of the right atrium, just below the SVC
- **Atrio-ventricular node (AV node):** situated in the wall of the inter-atrial septum (above and to the left of the opening of the coronary sinus); electrical impulses which have been conducted from the SA node through the atria are conducted through the AV node to the bundle of His

- **Bundle of His:** arises from the AV node; passes through the membranous part of the inter-ventricular septum; divided into right and left branches
  - **Right branch:** initially runs in the muscle of the septum then becomes sub-endocardial on the right side of the septum; reaches the anterior wall of the ventricle then divides into multiple sub-endocardial branches, supplying the right ventricle (branches are made up of Purkinje fibres)
  - **Left branch:** this reaches the endocardium of the septum then divides into multiple sub-endocardial branches (Purkinje fibres); Purkinje fibres make up the terminal sub-endocardial plexus

Blood supply of the heart

Blood supply of the heart by region

- Right ventricle – right coronary artery
- Left ventricle – left coronary artery
- Atrial arterial supply – variable
- Inter-ventricular septum – right and left coronary arteries

NB: There can be considerable variation from this general scheme.

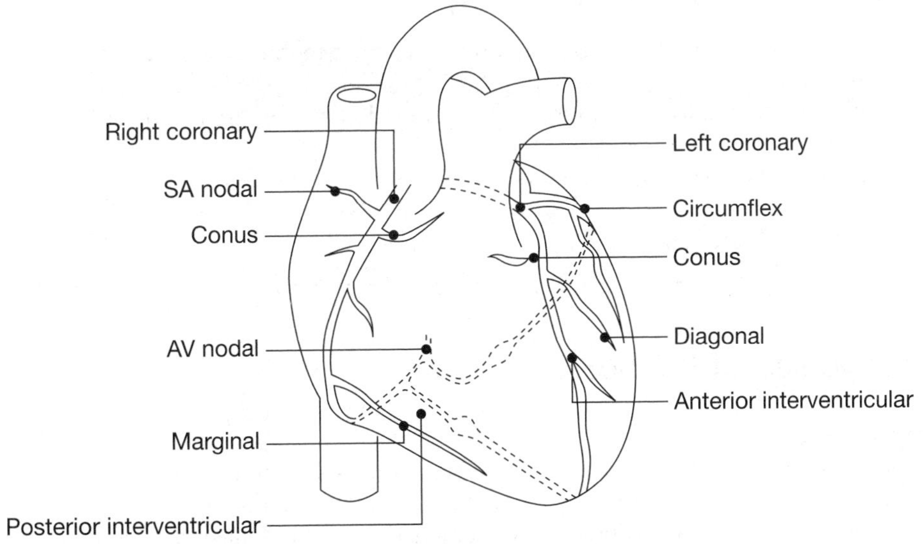

Figure 3.1g *Coronary arteries and their main branches, viewed anteriorly. Interrupted lines show the vessels on the posterior surface*

Blood supply of the heart by vessel

Right coronary artery

This arises from the right aortic sinus branches (passes between the right auricle and infundibulum of the right ventricle; downwards in the AV groove and backwards at the inferior surface of the heart).

Branches of the right coronary artery

Conus artery
SA nodal artery
Right marginal artery
AV nodal artery
Posterior inter-ventricular artery
Atrial and ventricular branches

Left coronary artery

This arises from the left aortic sinus (behind the pulmonary trunk; passes between the left auricle and infundibulum of the right ventricle).

Branches of the left coronary artery

Circumflex branch (direct continuation): continues in the AV groove supplying the ventricle
Anterior inter-ventricular artery (left anterior descending artery): most frequently discussed
SA nodal artery: supplies SA node in 40%
Conus artery
Ventricular branches

Great vessels of the heart

Ascending aorta

The proximal part is covered in a sleeve of serous pericardium (which it shares with the pulmonary trunk). There are three sinuses (bulges) in the proximal part – one above each aortic valve cusp. The right coronary artery emerges from the right sinus. The left coronary artery emerges from the left sinus.

Pulmonary trunk

The proximal part is covered in a sleeve of serous pericardium (which it shares with the ascending aorta). It passes backwards, divides into the right and left pulmonary arteries in the concavity of the aortic arch (in front of the left main bronchus).

3.2 CARDIOVASCULAR PHYSIOLOGY

In a nutshell ...

The **blood pressure** (BP) is regulated by the systemic vascular resistance (SVR) and the cardiac output (CO).

Peripheral vascular resistance depends on compliance of the blood vessels, predominantly the arterioles.

Cardiac output is measured by the stroke volume (SV) × heart rate (HR).

Stroke volume depends on venous return (Starling's law).

Systemic vascular resistance

Systemic vascular resistance depends on vascular compliance and the haemodynamics of blood flow.

Factors such as heart rate (HR) and stroke volume (SV) affect arterial pressure by altering the cardiac output, thus:

$$CO = HR \times SV$$

The less compliant the system is (with stiff arteries) the more work the heart must do to pump a given stroke volume. Compliance decreases with age when elastic fibres are partially replaced with collagen, and there is a decrease in the number of smooth muscle cells of the arterial walls.

Vascular compliance

The functions of the arterial system include blood distribution and conversion of pulsatile flow to steady flow (as this requires less work). This is accomplished by the elasticity in the vessel walls, known as compliance.

Mean arterial pressure (P_a) is derived from diastolic BP (P_d) and systolic BP (P_s) using the formula:

$$P_a = P_d + \tfrac{1}{3}(P_s - P_d)$$

ie Mean arterial pressure = diastolic pressure + ⅓ (systolic – diastolic pressure)

The pressure in arteries depends on both the rate of blood entering and the rate of blood leaving the system and the compliance of the vessels. Flow of blood through the vascular system requires a pressure gradient to be generated across the area where flow is to be established.

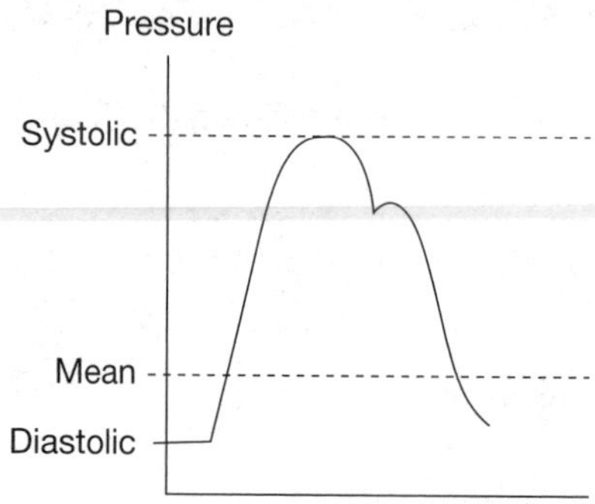

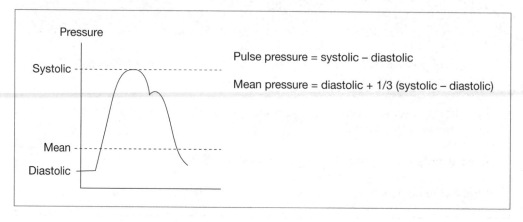

Figure 3.2a *The arterial pressure wave*

As in physics, Ohm's law states that for a current (I) to flow through a system with resistance (R), a potential difference (V) must be established across the ends of the system. The relationship V = IR is analogous to the vascular system. Pressure across the system is related to the flow or 'current' through the system (the cardiac output, CO) and the resistance to that flow (the systemic vascular resistance, SVR).

Hence, in the systemic circulation the pressure across the system is the difference between mean arterial pressure and right atrial pressure (P_{RA}, which is often approximated to 0).

$$P_a - P_{RA} = CO \times SVR$$

ie: Mean arterial pressure – right atrial pressure = cardiac output × systemic vascular resistance

Similarly, in the pulmonary circulation, the pressure gradient driving flow through the lungs is the difference between the mean pulmonary artery pressure (P_{pa}) and the pressure in the left atrium (P_{LA}), and is affected by the pulmonary vascular resistance (PVR).

$$P_{pa} - P_{LA} = CO \times PVR$$

ie Mean pulmonary artery pressure – left atrial pressure = cardiac output × pulmonary vascular resistance

Flow and vascular resistance

$$\text{Flow (Q)} = \Delta P/\text{Resistance}$$

$$\text{ie: Flow} = \frac{\text{pressure change across the vessel}}{\text{vascular resistance}}$$

where ΔP is the pressure change across vessel, therefore in the systemic circulation:

$$P_a - P_{RA} = CO \times SVR$$

(The same equation format can be applied to the pulmonary circulation.)

Flow in smooth vessels should be laminar, that is along the longitudinal axis, where it is governed by Poiseuille's law, thus:

$$\text{Flow} = \Delta P \pi \rho^4 / 8 \eta L$$

where η is blood viscosity, L is the length of the vessel segment, and *r* is the radius.

NB: There is strong dependence of flow on vessel radius; if the radius doubles, the flow will increase 16-fold for the same difference in pressure.

Blood viscosity is affected by:

- **Haematocrit levels:** conditions such as dehydration and primary or secondary polycythaemia raise the haematocrit levels. Haematocrit > 63% is enough to double the relative viscosity of the blood
- **RBC deformity:** conditions such as spherocytosis and sickle cell anaemia alter the ability of the red cell to deform as it passes through the capillaries, and this affects relative viscosity
- **Vessel radius:** cells tend to flow along the centre of the vessel to minimise friction with the vessel wall. Smaller vessels demonstrate increased friction
- **Low flow rates:** (eg systolic BP of > 50 mmHg) cause the RBCs to form rouleaux and stick together, thus increasing viscosity

If viscosity increases then flow rate decreases. Various conditions such as dehydration and polycythaemia both increase the haematocrit and thus the viscosity of the blood. An increase in pressure is therefore necessary to maintain the flow. There is a decrease in the apparent viscosity of blood when it flows in smaller vessels, so in small vessels there is a lower resistance to flow. Lower BP reduces the shear rate and therefore increases blood viscosity. Small arteries and arterioles provide the greatest resistance to flow in the systemic circulation by altering smooth muscle tone in their walls, so they are the main determinants of SVR.

The relationship between cross-sectional area and flow

Cardiac output is intermittent – the continuous flow in the capillaries is due to the elasticity of the aorta and branches. The flow changes from pulsatile to continuous while passing through arterioles. During diastole, continuous flow is maintained to the capillary bed by relaxation of the arterial elastic wall, previously stretched during systole. This 'capacitance' mechanism maintains the diastolic pressure, permitting continuous flow in the capillary bed.

The peripheral arterioles are more muscular and less elastic than the great vessels. They provide the greatest resistance (therefore the greatest pressure drop) in the arterial circulation.

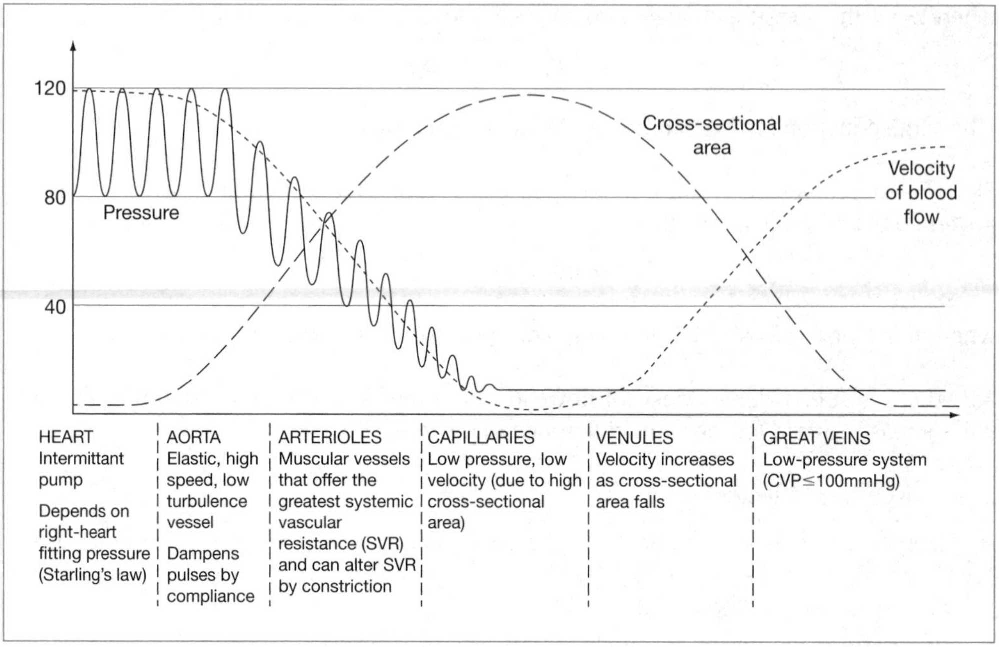

Figure 3.2b *Basic vascular physiology*

The peripheral vasculature is controlled predominantly by changes in the arterioles. The muscle layer of the media is intimately associated with the endothelial cell, allowing release of endothelial mediators to act locally. Control is achieved by a combination of intrinsic local and extrinsic systemic features.

- **Intrinsic mechanisms:** local mechanisms serve to match the flow through a capillary bed to its metabolic activity. Examples include the vasodilatation produced in response to products of metabolism, including CO_2, endothelial-derived relaxing factor (nitric oxide), lactic acid and H^+ ions. These lead to an increased blood flow
- **Extrinsic mechanisms:** systemic mechanisms involve the autonomic nervous system and hormones, and generally they are integrated with the whole cardiovascular system. Not only does this provide control over flow to specific beds but it will also control the total vascular resistance. The sympathetic nervous system releases noradrenaline (norepinephrine) as its transmitter, which acts at smooth muscle α-receptors to cause vasoconstriction

The balance between the two systems varies between tissues. Skin has a strong extrinsic component, whereas the brain has chiefly intrinsic autoregulation. Control is achieved by the arterioles, which contain abundant smooth muscle. This smooth muscle is intimately related to the endothelium, allowing agents released by the endothelium in response to bloodborne stimuli (eg hormones) to regulate its contraction. The baroreceptor reflex involves increased afferent nerve signals from baroreceptors in response to hypertension, leading to decreased output from the medullary cardiovascular centres, lowering BP. It is important for short-term control.

The greatest total cross-sectional area is at the level of the capillaries and this causes blood velocity to decrease considerably at this level. Slow flow and thin-walled vessels are ideal for transfer of substances between blood and tissues.

Capillary beds are arranged in parallel, allowing:

- Flow to each bed to be adjusted independently, according to metabolic needs (a large increase in flow to a particular area will be compensated for by a decrease in flow to other beds)
- Preferential direction of flow to certain vital areas if CO falls
- Overall SVR to be adjusted by increasing the resistance in many capillary beds
- Oxygenated blood to reach all capillary beds
- Certain individual beds to maintain blood flow locally, despite variation in CO (autoregulation)
- Feeding artery occlusions to affect only the particular bed

Total cross-sectional area and the number of vessels decrease on passing from the venules to the small veins to large veins and therefore velocity increases. Most of the blood volume of the systemic circulation is in the venous vessels which act as a reservoir and also to conduct the blood flow back to the heart.

Haemodynamics and stenosis

To maintain flow rate (volume per unit time) across stenoses, the velocity of the blood increases in the narrowed segment. Initial decreases in diameter have little effect due to effective compensation (by distal dilatation). With tighter narrowings laminar flow is lost

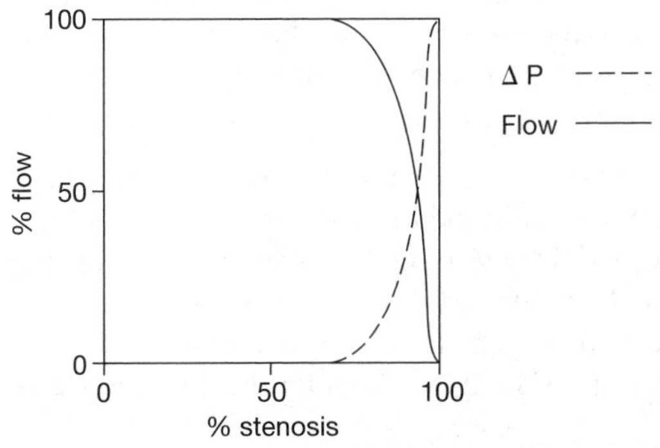

Note: when stenosis reaches 70% flow declines and pressure drop becomes significant

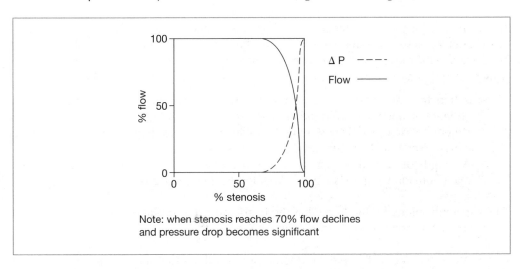

Figure 3.2c *Relationship of flow to degree of stenosis*

and turbulent flow occurs after the stenosis. This may be heard as a bruit as the energy dissipates. Turbulent flow increases wall pressure causing post-stenotic dilation.

The likelihood of turbulent flow can be estimated by calculating Reynolds' number N_R:

Laminar flow	$N_R < 2000$
Turbulent flow	$N_R > 3000$

Critical stenosis

Clearly, as the stenosis increases, a point is reached where flow can no longer be maintained, and the stenosis is now termed critical. This tends to occur at around 70% stenosis. As the resistance in the vessel is proportional to r^4 (where r is its radius; meaning the tighter the stenosis, the lower the flow) flow through the vessels will now sharply decline, and the pressure drops distally to try to maintain flow through the stenosis. This decreased pressure eventually becomes significant, leading to tissue ischaemia at times of exercise, which manifests as angina/claudication.

Physiology of heart muscle function and Starling's law cardiac output

Stroke volume

Starling's Law

Cardiac muscle cells (like skeletal muscle cells) are made up of sarcomeres. Sarcomeres contain thick filaments (myosin) and thin filaments (actin) as discussed previously in the section on muscle contraction in this chapter.

The filaments slide over each other (expending energy) and so shorten the sarcomere (therefore shortening of several sarcomeres is the mechanism by which the muscle cell contracts). The force that the muscle sarcomere can exert depends partly on the length of the sarcomere (which, in turn, is a reflection of the degree of overlap of the thick and thin filaments).

- When the sarcomere is very short the high degree of overlap interferes with contraction and the force is therefore reduced
- When the sarcomere is very long the relative lack of overlap means that less force can be exerted in between these two extremes
- A length of sarcomere exists where the overlap is high enough to produce maximum force but not so high as to interfere with force production

This has implications for the force that the heart can exert to pump blood (known as the Frank–Starling mechanism or 'Starling's law of the heart').

End-diastolic volume (EDV) refers to the amount of blood that the ventricle of the heart holds at its maximum (ie just before it contracts).

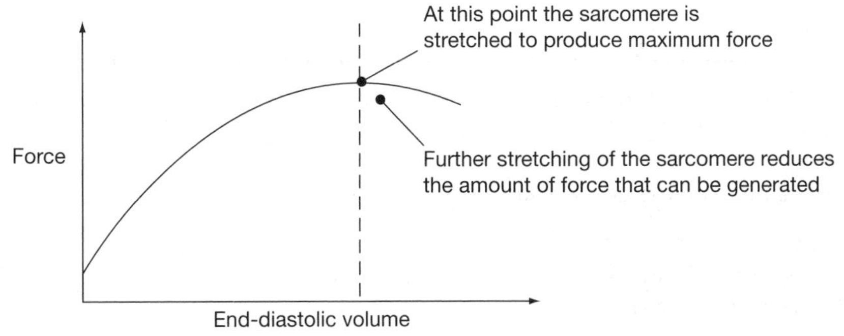

Figure 3.2d *End-diastolic volume (Starling's curve)*

The more blood in the heart (ie the higher the end-diastolic volume) the more the sarcomeres are stretched. Up to a point, increasing the amount of blood (by increasing venous return) increases the force the heart muscle can exert. Beyond a critical point, further increasing the amount of blood decreases the force the heart muscle can exert. Clinically EDV is difficult to measure but it can be inferred from CVP or wedge pressures. CVP is analogous to end-diastolic pressure of the right ventricle, which is analogous to EDV (assuming normal compliance and valve function). On the Starling curve, force is analogous to measured values of cardiac output or stroke volume.

Regulation of stroke volume

Stroke volume can be regulated by pre-load, cardiac contractility and after-load.

Pre-load

Pre-load is essentially the volume of blood available to fill the heart during diastole. This gives rise to end-diastolic ventricular wall tension (initial fibre stretch as in **Starling's law**). Pre-load is dependent upon:

- Venous filling time
- Diastolic filling time
- Atrial systole (ie in fibrillation)
- Myocardial/pericardial distensibility (compliance)

As pre-load increases, so does the force of contraction up to a certain point, after which increased pre-load causes a decrease in the force of contraction. Measured by CVP or PAOP.

Contractility

Force of myocardial contraction; determines cardiac output, SV and myocardial O_2 demand.

Increased by:

- Pre-load
- Nerves (sympathetic stimulation increases contractility as well as heart rate)
- Hormones (the following all increase contractility: adrenaline, thyroxine, glucagon)
- Drugs (inotropic)

The following all decrease contractility:

- Hypoxia
- Ischaemia and cardiac disease
- Acidosis and alkalosis
- Parasympathetic stimulation mainly by suppressing the SA node
- Electrolyte imbalance K^+, Ca^{2+}
- Reduced filling (Starling's law)
- Drugs (anaesthetics)

Measured indirectly via:

- Stroke volume and cardiac output
- Ejection fraction (echocardiography) (70%)

After-load
Ventricular wall tension required to eject stroke volume in systole.

Increased by:

- Aortic stenosis
- Raised SVR as in shock
- Increased ventricular volume (greater tension to contract, Laplace's law)
- Increased after-load increases cardiac work and oxygen consumption

Decreased by:

- Vasodilator drugs
- Vasodilator mediators as in septic shock

Heart rate

All heart muscle cells can depolarise, but the shape of the action potential varies between cells as discussed previously in section 2 of this chapter.

Cells of the SA and AV nodes, as well as the cells of the Purkinje conducting system have the ability to depolarise themselves (self-excitation: a process causing automatic rhythmical contraction) at regular intervals, thereby initiating a wave of depolarisation which passes throughout the heart. This ability is referred to as automaticity (pacemaking ability).

This slow spontaneous depolarisation of the membrane potential is due to slow inward calcium conductance. Repolarisation occurs following increased potassium conductance when the calcium channels close.

The cells of the SA node have the highest frequency of self-depolarisation, followed by the cells of the AV node, with the Purkinje system cells having the lowest frequency. The ventricular rate is around 40 b.p.m.

These cells have a long refractory period (a period following depolarisation during which any further depolarisation cannot take place). This means that the cells with the highest frequency of firing (the SA node) will therefore control the rate at which the entire heart depolarises (and hence controls the rate at which the heart beats). It follows that a denervated heart will continue to beat (eg this is seen after heart transplantation). Transplanted hearts increase rate via circulating adrenaline, but atropine (vagal block) has no effect on heart rate.

If the SA node cells fail to function, the cells with the next highest frequency (those in the AV node) will take over the pacemaking function of the heart. The SA node is normally slowed physiologically by vagal activity and accelerated by sympathetic hormones and innervation.

Conduction through the heart can be disturbed by disease processes (eg ischaemia, infarction) or by drugs (eg digoxin, adenosine).

Regulation of heart rate

The heart rate is controlled by the autonomic nervous system.

- **Sympathetic** nerve fibres (from C8 to T5) cause noradrenaline release at nerve endings, which acts on cardiac β-receptors, increasing heart rate and force
- **Parasympathetic** nerve fibres (in vagus nerves) cause acetylcholine release at nerve endings, acting on muscarinic receptors, causing a slowing of heart rate

Parasympathetic control predominates (therefore causing 'normal' heart rate to be 60–80, despite an intrinsic rate of 100 b.p.m.).

Control of the blood pressure

In a nutshell ...

- In the short-term blood pressure is controlled by neurological mechanisms with reflexes that can detect abnormalities and respond rapidly
- Long-term control and regulation of the blood pressure occurs by the regulation of blood volume by the kidney

Short-term regulation of BP

Short-term changes in blood pressure (a timeframe of seconds to minutes) are mediated by the autonomic nervous system.

Arterial BP sensors

Mean arterial pressure is monitored by baroreceptors primarily in the aortic arch and carotid sinus. They mediate rapid responses to changes in blood pressure (eg getting up from a chair) and their failure results in conditions like postural hypotension.

These are the sensors for two temporally different (but integrated) reflex pathways which act as feedback loops. Information from the baroreceptor is transmitted to the medulla oblongata where the vasomotor centre and the cardio-inhibitory control centre lie and the efferent response originates.

The vasomotor centre predominantly activates sympathetic nerves to increase the BP:

- Increases heart rate and contractility to increase CO
- Releases noradrenaline to cause vasoconstriction and venoconstriction which increases SVR and decreases hydrostatic pressure in the capillaries (favouring fluid resorption from the interstitium and thus volume expansion)

The cardio-inhibitory centre activates vagal parasympathetic nerves to slow the heart, reduce the cardiac output and decrease the blood pressure.

Increases in arterial pressure results in decreased sympathetic outflow to the vasculature (decreasing systemic resistance) and increased parasympathetic stimulation to the heart (decreasing the heart rate).

Decreased arterial blood pressure increases sympathetic outflow to the vasculature (increasing systemic resistance) and decreases parasympathetic stimulation to the heart (increasing the heart rate).

The range in which these two types of baroreceptor are active is slightly different: carotid sinus baroreceptors have a lower range of 60–180 mmHg and aortic arch baroreceptors detect higher pressures of 90–200 mmHg. Persistent elevation of the blood pressure results in re-setting of the baroreceptor range and blunting of the response.

Venous BP sensors

Baroreceptors located in the great veins, atria and pulmonary trunk are stretch receptors sensitive to changes in blood volume rather then pressure. Increased stretch of these receptors reduces sympathetic outflow and promotes vasodilation. Additionally, the Bainbridge reflex results in a decrease in heart rate when the stretch receptors in the right atrium detect higher blood volumes.

Chemoreceptors

Chemoreceptors found in the aortic and carotid bodies are predominantly sensitive to tissue oxygen and carbon dioxide levels. Low arterial pressure results in poor tissue perfusion and activation of these receptors which promote vasoconstriction in order to increase SVR.

Hormonal control of the BP

Catecholamines: sympathetic stimulation to the adrenal medulla results in the secretion of catecholamines (adrenaline/epinephrine and noradrenaline/norepinephrine) which cause increased heart rate, contractility and vasoconstriction

Antidiuretic hormone (ADH): is released from the posterior pituitary causing vasoconstriction and renal water reassertion to increase the blood volume.

Long-term regulation of the BP

Long-term changes in blood pressure (hours to days) are primarily mediated by humoral factors that control blood volume by regulating sodium and water retention. The reflex pathways are described below.

The renin–angiotensin–aldosterone axis

Decreased arterial BP is sensed as decreased renal blood flow by the juxtaglomerular apparatus (JGA) of the nephron. The JGA secretes renin, a proteolytic enzyme, which acts on pro-angiotensin as shown in Fig. 3.2e. High sympathetic outflow also causes an increase in renin secretion.

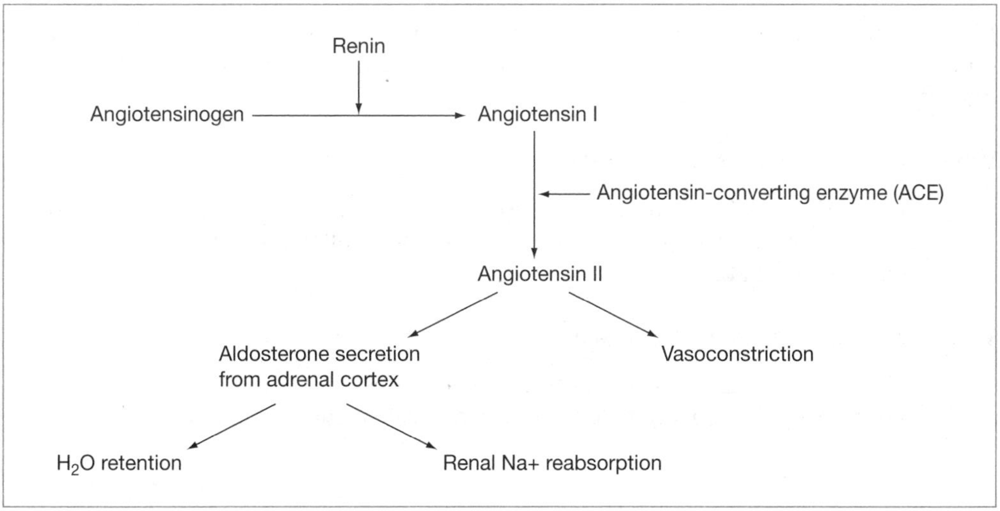

Figure 3.2e *The renin–angiotensin–aldosterone axis*

Natriuretic peptides

Blood volume changes also promote the release of atrial natriuretic peptide (ANP) from the right atrium. A second natriuretic peptide (brain natriuretic peptide, or BNP) is synthesised within the ventricles (as well as in the brain where it was first identified). BNP is apparently released by the same mechanisms that release ANP, and it has similar physiological actions. This peptide is used as a clinical diagnostic marker for heart failure. Natriuretic peptides are involved in the long-term regulation of sodium and water balance, blood volume and arterial pressure. This hormone decreases aldosterone release by the adrenal cortex, increases glomerular filtration rate (GFR), produces natriuresis and diuresis (potassium sparing), and decreasesrenin release thereby decreasing angiotensin II. These actions contribute to reductions in volume and therefore central venous pressure (CVP), cardiac output, and arterial blood pressure.

Pressure, flow, and volume changes in the heart: The cardiac cycle

Main features of the cardiac cycle

The cardiac cycle comprises the mechanical and electrical events during a single cycle of contraction and relaxation.

When left atrial pressure (LAP) exceeds left ventricular pressure (LVP) the left ventricle fills. Period of rapid filling:

- First third: diastolic rapid filling
- Second third: slow filling directly from venous system though atria
- Final third: atrial contraction (responsible for 25% filling)

In fast atrial fibrillation, ventricular filling and cardiac output is compromised particularly on induction of anaesthesia, hence every effort must be made to reduce the rate to < 100 prior to surgery.

When the left ventricle contracts, LVP rises:

- When LVP > LAP the mitral valve closes
- When LVP > aortic pressure the aortic valve opens, allowing blood to flow from the ventricle to the aorta

When LV is relatively empty and relaxing, LVP falls:

- When LVP < aortic pressure the aortic valve closes
- When LAP > LVP (again) the LV fills and the cycle begins again

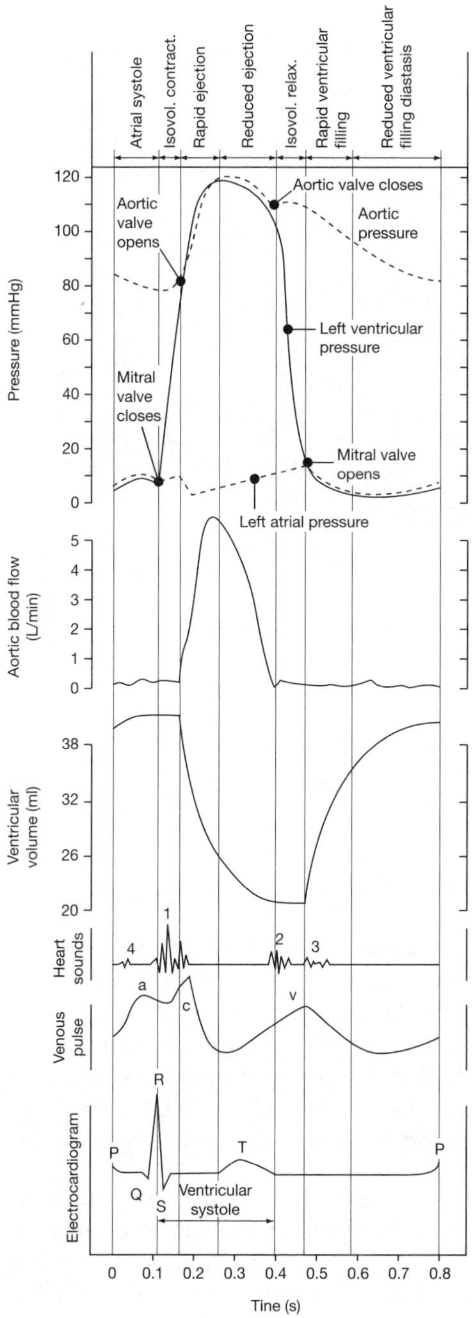

Figure 3.2f *Events in the cardiac cycle*

Normal values for aortic and intracardiac pressures

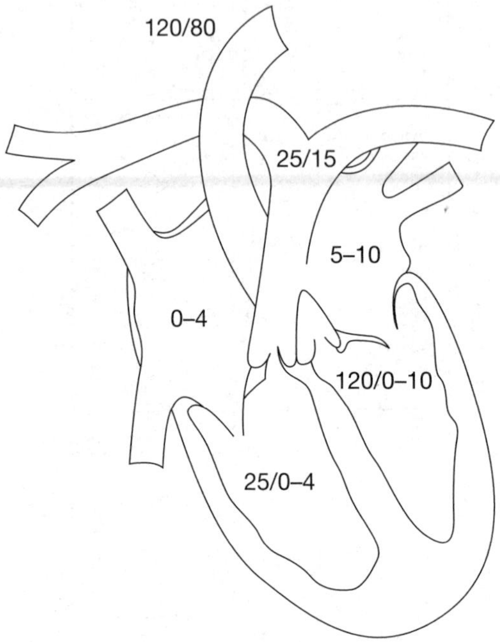

Figure 3.2g *Cardiac catheter measurements (as mmHg)*

The coronary circulation

The most important determinant of coronary blood flow and myocardial perfusion is aortic pressure. However, during systole, ventricular contraction causes compression of the coronary vessels, reducing or even briefly reversing the flow of blood to the myocardium. Most of the perfusion to the left ventricle therefore occurs in diastole, and so the diastolic aortic pressure is also important in coronary perfusion. The diastolic time is also important, hence at fast rates inadequate myocardial perfusion occurs. The direction of flow is from the outer surface inwards, therefore the sub-endocardial region is vulnerable to ischaemia.

Normally, autoregulation of coronary blood flow occurs by changes in the calibre of the coronary resistance vessels; this is in response to changes in myocardial activity and metabolic demand. It is thought to be mediated by the release of vasodilator metabolites. The coronary arteries are 'end arteries' thus occlusion will lead to ischaemia or infarction of the myocardium.

If, however, there is a slowly developing partial occlusion (eg due to atherosclerosis) a collateral circulation can develop to a degree, but this can never compensate for reduced flow through 'main' vessels.

3.3 THE ELECTROCARDIOGRAM AND CARDIAC CONDUCTION

Electrocardiography and cardiac conduction

The heart has three different types of excitatory tissue: atrial muscle, ventricular muscle and the specialised conducting system. The heart also has a large number of mitochondria. This means that energy for heart muscle function can be continuously generated via aerobic metabolism.

Cardiac muscle is striated and contains actin and myosin filaments which contract in the same manner as described for skeletal muscle. Depolarisation starts with an influx of sodium ions and slower voltage-gated calcium channels open at the same time. Repolarisation occurs with the influx of K^+ ions. The relationship between these ions and the action potential is shown in Fig. 3.3a.

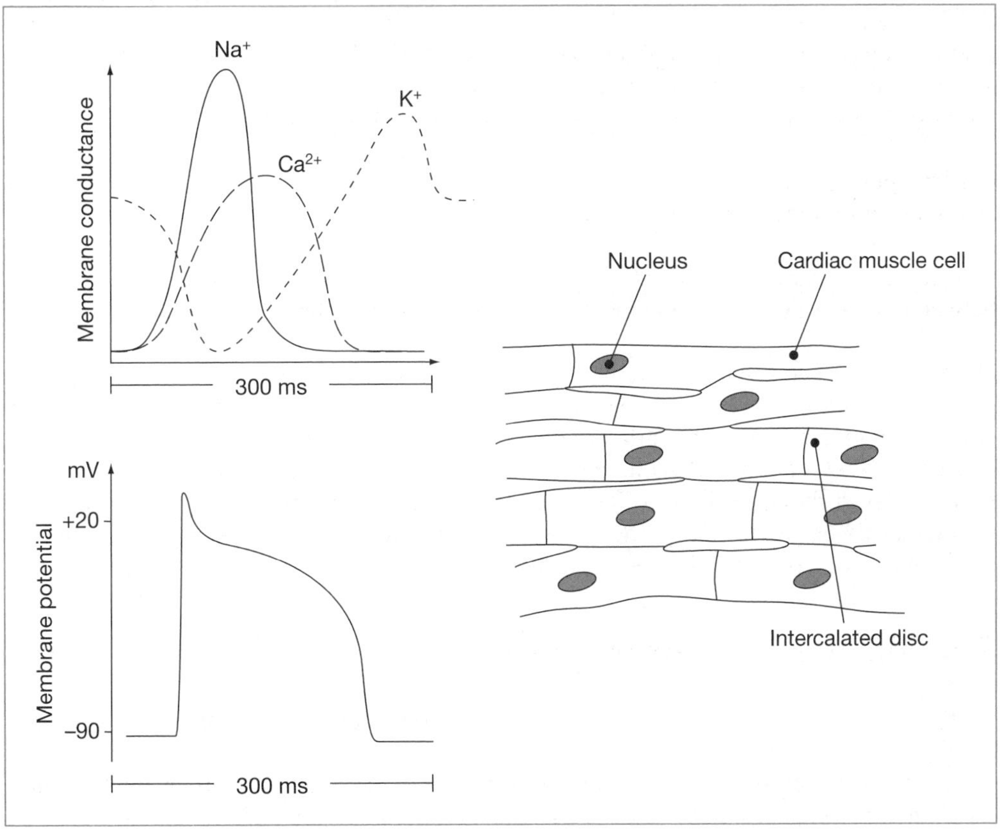

Figure 3.3a *The cardiac muscle showing (A) intracellular ion concentrations during depolarisation, (B) the action potential with characteristic plateau (maintained by Ca^{2+} ions), and (C) the muscle structure as a syncytium*

Rhythmical spontaneous depolarisation occurs in cardiac tissue. The sinoatrial (SA) and atrioventricular (AV) nodes of the heart have the highest rates of spontaneous activity but the cardiac muscle itself has intrinsic activity. No stimulus is necessary to cause depolarisation in these cells. This is because the cell membrane is relatively leaky to Na^+ ions. As Na^+ ions leak into the cell, the resting potential rises and depolarisation occurs spontaneously.

In addition to the release of Ca^{2+} ions into the sarcoplasm, large quantities of extra Ca^{2+} ions also diffuse into the tubules (tubules of cardiac muscle have a diameter 5 times greater than skeletal muscle, with a volume 25 times greater). Free intracellular calcium ions are the most important factor in regulating the contractility of the myocardium.

Increased intracellular calcium will **increase** the force of myocardial contraction

Decreased intracellular calcium will **decrease** the force of myocardial contraction

Many drugs that increase cardiac muscle contractile force involve increasing intracellular calcium. For example, cardiac glycosides inhibit the sodium pump and the myocyte responds by pumping out Na^+ in exchange for Ca^{2+}. This loads the myocyte with calcium and increases the force of contraction when the cell depolarises. Catecholamines also increase the calcium influx to the myocyte, whereas acidosis reduces it.

Cardiac muscle fibres are made up of individual cardiac muscle cells connected in series as a syncytium. Ions (and therefore current) can travel very easily through the intercalated disc between the cells. The heart consists of two separate syncytiums: the atria and the ventricles. These two syncytiums are separated by fibrous tissue and current passes between the two along the specialised conducting system of the AV bundle.

The SA node lies in the right atrium near to the SVC. Impulses are conducted through the atrial syncytium to the AV node which lies in the atrial septum. This has a slower rate of conduction to ensure that the atria are fully contracted in order to pump-prime the ventricles before they contract as well. The conducting system or bundle of His transmits the impulses in Purkinje fibres through the left and right bundles that ramify through the ventricular tissue. Abnormal pathways developing between the two syncytiums result in arrhythmias and Wolff–Parkinson–White syndrome.

The electrocardiogram (ECG)

- Records the sum of the electrical impulses generated by the heart during depolarisation and contraction
- Provides information on the rate and rhythm of heart contraction, as well as information on pathological processes (eg infarction, inflammation)
- A standard ECG consists of 12 'leads', best thought of as extensions of the direction of electrical flow from the heart, which can be measured. A positive deflection on the ECG (upwards) shows that depolarisation is conducted towards that electrode and vice versa

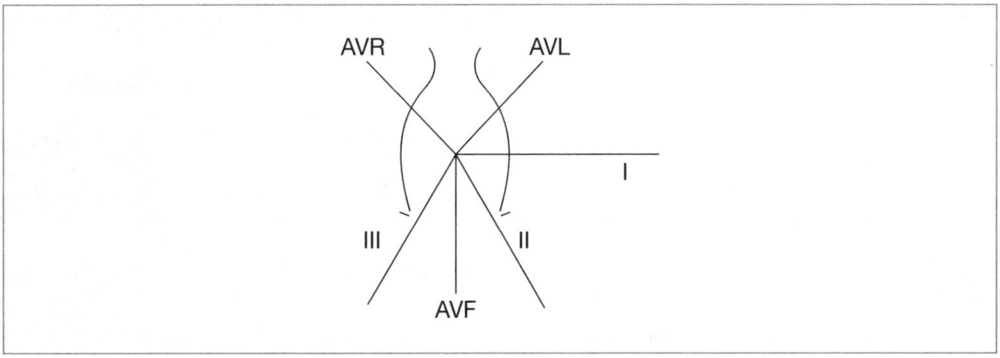

Figure 3.3b *12-lead ECG. The 6V leads look at the heart in a horizontal plane from the front and left side*

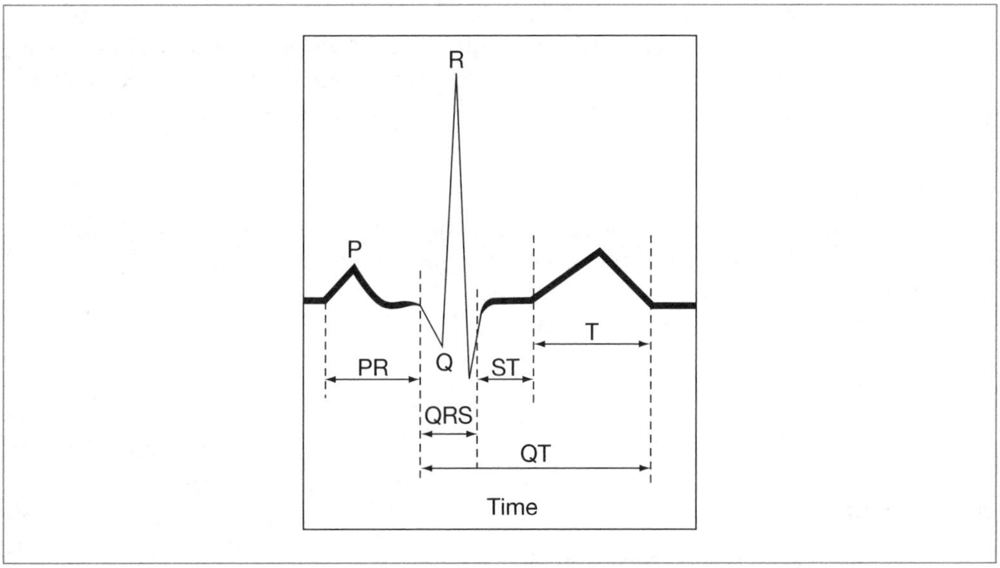

Figure 3.3c *The important deflections and intervals of a typical ECG*

The waveform produced by one (normal) heart contraction is shown. Different parts of the waveform have their own name and are related to different physiological actions occurring within the heart.

Parts of the ECG waveform and their normal dimensions

P wave

- Depolarisation of the atria
- < 2.5 mm height
- > 0.1 second duration
- Repolarisation is hidden within the QRS

QRS complex

- Depolarisation of the ventricles
- If first deflection is downwards it is called a **Q wave**
- First upward deflection (whether preceded by a Q wave or not) is called the
- **R wave**, and usually has increasing amplitude from V1 to V6
- First downward deflection after the R wave is called the **S wave**
- The QRS should be < 0.10 seconds (three small squares) in duration
- An S wave in lead I suggests right-axis deviation, an S wave in lead II suggests left-axis deviation. Normal axis is –30 to +90
- A wide QRS (> 0.12) occurs when depolarisation does not pass down the Purkinje fibres as in bundle branch block and complexes of ventricular origin (ectopics and 3rd-degree block)

PR interval

- Represents the (normal) conduction delay between the atria and the ventricles
- Should be three to five small squares (0.12–0.20 seconds)
- Greater than 0.2 seconds shows 1st-degree block
- A variable PR occurs in 2nd-degree blocks

T wave

- Represents repolarisation of the ventricles

ST segment

- The line between the S wave and the T wave
- Usually isoelectric (ie level with the baseline of the ECG)
- May be elevated acutely when myocardial infarction is present
- May be depressed when myocardial ischaemia is present

NB: The ST segment may be normal, despite presence of either infarction or ischaemia

Rhythm recognition

Rate
> 100: tachycardia
< 60: bradycardia

QRS width
< 0.12 sec: narrow complex (supra-ventricular origin)
> 0.12 sec: broad complex

Regularity
Regularly irregular: ectopics; 2nd-degree block
Irregularly irregular: atrial fibrillation

P-wave activity
Absent in AF, flutter, nodal, VT

P relations to QRS
Not in ventricular ectopics or complete heart block

3.4 CARDIAC FAILURE AND CARDIOGENIC SHOCK

Cardiac failure

The clinical features of cardiac failure are discussed in Chapter 6 *Peri-operative Care*.

Cardiac failure is the inability of the heart to supply adequate blood flow and therefore oxygen delivery to peripheral tissues and organs.

Coronary artery disease is the main cause of cardiac failure. Reduction in coronary blood flow and oxygen delivery to the myocardium results in hypoxia, which then leads to impaired cardiac function. Another common cause of heart failure is myocardial infarction. Infarcted tissue does not contribute to the generation of mechanical activity so the rest of the cardiac muscle must work harder to compensate for the loss of function. Valvular disease and congenital defects place increased demands upon the heart that can precipitate failure. Cardiomyopathies, myocarditis and chronic arrhythmias can also precipitate failure.

External factors precipitating heart failure include increased afterload (pressure load; eg uncontrolled hypertension), increased stroke volume (volume load; eg arterial–venous shunts), and increased body demands (high-output failure; eg thyrotoxicosis, pregnancy).

Cardiogenic shock

Pathophysiology of cardiogenic shock

Cardiogenic shock is sustained hypotension with tissue hypoperfusion despite adequate left ventricular filling. It is usually due to acute MI but may occur in sepsis syndromes, with drug toxicity, pulmonary embolism, or as part of multiorgan failure.

Myocardial ischaemia causes a decrease in contractile function, which leads to left ventricular dysfunction and decreased arterial pressure; these, in turn, exacerbate the myocardial ischaemia. The end result is a vicious cycle that leads to severe cardiovascular decompensation.

A systemic inflammatory response syndrome-type mechanism has also been implicated in the pathophysiology of cardiogenic shock. Elevated levels of white blood cells, body temperature, complement, interleukins, and C-reactive protein are often seen in large myocardial infarctions. Similarly, inflammatory nitric oxide synthetase (iNOS) is also released in high levels during myocardial stress. iNOS induces nitric oxide production, which may uncouple calcium metabolism in the myocardium resulting in a stunned myocardium. Additionally, iNOS leads to the expression of interleukins, which may themselves cause hypotension.

Symptoms and signs of cardiogenic shock

Cardiogenic shock is characterised by high cardiac filling pressures, high systemic resistance, and low cardiac output.

- Patients are usually in extremis
- LVF: florid pulmonary oedema and dyspnoea
- RVF: distended neck veins
- Haemodynamic compromise: hypotensive, tachycardic, pallor, with signs of poor cerebral and renal perfusion
- Signs related to underlying cause (eg arrhythmias, murmurs)

Management of cardiogenic shock

Cardiogenic shock requires critical care management.

- Ventilatory support with 100% oxygen (NIPPV may be appropriate)
- Inotropic support (adrenaline/epinephrine increases cardiac output and maintains peripheral vasoconstriction)
- Arrhythmia control
- If the systolic BP is good, pre-load can be reduced using nitrate infusions
- Acute myocardial ischaemia may respond to thrombolysis or emergency angioplasty
- An intra-aortic balloon pump may be inserted through the femoral artery as a holding measure

3.5 VENOUS ACCESS IN CRITICAL CARE

In a nutshell ...

Venous access may be achieved:

Peripherally: by insertion of cannulae into peripheral veins of the extremities (includes venous cut-down)

Centrally: by insertion of cannula through the peripheral system into a central large bore vessel

Peripheral venous access

In most patients requiring venous access for IV medication or fluids, a peripheral vein is the appropriate route. Peripheral venous cannulation may be a life-saving procedure in hypovolaemic shock.

Cannula sizes range from 12 G (the largest, for rapid infusion in hypovolaemia) down to 24 G (the smallest, for children).

NB: Flow is proportional to r^4 (where r is the radius of the lumen of the needle). High flow requires a large bore.

Indications and contraindications for peripheral access

Indications for peripheral venous access

- Fluid/blood infusion
- Blood sampling
- Drug administration
- Central venous line via peripheral route
- Peripheral venous feeding

Contraindications for peripheral venous access

- Local sepsis
- Puncture of potential A-V fistula sites in haemodialysis patients

Complications of peripheral venous access

- Infection
- Thrombophlebitis (usually chemical; eg erythromycin, cytotoxic agents)

- Accidental arterial cannulation
- Subcutaneous haematoma
- Extravasation (may just cause oedema, but cytotoxic agents can cause considerable tissue damage)

Common sites used for peripheral venous access

- Dorsum of hand
- Median basilic, median cephalic, basilic veins at antecubital fossa (avoid in haemodialysis patients)
- External jugular vein
- Femoral vein
- Long saphenous vein at the ankle (avoid in patients with coronary artery disease)
- Dorsum of foot
- Scalp veins in infants or neonates

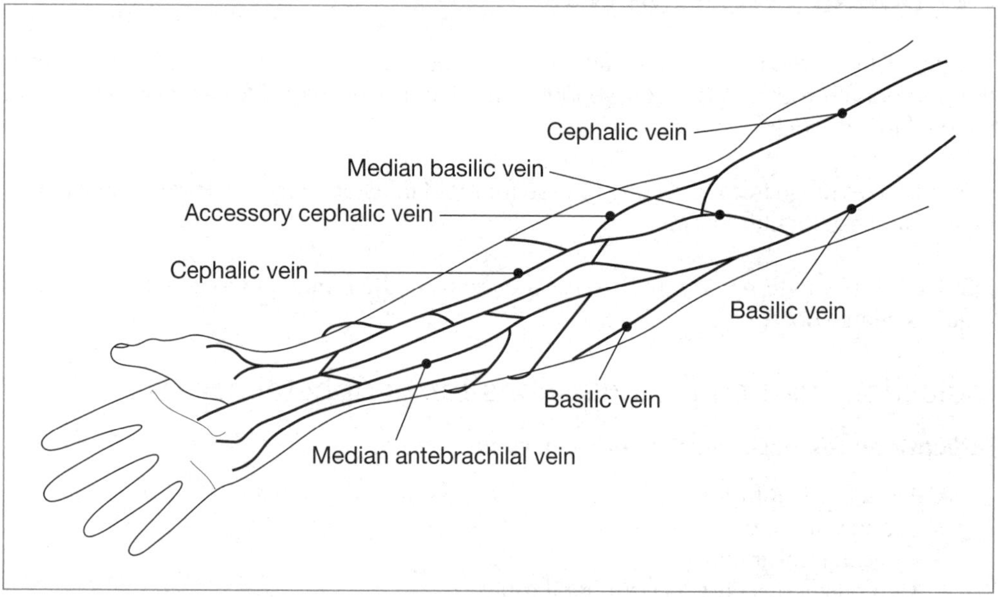

Figure 3.5a *Peripheral venous access – veins of the forearm*

Venous cut-down

Patients in hypovolaemic shock often have collapsed peripheral veins resulting in difficult cannulation. In such circumstances rapid access can be gained by open cut-down onto a vein and cannulation. The most common veins used for this are the antecubital veins and the long saphenous vein. Of the antecubital veins, the median basilic vein is most commonly used. It is found 2 cm medial to the brachial artery.

Procedure box: Venous cut-down

Indications

IV access in cases of circulatory collapse when attempts to establish peripheral venous access have failed

Useful in trauma, burns and children

Patient positioning

Supine, with medial side of the ankle exposed

Procedure

Prepare the ankle on the medial side with antiseptic and drapes

Infiltrate LA into the skin over the long saphenous vein (unless immediate access is required)

Make a transverse incision 1–2 cm anterior to the medial malleolus

Using blunt dissection, isolate the vein and free it from surrounding tissue

Ligate the distal end of the mobilised vein

Pass a tie around the proximal aspect of the vein

Make a small transverse venotomy

Dilate this with closed haemostatic forceps

Insert a large bore cannula and secure it with the proximal tie

Close the wound with interrupted sutures and apply a sterile dressing

Post-op

Standard wound care

Observe for infection

Complications

Haemorrhage due to lack of vascular control

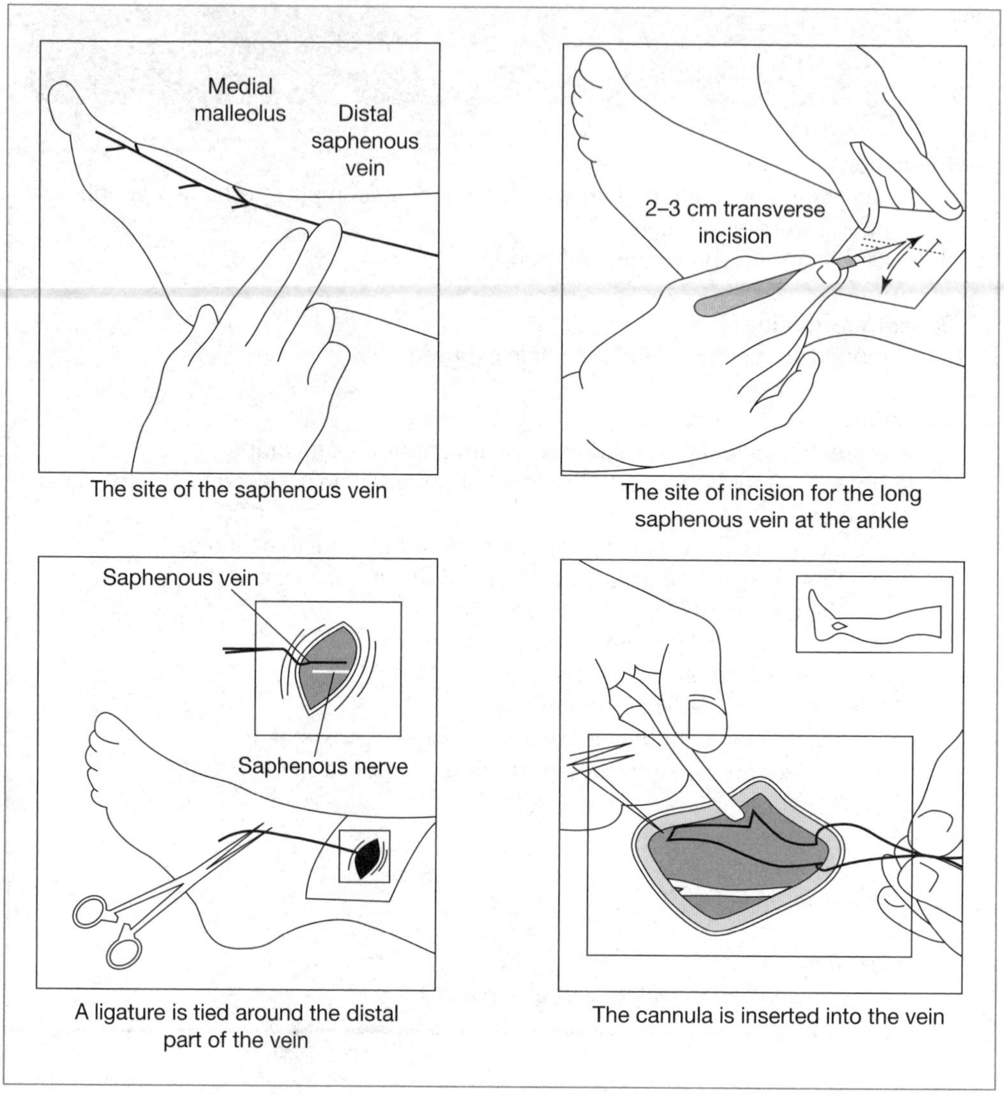

Figure 3.5b *Venous cut-down into long saphenous vein*

Central venous access

Central venous cannulation is a potentially dangerous procedure, particularly in a hypovolaemic patient, and should only be performed by (or supervised by) an experienced practitioner.

Central venous catheters may reach the SVC or right atrium via the basilic, cephalic, subclavian, external and internal jugular veins. The commonest sites are the subclavian and internal jugular veins. Insertion of catheters into the IVC via the long saphenous or femoral veins is associated with a high incidence of DVT and PE and should only be considered as a last resort.

Catheters may be introduced with the 'through cannula' technique, whereby a short plastic cannula is first introduced into the vein, thus:

- Needle introduced into vein
- Cannula advanced over needle and needle withdrawn
- Catheter inserted through cannula and cannula withdrawn

The Seldinger technique uses a flexible metal guidewire as an intermediate step to prevent the catheter coiling up on itself inside the vein:

- Needle introduced into vein
- Guidewire advanced through needle and needle withdrawn
- Catheter advanced over guidewire and guidewire withdrawn

Catheters may be Teflon or silastic – silastic catheters more expensive, but induce less reaction, are more flexible, and are most suitable for long-term central venous access. Wide-bore silastic catheters (single, double, or triple) (eg Hickman) are suitable for long-term parenteral nutrition or chemotherapy are introduced percutaneously or surgically and skin tunnelled (to reduce catheter-related sepsis) to an exit site on the chest wall.

Central venous anatomy

Catheters are usually inserted percutaneously, but may be placed under direct vision after surgical exposure of the vein.

The subclavian vein

The axillary vein continues as the subclavian vein as it crosses the outer border of the 1st rib behind the clavicle, and it ends behind the sterno-clavicular joint where it joins the IJV to form the brachiocephalic vein. It is closely related to the subclavian artery above and behind it and to the dome of the pleura below and behind it. The thoracic duct enters the brachiocephalic vein at its origin on the left and cannulation of the right side is therefore probably safer.

The internal jugular vein (IJV)

As the IJV runs down in the neck, it comes to lie lateral to the internal and common carotid arteries deep to sternomastoid muscle and joins the subclavian vein to form the brachiocephalic vein behind the sterno-clavicular joint. The vein may be punctured from three sites: the posterior border of sternomastoid muscle, the anterior border of sternomastoid muscle, and near its lower end between the two heads of the sternomastoid muscle – the first route is the most commonly used.

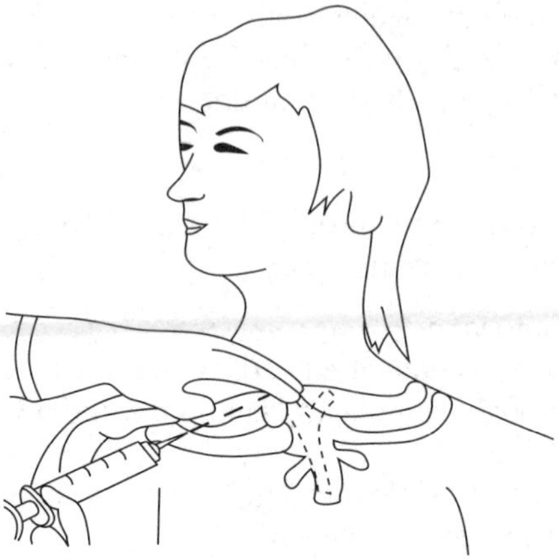

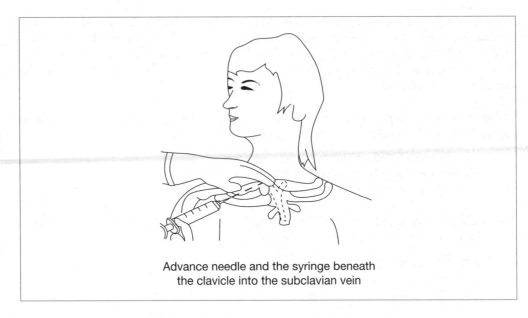

Advance needle and the syringe beneath the clavicle into the subclavian vein

Figure 3.5c *Access to the subclavian vein*

Insertion of central venous access

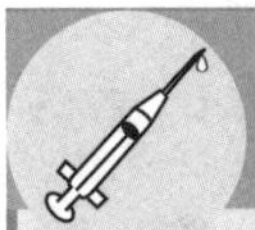

Procedure box: Central venous access

Indications

- Fluid infusion
- Drug infusion
- Cytotoxic drugs which would damage peripheral veins
- Inotropic drugs
- TPN (hypertonic solution would damage peripheral veins)
- Pacemaker electrode insertion
- Monitoring of central pressures (eg CVP, pulmonary artery pressure)

Contraindications

- Local sepsis
- Severe coagulation disorders

Patient positioning

- The patient should be supine, with arms by the side, head turned to the opposite side
- Prepare all your equipment and only then place the patient head down, just before you start the procedure

Procedure (Seldinger technique)

You will need:

- Skin preparation
- 10 mL of plain LA in a 10 mL syringe with a blue needle attached
- 10 mL of normal saline in a 10 mL syringe with a green needle attached (you must be able to differentiate between the syringe containing anaesthetic and the one containing saline)
- 10 mL of normal saline to flush the line at completion
- A CVP line kit complete with large-bore needle, guidewire, dilator and CVP line
- Small scalpel blade
- Silk suture and fixative dressings

Prepare the CVP line itself by opening all the taps on the three lumens and flushing the line through with normal saline to remove the air

Close all the taps except the lumen that the guidewire will emerge through (commonly marked with a brown bung)

Position your patient. Patients should be supine with a head-down tilt of 20–30 degrees to prevent air embolism. Make sure that you have prepared all equipment *before* tilting the patient, because the critically ill may not tolerate this position for long periods. The procedure should be performed under aseptic technique so glove and gown and drape the patient with sterile drapes

After infiltration of LA, and using the syringe filled with saline, introduce the green needle through the skin

Subclavian approach

Immediately below the junction of the lateral third and medial two-thirds of the clavicle. Advance the tip towards the supra-sternal notch, 'walking' the needle tip along the under surface of the clavicle.

Internal jugular approach

Palpate the sternocleidomastoid muscle and place the fingertips of your left hand on the pulsatile right carotid artery. You can gently displace the artery medially as you introduce the needle at the mid-point of the anterior border of the sternocleidomastoid muscle. Direct the needle tip away from your fingers (protecting the artery) and towards the ipsilateral right nipple of the patient. The needle should be angled at 30° to the skin surface.

Technique for line insertion for both approaches

Aspirate gently as the needle advances, until there is free aspiration of blood, indicating that the vein has been entered. You now know the depth and location of the vein

Attach the syringe to the large-bore needle and follow the track of the green needle with the large-bore needle until blood is aspirated easily

Leaving the large-bore needle in the vein, detach the syringe and advance the guidewire through the needle, checking that it advances freely, with no obstruction, then remove the needle over the guidewire

Make a small nick in the skin with a scalpel blade at the site of entry and dilate up the tract by passing the dilator over the guidewire

Railroad the catheter over the guidewire (you must always hold on to the distal part of the guidewire by the patient's neck until the proximal end emerges from the lumen of the catheter)

Check that the catheter advances freely with no obstruction, to its required length (usually about 20 cm)

Remove the guidewire, suture the catheter to the adjacent skin, and check that blood can be aspirated freely from all lumens. Flush the line with normal saline

Post-procedure

Take a CXR in expiration to exclude a pneumothorax and to check the catheter tip is in the optimal position (SVC or right atrium).

Complications of central venous catheterisation

Complications of insertion

- Pneumothorax
- Haemothorax (due to laceration of intrathoracic vein wall)
- Puncture of adjacent artery causing subcutaneous haematoma, A-V fistula or aneurysm
- Thoracic duct injury
- Brachial plexus damage
- Cardiac complications (arrhythmias, perforation of right atrium)
- Malposition of the catheter (eg into neck veins, axillary vein or contralateral veins)

Complications of use

- Catheter-related sepsis
- Catheter occlusion
- Catheter embolisation (due to migration of detached catheter)
- Central vein thrombosis

Subcutaneously implanted vascular access systems

These consist of a stainless steel (Port-a-Cath™) or plastic (Infuse-a-Port™) reservoir with a silicone septum buried in a subcutaneous pocket and connected to a silastic central venous catheter. Access to the reservoir is with a percutaneous needle which pierces the self-sealing septum without coring. Used for long-term antibiotics or chemotherapy.

Intra-osseous puncture

This is an emergency technique.

Procedure box: Intra-osseous puncture

Indication

Used in emergency situations in children aged 6 years or younger in whom venous access by other means has failed on two attempts.

Contraindications

- Local sepsis
- Ipsilateral fractured extremity

Complications

- Misplacement of the needle (this usually involves incomplete penetration of the anterior cortex or over penetration, with the needle passing through the posterior cortex)
- Epiphyseal plate damage
- Local sepsis
- Osteomyelitis

Technique of intra-osseous puncture

- Identify the puncture site – approximately 1.5 cm below the tibial tuberosity on the antero-medial surface of the tibia
- Clean and drape the area
- If patient is awake infiltrate the area with LA
- Direct the intra-osseous needle at 90° to the antero-medial surface of the tibia
- Aspirate bone marrow to confirm the position
- Inject with saline to expel any clot and again confirm the position; if the saline flushes easily with no swelling the needle is correctly placed
- Connect the needle to a giving set and apply a sterile dressing

Post-procedure

Discontinue as soon as reliable venous access has been established.

3.6 CARDIOVASCULAR MONITORING AND SUPPORT IN CRITICAL CARE

Non-invasive cardiovascular monitoring

The most important aspects of monitoring for the majority of patients are:

Pulse
Pulse character – palpable radial pulse suggests BP of > 90 mmHg
Capillary refill time – compress 5 seconds, usually < 2 seconds
Skin temperature (warm or cold)
Skin colour
Respiratory rate – increased
Urine output – 0.5 mL/kg minimum. Aim for 1 mL/kg
Mental state (anxiety, aggression, obtunded, coma)

Adjuncts to non-invasive monitoring

- **BP:** cuff width should be 40% of circumference of the limb. Systolic BP becomes inaccurate in shock, but mean arterial pressure (MAP) measured with automated devices is reliable
- **ECG:** 3-lead. Lead II is best as P wave is optimal for rhythm assessment and easier to see ischaemia
- **Pulse oximetry:** measures oxygen saturation by absorption of light wavelengths in fingertip. Demonstrates heart rate, perfusion and arterial Hb saturation. Normal around 97%; below 90% there is risk of severe hypoxaemia as steep part of oxygen dissociation curve. Inaccurate when cold peripheries, severe shock, nail varnish, and carbon monoxide poisoning

Invasive cardiovascular monitoring

CVP monitoring

Uses of central venous cannulation in the ITU include:

- **Monitoring:** CVP, passage of PA catheter
- **Infusion of drugs:** multi-lumen catheters usually used
- **Haemofiltration:** 8.5 Fr double lumen
- **Parenteral feeding:** tunnelled lines are best to reduce sepsis
- **Fluid challenge:** assess the response to a bolus of fluid (eg 250 mL)

Fluid challenge

The CVP is more useful as a trend in response to the rapid administration of 250 mL of colloid rather than as an absolute number. The fluid challenge assesses the compliance of the vascular system. The end point is return of normal BP and urine output or a filled vascular system. Overfilling with poor BP usually requires inotropic or vasopressor support.

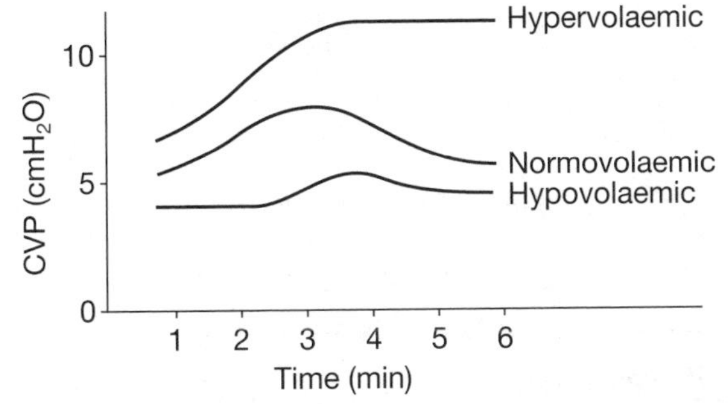

Figure 3.6a *Changes in CVP in response to an IV fluid bolus*

CVP lines are NOT normally used for initial resuscitation (eg in trauma) as placement of the line takes time, has complications, and fluid infusion through the line is slow compared to a big peripheral cannula. However a large-bore short cannula inserted centrally (such as a 12 or 14 G or a 8.5 Fr Swan introducer catheter) allows very rapid infusion.

Infection control

Risk of infection is least with subclavian, then internal jugular, and finally femoral. There is no evidence for routine changes of lines within 30 days unless there are local signs of infection. If systemic sepsis, then blood cultures should be taken from both the line and peripherally, if positive then remove line. Send the tip for culture. PA catheters should be removed after 5 days, and peripheral lines after 72 hours.

Transducer systems

CVP can be measured using a manometer, but electromechanical transducer systems are easier and more accurate and allow continuous measurement. They convert the mechanical energy of a pressure into an electrical signal by the changing of the capacitance or resistance through a flexible conductor.

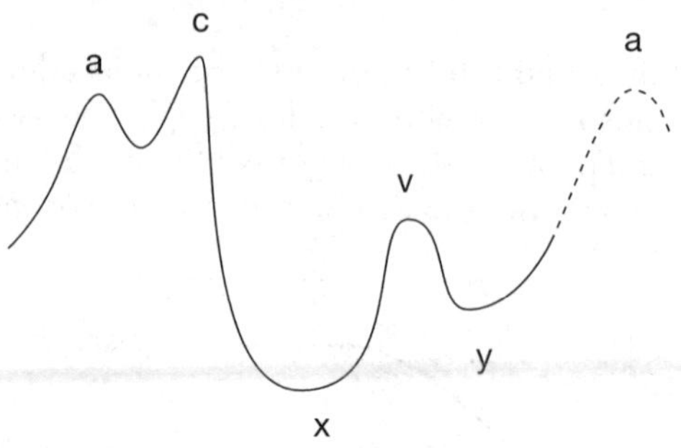

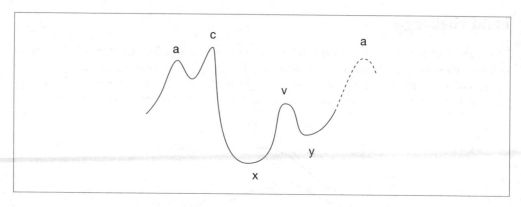

Figure 3.6b *CVP waveform*

Elements of CVP waveform

a	Atrial systole	AV valve open
c	Contraction of ventricle (carotid pulse)	AV valve closed
v	Filling of atria	AV valve closed
x	Ventricles relax	AV valve closed
y	AV valve opens	

The CVP waveform swings with respiration. In inspiration it dips if spontaneous breathing, and increases if ventilated (and vice versa).

Pulmonary artery catheter (Swan–Ganz catheter) monitoring

Generally, CVP (the pre-load of the right side of the heart) also fairly accurately reflects the pre-load of the left side of the heart. There are some situations where the CVP does not accurately reflect the left-sided filling pressures (eg pulmonary hypertension, right ventricular infarction, tricuspid valve disease).

In this situation, it is necessary to measure left atrial pressure. This is done by passing a pulmonary artery flotation catheter (a catheter with an air-filled balloon near the end) into a central vein and feeding it in (guided by the characteristic pressure waveforms of different parts of the central circulation) until it is 'wedged' in a distal branch of the pulmonary artery.

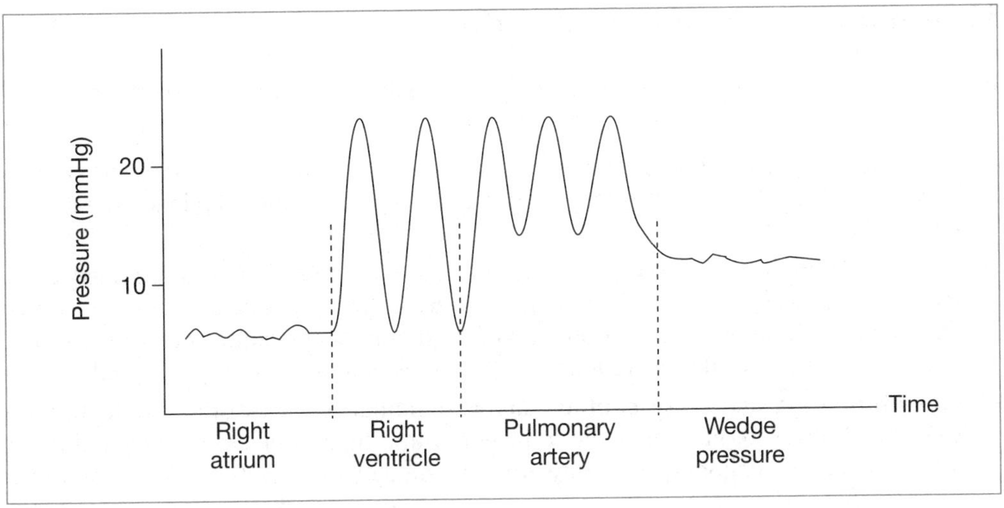

Figure 3.6c *Pressure waves as catheter is passed through the heart*

When wedged, the pressure distal to the balloon is a close reflection of the pressure in the left atrium. This pressure reading (pulmonary artery wedge pressure, PAWP) can be used in the same way as the CVP to guide fluid replacement. The balloon is deflated between readings to avoid pulmonary infarction.

It can be used to measure cardiac output by the thermodilution method (Fick principle) and, once this is known, it can be used with other cardiovascular measurements (CVP, PAWP, MAP, PAP) to calculate the SVR, PVR (pulmonary vascular resistance) and ventricular stroke work. A bolus (10 mL) of cold dextrose is injected and a thermistor at the catheter tip measures a temperature drop proportional to cardiac output. Knowledge of the cardiac output and SVR is sometimes useful in helping to determine if a critically ill patient who is in shock has a myocardial, hypovolaemic or septic (vasodilatory) cause, and for guiding inotrope therapy. Other measurements include oxygen delivery and consumption.

Fick principle (classically using oxygen consumption VO_2)

Cardiac output (CO) = $VO_2 / CaO_2^- - CvO_2$

$$\text{Organ blood flow} = \frac{\text{Amount of marker substance taken up by organ}}{\text{Concentration difference between supply and drainage}}$$

Measurement of cardiac output (CO)

Pulmonary artery catheters were the first reliable monitors for CO in the ITU. Once CO is measured the SVR can be calculated from data from an arterial line and CVP lines.

- **Continuous CO from PA catheter:** rather than using a cold bolus of fluid as indicator, a coil around the catheter warms the blood as it flows past and the drop in temperature is analysed continuously
- **PiC CO:** thermodilution from cold fluid injected via a CVP line and analysed via a modified arterial line containing a thermistor. By a double-indicator method it shows continuous CO, intrathoracic blood volume, and pulmonary extravascular lung water. From the latter two values the requirement for fluids or inotropes can be judged
- **Lithium dilution and pulse contour analysis:** similar to Fick's principle technique using small doses of lithium as the indicator with a lithium electrode attached to an arterial line. This calibrates the software, which calculates continuous CO by pulse wave analysis
- **Echo Doppler:** measures blood flow in the aorta via an oesophageal probe, hence gives indication of contractility and CO. Patients need to have a patent oesophagus and be sedated to use this technique. From the Doppler waveform, CO and contractility can be deduced
- **Echocardiography:** by visualisation of the ventricle by a trained operator shows filling, myocardial wall motion and ejection fraction (EF is normally 50–70%). May be used trans-thoracic or oesophageal

Arterial line monitoring

A 20 G cannula within an artery (usually the radial) allows optimal continuous measurement of arterial BP. It is also useful if multiple blood gas measurements are needed.

Complications of insertion of arterial lines

Haemorrhage/haematoma
Ischaemia
Aneurysm/AV fistula
Accidental drug injection
Infection
Thrombosis
Distal limb arterial occlusion

Cardiovascular support

In a nutshell ...

The principles of cardiovascular support in circulatory failure follow the **VIP rule**:
V entilate
I nfuse
P ump

Aim to maximise blood flow to vital organs by means of:
Appropriate fluid management
Drugs

Ventilate – Infuse – Pump (VIP)

Ventilate

- ABC rule of resuscitation
- Improve oxygenation and gas exchange
- Reduce O_2 demand to respiratory muscles, up to 30% of cardiac output
- Control acidosis by CO_2 control

Infuse

- Always ensure adequate filling prior to vasoactive support (Starling's)
- Fluid challenge using invasive monitoring
- Use of colloids as tighter dose response relationship

Fluids: The crystalloid–colloid controversy

Crystalloids

Consist of salt ions in water
Of the volume infused, about one-third stays intravascular and two-thirds pass to ECF, hence risk of tissue oedema
Examples: normal saline, Hartmann's solution
Advantage: ECF fluid deficit in shock is replaced

Colloids

Consist of osmotically active particles in solution
Expand plasma volume by volume infused

May leak into interstitium in capillary leak syndrome
Examples: Gelofusine™, Haemaccel™ (gelatine-based, half-life about 4 hours)
Dextrans (degraded dextrose; interfere with cross-matching)
Starches (long half-life in some cases; 10% solutions hyperoncotic hence increase plasma volume more than volume infused; some may have benefit in reducing capillary leak syndrome)
Albumin (pasteurised; suppresses albumin synthesis; normally some albumin leaks through the capillary membrane)
Blood (plasma reduced has haematocrit of about 70%)

A combination of crystalloids and colloids is probably the best approach.

Dextrose-containing fluids are not useful for volume replacement because they only replace water, which as the sugar is metabolised, re-distributes to intracellular and extra-cellular compartments. The dextrose allows water to be isotonic for IV infusion.

Potassium is replaced at a maximum rate of 20 mmol/hour in a monitored ITU environment. In hypokalaemic patients this reflects a large total intracellular deficit.

Magnesium replacement should be considered, aiming for a serum level of 1 mmol/L.

Volume expanding fluids should be considered separately from maintenance fluids. See section 2 of this chapter for further detail on maintenance of fluid balance.

Pump

The first priority in shock of any cause is to restore perfusion pressure; the second is to optimise cardiac output.

Blood pressure

- Aim for MAP > 60 or SBP > 90 mmHg (elderly people often require higher pressure to perfuse vital organs eg brain, kidney)
- An adequate pressure should maintain urine flow
- If SVR is low then a vasopressor such as noradrenaline (norepinephrine) is indicated to improve perfusion pressure
- Vasoconstriction may mask hypovolaemia, therefore closely monitor filling pressures and cardiac output

Cardiac output

- Drugs may be used to increase cardiac output by positive inotropic effect or for a specific effect on an organ system (eg renal and mesenteric blood flow is increased by dopexamine infusion at rate of 0.5–1 μg/kg/min. No evidence for prevention of renal failure)
- Monitor effect via DO_2, lactate, pH_i, urine output, cardiac output

Cardiac drugs

Inotropes: increase force of ventricular contraction (usually β effect)
Lusiotropes: enhance myocardial relaxation
Vasopressors: vasoconstrict blood vessels (α effect)
Vasodilators: vasodilate blood vessels (arterial, venous or both)
Chronotropes: increase heart rate (β effect)

Usually infused in μg/kg/min. Dose ranges and individual effects are unpredictable in the critically ill patient.

- **Adrenaline (epinephrine):** inotrope, vasopressor, chronotrope. Activates β-receptors, increasing intracellular cAMP. Low-dose β effects mostly, becoming more α at high doses. β_2 effects cause vasodilatation in skeletal muscle beds, lowering SVR
- **Dobutamine:** inotrope, vasodilator. Synthetic. Predominant β_1 effect increases heart rate and force of contraction, and hence cardiac output. Mild β_2 and α effects overall causing vasodilatation
- **Dopamine:** up to 5 μg/kg/min has dopamine receptor activity causing renal dilatation. 5–10 μg has mostly β inotropic effect. Above 15 mg has mostly α vasoconstrictive effect. Unpredictable ranges in different patients. Problems with dopamine include:
    - Gut ischaemia
    - Growth hormone suppression, immunosuppression
- **Dopexamine:** mesenteric and renal vasodilatation via dopamine receptors, and also has β_2 effects. Synthetic. Anti-inflammatory effect. May protect the gut against ischaemia in the presence of vasoconstrictors. Used at dose of 0.5–0.9 mg/kg/min for mesenteric protection
- **Noradrenaline (norepinephrine):** vasopressor effect predominates. Mild inotropic β_1. Increases SVR to improve perfusion pressure but may suppress organ and skin perfusion due to capillary vasoconstriction. Used to increase perfusion pressure in septic shock
- **Isoprenaline:** chronotrope used to increase heart rate in heart block while awaiting pacing. β_1 and β_2 effects
- **Phosphodiesterase inhibitors:** milrinone, enoximone. Increase intracellular cAMP by decreasing its breakdown. Increase inotropic and vasodilatation (inodilator and lusiotropic). Increased cardiac output, lowered PAOP and SVR, but no significant rise in heart rate or myocardial oxygen consumption
- **Vasodilators**
- **Hydralazine:** mostly arterial vasodilatation; to control BP
- **Nitroprusside:** arterial vasodilator with short half-life given as infusion
- **Nitrates:** venodilators, reducing pre-load

Cardiopulmonary bypass is used to support the cardiovascular system during certain types of surgery (eg cardiothoracic surgery and diversion of flow from the IVC and liver during transplantation). It is discussed in the *Cardiothoracics* chapter of Book 2.

3.7 CARDIOPULMONARY RESUSCITATION

International guidelines are produced by the European Resuscitation Council and were last updated in December 2005 – see http://www.resus.org.uk/. For latest guidelines liaise with your local Resuscitation Officer and obtain practical training. All hospital clinical staff must be proficient in basic life support (BLS).

In a nutshell ...

Cardiac arrest is defined as absence of a palpable pulse. It is classified as shockable or non-shockable.

Shockable cardiac arrest

Ventricular fibrillation (VF)
Pulseless ventricular tachycardia (VT)

Non-shockable cardiac arrest

Asystole, no electrical activity
Pulseless electrical activity (PEA) is an ECG rhythm compatible with a pulse, but pulse is absent (also referred to as electromechanical dissociation, EMD)

Common arrest rhythms

The commonest out-of-hospital cardiac arrest is VF due to ischaemic heart disease and myocardial infarction. This rhythm is treatable by defibrillation as rapidly as possible which stops the arrhythmia, puts the patient into transient asystole, allowing a sinus rhythm to re-start. The chances of successful defibrillation decline by 7–10% for each minute that the arrhythmia persists, as myocardial energy reserves are depleted.

The commonest in-hospital cardiac arrests are mostly asystole or PEA caused by continued cardio-respiratory deterioration. Recognition of the sick patient and early instigation of organ support such as oxygen, ventilatory and circulatory management, can prevent arrest and death.

Main causes of PEA cardiac arrest are the following 4 Hs and 4 Ts

H ypoxia	**T** ension pneumothorax
H ypovolaemia	**T** amponade
H ypothermia	**T** hrombo-embolism
H ypokalaemia, hyperkalaemia, hypocalcaemia	**T** oxicity

Important points in advanced life support (ALS)

- Check pulse and breathing:
  - A (Airway) Establish an airway and intubate to improve oxygenation and prevent aspiration
  - B (Breathing) Give oxygen and start ventilation
  - C (Compression) Start chest compressions at rate of 100/minute. Ratio of 30 compressions to 2 ventilations in single-rescuer and two-rescuer CPR. If intubated, chest compressions should be continuous
- Establish IV access and give adrenaline/epinephrine 1 mg by the IV route or 2–3 mg diluted to 10 mL via tracheal tube (causes peripheral vasoconstriction to improve coronary and cerebral perfusion). Repeat every 3–5 minutes
- Monitor ECG and consider the actions in the table below
- Continue chest compressions and administration of adrenaline/epinephrine every 3 minutes
- Return of spontaneous circulation (ROSC): ventilate if required, 12-lead ECG, CXR, blood gases, U&Es, FBC. ITU support

RECOMMENDED RESPONSES TO ECG RHYTHM ABNORMALITIES

Rhythm	Action
Ventricular fibrillation (VF) Pulseless ventricular tachycardia (VT)	Defibrillate 200 J, 200 J, 360 J Give amiodarone 300 mg (in 20 mL dextrose) for refractory shockable rhythms, followed by a further 150 mg and infusion at 1 mg/min for 6 h Lidocaine may be used as an alternative to amiodarone Vasopressin (40 units) may be used as an alternative to adrenaline/epinephrine Magnesium (8 mmol) should be given for refractory VF if there is any suspicion of hypomagnesaemia
Asystole (if there is any doubt that the diagnosis might be fine VF rather than asystole, treat as VF)	Atropine 3 mg IV or 6 mg via the tracheal tube (in a volume of 10–20 mL) can be given to provide total blockade of the vagus nerve
Pulseless electrical activity (PEA)	Check 4 Hs and 4 Ts for reversible causes – treat appropriately

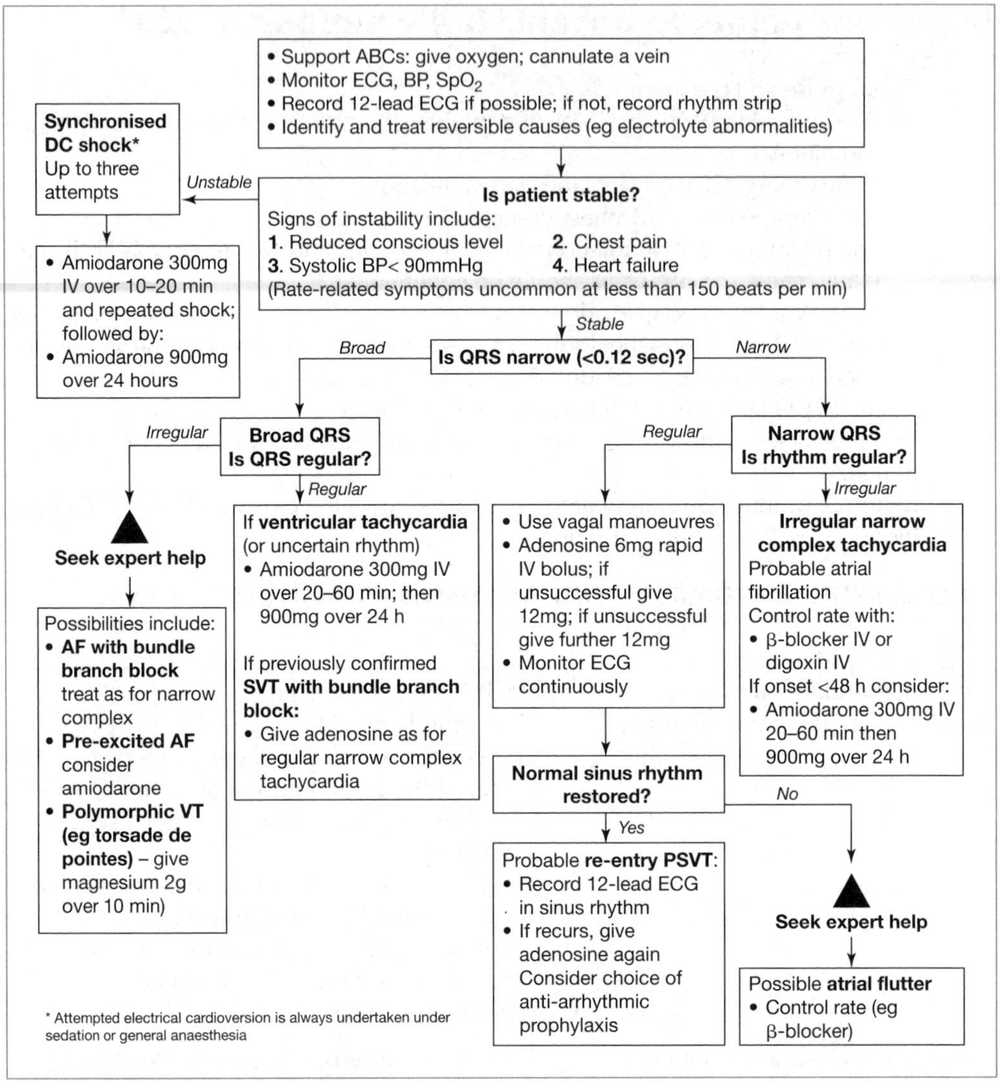
• Support ABCs: give oxygen; cannulate a vein
• Monitor ECG, BP, SpO2
• Record 12-lead ECG if possible; if not, record rhythm strip
• Identify and treat reversible causes (eg electrolyte abnormalities)
Is patient stable?
Signs of instability include:
1. Reduced conscious level
2. Chest pain
3. Systolic BP< 90mmHg
4. Heart failure
(Rate-related symptoms uncommon at less than 150 beats per min)
Unstable
Synchronised DC shock* Up to three attempts
• Amiodarone 300mg IV over 10–20 min and repeated shock; followed by:
• Amiodarone 900mg over 24 hours
Stable
Is QRS narrow (<0.12 sec)?
Broad
Narrow
Broad QRS Is QRS regular?
Irregular
Seek expert help
Possibilities include:
• AF with bundle branch block treat as for narrow complex
• Pre-excited AF consider amiodarone
• Polymorphic VT (eg torsade de pointes) – give magnesium 2g over 10 min)
Regular
If ventricular tachycardia (or uncertain rhythm)
• Amiodarone 300mg IV over 20–60 min; then 900mg over 24 h
If previously confirmed SVT with bundle branch block:
• Give adenosine as for regular narrow complex tachycardia
Narrow QRS Is rhythm regular?
Regular
• Use vagal manoeuvres
• Adenosine 6mg rapid IV bolus; if unsuccessful give 12mg; if unsuccessful give further 12mg
• Monitor ECG continuously
Normal sinus rhythm restored?
Yes
Probable re-entry PSVT:
• Record 12-lead ECG in sinus rhythm
• If recurs, give adenosine again
Consider choice of anti-arrhythmic prophylaxis
No
Seek expert help
Possible atrial flutter
• Control rate (eg β-blocker)
Irregular
Irregular narrow complex tachycardia
Probable atrial fibrillation
Control rate with:
• β-blocker IV or digoxin IV
If onset <48 h consider:
• Amiodarone 300mg IV 20–60 min then 900mg over 24 h
* Attempted electrical cardioversion is always undertaken under sedation or general anaesthesia

Figure 3.7a *Advanced life support – Tachycardia algorithm (with pulse) (from Resuscitation Council Guidelines)*

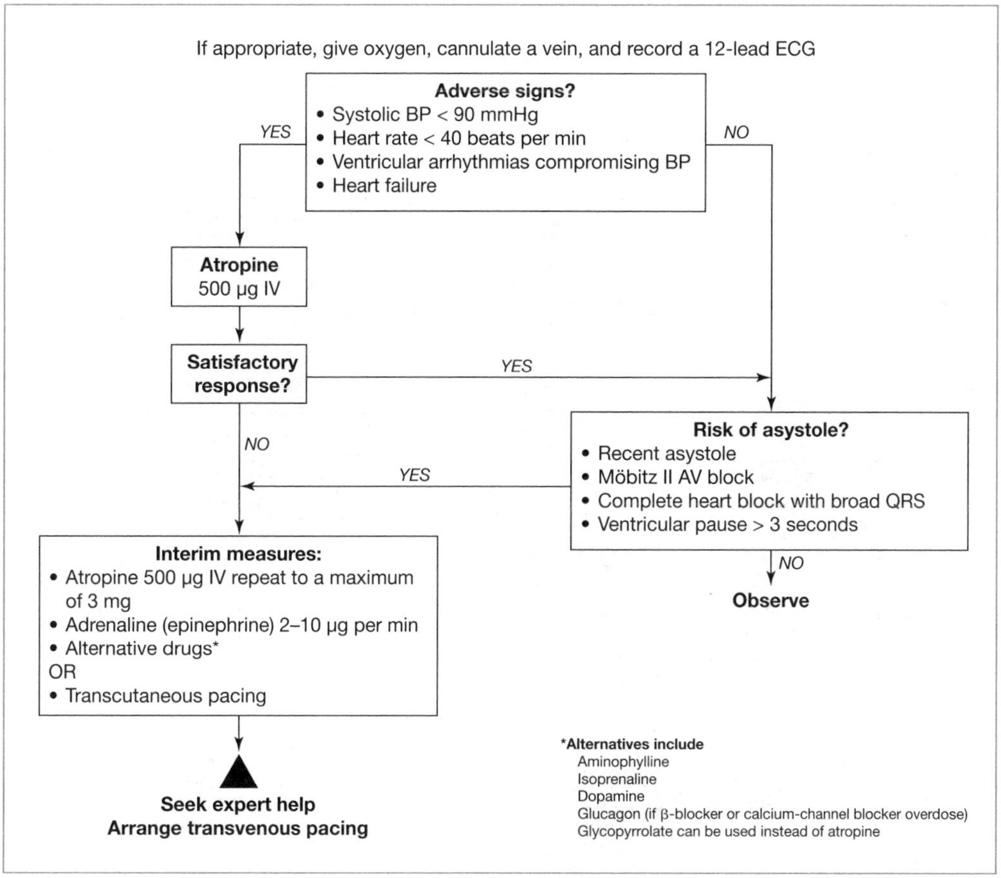
If appropriate, give oxygen, cannulate a vein, and record a 12-lead ECG
Adverse signs?
• Systolic BP < 90 mmHg
• Heart rate < 40 beats per min
• Ventricular arrhythmias compromising BP
• Heart failure
YES
NO
Atropine
500 μg IV
Satisfactory response?
YES
NO
Risk of asystole?
• Recent asystole
• Möbitz II AV block
• Complete heart block with broad QRS
• Ventricular pause > 3 seconds
YES
NO
Observe
Interim measures:
• Atropine 500 μg IV repeat to a maximum of 3 mg
• Adrenaline (epinephrine) 2–10 μg per min
• Alternative drugs*
OR
• Transcutaneous pacing
Seek expert help
Arrange transvenous pacing
*Alternatives include
Aminophylline
Isoprenaline
Dopamine
Glucagon (if β-blocker or calcium-channel blocker overdose)
Glycopyrrolate can be used instead of atropine

Figure 3.7b *Advanced life support – Bradycardia algorithm (includes rates inappropriately slow for haemodynamic state) (from Resuscitation Council guidelines)*

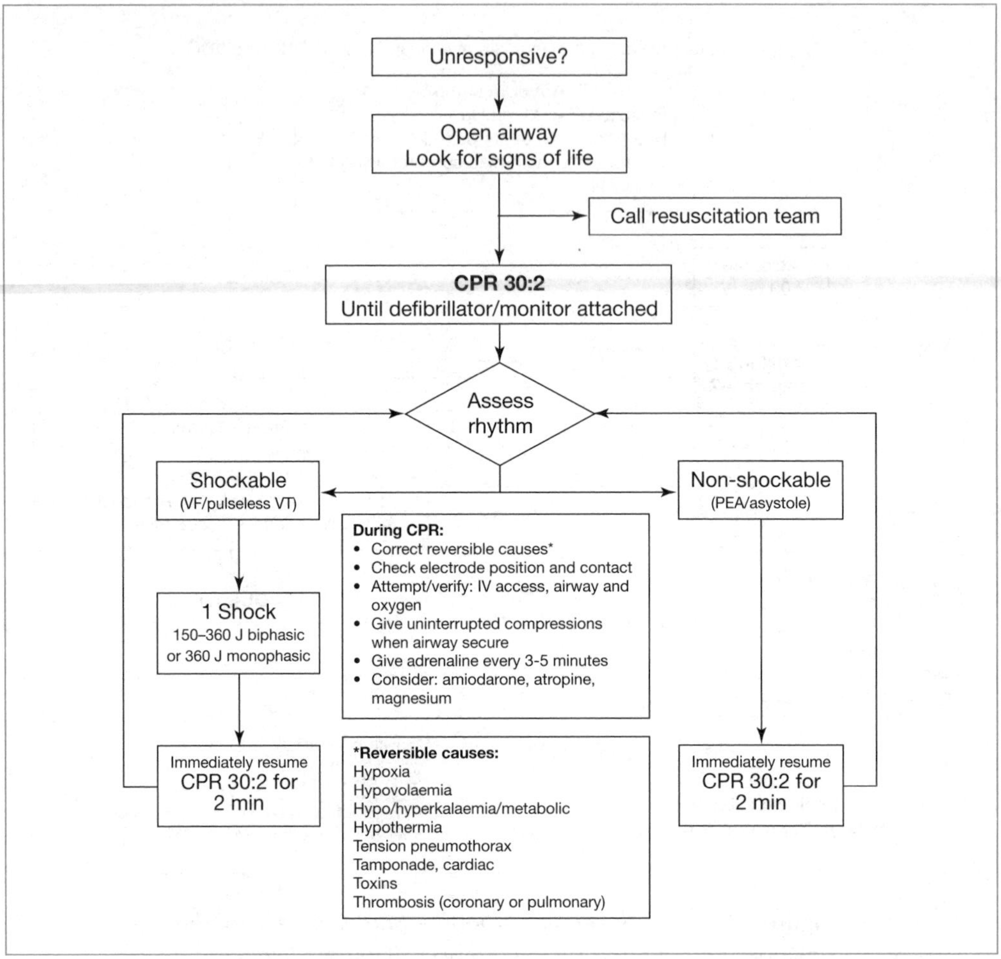

Figure 3.7c *Advanced life support – Adult advanced life support algorithm (from Resuscitation Council guidelines)*

Section 4

The respiratory system in critical care

4.1 ANATOMY OF THE THORAX AND LUNGS

Anatomy of the thorax

The thoracic cage

Sternum

This consists of three parts:

- **Manubrium:** jugular notch (upper concave margin); articulates with the clavicles, 1st costal cartilages and upper halves of 2nd costal cartilages; 1st costal cartilage joint is a primary cartilaginous joint (not synovial)
- **Body:** upper border is the manubrio-sternal symphysis, which is bridged by the 2nd costal cartilage; each lateral border has 5½ facets for articulation with costal cartilages 2–7
- **Xiphoid process:** posterior attachment of diaphragm; anterior attachment of rectus abdominus

Ribs

- **Head:** two facets for articulation with the two adjacent thoracic vertebrae (thoracic vertebra of the same number plus the one above) (NB: The 1st rib's head has just one facet for articulation with T1 only)
- **Neck:** the tubercle has one facet for articulation with transverse process of vertebra; the body continues anteriorly as the costal cartilage

Costal cartilages

- 1–7 articulate directly with the sternum
- 8, 9 and 10 run into one another and then into 7
- 11 and 12 float free

The intercostal spaces

Intercostal muscles

There are three muscle layers (as with the abdomen):

- **Outer:** external intercostal muscles (+ serratus posterior muscles and levator costae)
- **Middle:** internal intercostal muscles
- **Inner:** innermost intercostal muscles (+ transversus thoracis and subcostal muscles)

External intercostals

- Run obliquely downwards and forwards
- Replaced by the anterior intercostal membrane anteriorly

Internal intercostals

- Run downwards and backwards
- Complete anteriorly but replaced posteriorly by the posterior intercostal membrane

Innermost intercostals

- Cross more than one intercostal space
- Innermost layer includes transversus thoracis and subcostal muscles

Neurovascular bundle

- Between internal intercostals and innermost intercostals
- Under protection of the lower border of the ribs, hence drains or needles should always be sited above a rib

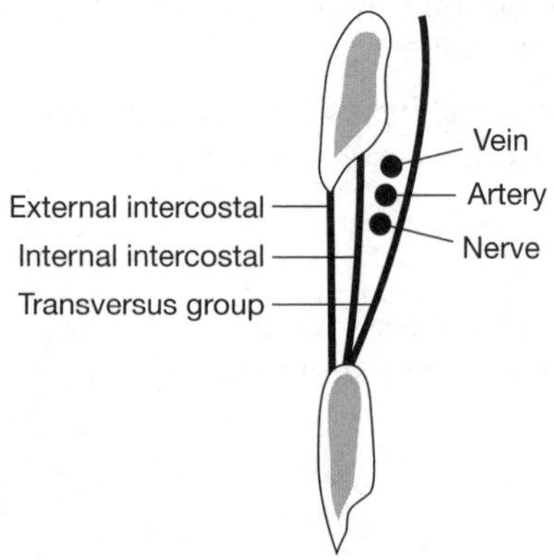

Figure 4.1a *Vertical section through an intercostal space*

Intercostal nerves

These derive from ventral primary rami of spinal nerves T1 to T11. There are three branches:

- Collateral branch
- Lateral cutaneous branch – anterior and posterior branches
- Anterior cutaneous branch

NB: The skin above the 2nd rib is supplied by supraclavicular branches of the cervical plexus, not by the 1st intercostal nerve.

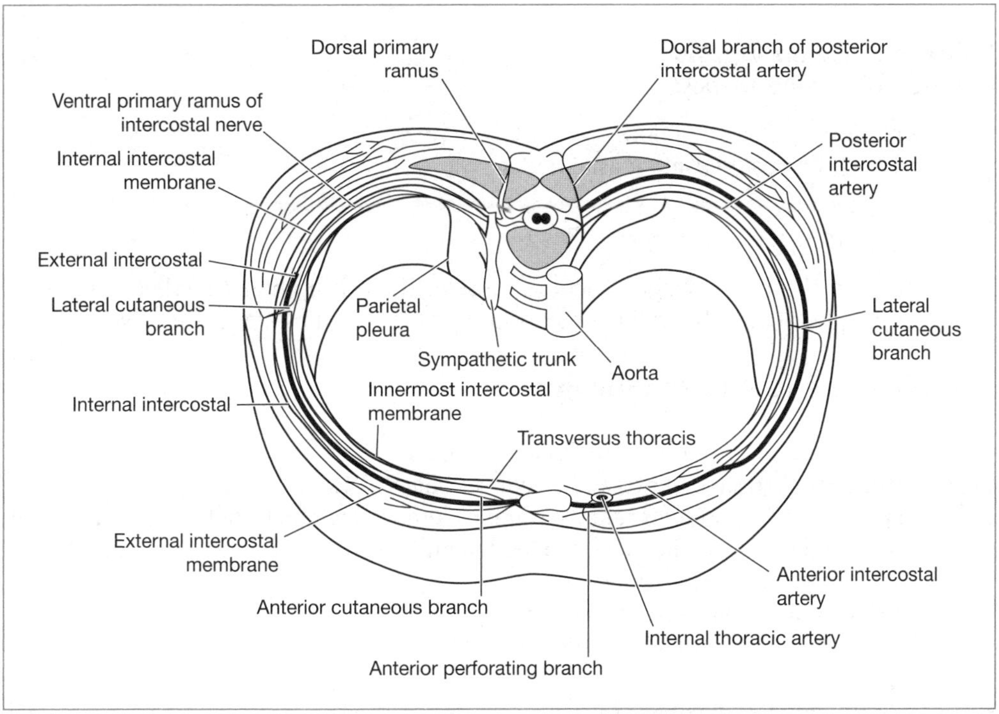

Figure 4.1b *Contents of an intercostal space*

Intercostal arteries

- Posterior intercostal arteries
  - Derived from the superior intercostal artery (from 2nd part of subclavian artery) in spaces 1 and 2
  - Derived directly from the descending aorta in spaces 3–11
- Anterior intercostal arteries
  - Derived from internal thoracic artery in spaces 1–6
  - From musculophrenic artery (continuation of above) in spaces 7, 8 and 9
  - Spaces 11 and 12 do not have an anterior intercostal artery

Intercostal veins

Each space has one posterior and two anterior veins. Posterior intercostal veins drain in different ways:

- Space 1: supreme intercostal vein
- Spaces 2 and 3: superior intercostal vein
- Space 4: either superior intercostal vein or azygos system
- Spaces 5–11: azygos system

Anterior intercostal veins drain into the internal thoracic or musculophrenic veins.

Intercostal lymph vessels

Drainage follows the arteries:

- Anteriorly: parasternal nodes
- Posteriorly: posterior intercostal nodes

The diaphragm

The diaphragm is a dome-shaped sheet of muscle. There is a central tendinous part and muscular peripheral part. The right dome (overlying the liver) lies higher than the left.

Attachments of the diaphragm

- **Sternal:** two slips of muscle to xiphoid process
- **Costal:** inner surface of ribs and costal cartilages 6–12
- **Vertebral:** right and left crura from upper lumbar vertebrae; right crus larger, from L1, L2 and L3; some fibres pass to the left and form a sling around the oesophagus; left crus from L1 and L2 only
- **Medial arcuate ligament:** thickening of psoas fascia
- **Lateral arcuate ligament:** thickening of lumbar fascia

Blood supply of the diaphragm

Intercostal arteries 7–11 and the subcostal artery supply the periphery. The main body is supplied by the right and left phrenic arteries (direct from aortic branches).

Nerve supply of the diaphragm

It is supplied by the right and left phrenic nerves (C3, C4 and C5) and the intercostal nerves (around the periphery).

Diaphragmatic openings

There are three main openings:

- **Aortic:** T12 level (behind the diaphragm and not actually in it)
- **Oesophageal:** T10 level (site of sliding hiatus hernia)
- **Vena cava:** T8 level (in the central tendon)

Other structures penetrating the diaphragm

- Phrenic nerves: right with the inferior vena cava, left through left dome
- Splanchnic nerves: with corresponding crus
- Sympathetic trunk: behind medial arcuate ligament
- Hemiazygos vein: left crus
- Superior epigastric vessels
- Lymph vessels

The trachea

This commences at the level of C6. It is held open by C-shaped 'rings' of cartilage. Trachealis muscle fills gap in the rings. It is divided into cervical and thoracic parts.

Cervical trachea

5 cm in length (but stretches during respiration).

Related structures are:

- Oesophagus (directly behind the trachea)
- RLNs (in the groove between the trachea and the oesophagus)
- Carotid sheath
- Thyroid (isthmus at 2nd, 3rd and 4th tracheal rings)
- Inferior thyroid veins
- Anterior jugular veins

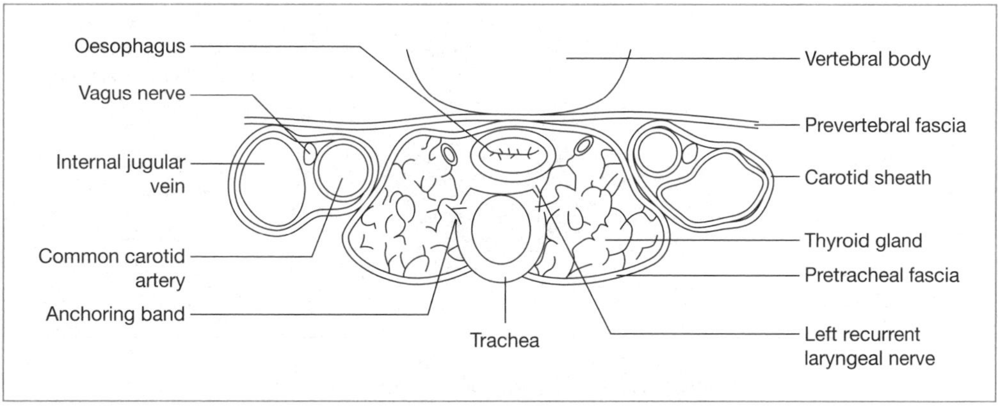

Figure 4.1c *Relations of the thyroid gland*

Thoracic trachea

5 cm in length (but stretches): begins at jugular notch of manubrium; bifurcates just below the manubrio-sternal angle (position is dependent on respiratory cycle).

Related structures are:

- Oesophagus
- Vagus and RLNs
- Manubrium
- Thymus
- Brachiocephalic veins
- Brachiocephalic trunk and common carotid arteries
- Pulmonary trunk and bifurcation
- Superior vena cava
- Azygos vein
- Cardiac plexus
- Tracheo-bronchial lymph nodes

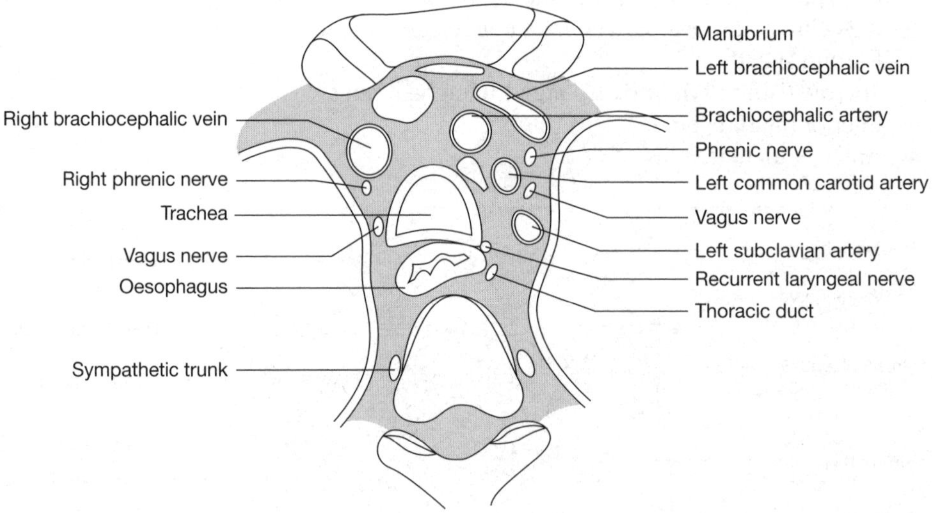

Figure 4.1d *Section of the mediastinum*

Blood supply of the trachea

It is supplied by the inferior thyroid and bronchial arteries.

Nerve supply of the trachea

The vagus and RLNs supply the mucous membrane. Parasympathetic (vagus) and sympathetic (upper ganglia of sympathetic trunk) supply the smooth muscle.

Lymph drainage of the trachea

This is by deep cervical and para-tracheal nodes.

The pleura

There are two layers separated by a small amount of fluid in a closed space. They couple the lungs and chest wall and allow the lungs to slide in the thorax during respiration.

Parietal pleura

- Outer layer covers the inside of the thoracic cavity
- Reflects around the root of the lung to be continuous with the visceral pleura

Visceral pleura

- The inner layer is firmly adherent to the surface of the lungs themselves
- The pulmonary ligament is a loose fold of pleura that hangs from the lung root allowing movement of the lung root during respiration

Nerve supply of the pleura

- Parietal pleura
  - Intercostal nerves
  - Phrenic nerves
- Visceral pleura
  - Autonomic innervation only

The lungs

- **Left lung:** two lobes separated by oblique fissure
- **Right lung:** three lobes separated by oblique and horizontal fissures

Lung roots

- Pulmonary artery lies superiorly
- Bronchus lies posteriorly
- Pulmonary veins lie inferiorly

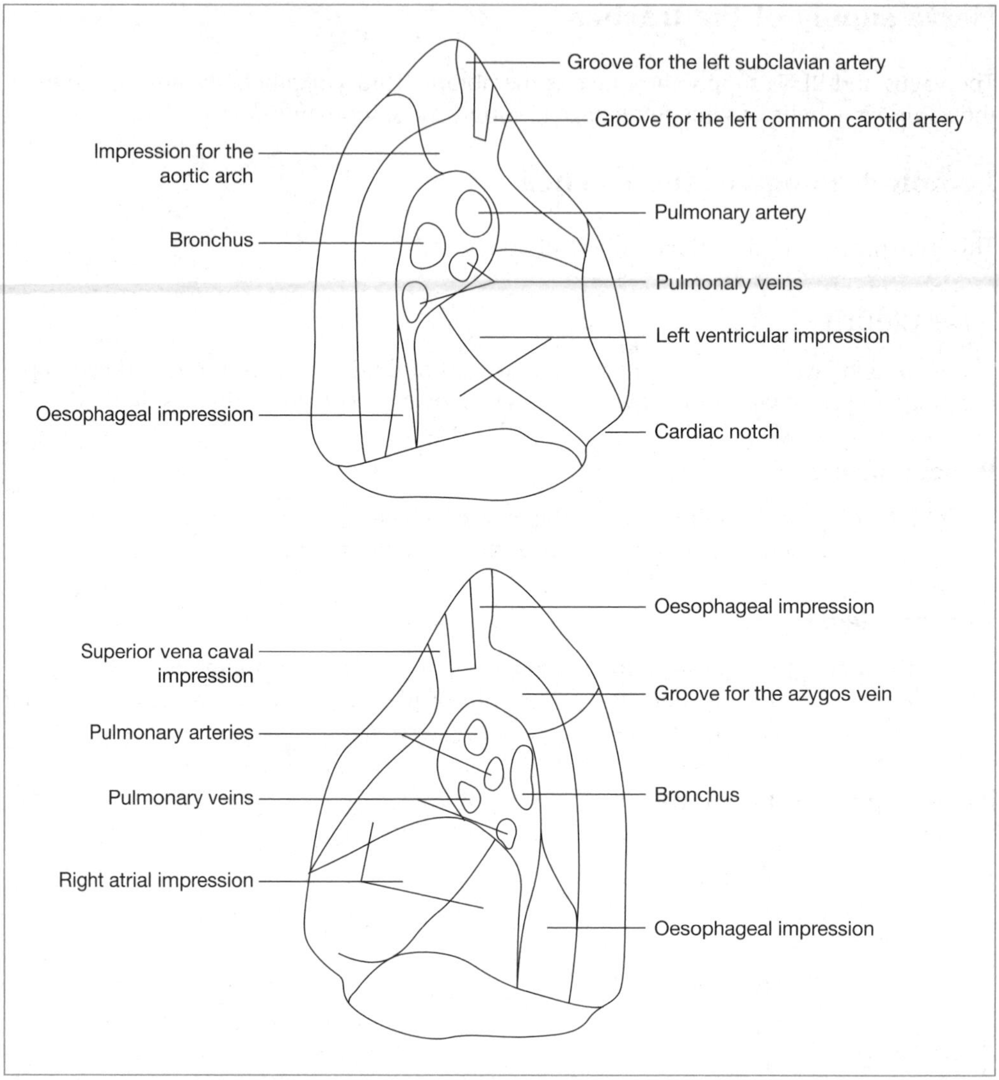

Figure 4.1e *Mediastinal surface of the right and left lungs*

Lobar and segmental bronchi

- The right (shorter and more vertical) and left main bronchi branch and become lobar bronchi, which branch and become segmental bronchi, which branch and become bronchioles
- Each lung has 10 bronchopulmonary segments: 5 per lobe on the left and 3 (upper), 2 (middle) and 5 (lower) for right lobes
- Each branch of a bronchus is accompanied by a branch of the pulmonary artery
- Blood supply to the bronchial tree is from its own small bronchial arteries

Pulmonary plexus

- From cardiac plexus
- Lies at hilum of each lung
- Supplies lungs with sympathetic and parasympathetic innervation

Surface anatomy of the thorax

- **Diaphragm** (in full expiration): extends from the 4th intercostal space on the right to the 5th rib on left
- **Pleura and lungs:** lung roots correspond to the level of the costal cartilages 3 and 4 (or T5–T7) at sternal edges

Remember 2, 4, 6, 8, 10 and 12 – they correspond to the relevant surface points that demarcate the lungs, as shown in the diagram.

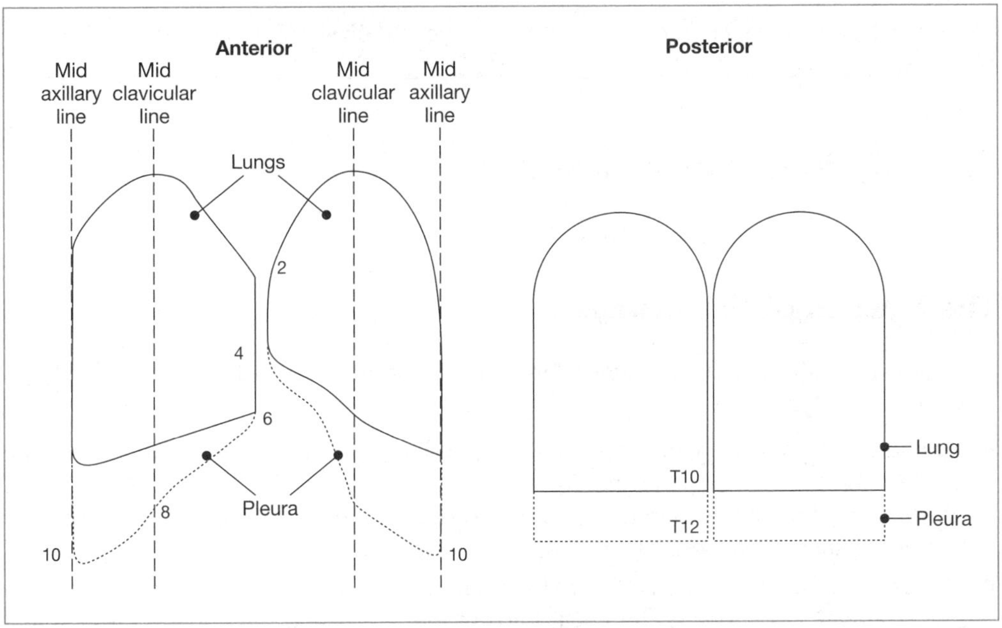

Figure 4.1f *Surface anatomy of the lungs*

4.2 RESPIRATORY PHYSIOLOGY

In a nutshell ...

The priority in treating critically ill patients is to maximise delivery of oxygen to the tissues (DO_2).

The **mechanics of ventilation** and the process of **gas exchange** determine the partial pressure of oxygen in the lungs.

The partial pressure of oxygen determines the **arterial oxygen content** and this relationship is described by the **oxy-haemoglobin dissociation curve.**

Arterial oxygen content × cardiac output = **oxygen delivery** to the tissues.

The physiology of ventilation

The mechanics of breathing

The function of the airways

Air passes through the larynx, trachea, bronchi and bronchioles to the alveoli. The functions of the airways are:

- **Conduits for gas passage:** the flow of gas depends on the pressure gradient between the alveoli and atmosphere and the compliance and resistance of the airways. Normal resistance is low but constriction and dilation of the airways occurs under autonomic control to alter airway resistance
- **Protection of the lungs:** air is filtered by nasal hair and the mucociliary escalator of the upper airway. Additionally the vocal folds of the larynx and the cough reflex protect against aspiration. The upper airways also warm and humidify the air

The action of inspiration and expiration

Muscles used in inspiration

- Diaphragm (main respiratory muscle)
- External intercostals
- Accessory inspiratory muscles
  - Scalenes
  - Sternocleidomastoid

  - Pectoralis
  - Latissimus dorsi

Action of inspiration

- The diaphragm contracts, flattening its domes
- The ribs swing up in a bucket-handle fashion, around their vertebral joints, pushing the sternum up and out, so increasing the cross-sectional area of the thorax
- Both of the above increase the thoracic volume leading to a reduced intrathoracic pressure. This is sub-atmospheric and so air flows passively into the lungs. Forced inspiration uses accessory muscles to further increase the intrathoracic volume and generate a higher intrapleural pressure

Muscles used in expiration

- Passive in quiet respiration as elastic recoil produces a positive intra-alveolar pressure
- Muscles of forced expiration: abdominal wall muscles; internal intercostals generate higher intra-alveolar pressures and drive air out

Action of expiration

- The diaphragm relaxes
- The lungs and chest wall recoil
- The thoracic volume reduces leading to a raised intrathoracic pressure causing airflow out of the lungs

Airway compliance

This is the 'elasticity' or 'stretchiness' of the lungs and it refers to the lungs and/or the chest walls.

$$\text{Compliance} = \text{change in lung volume} / \text{change in pressure}$$

A high or good compliance means that the lungs are easily inflated. Poor or low compliance means that the lungs are stiff, difficult to inflate and do not reach normal volumes. Poor compliance is caused by lung disease (eg pulmonary fibrosis, sarcoidosis, ARDS) or by disease of the chest wall (eg thoracic scoliosis).

Dynamic lung compliance is visualised by flow volume loops as shown in the diagram.

The surface tension in the spherical alveoli tends to cause them to collapse. To counteract this and minimise the additional work required to re-inflate collapsed alveoli, the pneumocytes produce surfactant which decreases the surface tension to that of a simple ionic solution.

Airway resistance

80% of total airway resistance is in the upper airways.

$$\text{Resistance} = \frac{\text{pressure}}{\text{flow}}$$

Where pressure = atmospheric pressure – alveolar pressure.

- Airway resistance is under smooth muscle control
- Parasympathetic innervation increases smooth muscle tone and hence resistance, thus ipratropium bromide (muscarinic antagonist) bronchodilates the airways
- Sympathetic innervation reduces it and so do sympathomimetics (eg salbutamol)
- Forced expiration increases airway resistance – due to increased intrathoracic pressure

The work of breathing

The work of breathing is usually only performed during inspiration as expiration is a passive phenomenon. It comprises:

- Work to expand lung against elastic and surface tension forces
- Work to overcome airway resistance (may be high in disease)
- Movement of the chest wall

Respiratory capacity

Respiratory capacity is dependant on the volume of gas moved and the respiratory rate at which this occurs.

Respiratory volumes

The amount of gas moved during respiration depends on age, sex, build and level of fitness. Spirometry measures functionally important changes in lung volumes.

Definitions used in spirometry

TV is tidal volume (0.5 L) – the volume of air moved in quiet respiration
IRV is inspiratory reserve volume (3 L) – the maximum volume inspirable following TV inspiration
ERV is expiratory reserve volume (2.1 L) – the maximum volume expirable following TV expiration
RV is residual volume (1.9 L) – the volume remaining in lungs after maximum expiration
FRC is functional residual capacity (1.9 L) – the is sum of ERV + RV (ie the volume in which gas exchange takes place)
VC is vital capacity (5.6 L) – the volume that can be expired after a maximal inspiratory effort
FVC is forced vital capacity
FEV_1 is forced expiratory volume – the volume expired in the 1st second of an FVC measurement
TLC is total lung capacity (6 L) – the sum of VC + RV
PEFR is peak expiratory flow rate – a cheap and easy measure of airway resistance

All of the above except RV (and hence TLC) can be measured by spirometry. To measure RV (or TLC) requires helium dilution methods or whole-body plethysmography.

NB: the above volumes are only meant as guides and relate to fit young adults.

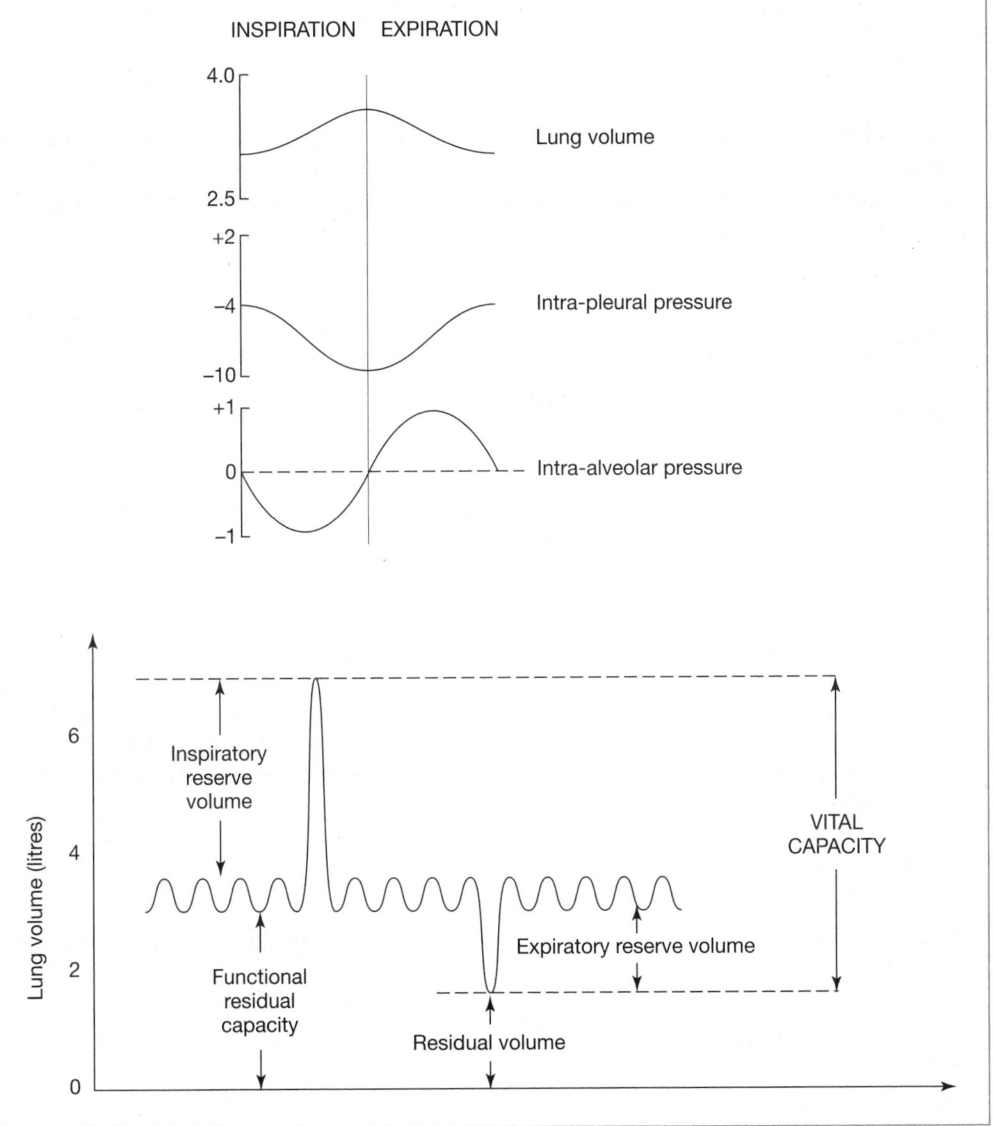

Figure 4.2a *Respiratory volumes and alveolar pressures*

Respiratory rate

The amount of air brought into the lungs per minute is the respiratory minute volume.

Minute volume = tidal volume × respiratory rate

Not all inspired air participates in gas exchange. Some occupies 'dead space'.

- Anatomical dead space: mouth, nose, pharynx, larynx, trachea, bronchi
- Alveolar dead space: volumes of diseased parts of lung unable to perform gaseous exchange
- Physiological dead space: anatomical dead space plus alveolar dead space

Because atmospheric pCO_2 is practically zero, all the CO_2 expired in a breath can be assumed to come from the communicating alveoli and none from the dead space. By measuring the pCO_2 in the communicating alveoli (which is the same as that in the arterial blood) and the pCO_2 in the expired air, one can use the Bohr equation to compute the 'diluting', non- pCO_2 containing volume, the physiologic dead space. Normal value is 0.3 litres.

Calculation of dead space

$$\text{Dead space /tidal volume} = \frac{\text{arterial } pCO_2 - \text{end tidal } pCO_2}{\text{arterial } pCO_2}$$

Dead space usually accounts for 150 mL but may be higher in disease states. Gas exchange depends on alveolar ventilation.

Alveolar ventilation rate = (tidal volume – dead space) × respiratory rate

Therefore any increase in dead space requires an increase in respiratory minute volume to achieve the same alveolar ventilation rate. This is very important in disease states with high physiological dead space and in patients on ventilators with high anatomical dead space (due to lengths of tubing).

The FEV_1: FVC ratio

The FVC gives an idea of the vital capacity. It is reduced in restrictive lung disease (eg fibrosis or collapse).

FEV_1 is the volume of gas expelled in the first second. It is reduced in obstructive airways as the gas cannot be forced out quickly.

- Normal value 0.7 (or 70%)
- Obstructive picture < 70%
- Restrictive picture > 70% or ratio stays the same

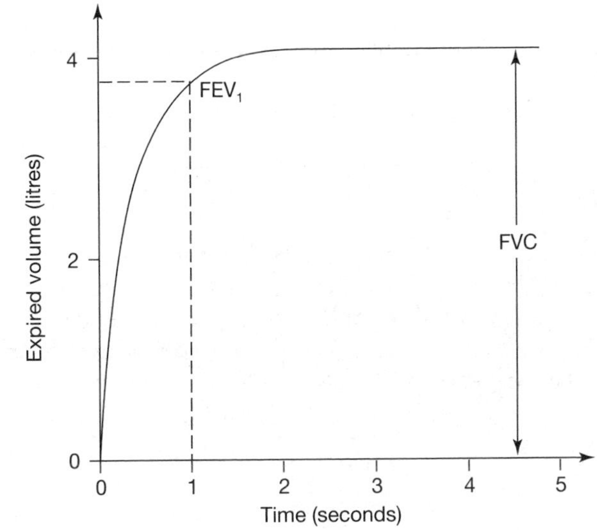

Figure 4.2b *The FEV_1: FVC ratio*

PEFR measurement indicates airflow resistance but is patient effort and technique dependant. The $PEFR_{25-75}$ is less subjective for objective assessment.

Control of respiration

In a nutshell ...

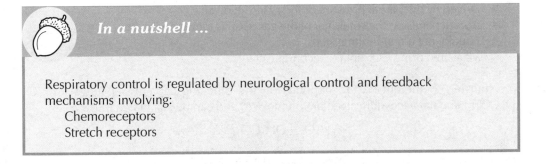

Respiratory control is regulated by neurological control and feedback mechanisms involving:

- Chemoreceptors
- Stretch receptors

Neurological control of respiration

Neurones controlling respiration are located in the medulla. Respiratory centres located nearby in the pons modify their activity. Inspiratory neurons have spontaneous rhythmical activity. Expiratory neurons are usually inactive unless forced expiration is required.

Chemoreceptors

Chemoreceptors detect chemical changes in the blood either due to changes in the partial pressure of oxygen or due to the local concentration of H^+ ions (which may be generated by dissolved CO_2 or metabolic products).

Chemoreceptors	
Central (medulla)	**Peripheral**
Detect changes in pH CO_2 crosses blood–brain barrier and dissolves in CSF Receptors detect the increase in CSF H^+ concentration	Carotid bodies via IX nerve (and less important aortic bodies via X nerve) Primarily detect changes in PaO_2 Less important detectors of changes in $PaCO_2$

Stretch receptors

In the Hering–Breuer reflex, negative feedback from lung stretch receptors as the lung inflates, causing termination of inspiration. These send inhibitory impulses through the vagus nerve to prevent over-inflation.

The physiology of gas exchange

Gaseous exchange

- Occurs by simple diffusion across the alveolar capillary interface
- Driven by the partial pressure of the gases involved
- Also depends on the solubility of the gas (CO_2 is more soluble than O_2)
- Usually not a rate-limiting step
- Measured using CO_2 uptake techniques

The transfer coefficient (kCO_2) depends on the diffusing capacity of lungs for CO_2 ($DLCCO_2$) and the accessible alveolar volume (VA) and can be calculated thus:

$$kCO_2 = DLCCO_2 / VA$$

The Ventilation–perfusion ratio (V:Q ratio)

Normal gas exchange requires adequate ventilation and perfusion. Usually the majority of alveoli will be both ventilated and perfused. There is some functional redundancy in the system and in the healthy state blood flow is diverted to the regions of the lung that are well perfused. This is a ventilation-perfusion match.

VQ ratio = alveolar ventilation rate/ pulmonary blood flow

If significant regions of the lung are perfused but not ventilated (ventilation-perfusion mismatch) then there is a decrease in the ratio with a tendency for a decrease in O_2 and CO_2 exchange and a gradual decrease on O_2 and increase in CO_2 in the arterial blood.

If significant regions of the lung are ventilated but not perfused there is an increase in the ratio and these regions add to the physiological dead space.

The oxyhaemoglobin dissociation curve

Oxygen is not very soluble in plasma and the majority of the oxygen is therefore carried bound to haemoglobin molecules. Most O_2 is carried by haemoglobin. A small amount of O_2 is dissolved in plasma and this is described by the PaO_2 value.

Haemoglobin readily binds oxygen at the capillary alveolar interface and releases oxygen at the capillary tissue interface. It is capable of changing its affinity for oxygen under these two different conditions because of the shape of the oxyhaemoglobin dissociation curve.

The haemoglobin molecule (Hb)

Molecular weight 66 500 kDa
Normal concentration 15 g/dL
Porphyrin ring attached to an Fe^{2+} ion
Binds four molecules of O_2 per molecule of haemoglobin
1 g of haemoglobin binds 1.34 mL of O_2 when fully saturated
O_2 saturation refers to the number of O_2-bound haem molecules expressed as a percentage of the total number available; it is measured by pulse oximetry

The relationship between O_2 saturation and PaO_2 is described by the O_2 dissociation curve. The sigmoid shape is formed because as each haem binds an oxygen molecule it increases its binding capacity at the other three sites in a phenomenon called 'cooperativity'. When all the sites are full the Hb is saturated and the curve plateaus. In the lungs as one molecule of oxygen binds to the haemoglobin it makes it easier for others to do so. When the haemoglobin reaches the tissues, the dissociation of one molecule of oxygen makes it easier for the remaining molecules to dissociate.

The Bohr effect

The Bohr effect describes the factors which alter the position of the oxyhaemoglobin dissociation curve. In the lungs CO_2 diffuses from the blood into the alveoli and the H^+ concentration falls. This pushes the curve to the left where the quantity of O_2 that can bind with the haemoglobin is increased, resulting in a higher saturation of the blood with O_2. When the blood reaches the tissues it absorbs the products of metabolism as CO_2 and this increases the H^+ concentration. The concentration of 2,3-diphosphoglycerate (2,3 DPG) increases with hypoxia and these factors shift the curve to the right which favours release of the O_2 molecules and delivers O_2 to the tissues at a higher O_2 partial pressure than would otherwise occur.

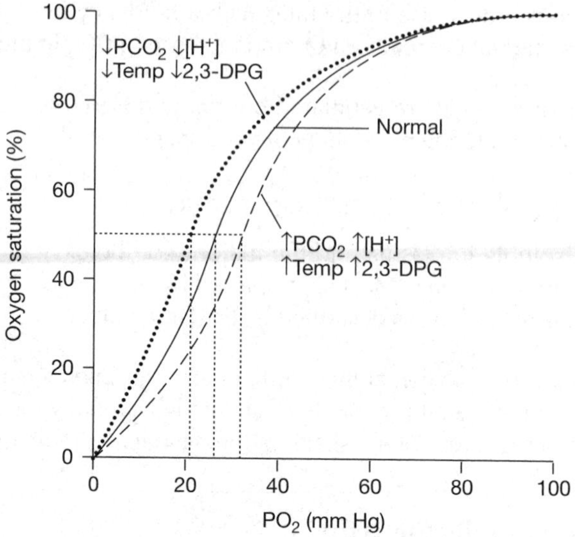

Figure 4.2c *The O_2 dissociation curve*

Factors that shift the curve

To the left – ie Increased affinity for O_2	To the right – ie reduced affinity for O_2
Decreased $PaCO_2$	Increased $PaCO_2$
Decreased H^+ concentration	Increased H^+ concentration
Decreased 2,3-DPG levels	Increased 2,3-DPG levels
Decreased temperature	Increased temperature
Increased fetal Hb (HbF)	
Increased carboxy-haemoglobin	

Hb has a much greater affinity (× 250) for carbon monoxide (CO) than for O_2 (so the Hb–CO curve is shifted far to the left). Myoglobin has only one haem molecule and so its curve is again far to the left.

Transport of CO_2

CO_2 is transported in three ways:

- Dissolved as free CO_2 in plasma (10%)
- Reacts with amine side groups of deoxy-Hb to form carbamino-Hb (30%)

- Reacts with H_2O of plasma to form $H^+ + HCO_3^-$ catalysed within the red blood cells by carbonic anhydrase. Inside the RBC the H^+ ions bind to the haemoglobin protein which acts as a buffer. In order to maintain electrical neutrality, the bicarbonate diffuses out of the red cells in exchange for chloride ions (**chloride shift**)

The Haldane effect reflects the observation that as the partial pressure of O_2 increases, the amount of CO_2 that is carried by the blood falls. This is because deoxy-Hb (venous) is a weaker acid than oxy-Hb and can hence carry more CO_2 in the carbamino-Hb form.

Oxygen delivery and consumption

Oxygen delivery

Oxygen delivery = Cardiac output × Arterial oxygen content

Oxygen delivery (DO_2) is the total amount of oxygen delivered to the tissues per unit time. It can be calculated using the formula:

$$\text{Oxygen delivery } (DO_2) = CO \times \{(Hb \times SaO_2 \times 1.34) + (PaO_2 \times 0.003)\}$$

In a 70 kg man:

Hb = haemoglobin (usually 15g/dL or 1.5g/mL)
SaO_2 = saturation of Hb with oxygen in arterial blood (usually 99% or 0.99)
PaO_2 = partial pressure of oxygen in arterial blood. The amount of dissolved oxygen (ie the PaO_2) is usually negligible compared to the amount carried by the haemoglobin. It is approximately 13 Kpa and 0.003 is the amount in mL of oxygen carried per kPa. However PaO_2 also affects SaO_2

So, arterial oxygen content (mL/min):

$= (1.5 \text{ g/mL} \times 0.99 \times (1.34) + (13 \text{ kPa} \times 0.003)$
$\cong 2 \text{ mL } O_2 / \text{mL of blood/min}$
$\cong 0.2 \text{ litres } O_2 \text{ per litre of blood/min}$

Cardiac output is approximately 5 litres/min. So oxygen delivery:

$\cong 5 \text{ litres/min} \times 0.2 \text{ litres/min}$
$\cong 1 \text{ litre/min}$

Oxygen consumption

Oxygen consumption is the oxygen content of arterial blood (CaO_2) minus the oxygen content of venous blood (CvO_2) multiplied by the cardiac output:

$$O_2 \text{ consumption} = (CaO_2 - CvO_2) \times \text{cardiac output}$$

where CaO_2 is the arterial content of O_2 and CvO_2 is the mixed venous content of O_2.

CvO_2 is measured by substituting mixed venous saturations (SvO_2 which is usually 75%) and PvO_2 (which is usually 4–5 kPa) into the equation for content. The values are measured directly via a blood-gas analyser with blood obtained from the tip of a pulmonary artery (PA) catheter. This provides true mixed venous blood. Some PA catheters have an oximeter at the tip to give continuous values.

CvO_2 is approximately 150 mL/litre and hence O_2 consumption is normally 250 mL/minute.

It can be seen that there is more oxygen delivered than is consumed, and consumption remains independent of delivery. There is an excess of supply over demand in healthy states. However, in low delivery states and in critical illness, oxygen consumption is initially supply-dependant.

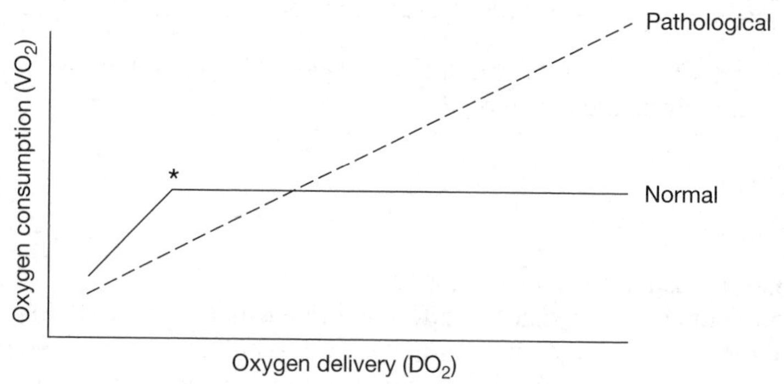

Figure 4.2d *VO_2/DO_2*

The oxygen extraction ratio (OER)

Under normal conditions, if oxygen demand is increased then supply is also increased (by increased ventilation and increased cardiac output). If the oxygen supply cannot be increased (due to cardiorespiratory disease or compromise) then the body will compensate for this lower oxygen delivery by redistributing blood preferentially to the tissues that need them and extracting more oxygen per mL of blood than before – ie the oxygen extraction ratio (OER) increases. This is called **physiological reserve**. Eventually reserve runs out and a critical point (point * on Fig. 4.2d) is reached – there just isn't enough oxygen to match supply, and anaerobic glycolysis takes place. This is known as **physiological dependence of VO_2** on DO_2 and it can be measured by an increase in arterial lactate concentration.

Oxygen extraction ratio

$OER = CaO_2 - CvO_2 / CaO_2 \times 100\%$

The plateau in VO_2 is maintained by increasing the extraction ratio for oxygen (OER). Blood flow is re-distributed to match local demand for oxygen mediated by the autonomic nervous system and nitric oxide. Any pathological effects that impact on the microcirculation impair the ability of the tissue to extract oxygen and the OER. This inability to extract oxygen, rather than an inability to deliver oxygen by means of the cardiorespiratory system, is likely to be the cause of reduced tissue oxygenation in critical illness.

Current approaches to goal-directed resuscitation are to maintain BP in order to adequately perfuse tissues (such as the kidney, thus maintaining urine output) and allow correction of acidosis.

From the equation for DO_2 it can be seen that methods of increasing tissue oxygen delivery include:

- Increasing cardiac output with fluids and inotropes
- Increasing saturations (SaO_2) with increased inspired oxygen concentration (FiO_2), PEEP and other ventilatory strategies
- Increasing haemoglobin with transfusion

Optimal haemoglobin concentration in critically ill patients is a compromise between oxygen carriage and perfusion. Perfusion is related to viscosity, which increases as the haematocrit increases. Usually when bleeding is not a risk then a haemoglobin of between 8 and 10 g/dL allows adequate oxygen delivery with good perfusion of narrow capillaries.

4.3 RESPIRATORY INVESTIGATIONS

The chest X-ray (CXR)

Interpretation of the CXR

On ITUs films are almost always AP views, therefore heart size is unreliable. They are also frequently supine films hence pneumothorax and effusions may not appear in the classical positions. CT scanning of the thorax can provide detailed information and ultrasound can help with isolation of effusions (and marking the site for drainage).

Remember

- Label (check patient details)
- Adequacy of film (exposure; thoracic vertebrae just visible)
- Attached equipment (ECG leads, CVP/PA line, NG tube)

- Heart size
- Mediastinum
- ET tube
- Hilar regions
- Diaphragm
- Lungs
  - Look for silhouette sign
  - Consolidation: air bronchogram, no volume change
  - Atelectasis: shift of fissures, decreased volume, compensatory hyperinflation
- Bones
- Soft tissues
- Special areas (apices, behind heart, look for pneumothorax)
- Effusions (may appear at apex in supine patients (transudate: protein < 30 g/dL)

Lung function tests

These tests measure for lung volumes, airway resistance and gas transfer.

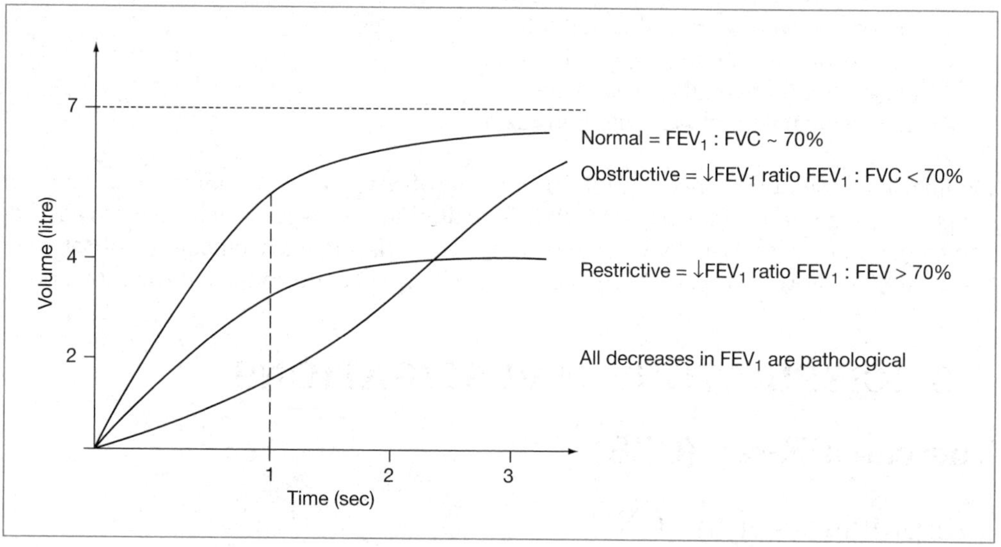

Figure 4.3a *Simple spirometry in obstructive/restrictive disease*

Flow volume loops

These loops help to characterise airflow obstruction as extra- or intrathoracic and measure severity – useful for work-up of neck/mediastinal masses.

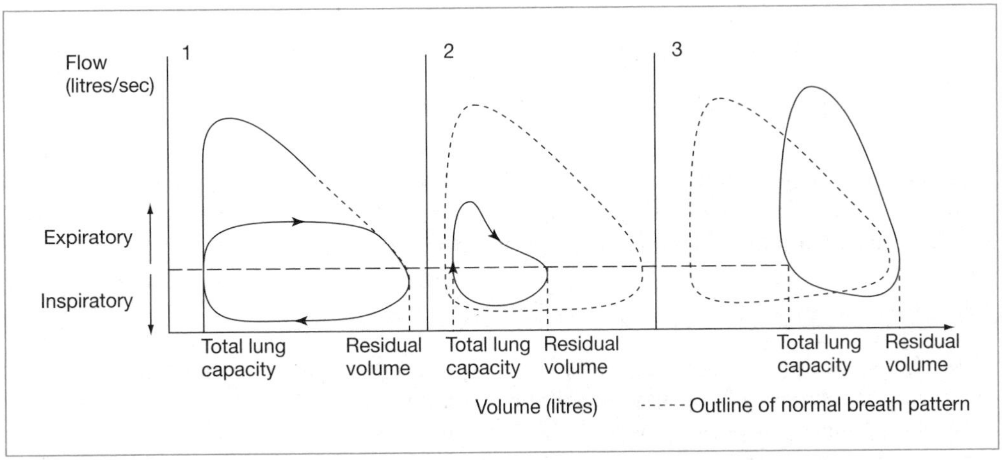

Figure 4.3b *Flow volume loops*

1. Tracheal/laryngeal obstruction
2. Obstructive lung disease
3. Restrictive lung disease

4.4 RESPIRATORY FAILURE

Definition and types of respiratory failure

The definition of respiratory failure is when pulmonary gas exchange is sufficiently impaired to cause hypoxia with or without hypercarbia: ie $PaO_2 < 8$ kPa or $PaCO_2 > 7$ kPa.

- **Type I respiratory failure:** this is low PaO_2 with normal or low $PaCO_2$. It is caused by diseases that damage lung tissue
- **Type II respiratory failure:** this is low PaO_2 with high $PaCO_2$. It is caused by ventilation being insufficient to excrete sufficient CO_2
  - Decreased ventilatory effort (eg exhaustion)
  - Obstructive airways disease
  - Inability to overcome restrictive airways disease
  - Failure to compensate for increased CO_2 production

Management of respiratory failure

- Exclude any airway problem and resuscitate as appropriate
- Give oxygen: in type I failure CPAP can improve PaO_2 if high-flow oxygen is inadequate
- Involve senior and ITU staff early for mechanical ventilatory support
- Take history (if possible) and examine thoroughly
- Regularly monitor ABGs

- Adjust inspired O_2 according to ABGs
- Give bronchodilators (nebulised or IV), steroids, and antibiotics as appropriate
- Ensure high-level supervision – HDU or ITU*
- Make repeated assessments

*Patients with a requirement of more than 40% oxygen to keep oxygen saturation of > 94% should be seriously considered for observation on HDU/ITU (a 'normal' oxygen mask, without a reservoir attached, can deliver at most about 40% oxygen).

Physiotherapy in respiratory failure

- Consider doxapram if respiratory effort is poor, but beware of exhaustion
- FRC is increased in upright and sitting positions
- Use patient positioning for postural drainage
- Percussion loosens secretions
- Bagging and suction removes secretions
- Tracheostomy or minicricothyrotomy aid suction in non-ventilated patients

NB: As students, we all seem to remember being told that high concentrations of inspired oxygen can ultimately stop a patient breathing in cases of hypoxic drive (low PaO_2 rather than raised $PaCO_2$ drives respiration in some patients with COPD). However, in reality this is unusual and the junior doctor should not be afraid to give an hypoxic patient high-flow oxygen when O_2 saturations are <90%. Respiratory depression in this situation does not occur immediately and delivery of oxygen is more important at this stage. These patients should be carefully monitored during O_2 therapy.

Investigation of respiratory failure

Alveolar oxygen gradient

This is a measure of lung ventilation (or physiological shunt). It compares the alveolar oxygen concentration and the arterial oxygen concentration to assess the efficacy of transport of oxygen from the alveolus into the blood.

The alveolar oxygen concentration (PaO_2) is a function of the barometric pressure (assumed to be at sea level, ie 101 kPa), the pressure of water vapour in the atmosphere (5 kPa) and the delivered concentration of oxygen (FiO_2).

The arterial concentration of oxygen (pO2) can be measured from the ABGs.

$$\text{Normal A–a gradient} = (\text{age} + 10) / 4$$

The A–a increases 5–7 mmHg for every 10% increase in FiO_2.

Calculating the alveolar–arterial (A–a) gradient

PaO_2 = inspired pO2 – ($PaCO_2$/RQ)

Where:

PAO_2 is the alveolar pO_2

Inspired pO_2 = (atmospheric pressure – saturated water vapour pressure) × FiO_2

$PaCO_2$ is close to $PaCO_2$ (when atmospheric pressure = 101 kPa and water vapour = 5 kPa)

RQ is the respiratory quotient (CO_2/O_2 = 0.8 for normal diet)

In healthy lungs, PAO_2 – PaO_2 (measured from blood gases) is around 10 kPa. This gap is known as the alveolar–arterial gradient (A–a gradient). This explains why the value for PaO_2 is about 10 less than for FiO_2, because account must be taken of CO_2 and water vapour in the lung. In diseased lungs the A–a gradient may be increased and is a useful indicator of hypoxaemia. The A–a gradient is normal in hypoventilation-related hypoxaemia, but decreased in VQ mismatch.

ITU specific pathologies that may result in respiratory failure

In a nutshell ...

Causes of respiratory failure in the ITU
- Respiratory infection
- ARDS

Specific respiratory infections in the ITU

Aspiration

- Current management depends on what is aspirated into the lungs. Look out for:
  - Particulate small airway obstruction
  - Acid damage to alveolar membrane
  - Possible infected material
- Management of aspiration
  - Observe, oxygen, physio. Ventilation if necessary
  - No antibiotics unless definitely infected material (as promotes resistant organisms)
  - Do not use steroids

Lung abscess

- Often caused by aspiration and hence anaerobic organisms
- Can be caused by: bronchial obstruction; pneumonia; infected pulmonary infarcts; haematogenous spread
- Treatment: antibiotics, postural drainage and physio. < 10% need surgical drainage

Opportunistic pneumonia

- Relatively common on ITUs
- May require bronchial lavage +/– trans-bronchial biopsy to identify organism
- Commonest infections are Gram-positive organisms but include Gram-negatives
- After use of antibiotics *Candida* may colonise and cause infection

Empyema

- Accumulation of pus in pleural cavity
- 50% caused by pneumonia, 25% post-surgical infections
- Gram-negative bacteria including *Pseudomonas* often found, as well as staphylococci
- Acutely low-viscosity fluid accumulates, then becomes more turbid with increased WCC; at this point a fibrous peel develops on the lung surface limiting expansion – after 6 weeks this peel becomes organised with fibroblasts
- Diagnosis from thorocentesis: pH < 7, low glucose, LDH > 1000 IU/litre and Gram-stain CXR and CT scan
- Treat with antibiotics and chest drain in the acute phase but if there is failure to respond then open formal surgical drainage may be required

Acute lung injury (ALI) and acute respiratory distress syndrome (ARDS)

Clinical features of acute lung injury

There is a spectrum of acute lung injury from mild to severe. Severe ALI is termed ARDS. ARDS is a term used to describe the respiratory component of SIRS or MODS (see section 8 of this chapter).

Lung injury causes an inflammatory response leading to damage to the alveolar capillary membrane and microcirculatory changes. This causes an increased pulmonary vascular permeability leading to thickened alveolar membranes and leakage of fluid into the interstitium and alveoli. This process may be the pulmonary manifestation of whole-body capillary leak syndrome in MODS. This gives poorer volumes, compliance and gaseous exchange capabilities of lungs. There are three areas of the lung in this condition:

- Collapsed solid lung with consistency like liver
- Ventilated and perfused lung (termed baby lung as much smaller than normal)
- Potentially recruitable alveoli – this is where ventilatory techniques may be beneficial

It may resolve with or without pulmonary fibrosis.

Diagnostic features of acute lung injury

- Pulmonary infiltrates on CXR
- PAWP is < 18 (hence infiltrates are not due to cardiac pulmonary oedema)
- Hypoxaemia with ratio $PaO_2/FiO_2 < 40$. ARDS criteria is severe hypoxaemia ie $PaO_2/FiO_2 < 27$
- A known cause (eg pancreatitis, aspiration, massive transfusion)

Other features include respiratory distress and decreased compliance.

Causes of ALI and ARDS

Direct	Indirect
Chest trauma	Sepsis
Aspiration	Hypovolaemia
Inhaled irritants (eg smoke)	Burns
	Pancreatitis
	Fat embolism
	Radiation
	DIC

Management of acute lung injury

General management

- Almost entirely supportive
- Treat underlying cause if possible
- Re-position patient (eg prone)
- Careful fluid restriction/diuresis
- Corticosteroids in fibrosis stage
- Trial of blind antibiotics (controversial)

Ventilatory management

Optimisation of oxygenation is achieved by:

- Increasing mean airway pressure
- Increasing FiO_2
- Increasing airway pressure:
  - Increased peak inspired pressure limited to about 34 cmH_2O
  - Increased PEEP
  - Increased inspiratory time, even so far as reversing the inhalation to exhalation ratio to 2: 1
- Increasing FiO_2: levels above 0.5 (50%) increase risk of oxygen toxicity, hence the above measures are used to minimise the inspired oxygen and targets of PaO_2 of 8 kPa and saturations of 90% are acceptable

The usual method is pressure control ventilation, with PEEP and sometimes reverse ratio. To limit the peak pressures a low tidal volume can be allowed hence the $PaCO_2$ can be allowed to increase (permissive hypercapnoea). The tidal volume should also be restricted to around 6 mL/kg as excessive volumes cause shear stress damage to the alveoli.

In severely hypoxaemic patients, nitric oxide maybe used to reduce the FiO_2 and improve oxygenation. The mainstay of therapy however is pressure support and PEEP to recruit collapsed alveoli and maintain them.

Ventilation in the prone position for periods of 4–8 hours may improve regional pulmonary V/Q matching and improve oxygenation. This is due to non-homogeneous distribution of damage, which tends to be in dependent lung. Despite this benefit in some patients there are risks of dislodging the endotracheal tube, catheters and other tubes.

Fluid balance: this is difficult as over-hydration is deleterious to injured lung but adequate cardiovascular performance is required. Judicious use of ventilation, fluids, and inotropes is needed.

Nitric oxide (NO) therapy

NO is a vasodilator that is formed naturally in almost all tissues (constitutive). It is also produced in excess in sepsis causing vascular dilatation.

When used clinically it is inhaled at a concentration of around 5–20 parts per million. Side effects include pulmonary toxicity due to nitric acid formation when oxidised. It causes vasodilatation in ventilated lung only, improving V/Q match thus preventing systemic vasodilatation and reversal of pulmonary hypoxic vasoconstriction. NO has very high affinity for haemoglobin, and combined this becomes methaemoglobin which deactivates NO and prevents systemic effects.

Outcome of acute respiratory distress syndrome

- 50–60% mortality
- Those who recover may be left with diffuse interstitial fibrosis but mostly have good outcome

Respiratory post-operative complications

Complications of non-thoracic operations

- Basal atelectasis/collapse
- Infection
- Pulmonary embolism
- Hypoventilation secondary to pain

Complications of thoracic operations

Patients at risk of complications:

- Elderly
- Smokers (IHD and COAD)
- Immobility post-operatively (increases risk of DVT/PE)

Causes of retained sputum:

- Pain and opiate drugs post-operatively reduce respiratory effort and cough
- Ciliary function is reduced (smokers)
- Requires excellent pain control: intercostal nerve block or ablation (in theatre); epidural; PCA; NSAIDs (beware of ulcers)
- Deep breathing exercises to be encouraged
- Requires careful monitoring and aggressive chest physiotherapy, mini-tracheostomy to suction secretions

Pneumonectomy

Leaves an empty hemithorax that fills with fluid and gradually solidifies.

Complications of pneumonectomy

- Tension pneumothorax
- Haemothorax (can be massive)
- Pulmonary oedema
- Empyema – often *Staphylococcus aureus* – requires drainage
- Bronchopulmonary fistula (patient starts coughing up fluid); requires moving patient onto side of operation, chest drain and surgical exploration unless small – rare but very serious

For further discussion see *Cardiothoracics* in Book 2.

4.5 RESPIRATORY MONITORING AND SUPPORT IN CRITICAL CARE

Airway

> ***In a nutshell ...***
>
> Management of a compromised airway is discussed in detail in Chapter 6 *Trauma*.
>
> Definitive airway management in critical care patients who are unable to maintain their own airway or who require invasive ventilation is intubation.
>
> **Nasal intubation** is preferred for paediatric ITU – there is an increased risk of haemorrhage in adults and risk of sepsis from sinus infection
>
> **Endotracheal** or **pretracheal intubation** is the mainstay of management

Nasotracheal intubation

This technique is contraindicated in the apnoeic patient and in patients in whom mid-face or basal skull fractures are suspected.

Guiding the tip of the tube into the trachea is achieved blindly by auscultation for the point of maximum breath sounds, which is not as reliable as visualisation of the cords using the orotracheal route. An alternative method is fibreoptic-guided insertion of the nasotracheal tube, but these endoscopes are costly and not widely available. This technique would seldom be advised in the acute trauma situation where speed and reliability are paramount.

Orotracheal intubation

Characteristics of the ET tube

- Internal diameter: 8–9 mm for males; 7–8 mm for females
- Length: 23 cm to teeth in males; 21 cm in females
- Checked on CXR level with lower edge of clavicle

The cuffed end:

- Creates a seal
- Helps prevent aspiration
- Can cause stenosis and tracheomalacia if high pressure (so pressure should be monitored)

Anaesthetic induction for intubation

This requires:

- **Skilled operator** trained in anaesthesia
- **Preparation of equipment**
- **Prevention of pressor response** on laryngoscopy with IV fentanyl or lignocaine/lidocaine especially if risk of raised ICP
- **Cricoid pressure:** application of pressure to the cricoid, the only complete ring cartilage in the airway, causes it to impinge onto the body of C6; this will prevent passive regurgitation once induced
- **Induction agent:** if haemodynamically unstable there may be a precipitous drop in BP; etomidate is reasonably cardio-stable, as is ketamine (which has the added value of bronchodilation)
- **Muscle relaxant:** suxamethonium has rapid onset (< 1 minute) characterised by fasciculations and is short acting; side effects include anaphylaxis and hyperkalaemia, especially following burns or in patients with paralysis, when cardiac arrest can occur

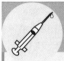

Procedure box: Endotracheal intubation

Indications

Unconscious patient who cannot maintain own airway (GCS < 8)
Where there is a risk of upper airway obstruction
Impaired gag reflex
To prevent rise in ICP (iatrogenic hyperventilation)
Requirement for mechanical ventilation (severe hypoxia or metabolic acidosis)
Anaesthesia for surgery
To enable suction of secretions

Contraindications

Severe lower facial trauma may be better managed with a surgical airway

Patient positioning

Supine with head in the 'sniffing the morning air' position
Unconscious or under GA

Procedure

Familiarise yourself with the technique and check all equipment before starting – laryngoscope, suction, ET tube (size 7–8 for females; 8–9 for males), Ambu bag, oxygen supply, assistant, muscle relaxant, sedation, IV access
Pre-oxygenate the patient with 100% oxygen for 3–4 minutes

Allow a maximum of 30 seconds for each attempt at insertion (hold your own breath!)
Slide the laryngoscope into the right side of the mouth, sweeping the tongue to the left
Place the tip of the blade in the groove between the epiglottis and the base of the tongue and draw the laryngoscope gently upwards (don't lever it on the teeth)
Directly visualise the vocal cords and slide the ET tube into the trachea
Check position of tube by auscultation of both lungs and the epigastrium
End tidal CO_2 monitors help verify correct position
Secure tube by tying in place (average length is 21–23 cm to teeth for females, 23–25 cm for males)

Hazards

Oesophageal intubation (a fatal complication if it goes unnoticed. If in any doubt as to the position of the tube, remove it, pre-oxygenate the patient and start again)
Tube too far down entering the right main bronchus
Airway damage or rupture

Post-procedure instructions

Always ensure that the tube is correctly positioned, allowing adequate ventilation of both lungs. If in any doubt or if the tube becomes displaced it may have to be removed and the procedure repeated.

Complications

Early (see *Hazards* above): damage to mouth and teeth; equipment failure; inability to intubate
Late: erosion; stenosis of the trachea and larynx

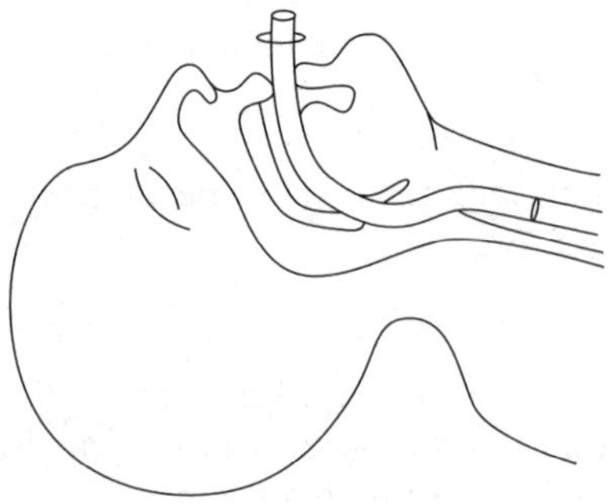

Figure 4.5a *Orotracheal intubation*

Alternative airways

- Emergency surgical airway: cricothyroidotomy
- Elective surgical airway: surgical tracheostomy
  - Percutaneous
  - Open surgical tracheostomy

For discussion of the emergency surgical airway see Chapter 5 *Trauma*.

Tracheostomy

An open surgical tracheostomy is slow, technically more complex, with potential for bleeding, and requires formal operating facilities. It is not appropriate in the acute trauma situation, but is better suited to the long-term management of a ventilated patient. It is performed when a percutaneous tracheostomy would be difficult (eg abnormal or distorted anatomy).

Percutaneous tracheostomy is also time-consuming and requires hyper-extension of the neck. In addition the use of a guidewire and multiple dilators make it an unsuitable technique in the acute trauma situation.

Procedure box: Percutaneous tracheostomy

Indications

Prolonged ventilation (reduces risk of tracheal stenosis from long-term intubation)
Aids weaning from the ventilator
Patients who are unable to maintain their own airway due to long-term disease (eg bulbar palsy)

Contraindications

Coagulopathy
Abnormal anatomy
Unstable patient

Patient positioning

Supine with the neck extended
Most are already intubated and ventilated under sedation or GA
The surgical area is infiltrated with 10 mL LA with adrenaline/epinephrine to reduce bleeding

Procedure

A bronchoscope is inserted into the trachea and the ET tube is withdrawn to the level of the cords by an anaesthetist

The tracheal stoma should be located between the 2nd and 4th tracheal rings and a superficial 2-cm horizontal incision is made at this level
A large-bore needle is inserted into the trachea through the incision and its location verified by aspiration of air through a syringe
A guidewire is passed into the trachea under direct vision by the bronchoscope
Lubricated sequential dilators are passed over the guidewire to enlarge the stoma to an appropriate size
A cuffed tracheostomy tube is passed over the guidewire and into the trachea. Once secure, the ET tube is removed completely

Hazards
Haemorrhage from subcutaneous blood vessels
Failure to cannulate the trachea

Complications

Early
Asphyxia
Aspiration
Creation of a false track
Subcutaneous/mediastinal emphysema
Haemorrhage/haematoma
Laceration of the oesophagus or trachea

Late
Vocal cord paralysis/hoarseness
Cellulitis
Laryngeal stenosis
Tracheomalacia

Mini-tracheostomy

A small tracheostomy tube may be inserted through the cricothyroid membrane – to aid suctioning of secretions and physiotherapy. This is not suitable as a definitive airway as the tube is not cuffed.

Mechanical-assisted ventilation

Indications and aims of mechanical ventilation

- Elimination and control of CO_2
- Improve oxygenation – reduces 'work' of respiration and therefore O_2 consumed

- Enables high levels of inspired O_2 to be administered
- Can open collapsed alveoli by raising pressure during inspiration and maintaining pressure during expiration

Complications of mechanical ventilation

- Airway complications (see above)
- Barotrauma (pneumothorax, pneumomediastinum, pneumoperitoneum, surgical emphysema)
- Cardiovascular – reduced venous return (high intrathoracic pressure)
- Increased pulmonary vascular resistance
- Gastric dilatation/ileus (gastric tube must be inserted)
- Accidental disconnection or wrong setting of ventilator
- Na^+ and H_2O retention – increased ADH and atrial natriuretic peptide
- Atrophy of respiratory muscles if no spontaneous effort
- Infection/pneumonia

Positive end-expiratory pressure (PEEP)

- Achieved by adding a valve to an assisted breathing circuit
- Expiratory pressure is not allowed to fall below a certain level (2.5–20 cmH_2O)
- Pressure prevents alveolar collapse at the end of expiration and recruits collapsed alveoli

Advantages: increases lung volumes and improves oxygenation. Can be used with the patient breathing spontaneously (see CPAP and BiPAP) or with mechanical ventilation.

Disadvantages: reduces physiological shunting, but further reduces venous return and increases barotraumas.

Continuous positive airways pressure (CPAP)

- Used in spontaneously ventilating patients (may or may not require airway management)
- If the patient is conscious and making respiratory effort this requires a tightly fitting mask to maintain positive pressure
- If the patient is not conscious or is tiring, intubation with a cuffed ET tube is required
- Same advantages and disadvantages as PEEP but also reduces respiratory effort
- Reduces cardiac work by reducing trans-mural tension

Bi-level positive airways pressure (BiPAP)

- Allows separate adjustment of the pressures delivered during inspiration and expiration
- Allows lower overall airway pressures to be used (reduces barotraumas compared to CPAP)

- Tolerated better because the high pressure corresponds to inspiration, and a lower pressure during expiration makes this phase easier for the patient
- May also have a spontaneous timed setting; if the patient fails to initiate a breath then the machine will initiate that breath for them

Intermittent positive pressure ventilation (IPPV)

Ventilators on ITU have a choice of mode and mandatory or spontaneous features; all have pressure limitation cut off and sophisticated alarms.

Controlled mechanical ventilation (CMV)

- Sets rate for breaths and breath volume either by volume or pressure control
- Allows no spontaneous respirations (eg as in anaesthetic ventilators)

Intermittent mandatory ventilation (IMV)

- Delivers 'mandatory' minute volume but allows patient to take spontaneous breaths between mechanical breaths
- Can be synchronised with spontaneous breaths **(SIMV)** thus preventing stacking of breaths. This occurs when a mechanical breath is imposed after a spontaneous one. Sensors in the ventilator detect the patient's own breaths. This is the main mode used in ITU

Mandatory-type ventilator features

This determines how breaths are delivered, either as a set volume or a set pressure.

Volume control

- Tidal volume to be delivered is set on the ventilator. Normal settings are 10 mL per kg. This is the usual mandatory type, however if compliance is poor the inspired pressure will be very high with risk of barotrauma. Therefore not suitable in ARDS and asthma

Pressure control

- An inspiratory pressure is set on the ventilator and tidal volume is dependent on compliance
- This type is used in ARDS; the inspiratory pressure is set to a value to achieve a satisfactory measured tidal volume but peak pressures are usually limited to 34 cmH_2O to avoid barotrauma

Spontaneous-type ventilator features

Pressure support

- This adjunct supports spontaneous breaths with a set pressure to increase their tidal volumes
- Allows very small breaths produced by the patient to be boosted to adequate volumes as an aid to weaning
- Sensitivity of breath detection can be altered via the trigger sensitivity and type
- Trigger for supported breaths is usually a drop in pressure, but flow triggering is more sensitive if required

Assist control (trigger) ventilation

- Uses patient's own respiratory rhythm to trigger delivery of a set tidal volume

Weaning from assisted ventilation

- Patient must have recovered from original problem requiring ventilation
- Conscious level, metabolic state, cardiovascular function and state of mind are to be considered (including normal phosphate)
- SIMV mode aids weaning with pressure support (PS). As the patient starts taking spontaneous breaths the SIMV rate is reduced until all breaths are spontaneous and supported by PS. PS is then reduced until the patient self ventilates without support
- The longer the time spent on a ventilator, the longer (more difficult) the weaning

Prior to extubation the patient may be placed on a T-piece, which allows oxygenation without support. CPAP is sometimes helpful.

The most successful method of weaning is with spontaneous breaths from the patient supported by pressure support.

Extubation

The patient must:

- Be able to breathe spontaneously indefinitely
- Have an effective cough reflex and be able to protect their airway
- Be conscious enough to co-operate

Other factors include adequate tidal volume without tachypnoea (ie respiratory rate/TV < 100).

Physiotherapy

It is essential that secretions are cleared in ventilated patients who cannot cough, especially those with pneumonia. Chest physio with suctioning should be carried out frequently.

Section 5
The renal system in critical care

5.1 RENAL PHYSIOLOGY

In a nutshell ...

The kidney has multiple functions.

Homeostasis of the extracellular fluid: control of water and electrolyte balance by plasma filtration followed by excretion and resorption of ions and water.

Excretion: elimination of waste products of metabolism (eg ammonium containing compounds) and foreign substances (eg drugs).

Metabolism: vitamin D hydroxylation and activation.

Endocrine: production of erythropoietin and control of the renin–angiotensin–aldosterone system.

Renal blood flow

The kidneys receive 20–25% of the cardiac output ie approximately 1200 mL/min (they represent only 0.5% of the body mass). This is called the renal fraction. The kidneys contribute to local control of renal blood flow by production of several hormones (eg renin, prostaglandins, nitric oxide and the kallikrein cascade).

Factors influencing renal blood flow include:

- Increased flow
  - Hormones (ANP)
  - Drugs (dopamine, dobutamine, captopril, frusemide)
- Decreased flow
  - Hormones (ADH, renin)
  - Anatomy (renal artery stenosis)
  - Drugs (adrenaline/epinephrine, noradrenaline/norepinephrine, β-blockers, indomethacin)

The nephron

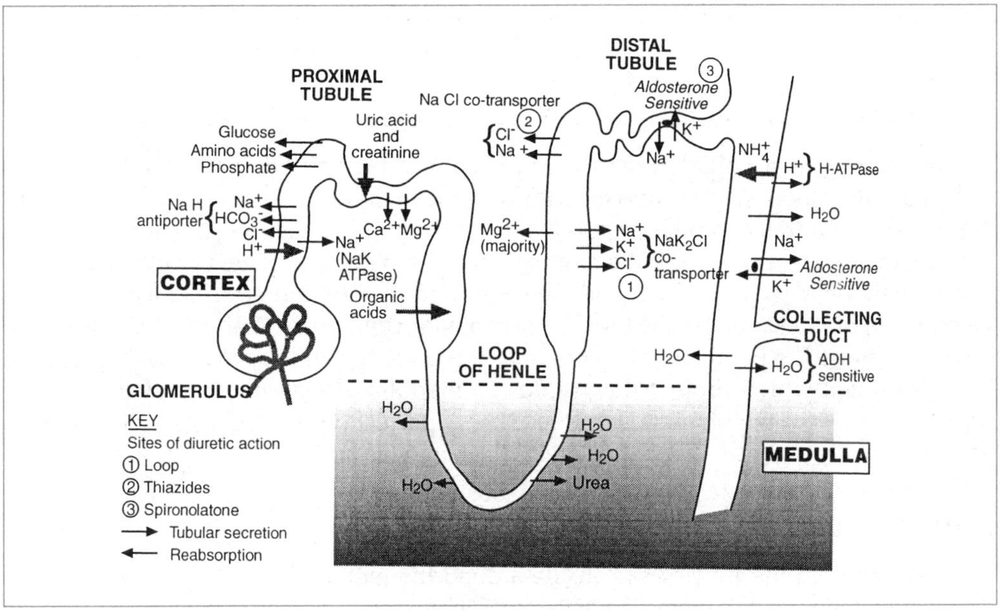

Figure 5.1a *The structure of the nephron*

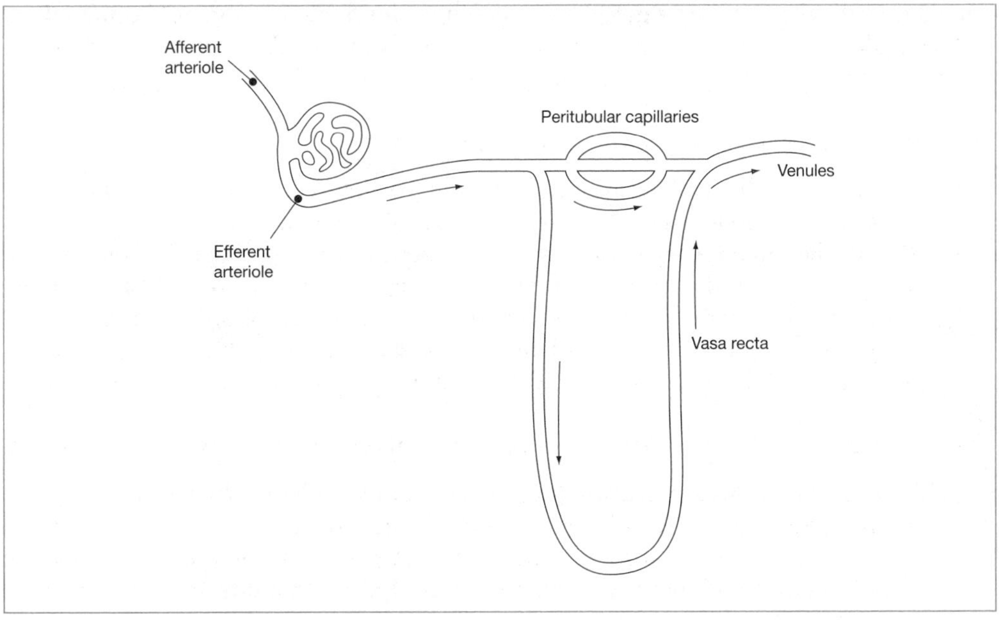

Figure 5.1b *The vasculature surrounding the nephron*

Each kidney has about 1 million functional units or nephrons arranged in parallel (see Fig. 5.1a). The nephron has two main regions – the glomerulus and the tubule. The glomerulus handles blood flow to the kidney and initial plasma filtration. The tubule further filters and processes the filtrate, reabsorbing water and solutes, and excreting others.

Structure and function of the glomerulus

The glomerulus is a coiled capillary bed nestling inside the Bowman's capsule. It is supplied with blood via an **afferent arteriole** and initial filtration of the plasma occurs through the fenestrated capillary endothelium and the basement membrane of the capillary. The major barrier to flow is the basement membrane. The total area available for filtration in the kidney is 1 m^2. The blood then passes to the **efferent arteriole** which forms a second capillary bed around the tubules (**peritubular capillaries**) to allow for reabsorption from the filtrate. The peritubular bed lies in the renal cortex and has long looping capillaries (vasa recta) which project down into the medulla along with the juxtamedullary nephrons. 1–2% of the blood flow to the kidneys passes through the vasa recta and flow here is relatively sluggish. Blood then drains back into the renal venules.

Structure and function of the renal tubule

This extends from the Bowman's capsule around the glomerulus to the collecting ducts (eventually drain into the ureter). Initially ultrafiltrate from Bowman's space drains through the podocyte 'foot' processes of the capsule into the **proximal convoluted tubule (PCT).** The PCT leads to the **loop of Henle**, which has both thin descending and ascending limbs followed by a thick ascending limb. Subsequently the **distal convoluted tubule (DCT)** joins the **cortical collecting duct**, which runs into the medulla forming the **medullary collecting duct.** At each stage the filtrate is progressively modified by secretion and resorption of water and electrolytes (see Fig. 5.1c).

There are two types of nephrons with different functions:

- **Superficial cortical nephrons** (80%): these have glomeruli lying close to the kidney surface and short loops of Henle reaching only the outer medulla
- **Deeper juxtamedullary nephrons** (20%): these have long loops of Henle which plunge deep into the medulla. They are accompanied by the vasa recta which are capillary loops derived from the efferent glomerular arterioles. The vasa recta are involved in a countercurrent system that maintains a high solute concentration in the renal medulla and are used to concentrate urine and thus preserve water

The ultrafiltrate is modified in the tubules by a combination of passive and active processes:

- Three sodium ions are **actively transported** out of the lumen by exchange for two potassium ions via an ATP-driven ion pump in the tubule wall
- This creates an electrical sodium gradient encouraging **simple diffusion** of sodium out of the filtrate. Other compounds such as glucose, chloride and some urea are also reabsorbed this way

- Sodium carrier proteins pull additional molecules (eg amino acids or glucose) into the cell with the sodium ions. This is called co-transport
- Water is drawn out of the tubules by means of passive osmosis

SUMMARY OF FILTRATE-MODIFYING ACTIONS WITHIN THE TUBULE

Nephron region		Resorbs	Secretes
Proximal convoluted tubule	Absorbs about 65% of filtrate Lined with a brush border of villi Extensive membrane area Many transporter molecules (both absorb and secrete)	Na^+, Cl^- H_2O HCO_3^- Glucose K^+ PO_4^{2-}	Organic acids and bases H^+ Some NH_4^+
Loop of Henle (descending)	No villi (site of simple diffusion)	H_2O	
Loop of Henle (ascending)	Thick portion has a brush border Site of active resorption	Na^+, Cl^-	
Distal convoluted tubule	Brush border Specialised 'brown cells' secrete H^+	Cl^-	H^+ NH_4^+ K^+
Collecting ducts	Specialised 'brown cells' secrete H^+	Na^+, Cl^- (Aldosterone) H_2O (ADH)	H^+ NH_4^+

Concentration and dilution of urine

The degree of urinary concentration is controlled by antidiuretic hormone (ADH; see *Renal hormones and their actions* below). In the absence of ADH, the ascending loop of Henle, the distal convoluted tubule, and the collecting ducts are relatively impermeable to water, so a higher proportion of the water in the filtrate is excreted. Concentration of urine is performed by the **countercurrent mechanism** and occurs in the long loops of Henle of the juxtamedullary nephrons and the vasa recta. The renal medulla has a very hyperosmolar interstitial fluid, maintained by active transport of NaCl. As the filtrate passes down the loop of Henle, water is drawn out by the high medullary osmotic pressure. In the ascending limb, additional sodium and chloride are actively transported out of the filtrate. Under the influence of ADH, the distal convoluted tubule and collecting ducts become highly permeable to water. This portion of the nephron passes through the hyperosmolar medulla, so allowing resorption of additional water and concentration of the urine.

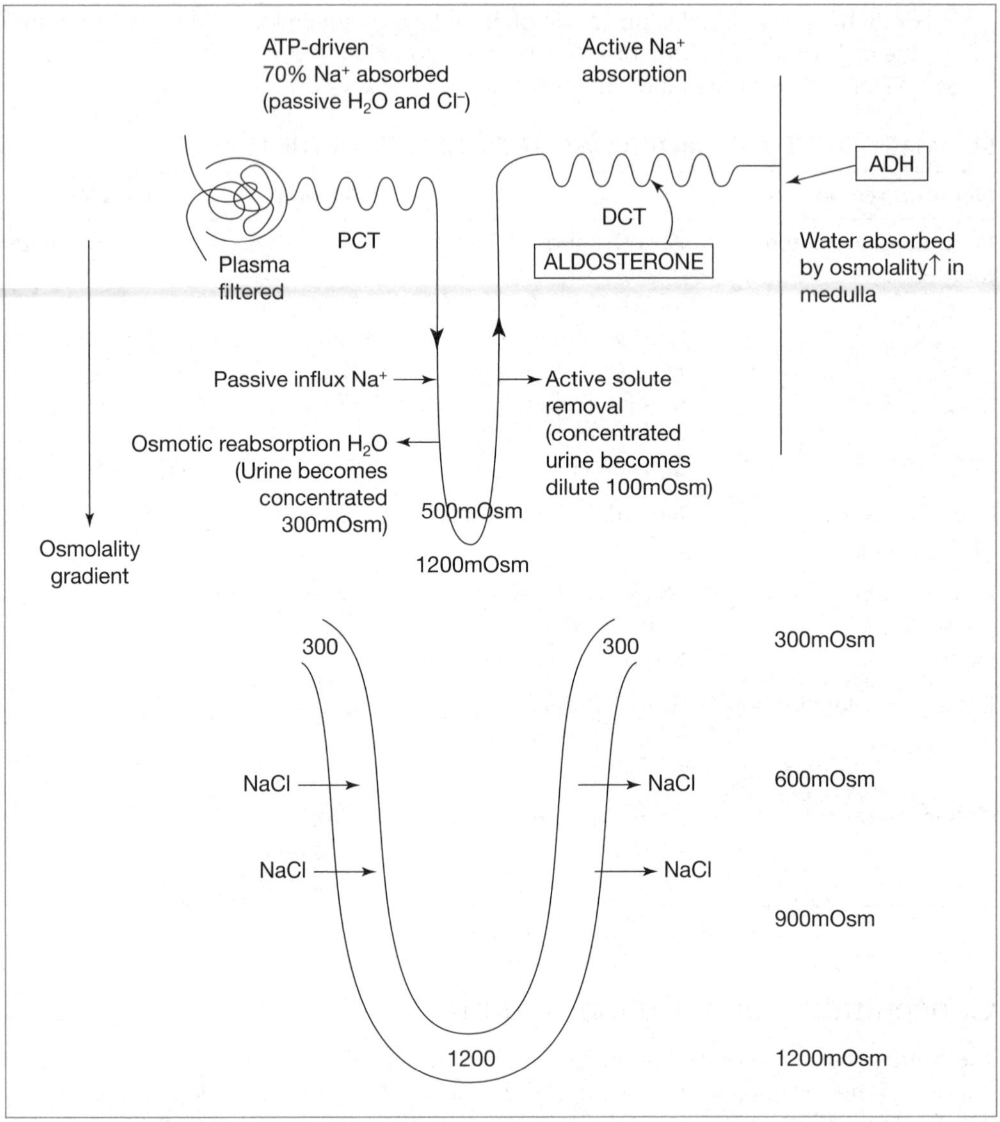

Figure 5.1c *Modifications of the filtrate in the renal tubule*

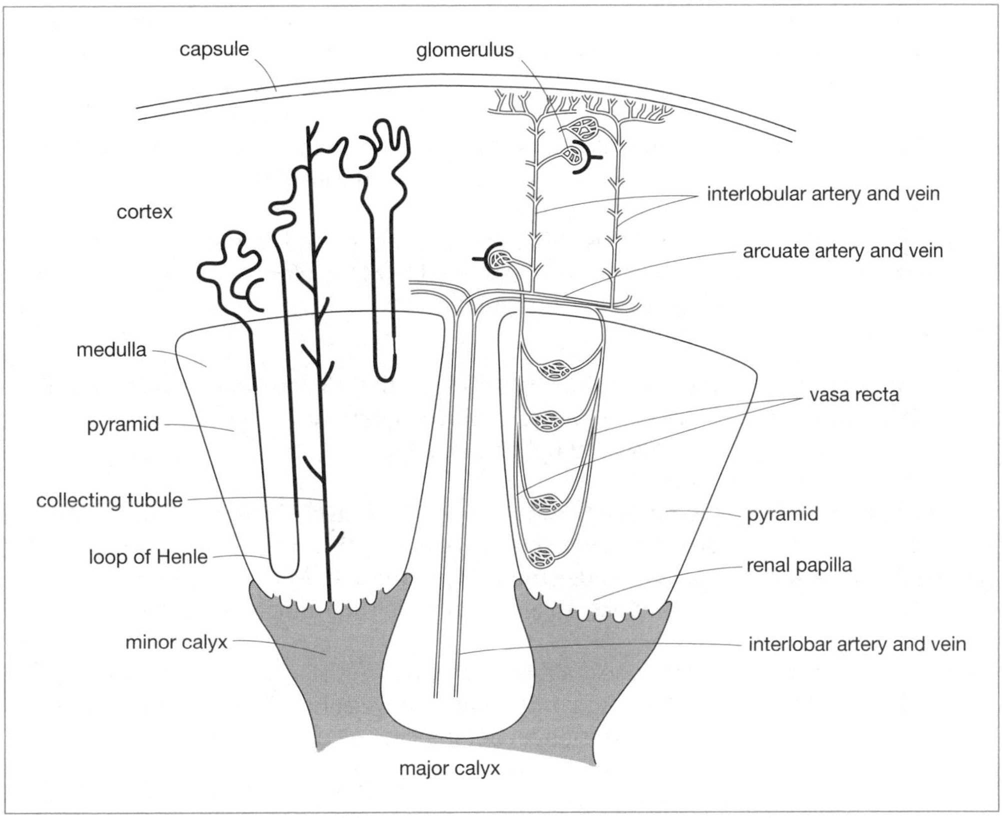

Figure 5.1d *Relationship between the tubule, cortex and medulla*

Glomerular filtration rate (GFR)

This is the net flow of filtrate across the basement membrane per unit time. It is the most sensitive indicator of renal function. There is great functional reserve within the human kidney, and plasma levels of urea and creatinine may be preserved despite massive loss of functioning nephrons. A representative value for GFR in adults is about 125 mL/minute or 180 litres/day. This value varies according to sex and body surface area.

GFR depends on:

- The difference in **hydrostatic pressure** between the glomerular capillary and the Bowman's space (fluid hydrostatic pressure is higher in the capillary promoting filtration of the plasma). Hydronephrosis causes an increase in the hydrostatic pressure of Bowman's capsule, reducing the difference between them and effectively reducing GFR

- The difference in **colloid osmotic pressure** between the glomerular capillary and the Bowman's space (the colloid osmotic pressure is that pressure exerted by the protein content of the fluid; here this is effectively the colloid pressure of the plasma because very few proteins are filtered into the Bowman's capsule – this opposes filtration)
- The **ultrafiltration coefficient** is a constant related to the area and conductivity of the basement membrane, may be altered in glomerulonephritis

As the glomerular capillary bed has an arteriole at either end (a unique situation) the hydrostatic pressure in the capillaries is determined both by afferent and efferent arteriolar resistance. This allows very precise regulation of capillary pressure and therefore glomerular filtration.

- **Afferent** arteriolar vasoconstriction decreases both GFR and glomerular plasma flow
- **Efferent** arteriolar vasoconstriction reduces glomerular plasma flow, and also increases glomerular pressure and therefore GFR

Autoregulation holds the glomerular filtration pressure relatively constant despite variation in mean arterial blood pressure over the range 80–180 mmHg. The mechanism for autoregulation is not completely understood. However it still occurs in denervated and isolated perfused kidney preparations, suggesting that it is intrinsic to the kidney.

If renal perfusion pressure increases, afferent arteriolar resistance also increases so that glomerular blood flow and GFR remain constant. Conversely, when blood pressure falls the afferent arteriole decreases in resistance, but the efferent arteriolar resistance increases to maintain GFR.

Juxtoglomerular apparatus (JGA)

Tubuloglomerular feedback is another mechanism by which GFR is regulated. This is negative feedback system whereby the GFR is inversely related to fluid delivery to the distal nephron. It is controlled by specialist cells in the **juxtaglomerular apparatus** (JGA). The JGA is located in the initial portion of the DCT where the DCT bends upwards, and is situated between the afferent and efferent arterioles of the glomerulus.

The JGA contains three cell types:

- Macula densa cells (cells of the tubule involved in feedback)
- Juxtaglomerular cells (smooth muscle cells of the arterioles which secrete renin)
- Extraglomerular mesangial cells

Measurement of glomerular filtration rate (GFR)

There are a number of ways of measuring GFR. Each requires the use of a solute that is:

- Detectable in plasma and urine
- Freely filtered by the kidney
- Not absorbed or secreted

- Not toxic
- Does not alter renal blood flow

This solute may be administered exogenously (eg inulin, which requires continuous infusion for steady plasma state) or may be produced endogenously (eg creatinine, which fulfils most of these requirements apart from a degree of tubular secretion).

Creatinine clearance therefore gives an approximation of GFR. To calculate GFR:

$$GFR = UV / P$$

Where V is the volume of urine produced, P is the concentration of the solute in the plasma, and U is the concentration of the solute in the urine.

The **filtration fraction** is the proportion of plasma filtered by the glomerulus. It is expressed as the relationship between GFR and renal blood flow and is normally about one-fifth of the value of GFR.

Renal blood flow (RBF) can be calculated if it is considered that renal plasma flow (RPF) is equal to the GFR, thus:

$$RBF = RPF / (1 - \text{haematocrit})$$

Diuretics

Diuretics work by increasing urine volume, This can be achieved either by increasing renal tubular excretion of sodium and chloride which draws water with it, or by giving an osmotically active substance such as mannitol.

Thiazides (eg bendrofluazide)

These act by inhibiting NaCl resorption in the DCT (thus exchanging urinary sodium loss for postassium loss) by acting on tubular ATPase ion pumps. Side effects include hypokalaemia, hyperuricaemia (alteration in the excretion of uric acid), glucose intolerance, and hyperlipidaemia.

Loop diuretics (eg furosemide, bumetanide)

These act by inhibiting the co-transport of sodium, chloride and potassium in the thick ascending loop of Henle. Potassium is lost in preference to sodium and so the hypokalaemic effect can be pronounced.

Potassium-sparing diuretics (eg spironolactone, amiloride)

These act as aldosterone antagonists and therefore prevent resorption of sodium in the DCT. These drugs do not cause the body to exchange sodium loss for potassium loss and therefore do not cause hypokalaemia. Care must be taken in the elderly not to cause hyperkalaemia.

Renal hormones and their actions

Antidiuretic hormone/arginine vasopressin (ADH/AVP)

This hormone is produced by the cells of the supraoptic nucleus of the hypothalamus and is stored in the posterior pituitary gland. It is released by a number of stimuli:

- Increased plasma osmolality (sensed by osmoreceptors in the brain)
- Decreased blood pressure (sensed by baroreceptors in the great vessels)
- Decreased circulating volume (stretch receptors and increased ANP)

Alcohol, opiates, prostaglandins, oestrogens and stress all decrease ADH secretion. ADH (AVP) acts to increase salt and thus water reabsorption in the DCT and to increase the permeability of the collecting system and thus increase the amount of water reabsorbed as the filtrate passes through the medulla. This concentrates the urine and reduces its volume.

Renin–angiotensin–aldosterone (RAA) system

Renin is produced and stored in the smooth muscle cells of the juxtaglomerular apparatus. It is released when arterial pressure falls. It has several intrarenal functions and acts enzymically on a plasma protein, angiotensin I.

Angiotensin I is quickly converted to angiotensin II by angiotensin-converting enzyme (ACE) in lung endothelium. Angiotensin II has three major actions:

- It is a powerful vasoconstrictor, increasing arterial pressure
- It acts directly on the kidney to conserve sodium and water and to decrease renal blood flow, which reduces urine volume, gradually increasing arterial pressure
- It stimulates the production of aldosterone by the adrenal glands

Aldosterone causes increased sodium retention by the kidney tubules, which expands the ECF compartment by causing retention of water.

Atrial natriuretic peptide (ANP)

Over-stretching of the atrial wall by high volumes is sensed by stretch receptors and results in the release of ANP into the bloodstream. This acts on the kidneys to increase sodium and water excretion and thus reduce blood volume by increasing urine output.

5.2 RENAL FAILURE

Renal failure

In a nutshell ...

Renal failure is defined as failure of the kidneys to maintain the correct composition and volume of the body's internal environment. Patients undergoing major surgery are at risk of developing renal failure, particularly in the post-operative period, where inadequate fluid rehydration is not uncommon.

Anuria is the absence of urine output. In most surgical patients, sudden anuria is more likely to be due to a blocked or misplaced urinary catheter rather than to ATN.

Oliguria is defined as a urine output of > 400 mL in 24 hours or > 0.5 mL/kg/hour. This is a much more likely presentation of impending renal failure in surgical patients than anuria. It is not uncommonly seen after inadequate fluid replacement.

Non-oliguric renal failure can also occur. It has a much lower morbidity.

Causes of renal failure

In a nutshell ...

Acute renal failure (ARF) is a rapid reduction in renal function (best measured by decrease in GFR or increase in serum creatinine) that may or may not be accompanied by oliguria. The abrupt decline in renal function occurs over hours or days.

The most useful classification system divides renal failure into pre-renal, renal and post-renal.

Causes of acute renal failure

Pre-renal causes

Volume depletion (eg haemorrhage, GI losses, dehydration, burns)
Abnormal fluid distribution, (eg sepsis, cirrhosis, CCF)
Local renal ischaemia, eg renal artery stenosis or prostaglandin inhibitors such as NSAIDs

Renal causes

Acute tubular necrosis (ATN) (eg sequelae to pre-renal, nephrotoxins)
Acute interstitial nephritis
Acute glomerulonephritis

Post-renal causes

Bladder outlet obstruction (chronic retention)
Bilateral ureteric obstruction (eg prostate cancer, bladder cancer, retroperitoneal fibrosis)

Pre-renal causes of renal failure

Under-perfusion of the kidneys is the commonest cause of renal failure in critical care.

Hypovolaemia is classified according to aetiology:

- Loss of whole blood (haemorrhage)
- Loss of plasma (burns)
- Loss of crystalloid (dehydration, diarrhoea, vomiting)

NB: As far as possible one should replace like with like, ie blood after haemorrhage or water (given as 5% dextrose) in dehydration. However, in many hypovolaemic patients, the priority is initially to rapidly replace lost circulating volume. This is with blood, or colloid, or isotonic crystalloid, such as 0.9% saline. The remaining fluid deficit can be made up more slowly with whatever fluid most closely resembles the fluid losses.

The typical mechanism is that hypoxaemia and hypo-perfusion reduce sodium absorption in the ascending loop of Henle, which is a high energy-consuming process. Hence the juxtaglomerular apparatus detects increased filtrate sodium concentration, and so reduces renal blood flow to conserve blood volume, resulting in reduced urine output. Appropriate treatment should reverse this process before ischaemic damage and ATN occurs.

Causes of pre-renal renal failure

Other causes of hypotension (eg drugs)
Septic shock
Anaphylactic shock
Endocrine shock
Low-output cardiac failure
Renovascular disease (eg renal artery stenosis)
Raised intra-abdominal pressure (abdominal compartment syndrome)
Renal artery emboli or trauma

Renal causes of renal failure

Intrinsic renal pathology:

- ATN due to prolonged ischaemia or tubular toxins, including drugs (eg gentamicin)
- Glomerulonephritis or vasculitis (eg SLE, polyarteritis nodosa, Wegener's granulomatosis)
- Goodpasture syndrome (anti-glomerular basement membrane antibodies)
- Interstitial nephritis, drugs
- Vascular lesions, hypertension, emboli, renal vein thrombosis
- Infections, pyelonephritis

Post-renal causes of renal failure

Obstruction to the flow of urine along the urinary tract:

- Pelvicalyceal: usually at PUJ (eg bilateral PUJ obstruction)
- Ureteric: luminal/intra-mural extrinsic obstruction; retroperitoneal fibrosis, stone
- Bladder/urethral outflow obstruction: urinary retention, high pressure or atonic bladder, urethral stricture, blocked catheter, cervical prostatic neoplasm

The most important causes of renal failure that must not be missed (because they are so easily treatable) are pre-renal, especially hypovolaemia/dehydration, and post-renal (particularly prostate or catheter problems). Also inadequate rehydration of a post-obstructive diuresis commonly results in pre-renal failure. See section 5.6 in Chapter 6 *Peri-operative Care* for guidelines and a scenario for post-operative management of acute renal failure.

Differentiating pre-renal and renal causes

This is initially on the basis of a history and examination. Where there is still a query as to the cause of renal failure, an analysis of the urine and serum biochemistry is performed. This is one of the simplest and most effective ways of differentiating pre-renal and intrinsic renal failure.

Urine analysis and serum biochemistry

Measurement	Pre-renal	Renal
Urinary sodium	Low: < 20 mmol/L	High: > 40 mmol/L
Urine		
Serum osmolarity ratio	> 1.2	< 1.2
Serum creatinine ratio	High: > 40	Low: < 20
Urine osmolality	> 500	< 350

Normal kidneys, in the presence of hypotension or hypovolaemia, will concentrate urine and conserve sodium (meaning that there will be less in the urine). If there is intrinsic renal pathology, the kidney will be unable to concentrate the urine or to conserve sodium.

The fractional excretion of sodium is normally < 1. In renal failure it is > 1 and can be used as a trend indicator.

Prevention of renal failure

- Prevention of hypotension or hypovolaemia
- Prevention of dehydration (especially in patients who continue to receive their 'normal' diuretic medication)
- Early treatment of sepsis
- Take care with potentially nephrotoxic drugs (eg NSAIDs, gentamicin): in all cases monitor renal function closely, substitute these drugs with non-nephrotoxic equivalents if there is any indication of deterioration in renal function

Presentation and management of renal failure

Assessment of acute renal failure

The main distinction is between renal and pre-renal causes. Post-renal causes are often clinically evident.

- History
- Examination
- Serum urea and creatinine
- Blood gases: a metabolic acidosis may occur
- Urinary measures of osmolality and sodium: these are helpful in distinguishing causes:
    - Pre-renal causes: high urinary osmolality and low urinary sodium
    - Renal causes: low urine osmolality and high urinary sodium

This is because there is a normal physiological response to the insults of pre-renal failure by concentrating the urine, but in renal causes the damaged tubules are unable to concentrate the urine in the normal manner.

- **Response to fluid challenge:** this may distinguish between pre-renal and renal causes. If no diuresis occurs with adequate fluid replacement, consider a renal cause
- **Bladder scanning for residual volume and catheterisation:** this diagnoses retention
- **Renal tract USS and Doppler:** these show renal blood flow, and evidence and level of hydronephrosis

Management of renal failure

The important steps in the management of oliguria are:

- **Exclude obstruction:** insert catheter or flush existing catheter, consider renal US
- **Correct hypovolaemia and hypotension:** may need CVP +/– PA catheter and assessment of response of CVP to fluid boluses. When optimally filled inotropes or vasopressor may be required to provide adequate perfusion pressure (perfusion pressure may need to be increased in hypertensives)
- **Fluid maintenance after resuscitation:** includes infusing volume equivalent to urine output each hour plus insensible losses (about 1000 mL/24h). Insensible losses will be increased in pyrexia
- **Treat the cause or any contributing factors:** eg stop NSAIDs and ACE inhibitors. Prostaglandin inhibition by NSAIDs causes renal vasoconstriction

In addition, various treatments are often used to try to reverse/prevent renal failure. Examples of such treatments are:

- **Frusemide:** either as a bolus or as a continuous infusion. An infusion of 5–10 mg/hour is more effective than bolus therapy (the principle being a frusemide-induced reduction of oxygen consumption by the nephron)
- **Dopamine or dopexamine:** cause stimulation of dopamine receptors.
- **Sodium loading with $NaHCO_3$** to reduce oxygen dependent sodium retention by the nephron
- **Mannitol:** increases urine output by osmotic diuresis. Does not prevent renal failure; some evidence of nephrotoxicity. Used successfully to reduce renal damage in jaundice and rhabdomyolysis. Beware that induced diuresis can cause hypovolaemia and reduce renal perfusion

However, none of these treatments have been proven to prevent renal failure, and the other measures shown above are much more important.

In established renal failure, artificial support may be required. This is commonly achieved by haemodialysis.

Other aspects to consider in a patient with impending or established renal failure are:

- Renal replacement therapy
- Hydration and fluid balance
- Optimisation of serum biochemistry
- Nutrition
- Treatment of infection
- Review of drug therapy

5.3 RENAL REPLACEMENT THERAPY

Indications for renal replacement therapy

- Hyperkalaemia (persistently > 6.0 mmol/L)
- Metabolic acidosis (pH < 7.2) with negative base excess
- Pulmonary oedema/fluid overload without substantial diuresis
- The need to 'make room' for ongoing drug infusions and nutrition, and to aid clearance of drugs already given (eg sedatives)
- Complications of chronic uraemia (eg pericarditis/cardiac tamponade)
- High urea (30–40 mmol/L)
- Creatinine rising more than 100 mmol/L/day

Methods of renal replacement therapy

CAVH	Continuous arterio-venous haemofiltration
CVVH	Continuous veno-venous haemofiltration
CVVHD	Continuous veno-venous haemodiafiltration
HD	Haemodialysis

In ITU, both haemofiltration and haemodiafiltration are commonly performed via a large-bore dual lumen central venous cannula (CVVH). As the flow of blood is both from and to the venous side of the circulation, a pump is required. The blood flow is in the region of 250 mL/min and alarms are incorporated to prevent air embolism. Anti-coagulation is needed and heparin is usually used as an infusion or prostacyclin if thrombocytopenia develops. Previously arterio-venous systems were used, but a large-bore catheter needs to be placed in an artery and filtration depends on arterial pressure. These techniques provide slow fluid shifts and maintain haemodynamic stability.

In haemofiltration the blood is driven under pressure through a filter (a semipermeable membrane). The 'ultrafiltrate' derived from the blood (which is biochemically abnormal) is disposed of, and is replaced with a replacement fluid. Small molecules such as sodium, urea, creatinine and bicarbonate pass through the filter with water (convection) but large molecules like proteins and cells do not. The usual volume of filtrate produced is 1–2 litres per hour and this volume is replaced with an electrolyte solution containing ions and buffer. The replacement fluid is buffered with lactate, acetate, or freshly added bicarbonate. (Bicarbonate is unstable in solution and lactate is metabolised by the liver to bicarbonate.) The system provides a clearance equivalent approximate to 10 mL/min and if solute clearance is inadequate then augmentation with dialysis can be used (CVVHD).

In haemodiafiltration (CVVHD) the dialysate augments clearance by diffusion by running an electrolyte solution on the outside of the filter. The clearance increases to about 20 mL/min. Fluid balance over 24 hours can be manipulated using these filters. If the patient is oedematous then 2 litres negative. If the patient is oedematous then removal of 2 litres may be appropriate and can be achieved by replacing 84 mL less per hour than is filtered.

In haemodialysis (HD) blood is pumped through the machine on one side of a semipermeable membrane, in a manner similar to haemofiltration. However, in HD dialysis fluid is also pumped through the machine, on the other side of the semipermeable membrane to the blood. The biochemistry of the blood equilibrates with that of the dialysis fluid, by diffusion, although some ultrafiltration also occurs.

HD tends to be more effective in terms of correcting acidosis and abnormal biochemistry in a short period of time. However, it is associated with more circulatory instability; continuous haemofiltration is often better tolerated in patients with pre-existing circulatory instability.

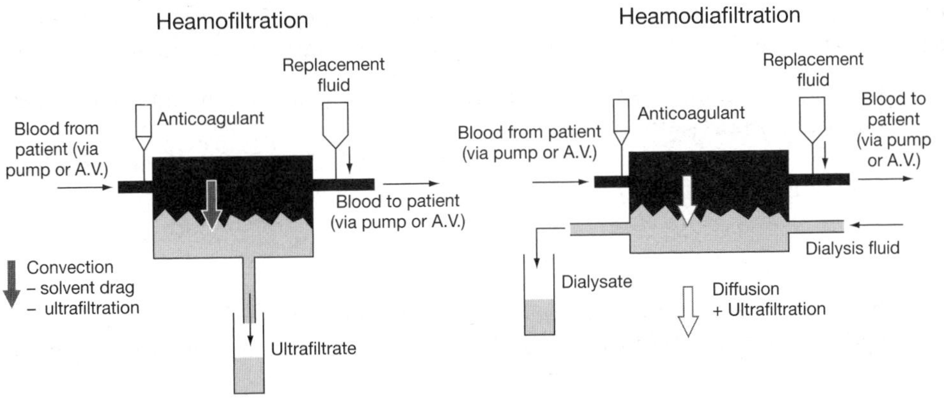

Figure 5.3a *Haemofiltration and haemodialysis*

Continuous ambulatory peritoneal dialysis (CAPD) is becoming more common. Fluid is instilled into the peritoneum by a special catheter (eg Tenckhoff catheter). The peritoneum acts as the dialysis membrane. Increasingly, this method is chosen by patients as they can perform it at home, but it is unsuitable for patients post-laparotomy on ITU.

Optimisation of serum biochemistry in renal failure

The following biochemical abnormalities commonly occur:

- Progressive rise in urea and creatinine
- Hyperkalaemia
- Hyponatraemia (due to relative water overload)
- Acidosis

- Hypocalcaemia
- Hyperphosphataemia
- Hyperuricaemia

The abnormalities requiring most urgent correction are hyperkalaemia and acidosis.

Treatment of hyperkalaemia

- 10 mL 10% calcium chloride IV (reduces risk of arrhythmia)
- 15 units IV insulin + 50 mL 50% dextrose
- Sodium bicarbonate infusion
- Salbutamol or other β-agonist

Neither insulin nor β-agonists or sodium bicarbonate reduce total body potassium. They increase intracellular potassium and so reduce the serum potassium. This reduces the risk of a fatal arrhythmia, but is only a short-term measure; haemofiltration/haemodialysis will be required medium/long term to prevent hyperkalaemia unless renal function improves.

- Calcium resonium: orally or PR (reduces total body potassium, but poorly tolerated orally and works slowly)
- Stop potassium-containing infusions (which may include TPN or enteral feed)
- Stop drugs such as potassium-sparing diuretics

Treatment of acidosis

- If artificially ventilated, increase the minute ventilation
- Sodium bicarbonate infusion (but this is controversial, may paradoxically increase intracellular acidosis, and is only a short-term measure)
- Artificial renal support

Nutrition in patients with renal failure

High-calorie diet needed, with adequate high-quality protein. Maximum of 35 kcal/kg/day (about 2500 kcal) plus 14 g nitrogen/day.

Treatment of infection in patients with renal failure

Infection and generalised sepsis may already be apparent as the cause or contributing factors in the development of renal failure. If the cause of renal failure (or other organ system failure) is due to sepsis it is unlikely to improve until the source of the sepsis is eradicated (eg intra-abdominal collection).

In anuric patients the catheter should be removed and not replaced until urine output has recovered, to prevent ascending urinary tract infection.

Review of drug therapy for patients with renal failure

All drug therapy given to patients in renal failure needs to be regularly and thoroughly reviewed.

- Drugs which may exacerbate renal failure or its complications (eg NSAIDs, ACE inhibitors, gentamicin and potassium-sparing diuretics) should be avoided
- Many drugs need dose adjustment to prevent overdosage because they, or their active metabolites, are excreted by the kidneys (this includes most antibiotics)
- If possible, serum drug levels should be checked and drug doses adjusted accordingly

Section 6

The gastrointestinal tract in critical care

6.1 GASTROINTESTINAL FAILURE

In a nutshell ...

Gastrointestinal failure may present in a variety of ways:

Failure to absorb feed
Ileus and functional obstruction (pseudo-obstruction)
Diarrhoea
Stress ulceration
Acalculous cholecystitis

The gut is also the site of bacterial translocation.

Mucosal integrity and GI function may be improved by fluid resuscitation and the judicious use of dopexamine or dopamine to improve splanchnic circulation and perfusion.

- **Stress ulceration** may be due to reduction in gastric and duodenal mucosal blood flow and may present with bleeding or perforation
- **Prolonged ileus** may compromise ventilation due to an increase in intra-abdominal pressure. It may respond to neostigmine or cisapride
- **Acalculous cholecystitis** occurs in the critically ill and is probably due to ischaemia (splanchnic hypoperfusion) with associated biliary stasis and retrograde infection from the bowel. It may progress to ascending cholangitis

6.2 BACTERIAL TRANSLOCATION

This is the passage of viable bacteria from the GI tract to sites that are normally sterile (mesenteric lymph nodes, peritoneal surfaces, and distant organs).

The gut has both metabolic and immunological functions and serves as a barrier to the numerous bacteria in its lumen. The barrier is intrinsically composed of the epithelial layer of the mucosa but its ability to exclude bacteria is aided by:

- Gastric acid
- Pancreatic enzymes
- Bile
- Mucus
- Bowel motility
- Gut-associated lymphoid tissue (GALT)

The epithelial layer is composed of enterocytes covered in a brush border, mucus and secretory IgA. Luminal bacteria have been demonstrated inside enterocytes and it is thought that this bacterial translocation is a normal phenomenon allowing the gut to 'sample' its contents and direct the activity of its immunological barrier. Sepsis occurs when this process is uncontrolled and bacteria cross the intestinal wall through the enterocytes (trans-cellularly) and through leaky tight junctions between cells (para-cellularly).

Factors predisposing to bacterial translocation

- Changes in the endogenous microflora
- Increases in the local concentration of a particular species (critical illness is associated with overgrowth of organisms, especially in the proximal GI tract which is relatively sterile in health)
- Reduced mucosal integrity
  - Ischaemia-reperfusion injury
  - Inflammation
  - Decreased luminal nutrition
- Reduction in immune status

Bacterial translocation is thought to occur in up to 15% of surgical patients, especially:

- Abdominal surgery
- Bowel obstruction of any cause
- Colorectal cancer
- Ischaemia, reperfusion injury
- Shock states

Septic complications are more prevalent in patients who have evidence of bacteria in mesenteric lymph nodes at laparotomy. Often the same bacterial species can be isolated from NG aspirates as septic foci, suggesting that translocation from the gut may be responsible for bacteraemia.

Enteral nutrition is thought to be important in these patients as certain luminal nutrients are important for enterocyte function (glutamine, alanine and anti-oxidants such as vitamin A). Luminal feeding also prevents mucosal atrophy and may reduce bacterial overgrowth.

6.3 GASTROINTESTINAL BLEEDING

Usually occurs from a source in the upper GI tract:

- Gastric or duodenal ulceration
- Oesophageal varices
- Aorto-enteric fistula
- AV malformations

The diagnosis and management of GI bleeding are discussed further in the section on the *Stomach and duodenum* in *Abdomen* (Book 2)

6.4 HEPATIC FAILURE

Definitions of liver failure depend on the relationship between the onset of jaundice and the subsequent onset of encephalopathy.

- Hyper-acute hepatic failure: < 7 days
- Acute hepatic failure: 7–28 days
- Sub-acute hepatic failure: 28 days to 6 months
- Fulminant hepatic failure: < 8 weeks

Many patients with hepatic failure will develop multiorgan failure and require critical care. Patients should be managed in a specialist centre with access to facilities such as transplantation.

For further discussion on the diagnosis and management of hepatic failure see the section on *Liver and Spleen* in *Abdomen* (Book 2).

6.5 PANCREATITIS

Pancreatitis may range on a scale from mild and self-limiting (eg after ERCP) to severe and combined with multiorgan failure requiring critical care facilities. Patients may deteriorate quickly and without warning (especially the elderly) and require regular repeated assessment.

Further discussion on the diagnosis and management of pancreatitis can be found in the section on *Biliary Tree and Pancreas* in the *Abdomen* chapter (Book 2).

Section 7

Neurological and psychological problems in critical care

7.1 INTRACRANIAL EVENTS

In a nutshell ...

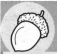

ICP is normally about 10 mmHg. It is considered critically high if it is > 24 mmHg.

Within the cranium are:
- Brain tissue
- Blood
- CSF

Any increase in one of these compartments causes a compensatory reduction in one or more of the others until compliance is lost and ICP rapidly rises.

Causes and effects of raised ICP

- Intracranial bleeding
- Cerebral oedema; head injury, liver failure, changes in osmolality
- Secondary brain injury; hypoxaemia, shock,
- Hypercapnia (CO_2 induced cerebral vasodilatation)

Raised ICP decreases cerebral perfusion pressure (CPP):

- CPP = MAP – ICP
- CPP of < 70 mmHg may lead to inadequate cerebral oxygenation

It is vital that CPP is maintained by ensuring an adequate MAP if ICP is raised. Hypotonic fluids such as dextrose are harmful due to osmotic changes in the brain, but isotonic fluids to optimise the BP should not be withheld. Vasopressors may be required to ensure an adequate CPP.

ICP monitoring

- Pressure transducer inserted through the skull
- Fibre-optic subdural transducer (easy to place)
- Ventriculostomy (more accurate, higher complications, but able to withdraw CSF if acute rise in ICP)

Cerebral blood flow monitoring

- Jugular venous saturation
- A catheter is placed retrogradely into the jugular vein with the tip lying at the base of the skull. Samples of blood or a fibre-optic oximeter tip measure the global oxygen saturation of blood draining from the brain. A low saturation implies poor perfusion and a higher saturation suggests increased blood flow

Taken in conjunction with ICP monitoring it can be helpful in determining therapy for raised ICP. If high cerebral blood flow then hyperventilation to a lower $PaCO_2$ of around 3.5–4 will reduce vessel diameter and hence ICP. If there is poor perfusion, then hyperventilation is harmful as perfusion is decreased to critical levels. Diuretics should be considered instead.

Other therapies for reducing ICP

- Nurse slightly head up
- Avoid cervical collars when ventilated
- Avoid tight tube ties round the neck and jugular CVP lines
- Ventilate to $PaCO_2$ around 4.0 kPa (over-ventilation leads to rebound increase in ICP)
- Mannitol causes transient decrease in ICP by osmosis and improved rheology, but it is transient with rebound increase (discuss with neurosurgeon first in head injuries)
- Keep sedated if ventilated, consider paralysis and care with suctioning

7.2 BRAINSTEM DEATH

The diagnosis of brainstem death

Definition of brainstem death

- Irreversible cessation of brainstem function
- In the UK, diagnosed by specific tests as follows

Pre-conditions for diagnosis of brainstem death

- Apnoeic coma requiring ventilation
- Known cause of irreversible brain damage (eg head injury, cerebral haemorrhage)

Exclusions from diagnosis of brainstem death

- Hypothermia (temperature below 35 °C)
- No depressant drugs (eg sedatives, opiates, muscle relaxants)
- No metabolic derangements (eg sodium, glucose, hepatic encephalopathy)

NB: Sodium is taken at the time of diagnosis because otherwise it may be difficult to normalise the value in diabetes insipidus.

Tests of brainstem death

These look for activity in the cranial nerves (CN).

- **Pupil responses:** CN2. No direct or indirect reaction to light
- **Corneal reflex:** CN5 and CN7. Direct stimulation with cotton wool
- **Pain reflex:** in facial distribution; motor. CN5 and CN7. Reflexes below the neck are ignored as they may be spinal reflexes
- **Caloric test:** instillation of cold water into the auditory canal, looking for nystagmus towards the stimulation. CN8, CN3 and CN6. Check canal is not blocked with wax first
- **Gag reflex:** CN9 and CN10
- **Apnoea test:** pre-oxygenate with 100% O_2 then disconnect from the ventilator. Insufflate oxygen into the trachea via catheter at 4 L/min. Observe for any sign of respiration for 10 minutes until $PaCO_2$ is above 6.65 kPa. May need to stop test if sats drop or becomes bradycardic and unstable

If the patient shows no response to the above tests then brain death can be diagnosed after two sets have been performed. Legal time of death is after the first set.

The tests are performed by two doctors, both 5 years post-registration, one of whom must be a consultant, and neither doctor should be a member of a transplant team. There is no set time between the two sets but at least 6 hours should have elapsed between the onset of coma and the first set.

Organ donation after brainstem death

The possibility of donation must be discussed with the relatives, usually after the first set of tests. If they agree to donation then the local transplant co-ordinator is contacted, who arranges viral and histocompatibility testing. They will come to the hospital and talk in detail with the relatives and liaise with the transplant surgeons. See Chapter 11 *Urology and Transplantation*.

7.3 PSYCHOLOGICAL ASPECTS OF RECOVERY FROM CRITICAL CARE

There are physical and psychological effects of a period spent in critical care.

Physical complications of critical care

- Reduced function due to disease process or pathology
- Muscle wasting and weakness
- Joint stiffness
- Nerve injuries or peripheral neuropathy
- Pressure sores
- Sleep disturbance and loss of diurnal rhythm
- Tracheal stenosis

Psychological impact of critical care

Do not underestimate the psychological impact of critical care. After recovery patients feel that they have lost a portion of their memory or their memory may be hazy and disjointed. They may recall pieces of conversation held around their bedside and have memories during periods of drifting in and out of consciousness. They often feel a loss of control. They may experience anxiety, depression and nightmares.

Some ITUs run a post-discharge clinic where patients can attend to talk about their experiences. Patient feedback may help the ITU to minimise the impact by altering practice.

7.4 DEALING WITH DEATH

See the section on *Surgery, Ethics and the Law* in Chapter 8 for discussion of general ethical issues in surgery.

Withdrawal of treatment

Over the duration of admission to the ITU and after a period of stabilisation and treatment it may become apparent that the patient will not recover.

Decisions may be taken that active treatment may be withdrawn, reduced or not increased. Withdrawal of supportive treatment such as inotropes, ventilatory support, or renal replacement therapy may be considered. Most units also have an upper threshold for certain types of treatment (eg inotrope doses) that represents what they consider to be maximal support.

In cases where there is a consensus from the medical and nursing staff that continued treatment would be futile, there is no medicolegal requirement to continue with treatment. This should be discussed in depth between the relevant family members and members of the medical and nursing teams caring for the patient.

Deaths that should be reported to the coroner

Report to the Coroner all deaths occurring:

- Within 24 hours of admission
- Related to surgery or anaesthesia
- In theatre
- Due to accidents and trauma (report all fractured neck of femur cases)
- Due to self or external neglect
- Due to poisoning or drugs
- Due to industrial or notifiable disease

If in doubt, discuss the case informally with the coroner's officer. They are an invaluable source of help and advice. You will need to tell them all the patient's details, the dates of admission and death, and give an outline summary of the case with suggested causes for completion of the death certificate.

It is very important that death certificates are filled in correctly as a great deal of epidemiological information is garnered from them and this has effects as far reaching as funding for service provision.

Section 8

Sepsis in critical care

8.1 SEPTIC SHOCK

Factors predisposing to sepsis in critical care

Factors predisposing to sepsis in critical care

Impaired barriers

Loss of gag reflex – reduced level of consciousness, drugs
Loss of cough reflex – drugs, pain
Ciliary function – high-inspired O_2, dry O_2, intubation
Gut mucosal barrier – ischaemia, change in gut flora (antibiotics)
Urinary catheters predispose to UTI
IV/arterial lines breach skin barrier

Impaired defences

Cell-mediated immunity
Humoral immunity
Reticulo-endothelial system
Caused by trauma, shock, post-op, sepsis itself, age, malnutrition, malignancy, splenectomy (humoral), immunosuppressive drugs

Gram-positive bacteria are the commonest cause of infection (eg staphylococci) and have taken over from Gram-negatives such as *Pseudomonas*, *Escherichia coli* and *Proteus*. Organisms such as *Actinobacter* are a particular problem on ITUs after use of broad-spectrum antibiotics or immunosuppression, as are fungal infections (eg *Candida* and *Aspergillus*).

Local antibiotic policy on ITUs should be formulated by collaboration with the microbiologist so that appropriate antibiotics for local organisms are used, as well as being based on culture and sensitivity.

Typical policies follow patterns such as:

Cephalosporin + metronidazole +/– gentamicin (renal toxicity)

↓

If unsuccessful

↓

Broad-spectrum anti-pseudomonals such as:
Piperacillin + tazobactam
Ciprofloxacin
Ceftazidime

or

Imipenem/meropenem

Antibiotic policy should be guided by culture and sensitivity of sputum, blood, wound and urine samples, but quite often these are not available, hence broad-spectrum agents are used. Take advice from your microbiologist.

- For MRSA: teicoplanin, or vancomycin (beware toxicity)
- For fungal infections: fluconazole followed by amphotericin if resistant or *Aspergillus*

Infection on ITUs

- Community acquired: tend to be sensitive organisms
- Nosocomial: tend to be resistant species
- Gram-positive are commoner, but *Pseudomonas* and other Gram-negatives still occur
- EPIC (European Prevalence of Infection in Intensive Care) study shown 21% infections acquired within ITUs

Septic shock

Classically high cardiac output, low systemic resistance, maldistribution of blood flow, and increased vascular permeability. There is suppression of contractility but tachycardia increases cardiac output. Vasodilatation results from NO production. Effects are induced by inflammatory responses but not always infection (eg pancreatitis).

Features of septic shock

- Pyrexia
- Tachycardia
- Warm skin/flushed or cold/mottled
- Hypotensive, low CVP
- Acidotic (lactic acidosis)

NB: NSAIDs and corticosteroids can mask pyrexia. Corticosteroids may also mask peritonitis.

Management of septic shock

Treat the cause and support organ function.

- High flow oxygen
- History (if available) and examination
- Urine, sputum, drainage (if appropriate) and blood cultures before antibiotics
- Broad-spectrum antibiotics whilst awaiting results
- CXR and relevant basic bloods
- Change catheter, IV/arterial lines (new sites if possible) unless newly inserted
- Send tips of removed lines for culture
- CVP (or PA catheter) and urinary catheters for monitoring shock/fluid balance
- Haemodynamic support (optimise intravascular volume)
- Increase perfusion pressure with noradrenaline/norepinephrine
- Monitor pH as a guide to optimal tissue perfusion
- Early enteral feeding or TPN if not possible
- Remember: prevention is better than cure

Complications of sepsis and septic shock

- Stress ulcers
- Pulmonary hypertension
- Hyper-catabolic state and hyperglycaemia
- Metabolic acidosis
- DIC
- MODS/MOF (multiorgan dysfunction syndrome and multiorgan failure)

Septic shock has approximately 50% mortality.

8.2 SYSTEMIC INFLAMMATORY RESPONSE SYNDROME (SIRS)

In a nutshell ...

Systemic inflammatory response syndrome (SIRS) is a disseminated inflammatory response that may arise as a result of a number of insults. It is described as a syndrome because the symptoms and signs can be produced by processes other than just infection.

Components of the inflammatory response:

- Oxygen free radicals
- Cytokines
- Macrophages
- Neutrophils
- Inducible intercellular adhesion molecules (ICAMs)
- Platelet-activating factor (PAF)
- Arachidonic acid metabolites
- Vascular endothelium
- Complement cascade
- Vasodilatation

The gut is thought to have an important role in the development of the syndrome and a 'two-hit' theory has been postulated.

Definitions in sepsis

- **Sepsis:** the body's response to infection, which includes two or more of the factors described in the box above
- **Severe sepsis:** sepsis with evidence of organ dysfunction or hypo-perfusion
- **Septic shock:** severe sepsis with hypotension (< 90 mmHg) despite fluid resuscitation
- **Septicaemia:** clinical signs and symptoms associated with multiplying bacteria in the bloodstream
- **Endotoxin:** toxin that remains within the cell wall of bacteria. It is heat stable. Lipid A conserved amongst different organisms acts to trigger various mediators responsible for sepsis
- **Exotoxin:** toxin actively secreted by bacteria, with specific effects according to organism
- **Carriage:** two consecutive surveillance samples of throat and rectum that are positive for micro-organisms

- **Colonisation:** presence of micro-organisms in a normally sterile organ without host response (eg blood, bladder, bronchi and CSF)
- **Infection:** microbiologically proven clinical condition with host response
- **Bacteraemia**: bacteria in bloodstream but not necessarily symptomatic or requiring treatment

Systemic inflammatory response syndrome (SIRS)

In a nutshell ...

SIRS is a harmful, excessive reaction of acute phase response. It is defined by two or more of the following:

- Tachycardia > 90 b.p.m.
- Respiratory rate > 20 breaths per minute or $PaCO_2$ > 4.3 kPa
- Temperature > 38 °C or < 36 °C
- WCC > 12 or < 4 × $10^3/mm^3$

Pathophysiology of SIRS

SIRS is a disseminated inflammatory response that may arise as a result of a number of insults:

- Infection and sepsis
- Ischaemia–reperfusion syndrome
- Fulminant liver failure
- Pancreatitis
- Dead tissue

Any localised injury stimulates an inflammatory response. This response involves recruitment of inflammatory cells (such as macrophages and neutrophils) to the area, release of inflammatory mediators (eg cytokines, IL-1, IL-6, IL-8, TNF-α), and changes in vascular permeability.

- These localised inflammatory responses are responsible for minimising further damage (eg from infection) and optimising conditions for healing
- Under certain conditions (eg major trauma) the extent of the inflammatory activity throughout the body is activated in an apparently uncontrolled manner, with an imbalance between inflammatory and anti-inflammatory responses
- The widespread activity of this systemic inflammation (SIRS) and activation of a mediator network is such that it damages organs throughout the body – initiating MOF

Important components of the inflammatory response

The inflammatory response is discussed in detail in Chapter 2.

Oxygen free radicals

- Occur after initial hypoxic injury and subsequent reperfusion (ie reperfusion injury)
- Mechanism involves the formation of xanthine oxidase during ischaemia from xanthine dehydrogenase which converts adenosine to hypoxanthine
- When oxygen becomes available the hypoxanthine is metabolised to uric acid via the enzyme xanthine oxidase and free radicals are formed in the process
- Cause direct endothelial damage and increased permeability

Cytokines

- Peptides released by various cell types which are involved in the immune response
- Produced by macrophages
- TNF: central mediator in sepsis, produces deleterious effects similar to effects of infection; pivotal role in host response
- IL-1: synergistic with TNF; initiator of host response; stimulates helper T cells
- IL-6/IL-8: reparative processes; production of acute phase proteins

Macrophages

- Phagocytosis of debris and bacteria
- Act as antigen-presenting cells to T lymphocytes
- Release inflammatory mediators, endothelial cells and fibroblasts

Neutrophils

- Migrate to inflamed tissue from the blood
- Release mediators
- Release proteolytic and hydrolytic enzymes, which cause vasodilatation, increased permeability, myocardial depression and activation of clotting mechanisms

Inducible intercellular adhesion molecules (ICAMs)

- Mediation of adhesion and migration of neutrophils through endothelium
- Induced by lipopolysaccharides (LPS) and cytokines

Platelet-activating factor (PAF)

- Released by neutrophils and monocytes
- Cause hypotension, increased permeability and platelet aggregation

Arachidonic acid metabolites

- Essential fatty acid
- Metabolised by cyclo-oxygenase to form prostaglandins and thromboxane, and by lipoxygenase to form leukotrienes

Vascular endothelium

- Increased permeability, allowing both inflammatory cells and acute-phase proteins from the blood to reach the injured (inflamed) area
- Complex organ in its own right, involved in vascular tone, permeability, coagulation, phagocytosis and metabolism of vascular mediators
- Nitric oxide: induced form stimulated by TNF and endotoxin via nitric oxide synthase; causes sustained vasodilatation
- Endothelin-1: powerful vasoconstrictor, increased in trauma and cardiogenic shock

Complement cascade

- Occurs in early septic shock via the alternative pathway
- Attracts and activates neutrophils

Vasodilatation

- Allowing increased recruitment of inflammatory cells from the blood

In the systemic inflammatory response syndrome, it is these changes in the vascular endothelium which, when widespread, cause circulatory failure and hypotension, contributing to MOF.

The 'two-hit' hypothesis and the role of the gut

The initial cellular insult (cellular trauma or shock states) sets up a controlled inflammatory response. A second insult is then sustained by the patient (eg repeated surgery, superimposed infection, bacteraemia or persistent cellular damage). This creates a destructive inflammatory response and results in loss of intestinal mucosal integrity, allowing translocation of bacteria and endotoxin into the portal circulation which further feeds back into the immuno-inflammatory cascade. See Chapter 2 *Infection and Inflammation*.

8.3 MULTIORGAN DYSFUNCTION SYNDROME (MODS)

Definitions of individual organ system failure

Cardiovascular failure (one or more of the following)

- Heart rate < 54 b.p.m. or symptomatic bradycardia
- MAP < 49 mmHg or (> 70 mmHg requiring inotropic support)
- Occurrence of VT or VF
- Serum pH < 7.24 with normal pCO_2

Respiratory failure

- Respiratory rate < 5 or > 49 breaths per min
- $PaCO_2$ > 6.65 kPa
- Alveolar–arterial gradient > 46.55
- Ventilator-dependent on day 4 in ITU

Renal failure

- Urine output < 479 mL in 24 hours, or < 159 mL in 8 hours
- Urea > 36 mmol/L
- Creatinine > 310 mmol/L
- Dependent on haemofiltration

Haematological failure

- White cell count < $1/mm^3$
- Platelets < 20×10^9/L
- HCT < 0.2%
- DIC

Neurological failure

- GCS < 6 in the absence of sedation

Gastrointestinal failure

- Ileus > 3 days
- Diarrhoea > 4 days
- GI bleeding
- Inability to tolerate enteral feed in absence of primary gut pathology

Skin failure

- Decubitus ulcers

Endocrine

- Hypo-adrenalism or abnormal thyroid function tests

Multiple system failures

Multiple organ dysfunction syndrome (MODS) may also be referred to as multiorgan failure (MOF) and is an important cause of death in intensive care. It refers to the process whereby more than one organ system has deranged function and requires support. Patients do not often die from single organ failure but from the development of MOF following the initial insult.

The degree of dysfunction can be difficult to quantify (eg dysfunction of the GI tract), or easily quantifiable (eg renal dysfunction, quantified by the degree of oliguria, serum biochemistry and acid–base status).

When assessing the degree of dysfunction, account must be taken of the support being provided for the organ system (eg for respiratory failure the concentration of inspired oxygen and ventilatory support must be considered when assessing arterial PaO_2).

MOF is a process that develops over a period of time, and can be in response to an initial severe stimulus (eg major burn, sepsis, multiple trauma, major surgery) or following several seemingly minor insults).

The development of MOF depends more on the body's response to a given stimulus rather than the stimulus itself. This may explain why different patients, with seemingly similar pathology or injuries, differ in their tendency to develop MOF.

Outcome of MOF

- In two-organ failure, mortality is in the region of 50% and increases to 66% on 4th day
- In three-organ failure mortality is around 80% on first day increasing to 96% if does not resolve
- In four-organ failure survival is unlikely

Pre-existing medical condition and age must be taken into account.

Treatment and prevention of MOF

The prognosis of established multiorgan failure is extremely poor (where three or more systems are in failure for more than 3 days, the prognosis is dismal).

The emphasis must therefore be on identifying at-risk patients early, and intervening quickly to prevent MOF.

In order to optimise the chances of recovery, the initial insult (eg intra-abdominal sepsis) must be treated if possible. Early nutritional support, particularly via the gut (enteral feeding) is increasingly being recognised as important in improving outcome.

Various anti-inflammatory treatments have been attempted, affecting different parts of the inflammatory response (eg anti-endotoxin antibodies, IL-1 antibodies), but in clinical trials none seem to have any effect on outcome. This is due to the complex and multiple pathways involved.

Chapter 8

Surgical Outcomes, Research, Ethics and the Law

Shireen McKenzie and Nerys Forester

Section 1
Clinical Governance

1.1 CLINICAL GOVERNANCE

In a nutshell ...

Clinical governance is essentially the combination of **risk management** and **quality control** (definition kindly passed on by Pete Cutting).

Risk management
- Error reporting
- Morbidity and mortality meetings
- Audit
- National guidelines

Quality control
- Completing the audit cycle
- Application of evidence-based medicine
- Patient feedback and satisfaction
- Personal professional development (appraisal and revalidation)

The Bristol enquiry brought to light failings within the NHS to set a national standard of care, and highlighted the lack of guidelines to assess the quality of care. This was the beginning of clinical governance.

The Department of Health (DoH) definition of clinical governance is:

> A system through which NHS organisations are accountable for continuously improving the quality of their services and safeguarding high standards of care, by creating an environment in which clinical excellence will flourish.

Aims of clinical governance

Clinical governance aims to produce the best possible patient care and places the responsibility for achieving this on the entire clinical team. It relies on a cycle of assessment, identification of areas for improvement, improvement and re-assessment (**audit cycle** or **reflective practice**).

It aims to implement evidence-based medicine and provide opportunities for research into improvements in practice.

It aims to reduce variation in quality of health care throughout the country.

Risk management

This was originally developed within the corporate sector to assess complications and minimise their recurrence and identify future potential risks. Risk management consists of:

- **Error reporting systems** in which **incident forms** are completed by any healthcare professional when anything goes wrong; they should be completed for 'near-miss' events as well as those events where mistakes occurred, thus helping to identify areas where future problems are likely (forms should not be used to apportion blame)
- **Morbidity and mortality meetings** held by MDTs
- **Record-keeping** as a tool for identifying potential or actual mistakes
- **Staff concerns** (there should be a forum for staff to voice concerns about current practices and suggest improvements)
- **Audit** to identify areas and extent of weak performance
- **Comparison** between individuals and organisations to produce guidelines to minimise risk (eg NICE, CEPOD)

Quality control

Quality control should cover every aspect of the patient's care. That includes access to treatment, treatment options, the right equipment and buildings, the right education for staff, the right audit tools, research availability, as well as:

- Completing the audit cycle
- Application of evidence-based medicine
- Patient satisfaction (focus groups and surveys)
- Personal professional development (aims to maintain good surgical practice by continually updating clinical and intellectual knowledge)

Personal professional development consists of two processes:

- **Appraisal** (a process that provides feedback on doctors performance, monitors continuing professional development and identifies shortcomings at an early stage, in order to ensure focused improvement)
- **Revalidation** (all specialists must demonstrate that they continue to be fit to practice in their chosen field; this is repeated every 5 years)

In both appraisal and revalidation clinicians must show continued professional development by compiling a logbook (for procedures), evidence of attendance at meetings, and of involvement in academic work, and appropriate training courses. These processes should enable all clinicians to uphold standards and accomplish the guidelines set out in the GMC's Good Medical Practice (2001).

Levels of clinical governance

Clinical governance is therefore achieved at the local level and the national level.

Local clinical governance

- Trust (audit cycle, morbidity and mortality meetings (M&Ms), risk management strategy)
- Personal (appraisal, re-validation, continuing professional development)

National clinical governance

National institute for clinical excellence (NICE)

- Set up in 1999
- Provides guidance on 'best practice', which is centred around evidence-based research and thorough audit (see http://www.nice.org/uk/

Healthcare Commission (formerly CHI, the Commission for Healthcare Improvements)

- Oversees recommendations set out by NICE
- Has a role in assessing NHS organisations, ensuring clinical governance is being achieved and reporting any failings within the trust
- Still has authority over foundation hospitals

National Confidential Enquire into Patient Outcome and Deaths (NCEPOD)

- Now comes under the umbrella of NICE
- Aims to review clinical practice in order to identify areas of potential improvement in the practice of surgery, endoscopy, medicine and anaesthesia
- Scottish audit of surgical mortality (SASM) is the Scottish equivalent of NCEPOD

1.2 DECISION MAKING

In a nutshell ...

The essence of medical practice is decision making:

- What information to gather
- Which tests to order
- How to interpret and integrate this information into diagnostic hypotheses
- What treatments to administer

There are four stages of decision making:

- Assessment and diagnosis (triage)
- Planning (strategy)
- Intervention (tactics)
- Evaluation (monitoring)

The basis of decision making

When treating an individual patient, medical decisions are based on different forms of knowledge.

- **Personal knowledge and experience**
- **Senior review**
- **Guidelines or protocols**

Personal knowledge

When faced with a complex situation in which there is doubt, a clinician will tend to consider a solution from past experience or look for answers in the literature (other people's past experience). This helps to form a set of 'decision rules' or protocols for dealing with a disease or condition. Information can be gleaned from reviews, research and meta-analyses (eg individual articles in journals, reports by the Cochrane Group).

There are two types of personal knowledge:

- Background knowledge about a disease or condition (applies to previous education and learning)
- Foreground knowledge about a disease or condition (applies to information gleaned from the individual patient's condition)

Senior review

Decision making can be guided by someone with more experience than you. This may be another doctor or an experienced member of an allied profession such as nursing, physiotherapy, dietetics etc.

Decision making is also affected by the facilities available to you. This includes personal abilities, abilities within your clinical team, facilities available at your hospital, facilities available in the vicinity or nationally. It may require the use of judicious referral.

Following and understanding the train of thought from someone with more experience should add to your personal knowledge of a disease, or condition, or treatment.

Protocols

Guidelines or protocols are developed by experts, based on their pooled experience and current knowledge, and they provide a framework for evaluating a case or situation that speeds up the decision-making process. They are also a helpful way to teach clinical decision making. Guidelines and protocols may be set by the individual surgeon, hospital, nationally or internationally.

Protocols may be expressed visually as algorithms. These show all the possible solutions and the sequence of steps made to reach each of those solutions. Thus algorithms create a picture of the diagnostic reasoning pathway – they organise a problem into events and decisions to be taken in a set order, and they act as a reminder of options that may have been overlooked. However, an algorithm can only be applied to a patient who falls within the specific clinical context explicitly described by the algorithm.

In constructing a protocol, the following must be taken into account:

- What type of protocol is needed (eg disease-based, symptom-based, or treatment-based)?
- Is the protocol evidence based, and what is the evidence?
- Who will be administering the protocol? What format is most suitable (eg narrative or flow diagram)?
- Which patients is the protocol for? (inclusion and exclusion criteria; indications for entering a patient into the protocol must be for specific clinical contexts)
- Are there any risks to the patient with the procedure and what is the risk–benefit ratio?
- Is the technique or procedure performed in a specified manner?
- What is the outcome measure?
- Has an audit been set up for the protocol? (Remember that the audit loop must be completed)

Traditionally, clinical decisions conform to initial pattern recognition (diagnosis aided by investigation) and implementation of a set method of dealing with the condition (treatment).

The stages of decision making

There are four stages in decision making:

- Assessment and diagnosis (triage)
- Planning (strategy)
- Intervention (tactics)
- Evaluation (monitoring)

Assessment and diagnosis (triage)

This involves using knowledge to recognise patterns in data collected about patients. We tend to start with a broad differential diagnosis, encompassing all diagnostic possibilities. Choosing when and where to limit data collection is important. Identifying which information was most relevant to the final diagnosis acts as a learning tool, helping add to our background knowledge.

Planning (strategy)

The differential diagnosis can be refined by planning and investigation. Clinicians use laboratory tests to help them make choices. Test results aid in narrowing diagnostic options and may identify patients who are likely to have occult disease. A test should generally be performed only if its results will aid in diagnosis or prognosis, or will affect subsequent management.

When planning tests it is important to understand how the results will be interpreted. Interpretation of test results requires an understanding of probability (see *Significance testing* in section 3.2). Tests may be interpreted differently by different clinicians, based on their own past experience. Tests are not perfect and are subject to a level of sensitivity and specificity. They may therefore give false-positive or false-negative results, providing misleading information. It is important to relate the result to the clinical picture.

Also consider that tests consume limited resources, may delay the initiation of treatment, may induce unnecessary treatment, or cause necessary treatment to be withheld, and may place the patient at risk for an adverse event from the test itself.

Intervention (tactics)

There may be many different treatment options and understanding the choice of one over the other and the likely outcomes is a result of education and experience. Determining a threshold for treatment involves assessment (often performed subconsciously) of the risk–benefit ratio for that patient.

Evaluation (monitoring)

Evaluation should occur continuously – anticipating, recognising and correcting errors as circumstances change. At the end of the process evaluation involves feedback. On a personal or departmental level, feedback is formalised as the audit cycle (section 2.2). Feedback allows for correction of mistakes and adds to learning by helping avoid error in the future.

1.3 ECONOMIC ASPECTS OF SURGICAL CARE

In a nutshell ...

Economic aspects can be subdivided into costs and consequences of surgery. These are expressed as:

- Cost–benefit analysis
- Cost–effectiveness analysis
- Cost–utility analysis

Health care consumes an increasing proportion of the total economy. Assessment of economic costs and benefits aims to determine and implement the most effective strategies. The interpretation of the cost–benefit ratio depends on perspective: the patient's perspective is different to that of the doctor, the healthcare provider, or policy makers. There is also variation in the cost–benefit ratio when prophylactic surgery is considered. Benefit gained in the present tends to be deemed as more important than benefits to be that will be gained in the future.

Economics can be divided into costs and consequences of surgery.

Costs of surgery

Costs can be classified as:

- Direct medical costs (eg personnel, drugs)
- Indirect medical costs (eg overheads such as administration, buildings)
- Indirect costs of lost productivity (eg days off work)
- Intangible costs (eg pain, fear, or suffering) that are difficult to quantify

Costs to the healthcare provider

- Personnel (surgical team, ward staff, theatre staff, support staff)
- Hotel costs (building maintenance, electricity, food)
- Drugs
- Laboratory tests
- Equipment (eg monitoring, theatre equipment)
- Disposables (eg syringes, dressings, theatre supplies)

Costs to the patient

- Lost earnings
- Out of pocket expenses
- Time

Costs to others

- Lost productivity (patients' employer)
- Lost time with family

Consequences of surgery

Positive consequences

- Relief from symptoms including pain
- Prevention of complications (morbidity and mortality)

Negative consequences

- Hospitalisation
- Operative risks (morbidity and mortality)
- Complications causing prolonged hospital stay
- Cosmetic result (scarring)

Economic assessment of intervention

Clinical **profit** is the gain expected from a clinical decision once the patient has paid the price of pain, disability, and financial loss while under treatment. The quality adjusted life year (QALY) combines survival with an adjustment for the quality of life experienced during those extra years (a value of 1 = full health and a value of 0 = death).

There are three methods for assessing the economics of an intervention.

- **Cost–benefit analysis (CBA):** all costs and benefits (including intangible costs like the value of lives lost or saved) are allocated a monetary value; CBA is calculated by the sum of the costs and benefits over a pre-specified time
- **Cost–effectiveness analysis (CEA):** this is expressed in 'health units' (eg lives saved or incidence of disease); it does not put a monetary value on life. It is useful for comparison of two strategies to prevent the same condition
- **Cost–utility analysis:** this integrates the quality of life by using the QALY; it is expressed as a monetary value per QALY gained

Section 2

Surgical outcomes and the audit cycle

2.1 SURGICAL OUTCOMES

In a nutshell ...

The outcome is the result.
The outcome may be positive or negative.
The outcome may be assessed after any action (at any time point in the process of diagnosis, investigation or treatment).

There are measures to predict outcome:

- Pre-operative scoring systems
- Research (randomised controlled trials and meta-analysis)

There are measures for recording outcome:

- Time (eg to recurrence)
- Mortality rates
- Economics (eg length of hospital stay)
- Subjective measures (eg patient satisfaction)

There are published outcomes giving national averages or target levels for positive outcome.

Definition of outcome

Outcome can also be categorised in terms of:

- **Physical health** – the difference from the physiological norm
- **Mental health** – anxiety or distress, quality of life, self-esteem
- **Social health** – ability to perform normal social roles

The outcome of an investigation, procedure, or course of a disease may be termed negative or positive. The outcome may be viewed differently in this respect by the clinician and the patient.

Positive outcomes refer to cure, increased survival times, and symptom relief.

Negative outcomes refer to death, complications and adverse events, sequelae resulting in loss of function and failed procedures.

Predicting outcome

A variety of clinical scales are used to aid prediction of surgical outcome. These include:

- American Society of Anaesthesiologists (ASA) grade (see Chapter 7 *Critical Care*)
- Acute Physiology and Chronic Health Evaluation (APACHE) (see Chapter 7 *Critical Care*)
- Physiological and Operative Severity Score for Enumeration of Morbidity and Mortality (POSSUM) (see Chapter 7 *Critical Care*). This scale also has modifications for sub-groups of major surgery eg for vascular surgery (v POSSUM) and the Portsmouth modification (p POSSUM)
- Glasgow Coma Scale (GCS)
- Trauma Severity Score

Research and meta-analysis of outcome measures can give an indication of the predicted outcome for specific patient groups (eg mortality rates for colorectal liver metastasis after chemotherapy and liver resection compared to mortality rates with chemotherapy alone).

Measuring outcome

Measurement of outcome may be **subjective** (eg patient satisfaction) or **objective** via measures such as:

- Time (time to cure; time to recurrence; time to symptom relief; time to readmission)
- Death (mortality: 30 days; 1 year; 5 years; 10 years)
- Complications
- Adverse events
- Economics (length of hospital stay)
- Delayed discharge

Patient satisfaction

This is multifactorial. It relies on a combination of results for the patient's physical, mental and social health. A treatment may not achieve a cure but may be regarded as having a positive outcome for the patient if there is relief from symptoms and alleviation of anxiety.

Published outcomes

It is important to compare like with like. Outcomes may vary between surgeons for a variety of reasons:

- Different surgical abilities
- Different available facilities and back-up (eg theatres, ITUs)
- Different case mix
  - Number of patients treated per year
  - Severity of disease treated
  - Patient co-morbidity

To compare outcomes, the patient mix should be standardised by factors such as:

- Cancer or disease stages
- Prediction scores (eg POSSUM)
- Demographics (eg age, sex, social class)

Published outcomes can be found in reports from large national and international audits (eg the Confidential Enquiry into Peri-Operative Deaths (CEPOD), the breast cancer screening audit database, and the Central Cardiac Audit Database (CCAD).

2.2 THE AUDIT CYCLE

In a nutshell ...

Audit is the collective review, evaluation, and improvement of practice with the common aim of improving patient care and outcomes. It is performed retrospectively.

Clinical audit is the process of quality control and forms a fundamental part of clinical governance.

Functions of clinical audit:

- Encourages improvement in clinical procedure
- Educates all members of the team
- Raises overall quality of clinical care
- Compares your practice with current best practice
- Provides peer comparison

Medical audit is doctors looking at what they do.

Clinical audit is interdisciplinary.

Comparative audit provides data from a wide group allowing comparison of individual results with national levels or averages.

Criterion audit is when results of the audit are compared with a pre-agreed standard, rather than against other groups in the audit.

Audit requirements of College

- Audits are carried out in each surgical discipline
- Everyone must attend (all disciplines)
- One consultant is responsible for the audit programme
- Audits must be undertaken regularly
- Records and minutes of meetings must be kept

Data collection for audit

Regular audit of the medical notes is required.

- Data should investigate:
  - Access of patients to care (eg waiting time, cancellations)
  - Process (eg investigations)
  - Outcome (eg deaths, complications)
  - Organisation of hospital and resources
  - Financial implications
- The audit process should be consultant-led and the consultant has to be in attendance

Minutes of meeting must include:

- Who attends attended
- Topics discussed
- Conclusions and recommendations
- Date for reviewing the topic
- Action to be taken on unresolved topics

Evidence of regular audit meetings is mandatory for educational approval of training posts.

Audit of structure, process or outcome

- **Structure** refers to the availability and organisation of resources required for the delivery of a service (eg resources can include staff, equipment, accommodation)
- **Process** refers to the way the patient is received and managed by the service from time of referral to discharge
- **Outcome** means the results of clinical intention

Constructing an audit

Standard is the best practice.

- **Indicator** is the thing to be measured
- **Target** refers to what would be the desired result
- **Monitoring method** encompasses the method of data collection, who is collecting it, and the frequency of collecting it

The audit process is a cycle as shown in Fig. 2.2a. This is an important concept as implemented changes should always be re-assessed and compared to the national standard and previous assessment within the department.

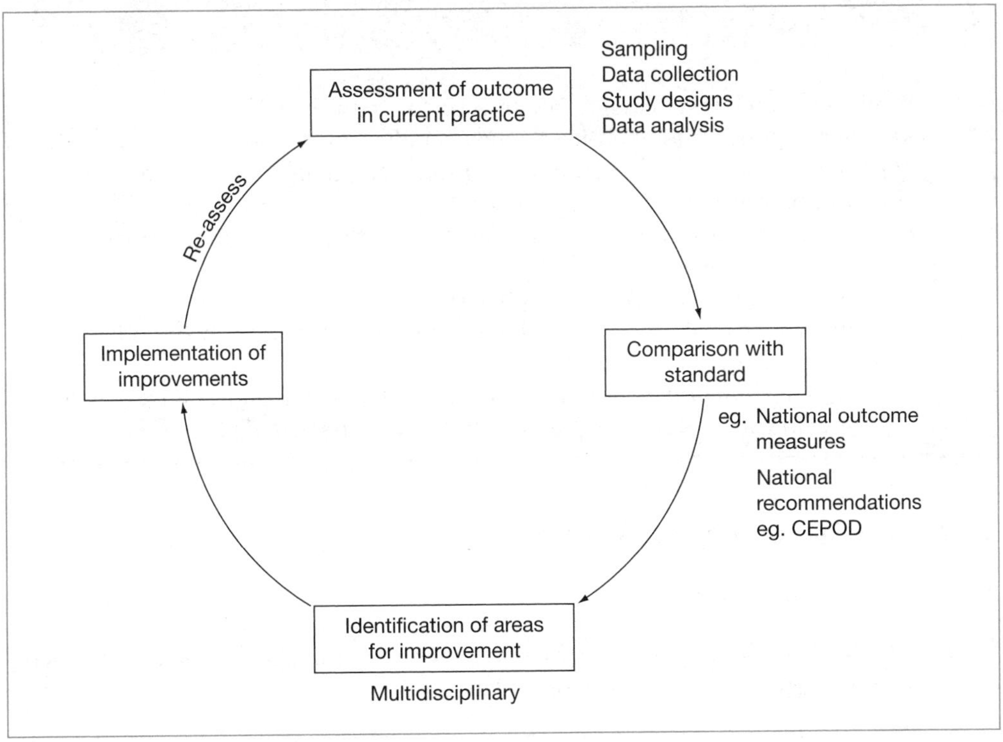

Figure 2.2a *The audit cycle*

Section 3
Surgical research and statistics

3.1 SURGICAL RESEARCH

In a nutshell ...

Surgical research is systematic investigation to establish fact
Research is used to forward basic understanding of disease processes, in the improvement of surgical outcomes, or in surgical training to teach the basics of critical appraisal
Research should also be applied to clinical practice in the form of evidence-based medicine (EBM)
As a surgical trainee you should be able to:

- Read, understand and critique the literature in order to apply the principles of evidence based medicine
- Appreciate the principles of how to set up, design and fund a clinical study
- Write up your research for publication in a peer reviewed journal

The hierarchy of evidence

All research starts with a **hypothesis**.

Evidence for the hypothesis can be regarded as a spectrum from the anecdotal to the rigorously tested. This generates a hierarchy of evidence:

Case reports

↓

Case series

↓

Cross-sectional surveys
(observational studies that assess prevalence across a given population, which may be performed by questionnaire or interview with participants or by review of case notes)

↓

Retrospective studies
(observational studies that test hypotheses on aetiology or treatment of disease)
↓
Prospective studies
(observational studies that test hypotheses on aetiology or treatment of disease)
↓
Randomised controlled trials (RCTs)
(studies that test hypotheses on the treatment of disease)
↓
Systematic review of RCTs
(may include meta-analysis)

There are advantages and disadvantages to different study designs. The gold standard is regarded as the randomised control trial. Studies lower down the hierarchy of evidence are usually performed to establish enough evidence to justify the cost and time-consuming nature of more rigorous testing. These studies also enable the investigator to refine the hypothesis as the evidence mounts.

Blinding

This refers to the process by which the person assessing the outcome remains unaware of the groups to which the participants have been allocated. The more people blinded to the treatment group (participants and assessors), the less likely is the introduction of observer bias. Double-blinding means that both the participant and the assessor are unaware of the treatment group.

Controls

A control group is a group of participants that is not exposed to the risk factor or treatment being studied. The control group must have similar characteristics to the treatment group to avoid introducing bias. This is called 'matching' and controls for differences between the two groups in terms of age, sex, socio-economic factors, and other risk factors, for example. Matching aims to ensure that any differences seen are due to the factor being studied and are not influenced by other parameters.

Meta-analysis

This is a cumulative statistical test that pools the results from all the studies that have been conducted to answer a specific question. Often the difficulty with medical research is the existence of multiple, small studies, possibly with conflicting or inconclusive results. Meta-analyses and systematic reviews are processes used to combine relevant studies into one larger, more precise study with a single overall result.

Meta-analysis is a mathematical tool that increases the power and precision of research already performed. It is useful for detecting small but clinically important effects (eg the benefits of thrombolysis in MI). While meta-analysis is the method used to combine studies, it is preceded by a systematic review or search for all relevant studies.

The Cochrane Collaboration provides support for authors undertaking a systematic review. It ensures a thorough search of the available literature and helps authors to avoid missing published (and even unpublished or on-going) works. A systematic review searches the literature in a methodical way, with strictly defined inclusion and exclusion criteria.

Evidence-based medicine (EBM)

There is an increasing demand from both patients and clinicians for health care based on the best available evidence. There is a tremendous volume of published research out there and clinical practice tends to lag behind the research data.

What is EBM?

In a nutshell ...

Evidence-based medicine (EBM) is the application of the best research evidence to your clinical practice. It is therefore a set of strategies for keeping your clinical practice up to date.

It involves:

- Asking an answerable clinical question
- Tracking down the best evidence
- Critical appraisal of the evidence
- Applying the evidence to clinical practice

The best research evidence involves the integration of aspects of:

- Patient values and expectations
- Clinician experience
- Audit
- Published research

Published research follows a hierarchy of evidence as outlined previously. However, research may be applicable to your own practice only if the patient groups are similar.

The practice of EBM can be broken down into the following steps:

- Ask an answerable question
- Track down the best evidence in order to answer that question
- Critically appraise that evidence
- Use that evidence in your clinical approach or management of individual patients
- Evaluate the effectiveness of applying that evidence (in individual cases and across your practice as a whole)

This structure is based on the recommendations of Professor David Sackett, formerly of the Oxford Centre for EBM.

Asking an answerable question

Clinical questions may be **background questions**, such as general questions about disease incidence or pathology, questions about disease progression or prognosis, etc.

More importantly, clinical questions may be very specific and applicable to individual patients, ie **foreground questions**. For example, in a 40-year-old woman with early breast cancer what is the best combination of post-operative chemotherapeutics (monotherapy versus polytherapy) to prolong survival?

Clinical questions tend to fall into four categories:

- Diagnosis and screening
- Prognosis
- Causing harm (or side effects)
- Treatments

It is helpful to write down the clinical question that you want to answer and then divide it into these four parts (PICO):

P The **P**atient or problem eg early breast cancer
I The proposed **I**ntervention or treatment eg monochemotherapy
C The **C**omparative treatment eg polychemotherapy
O The **O**utcome eg survival

Tracking down the best evidence

Tracking down the best available published evidence basically involves literature searching. You should be familiar with on-line methods of searching for literature (and hospital librarians are often invaluable in performing searches or teaching search strategies).

Useful sources of evidence currently available include:

- Databases such as *PubMed* or *Medline* (http://www.pubmed.org/) or the TRIP database (http://www.tripdatabase.com/)
- Systematic reviews from the *Cochrane Collaboration* (www.cochrane.org/)

- Appraised studies from the *Evidence-Based Medicine Journal* (http://www.evidence-basedmedicine.com/) and the clinical evidence website (http://www.clinicalevidence.com/)

The best evidence depends upon the question you are asking.

Questions about **diagnosis** are best answered using cross-sectional studies
Questions about **harm** or side effects are best answered using a cohort study
Questions about **prognosis** are best answered using cohort studies
Questions about **treatment** are best answered using RCTs or systematic reviews

Critical appraisal of the evidence

In a nutshell ...

Critical appraisal essentially means **satisfying yourself** and **justifying to others** that evidence has sufficient validity to be applicable to your patients or questions.

Critical appraisal of a paper can be performed using the mnemonic RAMBOS:

R andomisation
A scertainment
M easurement
B linding
O bjective
S tatistics

The hierarchy of evidence outlines important factors in the design and performance of different clinical studies. A systematic method for undertaking critical appraisal (ie quantifying validity) is outlined below.

Was the study randomised?

Randomisation is important in trials related to comparison between treatments. This is often done by computer but may be done by allocating numbered envelopes.

Look to see whether the randomised groups had similar demographics at the start of the trial (this shows that the randomisation has roughly worked).

Are there any differences between the groups (ie bias) and (if there are) which treatment will these differences favour?

How did the study ascertain the outcome?

Was the outcome measurement sensible and valid? How methodologically sound is the study?

Appraising the methodology

Appraisal of the evidence requires an understanding of the following:

- Study hypothesis
- Selection process
  - Which patients were chosen and why
  - Whether there are any sampling errors
  - Whether the study has any bias (error that does not occur by chance)
  - Number of participants should be determined by a power calculation at the start of the study
- Study design (eg prospective study or RCT)
  - Is the study methodologically sound?

If the study relates to a **diagnostic test** it should include:

Participants with and without the condition being tested
Participants at all stages of the disease
A definitive test performed separately to establish disease status for comparison

If the study is a **cross-sectional survey** it should have:

Validation by pilot study
Appropriate type of survey to answer the question
Response rate > 60%

If the study is a **prospective study** it should include:

A matched control group not exposed to risk factor or treatment
A degree of exposure to the risk factor (eg cigarette smoking in pack years)
A specific and measurable outcome
Contribution of other prognostic risk factors to the one being studied
Sufficient follow-up

If the study is a **retrospective survey** it should use:

A definitive method for retrospective identification of the factor to be studied
Control subjects who had the same opportunity of exposure to the risk factor as the study group

If the study is a randomised controlled trial **(RCT)** it should:

Have strict inclusion and exclusion criteria
Be randomised according to accepted practice
Be double-blinded (during trial, and for subsequent data analysis if possible)
Ensure that all other treatment of the two groups is equal

If the study is a **systematic review** it should:
Perform a thorough search for all studies eligible for inclusion
Include assessments by more than one assessor
Only include properly randomised studies

All studies suffer from loss to follow-up. Up to 5% loss to follow up leads to little bias. If more than 20% of patients were lost to follow-up this affects study interpretation. How were the results from patients lost to follow-up managed? Acceptable methods for managing loss to follow-up include either excluding all missing values from the subsequent analysis or carrying forward the last known measurement.

How was the outcome measured?

Both treatment groups must have the outcome measured in the same way otherwise this is a source of bias and therefore error.

Was the study blinded?

Error can be minimised by ensuring that neither the participant nor the researcher know which treatment group the participant has been allocated to (double-blinding). Sometimes this is not possible. However, ideally the person tasked with interpretation or data analysis should remain blinded to the treatment group.

How objective was the outcome measurement?

Objectivity is important. Factual data such as survival times, blood test results or disease recurrence are more objective than patient allocated scores or scales such as worse, the same, better. Also consider the potential of the placebo effect.

Were the statistics used appropriate, and what do they tell you?

Statistics are discussed in detail in section 3.2. Statistics essentially are a method for assessing the role of chance in reaching the result. Look for clinically meaningful measures:

- Diagnosis: likelihood ratios
- Prognosis: proportions and confidence intervals
- Treatments: absolute and relative risk reduction; numbers needed to treat

Applying evidence to clinical practice

Everyone is busy and finding the time to search for evidence is not often high on the priority list. It may be helpful to keep a note of the answers you find to common questions. It is also helpful to think about how you might communicate medical evidence to patients when you are explaining diagnoses, prognoses and treatment options.

Development of clinical projects

Study design

- What is the hypothesis?
- What is the aim (eg basic knowledge, improving care)?
- What is the current evidence in the literature?
- How will you test the hypothesis?
- How will you select patients to provide a representative sample and to avoid bias?
- What are the inclusion and exclusion criteria?
- How large will the study need to be to be statistically valid (power calculations)?
- What data will you collect?
- What statistical tests will be used in data interpretation?

Additionally:

- Will you require ethics committee approval?
- How will the study be funded?

Study protocol

The study protocol should be written out in full, clearly stating the study design (including all the factors outlined above). The evidence from the current literature should be summarised and referenced. Patients should be given verbal and written information and all patient information sheets should be included in the protocol.

Ethics committees

In a nutshell ...

Ethics approval is always needed for ANY studies involving humans. Ethics will want to see evidence of:

- Study aim and hypothesis
- Risk–benefit analysis
- Informed consent
- Patient confidentiality
- Procedures for use of human tissue (if relevant)

Ethical approval will always be required for studies involving patients, staff, or animals. The study protocol should be submitted to the local ethics committee who have a statutory requirement to oversee research.

The local ethics committee (LREC) is supervised by the main ethics committee (MREC), which is supervised by the central ethics committee (COREC).

The key ethical principles for human research are:

- Respect for autonomy (to ensure informed freedom of choice)
- Beneficence (to do good)
- Non-maleficence (to do no harm)
- Justice (to give fair and equal treatment without bias)

Ethics committees will need to be satisfied that you have taken into consideration the following factors:

- **Risk–benefit ratio**
  - Is the risk to the research subject justified by the potential benefit of the research?
  - The value of the individual outweighs the principle of 'the good of society'
- **Informed consent**
  - Patients should be competent to consent (special cases for children; vulnerable people eg those with learning difficulties, those who are unconscious or who are suffering from confusional states)
  - Verbal and written information should be given to all participants
  - There should be an opportunity for patients to get their questions answered
  - Patients should receive full disclosure on risks of participation
  - Ideally patients should be given time to assimilate information (often 24 hours) before the giving of consent
  - Written consent should be given by the patients, and signed and dated
  - Patients should be aware of their right to withdraw at any time and for any reason without compromise to their further care
- **Patient confidentiality**
  - Assure anonymity
  - Consider adequate data storage
- **Use and storage of human tissue** (if required)
- **Aims of the study and their subsequent application**

Research funding

Options for funding include:

- University funds
- Trust funds
- Research Grants (eg Royal College of Surgeons, Medical Research Council)
- Charities (eg the Wellcome Trust, disease specific foundations)
- Drug or pharmaceutical companies

It is important that funding does not produce a conflict of interests. The researcher should be free to design, implement and run the project without undue influence from the funding body. This particularly applies to the interpretation of results if funding comes from the commercial sector.

Research paper writing

Paper content

The paper should include abstract, introduction, methods, and results sections, and a discussion. All data belongs in the results section.

The discussion is often the hardest part to write, but it can be structured as follows:

- A short summary of the main findings
- A comparison to other findings in the literature
- A short critical appraisal of the study pointing out its strengths and weaknesses
- An indication of the future direction of the research

Tables and figures

Use tables and figures that are informative and economical with space; this is a much more visually pleasing way to display information than large blocks of text. However, certain journals have limits on the number that may be included (they are expensive to publish) so do combine figures if possible.

Each figure should have a legend that is fully explanatory of the figure (whereby if the figure was separated from the text you should still be able to interpret the figure using only the information written in the legend).

Tables can have footnotes. You can use these to indicate the important points outlined in the table or the statistically significant values.

References

Cross-reference statements in the text with the current literature and always read all papers that you use as a reference! Reference-managing computer programmes are very helpful (eg EndNote™ or Reference Manager™) and will often contain templates for different journal styles.

Think ahead to the destination publication and look at the way its articles are structured. If you structure and write yours in the style of that publication it will save you time in the long run.

3.2 BASIC STATISTICS

In a nutshell ...

Stats are important:

To practise evidence-based medicine (investigations and treatments)
To correctly plan and execute meaningful research

In order to get the best out of statistics:

- Think about study types and design at the beginning (type, bias, tests to use)
- Categorise data: this choice then determines the pathway taken for subsequent statistics to be performed
    - Nominal
    - Ordinal
    - Metric
- Identify the measure of location: the mode, mean, or median
- Measure the spread of data
    - Range and interquartile range
    - Standard deviation
    - Standard error and confidence intervals
- Test for the normal distribution of the data (normal vs skewed)
- Decide whether you need a parametric or non-parametric test
- Test for significant differences (null vs alternate hypothesis)

The increasing practice of evidence-based medicine and investigation into the appropriateness of clinical therapies requires a sound understanding of statistics, what they can be used for, and what they actually mean. In addition, most surgeons will be involved in conducting clinical research throughout their career, and prior knowledge of statistics and research methodology is fundamental to the ability to construct well-designed trials or experimental questions which will allow appropriate data handling and interpretation.

Study types and design

There are two main types of epidemiological study design. These have been discussed in the previous section. They are categorised as:

- Observational studies
- Experimental studies

Observational studies can be descriptive or analytical. Analytical studies include case–control studies, cohort studies and cross-sectional analyses.

Experimental studies are the randomised controlled trials (RCTs).

SUMMARY OF THE FEATURES AND LIMITATIONS OF DIFFERENT STUDY TYPES

Type of study	Main features	Limitations of method
Case–control	Retrospective analysis Compares group of patients with disease to group without disease to obtain details about previous medical history/lifestyle Defines risk factors for disease First case–control study showed relationship between smoking and lung cancer (eg Doll 1994)	Useful for rare diseases and those with long latent periods Disadvantages are retrospective data collection and potential bias, and no information about disease incidence
Cohort	Observational study Prospective Monitors disease development in subjects without disease over time Gives disease incidence Example is Framingham Heart study	Accurate and precise information about disease development Good for temporal associations between exposure and disease Needs large numbers over long period of time
Cross-sectional	Observational study Determines presence or absence of disease in a group of subjects Gives disease prevalence	No comparative element Unable to determine cause or effect
Randomised controlled trial	Gold standard of all treatment studies! Intervention study Groups differ in treatment or intervention Equal spread of confounders (eg age, sex, social class) Single blind: patient unaware of treatment group Double blind: patient and investigator unaware of treatment group (difficult in surgery!)	Best way of determining treatment benefit Bias should be eliminated by randomisation (which is simple, by random number generation, stratified to ensure equal distribution of important factors across treatment groups, or blocks, to ensure patient numbers are equal within treatment groups)

Incidence is the rate of occurrence of a new disease within a population.

Prevalence is the frequency of a disease in a population at any given time.

Significance testing

In order to determine whether or not the data you have collected between two or more groups is significantly different, a variety of statistical tests are available to test the hypothesis or study question. Usually, this is constructed in the form of the **null hypothesis**, which states that no difference exists between the two populations sampled. The subsequent tests either prove or disprove this hypothesis.

If our tests disprove the null hypothesis (or show it is very unlikely), this means we accept the **alternative hypothesis**, that a difference between the two groups does exist, and that this relationship has not been found by chance. With all statistical tests, the null hypothesis is tested by calculating a *p* value (or equivalent). The ***p* value** is the **probability** that the null hypothesis is true. Hence if the *p* value is very small, the null hypothesis is less likely to be correct. We are usually willing to accept that we will get the answer 'wrong' 5% of the time – that is a *p* value of 0.05 or lower would mean that the null hypothesis was false, and that the alternative hypothesis was true.

To test our hypotheses, a number of different statistical tests are available; correct usage depends on our knowledge of the type of data collected. To determine which test we should use, we need to ask:

- Is the data metric or categorical?
- Is it normally distributed?
- Is the data from separate groups, from paired groups, or from multiple (> 2) groups?

Types of data

Fundamental to all research is the type of data collected in a study. There are three types:

- Nominal (eg ethnic group, sex, blood group)
- Ordinal (eg scales like Apgar, GCS)
- Metric (eg height, weight, BMI, parity)

Nominal and ordinal data are **categorical** variables, and differ in the fact that nominal data cannot be put into a logical order, whereas ordinal data can. However, when considering ordinal data, when the data sets are placed in order the differences between them are not equal – for example a GCS of 8 is not twice as good as a GCS of 4. A common mistake is to interpret such data as if it is metric data; ordinal numbers are not real and so they do not obey mathematical laws (eg GCS cannot be averaged).

In **metric** data, the numbers represent values with units and relate to one another. Metric data can be continuous – where the number of possible values is infinite (eg weight) – or discrete – where there is a finite number of values, usually whole numbers (eg number of days to discharge, number of subjects in group, number of post-op deaths).

Once the type of data collected has been identified, the data set needs to be described in terms of:

- Location, or central tendency
- Spread, scatter, or dispersion

The way in which the data is described depends on the type of data you are describing!. In addition, the type of data also determines the statistical tests you can subsequently apply.

Measures of location

There are three measures of location:

- Mode
- Mean
- Median

The **mode** describes the most commonly occurring (most frequent) value within a data set. It is used to describe categorical variables (eg blood group), (nominal data).

The **mean** is the average value within a data set (eg the average height or weight of a group of individuals). It can **only** be used with metric data.

The **median** is the middle value obtained within the data set after the values have been ordered or ranked. It can be used with ordinal data (eg GCS) but not with nominal data. It can also be used with metric data, and may be appropriate to do so when a data set is skewed (eg study with groups at extremes of age, data not normally distributed).

Measures of spread

Measure of spread of a data set provides information about the number of individuals sampled and the range of values measured within a study:

- Range or interquartile range
- Standard deviation

As before, the measure of spread used to describe the data depends on the data type and measure of location used to describe it.

The **range** is the smallest to highest value obtained in the study. It can be used with both ordinal and metric data, often given when the median value is used.

The **interquartile range** describes the data spread in terms of four 'quartiles', that is the data set is divided equally into four. The first 25% of values lie in the first quartile, with the median being the middle or 50th quartile. The interquartile range is represented by the numbers that are the 25th quartile to the 75th quartile. This way of expressing data is very sensitive to outlying values, and gives an indication of how large or small the range is that the middle value lies within.

The **standard deviation** (SD) describes the spread of the mean. It is a measure of the average distance of the individual data values from their mean – ie the variability between individuals of the factor measured.

- It can only be used to describe metric data
- The wider the spread of the values measured, the greater the distance from the mean, and so the greater the standard deviation
- Outliers have a marked effect on standard deviation
- Mathematically, standard deviation is calculated as the square root of the sum of the squares of each of the differences of each observed value from the mean value (often referred to as the square root of the variance)
- Standard deviation can be used to see if the data is normally distributed

If the values obtained are normally distributed, then 95% of these values will lie within 2 (more accurately 1.96) SDs on either side of the mean, with 99% of the values within 3 SDs on each side of the mean. Hence, if you cannot fit 3 SDs between the mean and the minimum or maximum value then the data distribution is not normal, and further hypothesis testing of these values should not use parametric tests of significance.

The **standard error** (SE) of the mean reflects the fact that your set of measurements only samples part of the population that you could have studied (for example, only some of the blood pressure of people with or without hypertension), and so is unlikely to determine the population value exactly. It is the reliability with which the mean data value you have calculated for your data set reflects the actual mean value for the population. It therefore reflects the size of the sample studied, with large samples giving a more accurate estimation of population mean than smaller samples. Mathematically, it is derived as the standard deviation divided by the square root of the number of subjects sampled.

Hence, standard deviation describes the spread of measurements, while standard error of the mean tells us how good our estimate of the mean population value is.

The standard error of the mean is more useful when converted to a **confidence interval** (CI), a range of plausible values between which you can have a degree of confidence that the true average value for the population you have sampled will lie. This depends on the number of subjects sampled and the confidence level with which you need to know the mean value. Usually this is acceptable at a 95% CI – ie the values within which the true population mean would be found 95% of the time (also described as the mean 1.96 times the standard error of the mean).

Confidence intervals are of particular value in a clinical setting. They can be used when comparing the means of two groups (eg treated versus untreated). If the confidence intervals overlap, the two groups cannot be significantly different as it is possible the true population means could be the same.

The normal distribution

If you study the frequency distribution of a data set, the majority of biological data can be described by a bell-shaped curve, which is symmetrical about the mean – height or weight, for example. Only metric data can be truly described as normally distributed.

Tests of normality can be applied to data sets to calculate whether or not the values collected are normally distributed (Shapiro Wilks and Kolmogorov Smirnov tests). The normal distribution is fundamental to hypothesis testing, as normally distributed data can be analysed using **parametric** tests, while non-normally distributed data must be analysed using **non-parametric** tests (which are also used for ordinal categorical data, and work by ordering or ranking the values obtained).

Sometimes a data set may show a **skewed** distribution, with higher frequencies of values occurring at the extremes of the values measured. These data sets may be 'transformed to normality' using mathematical functions (eg logarithmic transformations) after which parametric tests can be used on the transformed data set (remembering to transform the data back when the analysis is complete!).

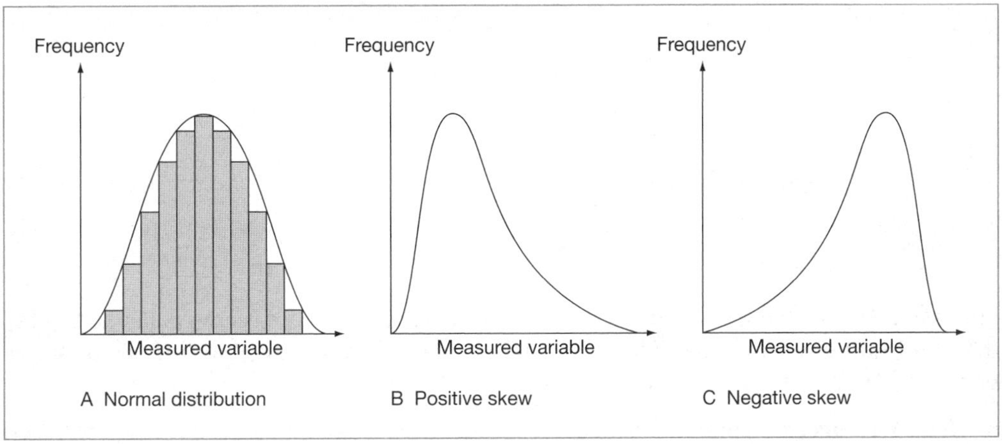

Figure 3.2a *Data distribution – normal and skewed*

Selecting an appropriate statistical test

Once you have described your data set, tested for normality if appropriate, and decided whether you need parametric or non-parametric statistical tests, the flow diagram in Fig. 3.2b can be used to determine the correct test to use.

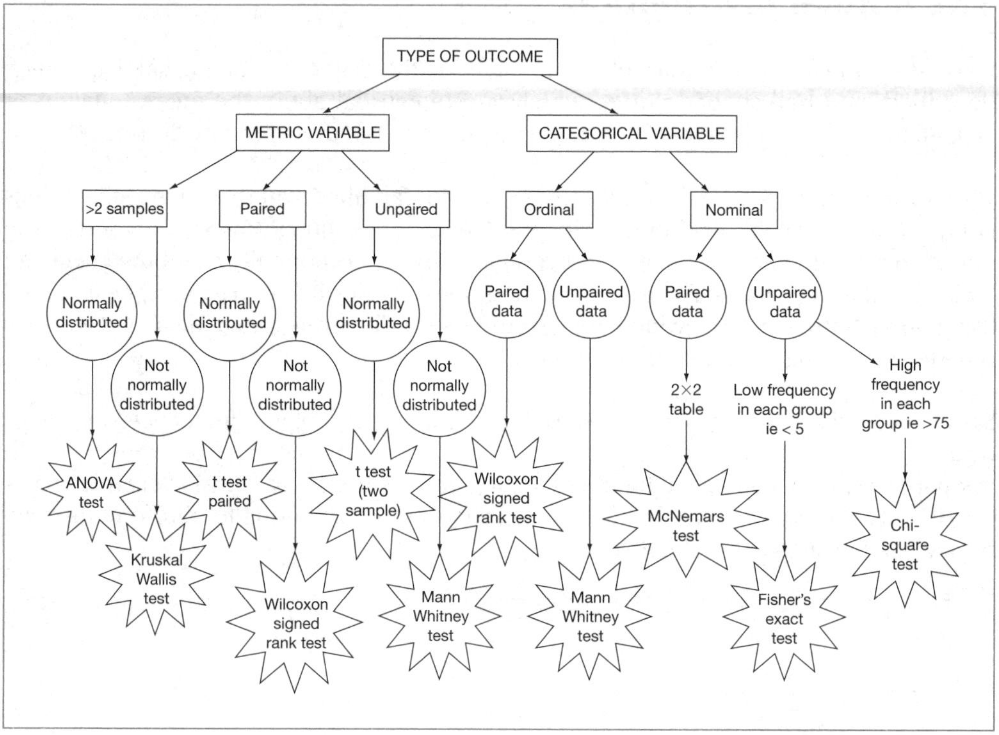

Figure 3.2b *Selecting the right statistical test for your data*

However, even with the selection of the correct statistical test there is always the possibility that the result given may be incorrect – due to chance. In statistical testing two types of error are possible: type 1 and type 2.

- **Type 1 errors (α errors):** a false-positive result – ie we state there is a difference when there is none; this error decreases with the *p* value and is usually accepted at 0.05 (a 95% chance that the difference observed is correct)
- **Type 2 errors (β errors):** a false-negative result – ie we state there is no difference when there actually is one. This error usually occurs with small sample sizes, and is less important than type 1 errors; it is usually accepted to be 0.2 (a 20% chance that any actual difference between the groups will be missed) or less

These errors can be used to calculate the **power** of a study, so that it can be correctly designed to minimise the risk of a study missing a true difference of clinical importance. The power of a study is $1 - \beta$, which is the chance of not getting a false-negative result.

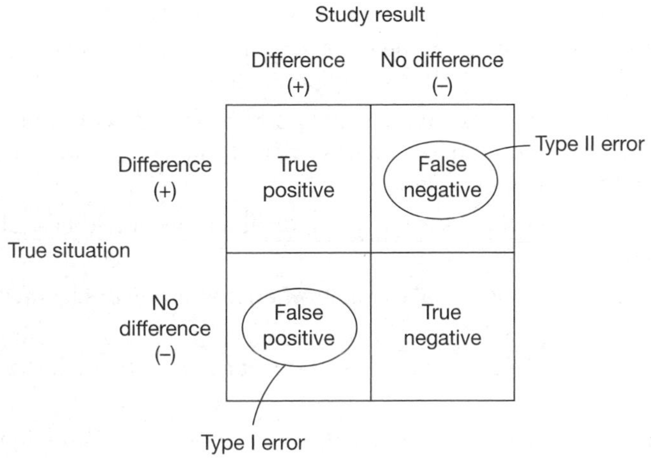

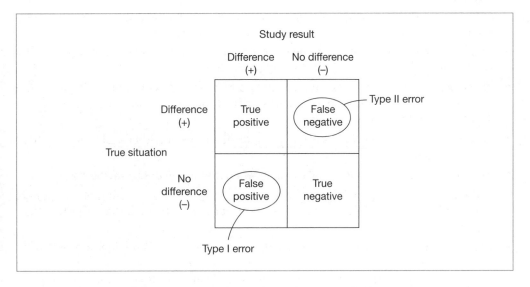

Figure 3.2c *Study results and power calculations*

Power calculations are used to calculate the number of samples needed within each group to show a true difference between groups, should one actually exist. They depend on the type of data collected and can be calculated mathematically, or using a normogram. They need to be done before you start the study, and require a prediction of what magnitude of difference between the groups you would consider to be clinically relevant. A statistician would be a useful friend while attempting such calculations!

Bias and confounding

As well as effects due to chance, studies may also be subject to the effects of bias and confounding.

Bias is the distortion of the estimated effects due to a systematic difference between the two groups being compared. There are many types of bias, either due to the selection of patients (eg putting all the patients with high BP in the non-antihypertensive treatment group), or due to collection or recall of information collected in the study.

Types of bias

- **Observer bias:** may occur when measurements are made. Such bias can be intra-observer (ie the same person measures a quantity differently each time) or inter-observer (ie different observers measure the same quantity differently, whereby agreement – or lack of it – is measured by a kappa coefficient)
- **Selection bias:** may occur when the study population is drawn from participants who are not wholly representative of the target population
- **Prevalence bias:** may arise when the study population is drawn from participants who are part of a special sub-group of the disorder of interest (ie not representative of all those at risk in the target population)
- **Recall bias:** this is the effect on the study of different individuals' abilities to recall events correctly
- **Information bias:** concerns mistakes made when measuring or classifying data
- **Publication bias:** even with a perfectly designed trial, research ultimately suffers from publication bias because positive studies are more likely to be published than negative ones
- **Confounding** occurs when the effect or outcome you are studying is affected by another variable, such as sex, socioeconomic class, or age. This is usually controlled for in a study by randomisation, mathematical modelling, or stratification of data

Statistical error

This occurs when multiple statistical tests are used, for example, to compare a control group to several different patient groups. It should be remembered if you do a test 20 times, then one time out of 20 (5%) it will be significant by chance. If using multiple tests on data sets a correction factor must be applied to the *p* values obtained to reflect this possibility, or you should choose a test designed for $n > 2$ groups, which have correction factors available as post hoc tests (eg Bonferroni correction, Tukey test).

Correlation and regression analysis

The strength of an association between two variables can be assessed by means of a scatter plot.

Correlation is the most widely used measure of association between two variables. It does not imply causality – ie that one variable causes the change in the other variable. The strength of the association depends on how close the measured points lie to the line of best fit between the data points. If all points fall exactly on the line there is perfect correlation, reflected by a correlation coefficient of 1. A correlation coefficient of 0 means no association between the variables exists. The association between the variables may be positive (as one increases so does the other) or negative (one increases as the other decreases). To use Pearson's correlation coefficient each data set compared should be normally distributed, otherwise Spearman's coefficient should be used.

Linear regression is used to determine the nature and direction of a causal relationship between variables. It allows generation of a mathematical model which uses the value of 1 or more independent variables to predict another (eg using age, smoking status, and waist size to predict systolic BP). The strength and significance of each independent variable within the model can be calculated and used to determine factors that significantly affect the variable of interest.

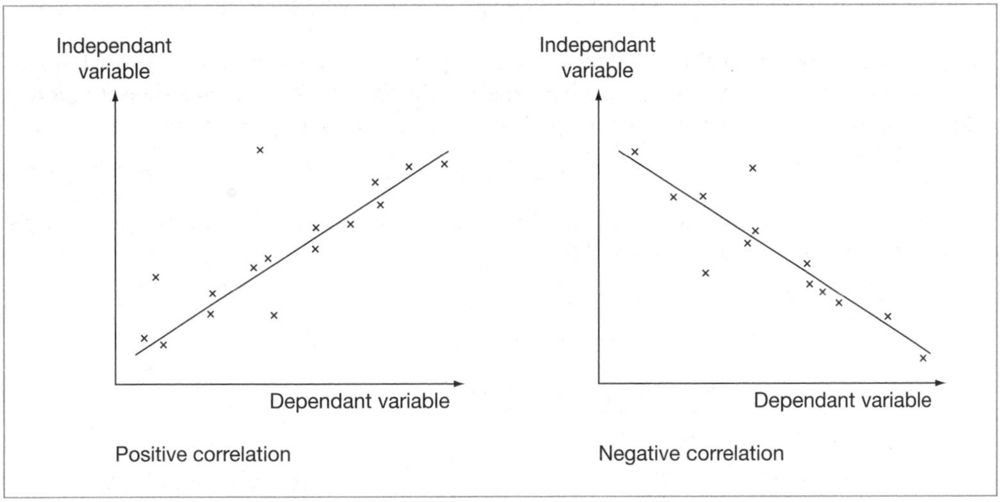

Figure 3.2d *Positive and negative correlations*

Survival analysis

Survival analysis is often used in medicine, where a recognised end-point can be measured. This can be death, limb loss or salvage, or joint replacement failure, for example, with the time to occurrence and cumulative frequency of the number of patients reaching the end-point in question documented. This information allows you to plot a survival curve (eg a Kaplan–Meier curve). Difficulties with this type of analysis include: losses to follow-up, and patients who opt out of the research programme. All patients originally included in the study should be included in analysis on an 'intention to treat' basis, with the worst-case scenario applied to losses to follow-up (that is, assume all losses are worst outcome measures).

Sensitivity and specificity of a test

The ability of a test to predict the presence or absence of a disease can be measured using sensitivity and specificity.

- **Sensitivity** is the ability of a test to correctly identify people with the condition (true positives). Therefore, a highly sensitive test (Sn) has a high rate of detection of the disease or condition. The false-negative rate is therefore low, so if the test is negative it effectively rules the diagnosis 'out' (remember **SnOUT**)
- **Specificity** reflects the ability of a test to correctly identify people without the condition (true negatives). Therefore, a highly specific test (Sp) has a low false-positive rate, so if the test is positive it effectively rules the diagnosis 'in' (remember **SpIN**)

The **positive predictive value** of a test is the proportion of patients the test identifies as having the condition who actually do have the condition, whereas the **negative predictive value** is the proportion of patients the test identifies as not having a condition who do not have the condition.

These concepts are easier to visualise after constructing a **2 × 2 table** of the possible outcomes of a test to diagnose a condition.

		DISEASE		
		PRESENT (+)	ABSENT (–)	
TEST OUTCOME	POSITIVE (+)	a = True	b = False	$\frac{a}{a+b}$ = Positive Predictive Value (PPV)
	NEGATIVE (–)	c = False	d = True	$\frac{d}{d+c}$ = Negative Predictive Value (NPV)
		$\frac{a}{a+c}$ Sensitivity	$\frac{d}{b+d}$ Specificity	

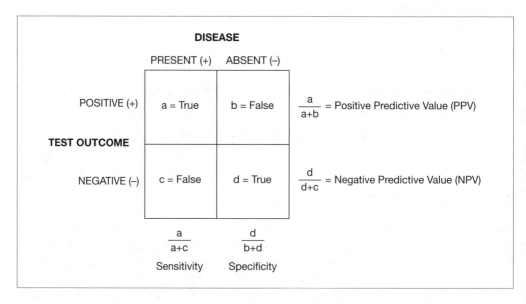

Figure 3.2e *2 × 2 table for the calculation of sensitivity and specificity*

Section 4
Ethics

In the society in which we practice medicine today, it is increasingly important to be aware of the legal implications of our clinical decisions. This is essential, not to practice defensive medicine, which could potentially hinder the treatment of our patients, but to safeguard high standards and to ensure the safety and well-being of patients under our care.

The law is shaped by the application of precedent, namely the decisions taken during previous similar cases. Although the legal boundaries set out are clear, there will always be a struggle between law and morality. It is important to know and understand these laws and to find an even balance.

4.1 DUTY OF CARE AND STANDARDS OF CARE

In a nutshell ...

Duty of care is defined as the legal duty to ensure that the patient receives proper treatment in the proper manner (to do what is best for the patient).

Standard of care is the quality of treatment that can be expected to have been given at a particular date in time.

All healthcare professionals are subject to the duty of care. Once responsibility for a patient has been accepted, then the healthcare professional has a duty to continue that care until the responsibility can be passed on to another professional.

This standard of care emphasises that it is important to stay up to date with current practice.

The standard of care is the same regardless of level of training (eg an SHO performing an operation must meet the basic standard of competence as a consultant performing the same operation – inexperience is not a defence against failing the standard of care).

4.2 CONFIDENTIALITY

In a nutshell ...

Confidentiality is the undertaking not to divulge personal information without consent.

Consent may be:
- Written or verbal
- Implied or informed

Consent is not required for disclosure in cases of:
- Notifiable disease
- Public Interest
- Prevention of harm to the patient or a third party

Respect and protect confidential information.
(GMC 2001)

Confidentiality stems from Hippocrates' practice where he vowed to keep his consultations as 'sacred secrets'. This maxim ensures trust in the relationship between a doctor and patient and results in the revelation of information that could possibly assist with diagnosis and treatment. It is the duty of the clinician to interpret each case individually.

Disclosure of patient information

Disclosure of patient information with consent

Consent may be implied or informed.

- **Implied consent** (sharing information between medical teams): it is impossible to provide the best care for patients without divulging their history to the associated team. Most patients expect to have their case discussed within and between medical teams. This should be re-affirmed verbally so that they have implied their consent. The same applies to the use of their information in audit, as they have the option of declining any sharing of information
- **Informed consent** (insurance companies/research/police): either written or verbal consent is required if a third party such as an insurance company requests information regarding a patient. This also applies to the police and solicitors who cannot obtain confidential information about a patient without their consent. The only exception is when a judge or court requests the information. In that instance you should reveal only the confidential information that is immediately relevant to the question asked

Disclosure of patient information without consent

In certain circumstances, consent for the disclosure of patient information is not required. Notwithstanding, wherever possible the patient should be informed of the intention to disclose. If the patient objects, disclosure can continue, but the patient's objections should be documented.

Consent is not required in the following situations:

- **Notifiable diseases** (eg TB, hepatitis A, B, non-A, non-B, HIV, malaria, *Salmonella*): these diseases must be reported to the Department of Public Health
- **Prevention of harm to the patient or third party:** the level of the risk has to be assessed by the clinician at that time, even if there is only a potential of harm occurring
- **In the public interest:** if you receive confidential information that if reported to the appropriate authorities would prevent harm or benefit the public, the need for disclosure outweighs the right of privacy; however the general principles still stand and the patient should be informed and consent obtained if possible

In all of the above cases one should only reveal **relevant** information to stay within the legal bounds of confidentiality.

Confidentiality and teaching

For our profession it is essential to use clinical cases for teaching, thus breaching elements of confidence. All patients should be informed that their case might be used for teaching purposes. Where possible all identifying data should be removed and the case made anonymous.

Confidentiality after death

We have the same legal obligations to maintain the confidentiality of deceased patients as we do with those still alive. Any previous declarations made before death pertaining to disclosure must be upheld.

There may be a conflict between the law and moral issues and this may cloud decisions. If in doubt it is essential to obtain advice from seniors, the GMC, or your medical defence organisation.

4.3 CONSENT

In a nutshell ...

Patients have a right to information about their condition and the treatment options available to them. Informed consent should be sought before investigation, treatment, screening, or research.

Competency to consent must be shown:
Competent: informed consent (written or verbal)
Incompetent: temporary, transient, permanent

Every human being of adult years and sound mind has a right to determine what shall be done with his own body; and a surgeon who performs an operation without his patient's consent commits an assault.
(Justice Cardoza, Schloendorff vs Society of New York Hospital 1914)

Consent encompasses human rights, ethics and medical law. Every patient has the right of autonomy over his or her body. **Trespass** refers to intentionally touching another person without their consent. Failure to provide informed consent could lead to a civil case for **battery**.

The mental capacity of the patient must be established before determining the appropriate consent required.

Competence to consent

In order for a patient to be deemed mentally competent they should have the ability to:
Understand the information given to them
Retain the information received
Contemplate the information

As the clinician, one must decide whether the above criteria have been met. One way to determine this is to ask the patient what they understand from what has been discussed (can they repeat it back to you in their own words?) and if they have any further questions. This way a level of understanding can be established.

It is also important to be aware that in the light of bad news or anxiety, decision-making and understanding can be impaired – regardless of intelligence. Each patient must be assessed individually and the information pitched at an appropriate level. Once a patient is deemed competent they are legally entitled to informed consent.

Informed consent

Informed consent should include:

- **Details of the diagnosis and prognosis**, and the prognosis if the condition is left untreated
- **Options for management** of the condition, including the option not to treat
- **A detailed explanation of the proposed procedure(s)**: including subsidiary treatment such as pain relief
- **Side effects and complications:** What the patient may experience during or after the procedure, including common (incidence > 1%) and serious side effects or complications
- **Risks and benefits:** for each treatment option
- **The name of the doctor(s)** who will have responsibility for treatment
- A reminder that patients may change their minds and/or seek further opinions
- An opportunity for patients and relatives to ask questions

Ideally the clinician performing the treatment should obtain consent. If this is not possible then consent should be obtained by a suitably qualified person with sufficient knowledge of the proposed investigation, treatment and risks. Informed consent can be verbal, or written, although it is always better to have a written record that consent has been obtained. Patient-advice leaflets and visual aids are a useful adjunct to obtaining consent.

In reality a lot of patients find it difficult to assimilate all this information and it is common to hear them say 'Whatever you think is best, doctor'. This poses a dilemma (legal vs moral) for the clinician. The patient can be offered (without coercion) advice on the most favourable treatment option and the major complications associated with this should be discussed.

Refusal of treatment

Once the necessary information, as outlined above, has been relayed to a competent patient, the patient is still legally entitled to refuse treatment/diagnosis even if the potential condition is life-threatening. This is a morally difficult path for a clinician to take. However failure to do so is a breach of the patient's autonomy and one could be liable for a charge of assault.

For example, consider a Jehovah's Witness patient. For followers of this faith receiving a blood transfusion is considered to be a mortal sin. If such a patient who is competent declines blood transfusion or blood products these wishes should be respected even in a life-threatening situation. The scope of this subject is vast, however it is worth discussing with the patient which products they are willing to have in case of an emergency, as in practice this

can vary (see Royal College of Surgeons guidelines on The Jehovah's Witness patient, found at http://www.rcseng.ac.uk/services/publications/docs/jehovahs_witness.html/).
While patients can refuse a procedure or operation, they cannot demand a procedure that is considered to be medically inappropriate.

Consent in research and clinical trials

Informed consent is not only required for procedures. It is also legally required for entering patients into clinical trials or for the pathological use of tissue (section 63 of the Human Tissue Act 1983). As with clinical procedures, the consent is not informed unless:

- Information has been provided about the clinical trial/pathological use of the tissue
- The patient is aware of the implications of the trial compared with the conventional treatment and whether there is a potential change of their prognosis
- If information is withheld, the patient's consent is not informed and recruitment is therefore illegal

Verbal and implied consent

Verbal consent

A signature is usually required from the patient to confirm an understanding of the intended procedure and a willingness to continue. The clinician's signature signifies that the consent has been informed.

In certain circumstances where a patient is unable to sign (eg physical disability, or still conscious before an emergency procedure but debilitated) verbal consent is legal. However, another healthcare professional should be present as a witness. The name, position, and signature of this person should be documented, as well as the reason for verbal consent.

Implied consent

The majority of the working day could be taken up with obtaining written consent for every minor examination or procedure carried out within the hospital! Therefore, in cases where there are no major complications, there is the concept of implied consent. For example, after the intended procedure has been explained to the patient, the action of offering an arm for venepuncture or undressing for an examination is known as implied consent. The patient has used his/her autonomy in order to allow you to proceed.

The patient who is unable to consent

The incompetent patient

Patients do always not fit into the categories outlined here and much of the assessment is down to the individual clinician. However there are some broad categories that can be of help.

Temporary mental incompetence (eg young children)

The term incompetence is probably inappropriate in this situation, but is used to imply that young children of a certain age do not have the appropriate mental reasoning for development of informed decisions. This is not true of all children.

Under 16 years of age

This is a difficult area because the legal age of consent does not always coincide with the age of mental competence. The legal age of consent is 16. However if a child younger than 16 displays competence (an understanding of their condition, the ability to remember the information, and the logic to ask appropriate questions regarding this topic) they can legally consent to treatment – even if their parents refuse. These children are known as Gillick competent (mature minor) after the Victoria Gillick case (Gillick v West Norfolk and Wisbech Area Health Authority 1985).

Gillick-competent patients can accept treatment without being over-ridden by their parents. However, if they refuse treatment the converse is true and the parents can consent to treatment. If both the child and the parents refuse treatment in a life-threatening case, the court should be consulted if time allows.

16–18 years of age

The family law reform act of 1969 states that consent for any medical, surgical or dental procedure for diagnosis or treatment can be performed with the consent of the minor (aged 16–18) and consent of the parent/guardian is not required.

However even in this age group, if life-threatening treatment is refused they require the consent of their parents. Where possible, all treatment options should be discussed and the views of the competent minor should be considered, along with those of the parents and clinician in the decision making process.

Transient mental incompetence (eg the unconscious patient)

The relatives of the patient are unable to consent on behalf of the patient (their agreement should be sought without breaching confidentiality, but their signature on a consent form is invalid). Therefore, the clinician must, in this situation, act in the best interest of the patient. The law that allows this action is the **doctrine of necessity**, whereby procedures can be undertaken in an emergency without consent if:

- There is a necessity to act while the patient is unable to communicate
- The action to be taken is consistent with the action that a reasonable person would take given the circumstances
- The action is in the best interest of the assisted person

In summary, as long as the actions taken in the 'best interest of the patient' in an emergency situation are those that a colleague of equal standing would take in the same situation, there should not be a problem with a lack of consent.

The only time that this may not apply is when a patient arrives conscious and expresses certain wishes regarding treatment before becoming unconscious. This is known as an **advanced refusal** (advanced directive/living will), which is not as common in the UK as it is in the USA. If the patient was mentally competent before unconsciousness, the conscious wishes must be legally adhered to.

Permanent mental incompetence

This includes psychiatric illness, mental disability, and persistent vegetative state (PVS).

A psychiatric illness or mental disability does not automatically render a patient incompetent to consent and these patients require individual assessment. The Mental Health Act 1983 – whereby a patient can be detained for a mental disorder – states that consent should be obtained for certain procedures. In cases of psychiatric illness or mental disability when competence cannot be demonstrated, the clinician must act in the best interest of the patient with respect to appropriate treatment.

Persistent vegetative state (PVS)

Death can now be characterised by the irreversible loss of function of the brainstem, leading to loss of spontaneous respiration. In PVS there is lack of awareness, of physical activity, and of cognitive function, although spontaneous respiration still occurs. Consequently these patients are unable to consent and the clinician must act in their best interest with respect to appropriate treatment.

> **Diagnostic criteria of persistent vegetative state (PVS)**
>
> Several criteria have to met before the diagnosis of PVS can be confirmed (Medical Ethics Committee of the BMA):
>
> - Rehabilitation must continue for 6 months
> - PVS cannot be confirmed until 12 months after trauma
> - PVS diagnosis needs to be confirmed by two other doctors

Recovery is extremely unlikely. Physiotherapy is necessary to prevent chest infection and complications of immobility, and as long as enteral feeding is continued the patient might exist in this state for years. There is, therefore, a moral conundrum as to what constitutes the patient's best interests, and decisions about treatment should be taken after discussion with, and preferably with full agreement from, the relatives.

4.4 OTHER ETHICAL AND LEGAL ISSUES

Negligence

In a nutshell ...

Negligence is a breach in the duty of care that results in damage to the patient.

Gross negligence is a breach in the duty of care of such recklessness that it is considered to be a criminal offence.

Incompetence is a breach in the duty of care that does not result in damage to the patient.

Recognise the limits of your professional competence.
(General Medical Council 2001)

Negligence is measured by the **reasonable man test** defined by Baron Alderson in 1856, thus:

> Negligence is the omission to do something which a reasonable man, guided upon those considerations which regulate the conduct of human affairs would do, or doing something which a prudent and reasonable man would not do.

As surgical trainees, we act under the responsibility of our trainers, but this does not mean that we are not responsible for our own actions. 'I was told to do it' is not legally defensible. Each consultant has overall responsibility for the patient (and so should remain informed) and each junior has a responsibility to perform in line with the expected standard of care.

There is a sequence of events that lead to negligence. A duty of care exists towards our patients and once this responsibility is accepted it must be carried out to the highest standards possible. The offence of negligence is where a breach of this duty has occurred and damage results as a consequence of this breach. This is liable to court action. If the breach entails extreme recklessness or carelessness then this is a criminal matter and is **gross negligence**.

In the event that a breach of duty occurs and damage cannot be legally proven, this is **incompetence** in practice and the GMC or the local health authority can still undertake to discipline those involved.

Euthanasia

In a nutshell ...

Euthanasia is the act of taking life to relieve suffering.
(Concise Oxford Medical Dictionary 1990)

Although the definition may appear perfectly acceptable, this act is illegal in many countries and is regarded as murder. Patient autonomy and wishes are of great importance, but even if a patient who is suffering requests an end to their life, in the UK we legally cannot comply with that wish.

To what extent can suffering be relieved?

It is within the boundaries of the law to administer analgesia to alleviate pain. If, as an indirect consequence of administering the analgesia, the anticipated death is expedited by an insignificant period, it is implied that the intention would be to alleviate pain and suffering, and not to cause death.

If death is approaching and a drug is administered to deliberately hasten death, this is illegal euthanasia. This does not apply to omission of treatment. For example, in the case of Airedale NHS Trust vs Bland 1993 the hospital, consultant and parents applied for legal permission to withdraw enteral feeding from a patient with PVS which would inevitably lead to death. The taking of this action was approved by the court; however this death could not be accelerated by the concomitant use of medication.

NB: Legislation passed in 1993 makes euthanasia/assisted suicide legal in the Netherlands; however, certain legal requirements must be met.

Whistle blowing

> *Act quickly to protect patients from risk if you have good reason to believe that you or a colleague may not be fit to practice.*
> (General Medical Council 2001)

The phrase whistle blowing perhaps has negative connotations. The ultimate aim of bringing failings to light is to protect patients. Inappropriate or substandard practice should be reviewed with the aim of adjusting practice or providing additional training for improved professional development.

Approach a senior for advice, such as the lead clinician, educational supervisor, or postgraduate dean. The intention is not to produce an overly defensive medical culture, but in a professional and delicate manner to aim to help an under-achiever to improve through re-education. Everyone has to reach the same standard of care.

Clinical freedom

In the current professional climate, with litigation in the back of many clinician's minds, it appears that 'clinical freedom' may be a misnomer. Current legislation and guidelines should not pose boundaries, but provide a structure to expand new concepts in clinical and academic practice, while constantly upholding the duties set out by the GMC. Thus, by adhering to current and evolving practices, the NHS will maintain its standards of care for patients and competence of its clinicians.

Chapter 9

Vascular

Sam Andrews and Nerys Forester

Section 1
Investigation of vascular disease

1.1 PRINCIPLES OF VASCULAR SURGERY

In a nutshell ...

Vascular disease includes:
- Arterial disease: occlusive, aneurysm, carotid, trauma
- Venous disease: thromboembolic, varicose veins, leg ulcers
- Lymphatic diseases

Also included are miscellaneous conditions traditionally treated by vascular surgeons:
- Vasospastic disorders
- Thoracic outlet syndrome
- Hyperhidrosis
- Amputations
- Vascular trauma (see *Trauma* chapter)

Vascular interventions are performed:
- To improve or restore arterial flow (eg angioplasty, stenting, bypass)
- To prevent vascular catastrophe (eg carotid endarterectomy, aneurysm surgery)

The main principles of vascular surgery are to first gain proximal and distal control of flow and then correct the vascular abnormality. These principles can be applied equally well to peripheral vascular disease (PVD), carotid surgery, aneurysm or vascular trauma.

Vascular physiology is covered in Chapter 7 *Critical Care*.

1.2 VASCULAR INVESTIGATIONS

In a nutshell ...

General vascular investigations, eg blood tests, CXR, etc.

Specific vascular investigations:
- Ankle brachial pressure index (ABPI)
- Duplex Doppler Ultrasound
- Angiography
- Contrast angiography
- Digital subtraction angiography
- CT and MR angiography
- Venography
- Lymphoscintography
- Radio-isotope imaging

General vascular investigations

As vascular disease is a multisystem disorder all vascular patients require a general work-up with modification of vascular risk factors. In addition, those requiring complex vascular procedures may require other specific investigations.

- FBC looking for:
  - Anaemia
  - Polycythaemia
  - Concurrent infection
- Clotting
  - Especially if anticoagulated
  - Excludes pro-thrombotic states
  - Baseline before heparinisation or warfarinisation
- U&Es (for renal function)
- ESR (for vasculitides)
- Random or fasting blood glucose (to exclude diabetes)
- Fasting lipids
- Urinalysis
- CXR (often smokers)
- ECG (co-existing cardiovascular disease is common in arteriopaths and has implications for surgery)
- Echocardiography or exercise ECG in high-risk cardiac patients

Specific vascular investigations

Ankle brachial pressure index (ABPI)

ABPI is used to assess the blood supply to the lower limb. It is simply a measure of BP in the foot, which is usually roughly equal to that of the arm. Hence, this absolute pressure in the foot can be compared with the brachial systolic BP to provide the ankle brachial pressure index (ABPI).

$$\text{ABPI} = \frac{\text{foot artery occlusion pressure}}{\text{brachial systolic pressure}}$$

Procedure box: How to perform an ABPI

Place a BP cuff around the calf
Use a handheld Doppler probe to find the dorsalis paedis or posterior tibial artery signal
Inflate the cuff, noting the pressure at which the signal stops
Release the pressure, confirming that the signal returns at the pressure noted
This is the occlusion pressure
Take the blood pressure at the brachial artery in the normal way
Compare the systolic BP recorded in the arm with the occlusion pressure recorded in the foot. If they are the same, the ABPI is 1 (normal ABPI is 0.9–1.1)
If peripheral circulation in the lower limb is reduced, the BP in the foot is low and the ABPI is low

ABPI may be used to confirm the presence of PVD and as a baseline measure before investigation.

The following ABPI values imply:

> 1.1	Calcified or incompressible vessels (eg in diabetes or renal failure)
0.7– 0.9	Mild ischaemia
0.4– 0.7	Moderate ischaemia
< 0.4	Severe peripheral (critical) ischaemia

Duplex Doppler ultrasound (US)

Duplex Doppler US is used for:

- Assessment and monitoring of arterial blood flow
  - Carotid disease
  - PVD
  - Graft surveillance
- Abdominal aortic aneurysm (AAA)
  - Assessment
  - Monitoring
  - Screening
- Renal disease
  - Renal artery stenosis
- Venous disease
  - Demonstrates reflux in varicose veins (with reverse flow in veins following calf compression)
  - Useful to mark varicose vein perforators in redo surgery
  - Diagnosis of DVT (veins non-compressible with Doppler probe)

There are two aspects to Duplex Doppler US (bi-modal system):

- Grey-scale US: visualises the vessel, vessel wall, plaque, lumen and measure degree of stenosis in mm
- Doppler US: uses the Doppler principal to measure the blood velocity, which is proportional to the degree of stenosis of the vessel

Duplex Doppler US as an investigation for vascular disease

Advantages of Duplex Doppler US

Cheap
Non-invasive
Accurate measurement of stenosis
Colour image shows direction of blood and turbulent flow

Disadvantages of Duplex Doppler US

Operator dependent
Views may be obscured by bowel gas
Poor images in calcified vessels
Not good for near occlusions

Contrast angiography

Traditional contrast angiography is performed by introducing a radio-opaque dye into a vessel and taking X-ray images. BEWARE: contrast is nephrotoxic. Most radiology departments have a protocol for a renal protection regimen based on the patient's creatinine level. In pre-existing severe renal impairment imaging may be performed using a stream of small bubbles of carbon dioxide. This protects renal function but compromises the quality of the images obtained.

Uses of contrast angiography

- Assessment of arterial disease in most areas (especially upper and lower limb, abdomen and thorax)
- Emergency assessment of vascular crises, such as:
  - Acute ischaemia
  - Lower limb embolus
  - Brachial artery occlusion
  - Differentiates mesenteric ischaemia due to arterial occlusion (will show abrupt cut-off in superior mesenteric artery circulation) from vein thrombosis (will show delayed contrast passage)
- Renovascular disease
  - Renal artery stenosis
  - Fibromuscular hyperplasia
- Calibrating angiograms to assess suitability of AAA endovascular repair

Classification of contrast angiography

- By method of administration (eg intra-arterial, intravenous)
- By route of administration (eg trans-lumbar, trans-femoral, trans-brachial)
- By area to be imaged (eg carotid, visceral, femoral)
- By method of image processing (eg traditional, digital subtraction, CT, MR)

In intra-arterial angiography, the contrast is introduced by direct arterial puncture via a catheter which is directed proximal to the area to be imaged (eg femoral puncture to release contrast into the aorta to image the iliac and femoral vessels).

Intra-arterial angiography

Advantages of intra-arterial angiography

Small volume of contrast required
Good quality images (especially below knee where Doppler imaging is less useful)
Allows concurrent treatment (angioplasty or stenting)

Disadvantages of intra-arterial angiography

Arterial wall damage (may cause bruising, false aneurysm, dissection)
Contrast reactions (including anaphylaxis)
Distal embolisation
Groin haematoma

Digital subtraction angiography

Digital subtraction is a process which enhances the images obtained with contrast angiography. The pre-angiography image without contrast is subtracted from the post-angiography image with contrast to leave just an outline of the lumen of the vessel. This can be via intra-arterial (IADSA) or intravenous (IVDSA) injection of contrast.

IADSA is the most accurate investigation for imaging the arterial system. However, IVDSA is less invasive and does not require arterial puncture. The contrast is introduced via a central vein and delayed images are produced to show the 'arterial phase' and are digitally subtracted from pre-contrast images to produce better views.

Intravenous digital subtraction angiography (IVDSA)

Advantages of IVDSA

Less invasive: no arterial puncture

Disadvantages of IVDSA

Poor quality images (obscured by bowel gas)
Large volume of contrast required
Some contrast materials nephrotoxic
Patients must be able to stay very still throughout both procedures

CT and MR angiography

Multislice computed axial tomography (CAT) and MR angiography (MRA) are now becoming the mainstays of vascular investigation. Computer generated 3-D images can be produced, and detailed image reconstruction performed. MRA is a specific application of MRI, producing angiogram-type images without need for contrast, utilising blood flow through the vessel to create images.

Advantages of CT and MRA

Quick
Non-invasive
No radiation dose for MR

Disadvantages of CT and MRA

Relatively expensive
Operator dependent
MR precludes patients with metal implants
Picture degeneration in CT of patients with metal implants
Does not allow concurrent angioplasty and stenting
Variable image quality at present

Venography and MR venography

Venography uses contrast to image the venous system, either ascending venography (contrast injected into foot vein) or descending venography (contrast injected into groin ie femoral vein). The technique has been largely replaced by Doppler US scanning. However, it is occasionally used to differentiate primary from secondary venous insufficiency, or to diagnose below-knee DVT, when USS cannot adequately demonstrate the calf veins.

Magnetic resonance venography (MRV) is a specific application of MRI that can be performed with or without gadolinium contrast. It is effective for evaluating diseases of larger veins (eg thrombus vena cava, identification of obstruction or occlusion of the brachiocephalic, subclavian, and jugular veins, venous sinus thrombosis, pelvic circulation). MRV has not been established as superior to Duplex US for diagnosis of DVT.

Imaging of the lymphatics

Lymphoscintography is now the main investigation to image the lymphatic system. Radio-labelled colloid is injected into web spaces between 2nd and 3rd toes and images obtained with a gamma camera.

Radio-isotope imaging

Radio-labelled fibrinogen is occasionally used in diagnosis of thrombotic venous disease (eg DVT). Radio-labelled white cell scans may be used for assessing graft infection instead of CT scanning.

Section 2
Aneurysms

In a nutshell ...

An aneurysm is a pathological, permanent, segmental dilatation of an artery to > 1.5 times its normal diameter. In the western world arterial aneurysms are usually due to atherosclerosis. Aneurysms have clinical implications because of their ability to rupture, leak or embolise.

Rupture of the abdominal aortic aneurysm is a common cause of sudden death and the risk of rupture increases with the size of the aneurysm. For this reason surgery is considered for all symptomatic abdominal aortic aneurysms, for those of > 5.5 cm in diameter, and those that are expanding at a rate of > 1 cm per year.

Other arteries may become aneurysmal but are less common .

2.1 ANATOMY OF ARTERIES

In a nutshell ...

Two types of artery
- Elastic
- Muscular

Three histological layers
- Tunica intima
- Tunica media
- Tunica adventitia

Structure of arteries

There are two types of artery:

- **Elastic** conducting arteries (eg aorta) which expand to take the forward blood flow of systole and use this stored energy to recoil during diastole (this provides constant blood flow)
- **Muscular** distributing arteries (eg femoral artery) which taper as the media thins down to a few layers of vascular smooth muscle cells and become arterioles

Microscopically, arteries consist of three layers:

- **Tunica intima:** innermost layer; composed of a single layer of endothelial cells which are orientated in the direction of flow and have a role in both coagulation and vasomotor tone
- **Tunica media:** middle layer; composed of elastin and collagen fibres with vascular smooth muscle cells which function either to control vasomotor tone or to synthesize the structural proteins of the vessel wall
- **Tunica adventitia:** outermost layer of connective tissue

Elastic arteries have a high amount of elastin and collagen in the media, with relatively fewer smooth muscle cells (which predominate in muscular arteries). The media is an important structure in the arterial wall, and abnormalities within the media of the vessel are pathological in aneurysmal disease.

Anatomy of the aorta

The aorta has thoracic and abdominal components. Aortic wall histology changes rapidly as the aorta descends past the renal arteries, with the thoracic aorta having > 30% elastin compared to < 20% in the abdominal section.

Thoracic aorta

The **ascending thoracic aorta** is 5 cm long, beginning at the base of the left ventricle. The sinuses of valsalva are three bulges in the wall of the ascending aorta just above the aortic ring – these give rise to the right and left coronary arteries.

The **aortic arch** starts behind the right margin of the sternum and gives rise to the brachiocephalic, left common carotid and the left subclavian artery. It ends at level of T4.

The **descending thoracic aorta** lies in the posterior mediastinum extending between T4 and T12. Gives branches to pericardium, lungs, bronchi, oesophagus, intercostal and phrenic arteries.

For a detailed discussion of the pathology and surgery of the thoracic aorta see the chapter on *Cardiothoracics* in Book 2.

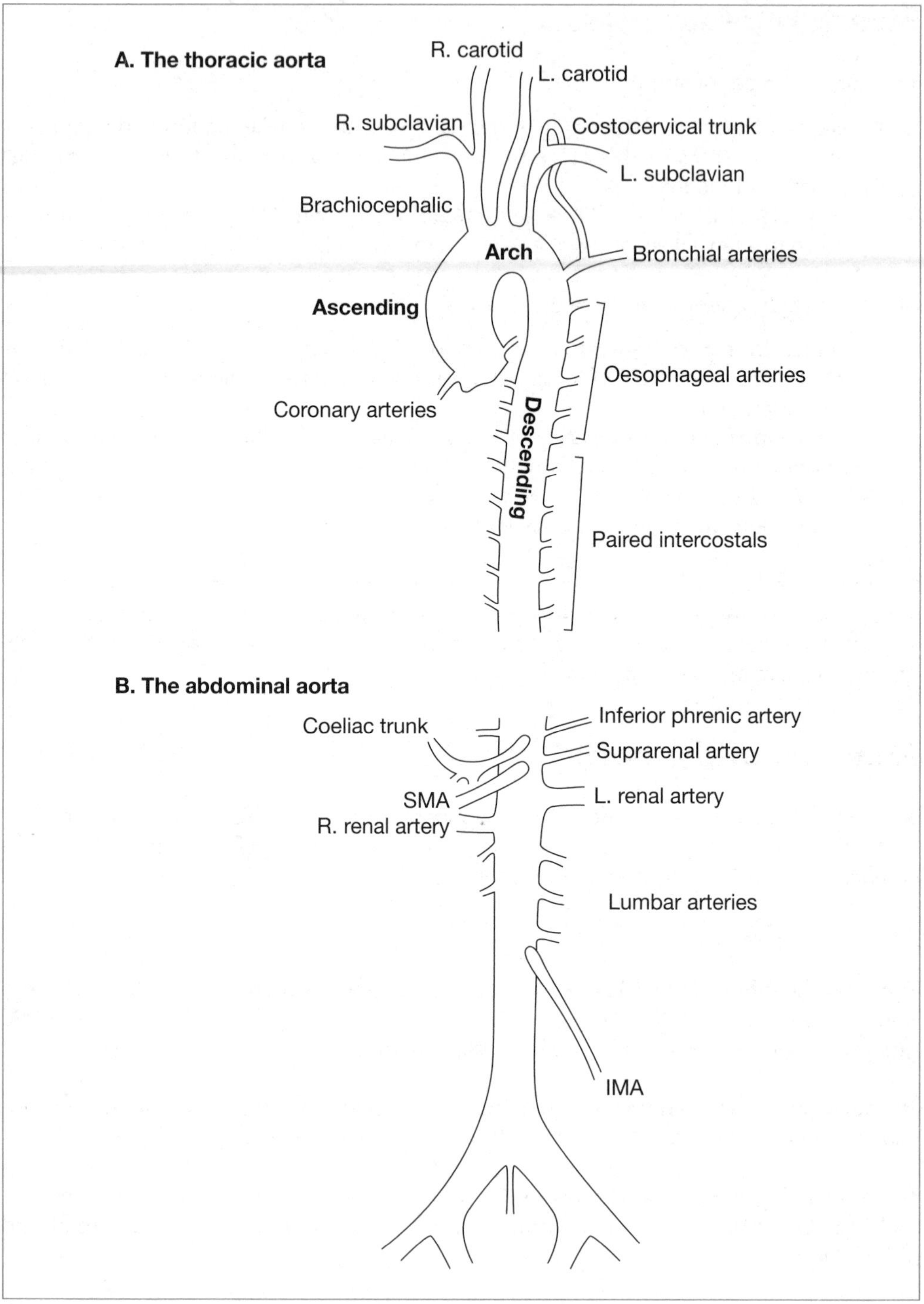
A. The thoracic aorta
R. carotid
L. carotid
R. subclavian
Costocervical trunk
L. subclavian
Brachiocephalic
Arch
Bronchial arteries
Ascending
Oesophageal arteries
Coronary arteries
Descending
Paired intercostals
B. The abdominal aorta
Coeliac trunk
Inferior phrenic artery
Suprarenal artery
SMA
L. renal artery
R. renal artery
Lumbar arteries
IMA

Figure 2.1a *The aorta*

Abdominal aorta

The abdominal aorta enters the abdomen between the diaphragmatic crura anterior to the T12 vertebra, as a continuation of the thoracic aorta. It descends on the vertebral bodies until its bifurcation at the level of the body of L4 vertebra where it bifurcates into the common iliac arteries, with a small median sacral artery between. It is crossed anteriorly by the splenic vein, body of the pancreas, 3rd part of the duodenum, and the left renal vein. On its right lie the IVC, the right ureter, and the azygos vein. On its left lie the left sympathetic trunk, and the left ureter.

Branches of the abdominal aorta

3 paired visceral branches

- Suprarenal (adrenal)
- Renal
- Gonadal

3 unpaired visceral branches

- Coeliac axis
- SMA
- IMA

Parietal branches

- 1 pair inferior phrenic
- 4 pairs lumbar, plus median sacral artery (variable)

(NB: the artery of Adamkiewiecz arises from lumbar arteries as the main blood supply to the spinal cord; high aortic surgery can cause spinal cord ischaemia).

2.2 PATHOLOGY OF ANEURYSMS

In a nutshell ...

An aneurysm is a pathological, permanent, segmental dilatation of an artery to > 1.5 times its normal diameter. The upper limit of the normal aorta is considered to be 2 cm, ie it is aneurysmal at 3 cm. Mechanical factors are very important in progression of aneurysm. According to **Laplace's law** any increase in vessel diameter will increase wall tension, causing continued arterial dilatation, and eventually rupture.

Aneurysms may be classified as:

- **True aneurysms:** dilatation of an artery involving all layers of arterial wall
- **False aneurysms:** pulsatile, expansile swelling due to a defect in an arterial wall, with blood outside the arterial lumen, surrounded by a capsule of fibrous tissue or compressed surrounding tissues

True aneurysms may be fusiform (spindle-shaped) or saccular (bag-like weakness in part of the arterial wall).

Other descriptions of abnormal arteries:

- **Tortuous:** increase in length of an artery causing curvature between two fixed points
- **Arteriomegaly:** generalised dilatation or lengthening of arteries

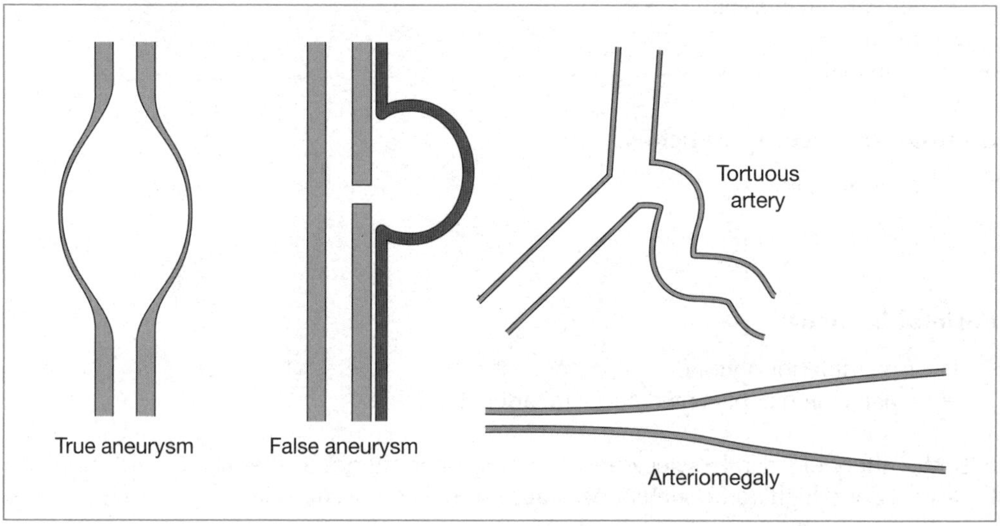

Figure 2.2a *Aneurysm types*

Aetiology of aneurysms

- **Degenerative** (**atherosclerotic**)**:** this is the commonest cause, due to inflammation and proteolysis in the substrata of the tunica media
- **Inflammatory:** possibly a more severe form of degenerative AAA. It is characterised by variable degrees of inflammation in aneurysm wall, causing adhesion to adjacent structures (especially duodenum, small bowel, ureters), and it is related to (sometimes associated with) retroperitoneal fibrosis (with symptoms of ureteric obstruction and CRF). Usually it presents with abdominal pain, weight loss and a raised ESR. Management is conventional or endovascular repair but surgery may be more challenging due to inflammation and fibrosis

- **Congenital:** eg Berry aneurysms of the cerebral circulation
- **Mycotic:** these can be from endogenous sources (eg infected emboli in endocarditis) or from exogenous causes (eg from infected needles in IV drug abuse)
- **Infective:** these are commonest in syphilitic aneurysms (often affecting the arch of the aorta and descending aorta). Syphilitic aortitis is rare now because of increased use of antibiotics in primary and secondary syphilis
- **Traumatic:** damage to the arterial wall can be from blunt or penetrating injury (including iatrogenic) and can result in true or false aneurysm formation
- **Connective tissue disorders:** tend to present young at 40–50 years or with a family history eg Marfan syndrome, Ehlers–Danlos syndrome, tuberous sclerosis, Takayasu's arteritis
- **Post-stenotic:** due to altered vessel haemodynamics

2.3 ABDOMINAL AORTIC ANEURYSM (AAA)

In a nutshell ...

The infrarenal abdominal aorta is the commonest site for atherosclerotic aneurysm. Ruptured AAA is the 13th commonest cause of death in the western world.

- Size is the most important risk factor for rupture, although rate of expansion is also significant
- 75% present as an asymptomatic incidental finding on imaging
- Symptomatic aneurysms are usually expanding rapidly or leaking and need prompt repair
- Treatment is surgical replacement with a graft or endovascular stenting
- Elective repair has a mortality rate of 5% and is offered to fit patients with an aneurysm of > 5.5 cm diameter or expanding at a rate of > 1 cm per year
- Elective surgery aims to avoid future rupture
- Most patients with ruptured aneurysms die before reaching hospital, and of those operated on 50% will die during or within 30 days of surgery

Demographics of AAA

- 6M to 1F
- Affects 1 in 20 (5%) men aged > 65
- Incidence increases with age (6% of 65–74 men; 9% of > 75 men)
- Risks include smoking, hypercholesterolaemia, male sex
- Family history (12-fold increased occurrence in 1st-degree relatives)
- 95% infrarenal; 5% suprarenal
- 30% involve iliac arteries

Natural history of AAA

The natural progression of an AAA is to expand and rupture.

Size is the most important risk factor for rupture. An increase in size by 10% per year or more also significantly increases risk. Smaller aneurysms expand more slowly than larger aneurysms. Not all growth is linear and there may be periods where expansion accelerates or stops altogether.

Rates of rupture taken from a non-operated series are:

- 4% per year if < 5 cm
- 7% per year if 5–6 cm
- > 20% per year if > 6 cm

There is some value in risk factor modification to reduce growth rate (eg decrease BP, prescribe statins).

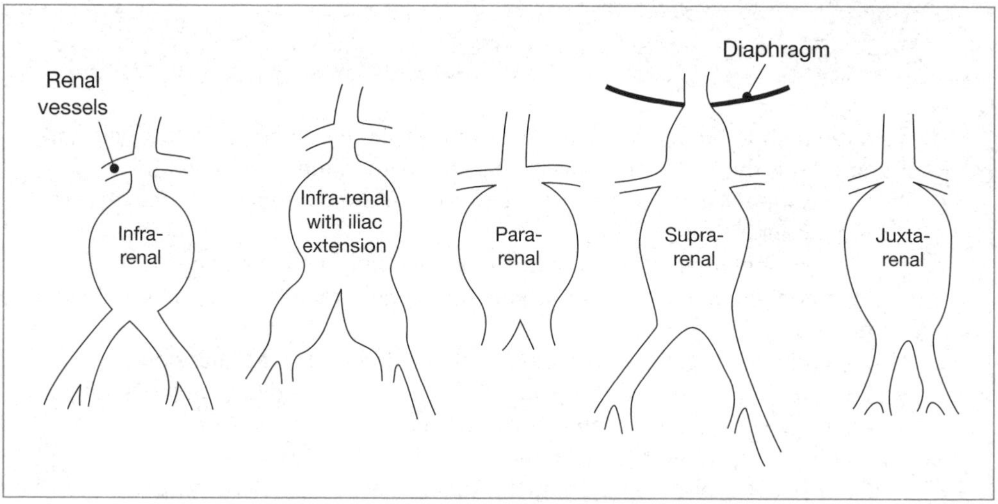

Figure 2.3a *Abdominal aortic aneurysm types. All AAA may extend into the iliac vessels. Suprarenal AAA may extend into the chest as a thoraco-abdominal aneurysm*

Presentation of AAA

- **Asymptomatic:** usually incidental finding in clinical or radiological examination. 75% present this way
- **Pain:** this is central abdominal and may radiate to the back. This is a sign of expansion or, if sudden and acute, potential rupture

- **Rupture:** this is the most devastating presentation. There is a 95% mortality overall, and 50% mortality in those who reach hospital alive. The patient typically presents with a hypotensive episode or collapse associated with severe central abdominal pain radiating to the back and the flanks. An aneurysm commonly ruptures the postero-lateral wall causing a retroperitoneal haematoma. This may be seen as bruising in the flanks or it may track down into the scrotum. Occasionally rupture may form a temporarily contained haematoma. Co-existing COAD is a known risk factor for aneurysm rupture
- **Shock**
- **Embolisation:** thrombi/atheroma from the aneurysm may give rise to acute limb ischaemia or small areas of distal infarction (trash foot)
- **Other:** AAA can rarely present with acute thrombosis or fistulation into surrounding structures (eg IVC, duodenum, terminal ileum)
- **Screening:** this is being evaluated in some regions. A single US at age 65 will pick up most AAAs and negative scans at this age may rule out future aneurysmal change. Larger AAAs can be referred for surgery. Smaller AAAs can be entered into a surveillance programme

Pre-operative investigations for AAA repair

- Bloods
  - FBC
  - U&Es (for concurrent renal failure)
  - Blood sugar
  - ESR (may be elevated in inflammatory aneurysms)
  - Cross-match 6 units
- ABPI: to assess co-existing PVD and document pre-operative state in case of trash foot post-operatively
- CXR
- ECG and echocardiogram
- Lung function tests: to aid anaesthetic assessment
- US: usually used as a screening tool
- CT: this is mandatory for elective aneurysm surgery, allowing assessment of proximal neck anatomy, iliac extension, inflammation and other possible intra-abdominal pathology (these patients are often elderly and an occult tumour is occasionally found)
- Arteriography: this is not currently part of standard elective AAA work-up, but is necessary before endovascular repair

In ruptured AAA there is often insufficient time for full pre-operative investigations. Minimal requirements for an emergency aneurysm repair include IV access × 2, basic bloods, cross-match 10 units and portable CXR. A CT scan may be required to confirm the diagnosis but bear in mind that unstable patients should not be taken to CT.

Elective repair of AAA

Elective repair is offered to patients whose aneurysms have maximum diameter of > 5.5 cm and who are fit enough to withstand surgery, to prevent continued expansion and rupture. Following the recommendations of the **UK Small Aneurysm Trial**, surveillance screening is offered to patients with asymptomatic small aneurysms of < 5.5 cm. Surgery is considered for all symptomatic AAAs, those of > 5.5 cm, and those that are expanding at > 1 cm per year.

Elective infra-renal aneurysm repair has a mortality rate of about 5%. Emergency aneurysm repair has a mortality rate of around 50%.

Op box: Open abdominal aortic aneurysm (AAA) repair

Indications

Elective repair if diameter > 5.5 cm or expanding at rate of > 1 cm/year; urgent repair if the aneurysm is undergoing rapid expansion or the patient presents with pain; emergency repair for rupture.

Pre-op

- Appropriate pre-op assessment and management (eg antihypertensives, smoking cessation)
- GA with an ET tube, central line, arterial line, epidural catheter, and urethral catheter
- Prophylactic antibiotics and thromboprophylaxis
- Consent with complications and hazards in mind

Positioning

Supine.

Incision

Usually mid-line longitudinal incision. Some use a transverse incision.

Procedure (summarised)

- Enter abdominal cavity, retract bowel, and duodenum to right
- Divide posterior peritoneum and dissect aneurysm
- Define proximal neck of aneurysm and distal extension (may be into iliacs)
- Administer IV heparinisation
- Apply aortic clamps (distal then proximal) and secure before opening aneurysm sac
- Over-sew lumbar arteries and IMA if they are patent
- Repair with either inlay tube graft, or Y-graft (trouser) if iliac arteries involved
- Achieve haemostasis; close aneurysm sac over the graft

Intra-operative hazards
Beware abnormal anatomy affecting the renal vessels; duodenum and ureters lie close to an aneurysmal sac (and may be involved if inflammatory aetiology).

Closure
Standard abdominal closure for laparotomy (in emergency cases a mesh may be required to close to prevent abdominal compartment syndrome).

Post-op instructions
ITU for post-op care.

Complications of AAA repair

Elective peri-operative mortality is 3–5%.

Immediate complications of AAA repair

- Haemorrhage (primary)
- Distal embolisation (ischaemic leg, trash foot)

Early complications of AAA repair

- Haemorrhage (reactive, secondary)
- MI
- Renal failure (especially if proximal clamp above renal vessels)
- Multi-organ failure, DIC, ARDS
- Colonic ischaemia
- Pneumonia, ARDS
- Stroke
- DVT, PE
- Paraparesis due to spinal ischaemia (lumbar vessels over-sewn)

Late complications of AAA repair

- Late graft infection (causing graft thrombosis, false aneurysm formation, or rupture)
- Aorto-enteric fistula
- Anastomotic aneurysm

Endovascular AAA repair (EVAR)

EVAR is a new modality of treatment of AAA, for which 35–40% of AAAs are suitable. A prosthesis consisting of a vascular graft with an integral metallic stent is introduced via a catheter through a femoral arteriotomy. It is advanced over a guidewire under fluoroscopic control into the aneurysm. The 'stent–graft' is then positioned such that when the stents are expanded (usually by balloon catheters) the aneurysm is excluded from the circulation and thus is no longer at risk of rupture.

Stents can be straight or Y-shaped, with one or two iliac limbs. EVAR requires detailed pre-op assessment with calibrating angiograms to assess graft proximal fixation point (minimum of 1–1.5 cm below renal arteries) and often pre-op embolisation of any vessels (eg lumbar vessels) feeding into the aneurysm sac.

Advantages of endovascular repair

- Avoids large chest/abdominal incisions
- No aortic cross-clamping and physiological insult
- Reduced blood loss
- Potentially shorter anaesthetic

Disadvantages and complications of endovascular repair

- High cost
- Long-term results unclear (device failure possible)
- 'Endoleak' (two main types: type I is a leak at proximal or distal attachment site; type II is a failure to adequately exclude vessels feeding into the aneurysm sac)
- Distal embolisation
- 'Stent–graft' migration
- Femoral false aneurysm (at groin puncture site)
- Renal failure (as large volume of contrast required)

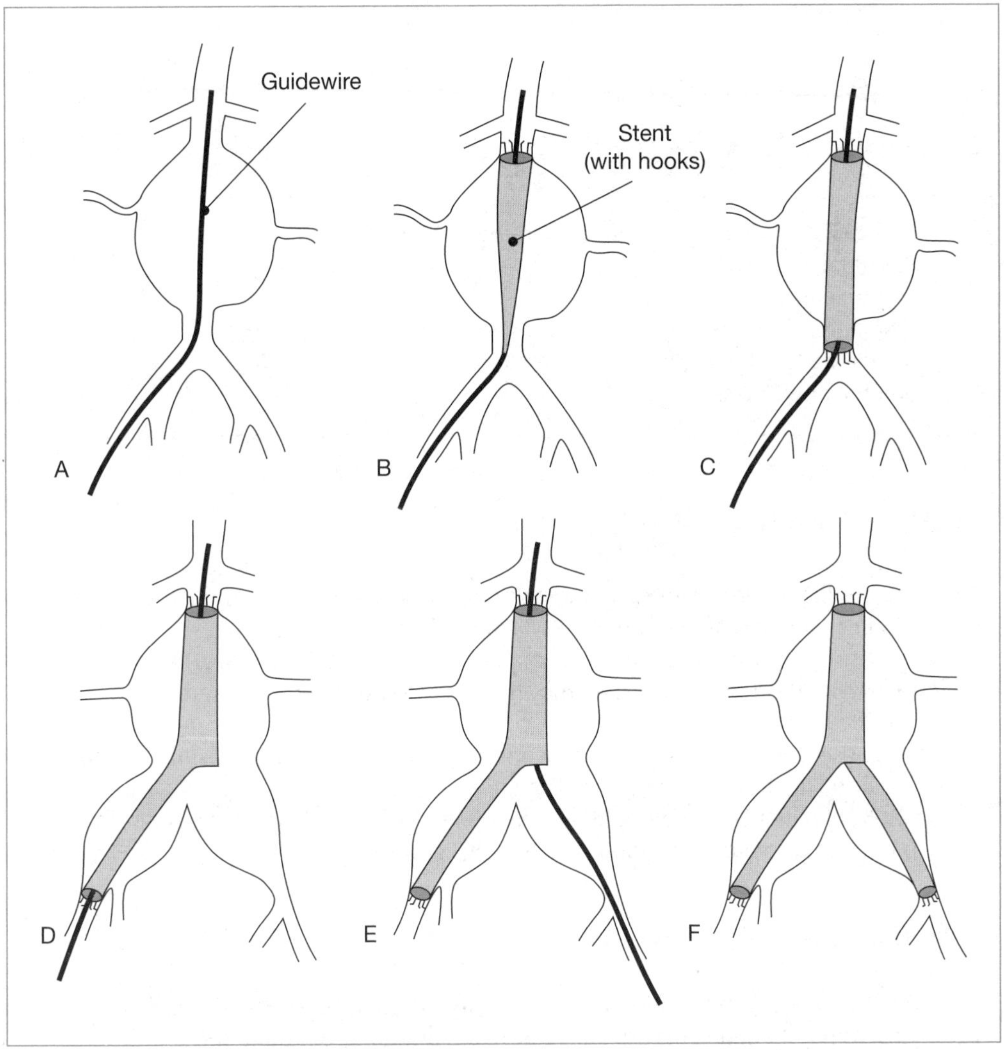

Figure 2.3b *Deployment of endovascular devices*
(A) A guidewire is passed from a femoral puncture site through the common iliac artery and across the lumen of the AAA to infrarenal aorta of normal diameter.
(B) The proximal end of the stent is deployed by balloon angioplasty.
(C) The distal end of the stent is deployed by balloon angioplasty.
(D) If a bifurcated graft is required the first component is inserted through the right femoral puncture over a guidewire.
(E) A second guidewire is introduced through the left femoral artery and navigated into the lumen of the first stent.
(F) The second component of the graft is deployed.

2.4 PERIPHERAL ANEURYSMS

In a nutshell ...

Aneurysmal disease may be generalised involving:
Popliteal aneurysms
Femoral aneurysms
Iliac aneurysms
Visceral artery aneurysms
Splenic aneurysms

Popliteal aneurysms

- The popliteal artery is the 2nd most common site of atherosclerotic aneurysms
- Popliteal aneurysms account for 70% of peripheral aneurysms
- Occasionally they present with expansile swelling, but more commonly with aneurysm thrombosis or distal emboli leading to peripheral ischaemia
- Rupture is rare
- Diagnosis confirmed by USS/CT or arteriography (also assesses distal vasculature)
- Repair by ligation and vein bypass graft
- > 30% of patients with a popliteal artery aneurysm will also have an AAA (remember to request a screening abdominal US in this group)

Femoral aneurysms

- These can occur in isolation but are usually part of a generalised arterial dilatation
- Most femoral aneurysms are false following arterial groin puncture
- Often they are symptomless and rupture rarely
- Occasionally they are a source of distal emboli and may thrombose
- Repair is by insertion of prosthetic graft or reversed saphenous vein
- Infected chronic femoral aneurysm due to IV drug abuse is becoming more common and is difficult to treat because prosthetic grafts invariably become infected

Iliac aneurysms

- The majority of these are found associated with an AAA
- Isolated aneurysms are rare (2%) and most of these involve the common iliac
- Rupture can occur

Visceral artery aneurysms

- Aneurysms can also occur in the renal, coeliac or mesenteric arteries
- Often they are asymptomatic but may present with rupture

Splenic aneurysms

Splenic aneurysms represent 60% of visceral artery aneurysms. The prevalence is 1–10% in autopsy studies. They are usually saccular, isolated and found in the middle or distal splenic artery. They are most common in middle-aged women but 10% are associated with AAA.

Presentation and treatment

- 80% asymptomatic; 20% cause left upper quadrant pain; 2–10% rupture
- Signet ring calcification may be seen in the left upper quadrant on plain AXR in 70% of cases
- Treatment options include simple ligation, resection with bypass or embolisation

Section 3
Lower limb ischaemia

3.1 ANATOMY OF THE LOWER LIMB ARTERIES

In a nutshell ...

Knowledge of the vascular anatomy of the lower limb is important for both diagnosis and reconstructive surgery.

- Iliac arteries
- Femoral artery
- Femoral triangle (see *Abdomen* chapter in Book 2)
- Popliteal artery
- Anterior tibial artery
- Posterior tibial artery
- Peroneal artery

Iliac arteries

Common iliac artery

- The aorta divides into the common iliac arteries to the left of the mid-line at the level of the body of the fourth lumbar vertebra
- The common iliac arteries pass downwards and laterally to bifurcate into external and internal iliac arteries in front of the sacroiliac joint
- There are usually no branches of the common iliac artery
- The ureter passes in front of the common iliac artery at the level of the bifurcation

External iliac artery

- Commencing at the bifurcation of the common iliac artery, the external iliac artery travels downwards and laterally to pass under the inguinal ligament at the mid-inguinal point, where it becomes the femoral artery
- The branches are the inferior epigastric and the deep circumflex iliac artery

Internal iliac artery

- Commencing at the bifurcation of the common iliac artery, the internal iliac runs inferiorly to lie opposite the upper margin of the greater sciatic notch where it divides into an anterior and posterior trunk
- The internal iliac artery lies between the internal iliac vein (posteriorly) and the ureter (anteriorly)
- The anterior and posterior trunks of the internal iliac artery supply the pelvic organs, perineum, buttock and anal canal

Femoral artery

- Arises from the external iliac artery
- Crosses the inguinal ligament and enters the thigh at the mid-inguinal point (half-way between symphysis pubis and anterior superior iliac spine)
- Lies in femoral triangle, lateral to femoral vein, medial to femoral nerve (see *Abdomen* chapter in Book 2) where it gives off the following branches:
  - Superficial circumflex iliac
  - Superficial epigastric
  - Superficial and deep external pudendals
  - Profunda femoris
- Descends almost vertically through the femoral canal to enter the adductor canal. The adductor canal is also known as the subsartorial or Hunter's canal. It is an important landmark for bypass grafting as it contains the femoral artery and vein, saphenous nerve and nerve to vastus medialis. The boundaries of the adductor canal are:
  - Vastus medialis
  - Adductor muscles
  - Sartorius (the roof)
- The femoral artery then enters the popliteal fossa via the adductor hiatus in the adductor magnus, to become the popliteal artery
- The profunda femoris is the largest branch of the femoral artery. It arises posteriorly or posterio-laterally before descending medially to enter the adductor compartment. It gives off the medial and lateral circumflex femoral branches then three perforators, before ending as the fourth perforator

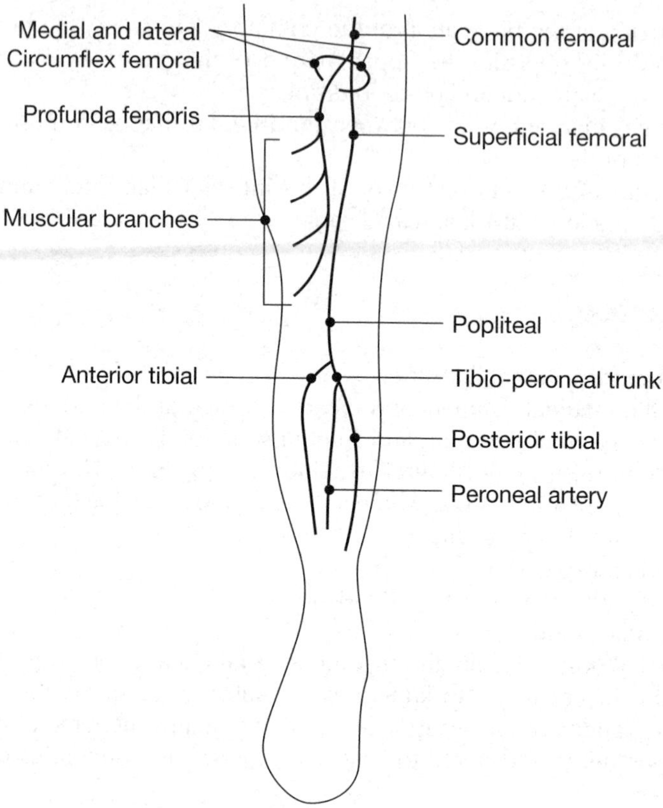

Figure 3.1a *Arterial supply of the lower limb*

Popliteal artery

- Arises from femoral artery as it enters the popliteal fossa (bounded by semimembranosis and semitendinosis above and medially, gastrocnemius below, popliteus in floor)
- It is the deepest structure in popliteal fossa (tibial nerve is the most superficial)
- Lies medial to popliteal vein
- Ends at the lower border of the popliteus muscle by dividing into anterior tibial and tibioperoneal trunk (gives rise to posterior tibial and peroneal arteries)

Anterior tibial artery

- Enters the anterior compartment of the leg via an opening in the interosseous membrane
- Descends with the deep peroneal nerve

- Enters the foot under the extensor retinaculum to become the dorsalis pedis artery
- Extensor hallucis longus (EHL) tendon lies medial, and the extensor digitorum longus (EDL) tendons lie laterally
- Surface markings: from mid-point between the tibial tuberosity and fibular head to mid-way between medial and lateral malleolus

Posterior tibial artery

- Passes deep to soleus and gastrocnemius
- Tibial nerve is initially medial but crosses posteriorly to lie on the lateral side
- Passes through tarsal tunnel (with tibialis posterior muscle, FDL, FHL and tibial nerve)
- Passes behind the medial malleolus and divides into the medial and lateral plantar arteries
- Supplies the posterior compartment structures of the lower leg

Peroneal artery

- Arises near the origin of the posterior tibial artery and descends behind the fibula
- Numerous perforating branches supply the lateral compartment of the leg before ending at the ankle

3.2 PATHOLOGY OF PERIPHERAL VASCULAR DISEASE (PVD)

In a nutshell ...

PVD describes occlusive vascular disease to the limbs. Lower limb PVD is much more common than upper limb

Atherosclerosis with thrombosis is the most common cause of PVD, with vasculitides, connective tissue diseases and thrombo-embolic disease occurring less frequently

Peripheral vascular disease is more extensive in diabetic patients

In people aged 50–75 years, 30% of the UK population has detectable occlusive disease, with about 15% of these being symptomatic

Atherosclerosis

In a nutshell ...

In the western world, complications of atherosclerosis cause more deaths per year than any other pathological process. Atherosclerosis is less common in the Far East and Africa where vasculitis is more common.

The most important risk factors are smoking, hypertension, diabetes and hyperlipidaemia.

A plaque initially develops as a fatty streak. There are two main hypotheses as to how it progresses: the injury hypothesis and the macrophage hypothesis.

A plaque comprises a fibrous cap, intra-intimal core, and basal region.

Complications include **thrombosis** and **embolism**.

Sequelae include vessel stenosis or occlusion.

Definition of atherosclerosis

- Focal intimal accumulation of lipids and fibrous tissue associated with smooth muscle proliferation
- Develops as a plaque beneath the endothelium
- In large and medium-sized arteries

Risk factors for atherosclerosis

- Smoking
- Hypertension
- Diabetes
- Male sex
- Hypercholesterolaemia
- Hypertriglyceridaemia
- High-fat diet
- Family history
- Obesity
- Old age
- Homocystinaemia

Development of atherosclerosis

The initial lesion is a fatty streak composed of a collection of lipids. Macroscopically these are seen as small raised dots on the endothelial surface of the blood vessel. These dots coalesce over time to form streaks. Such lesions have been recognised in children as young as 1 year. Two main theories concerning the development of atherosclerosis exist; the response to injury hypothesis, and the macrophage hypothesis.

- **Response to injury hypothesis:** intimal damage may lead to monocyte and platelet adherence to endothelium, and migration into the vessel intima. Hypertension, shear stress, turbulent flow and chemical damage (eg nicotine and hyperlipidaemia) have all been implicated in causing the intimal damage. Once inside the intima, localised inflammation and disruption of the endothelium encourages further platelet adhesion, leading to the release of thromboxane and platelet-derived growth factor (PDGF). This promotes smooth muscle migration into the developing plaque. Inside the intima, monocytes become macrophages, able to scavenge molecules such as lipid to become foam cells
- **Macrophage hypothesis:** lipids (especially modified lipids such as oxidised LDL, increased by smoking) collect within macrophages derived from blood monocytes beneath the overlying endothelium. They may break down at the plaque base leading to the formation of a lipid-rich pool, and secretion of cytokines and toxic metabolites propagate the disease process

Structure of atherosclerotic plaques

- Superficial fibrous cap
- Intra-intimal area with accumulations of lipids, smooth muscle cells and macrophages/foam cells
- Basal zone with lipid accumulations and tissue necrosis

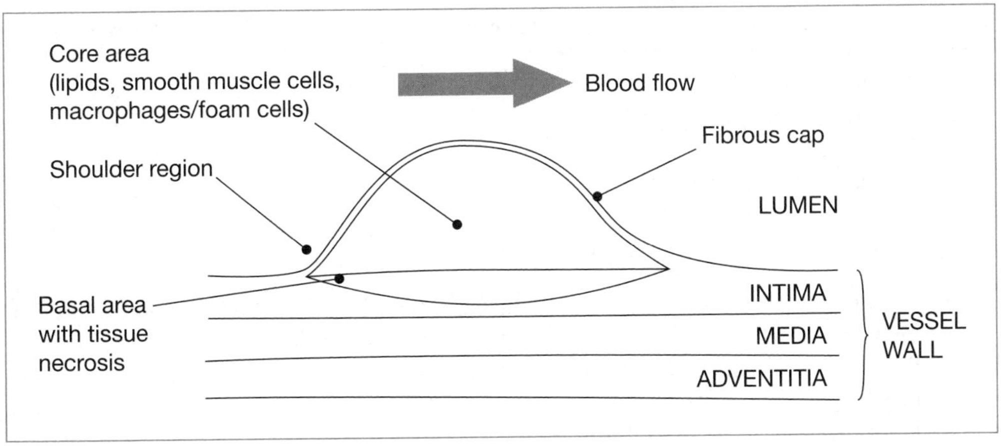

Figure 3.2a *The atherosclerotic plaque*

Complications of atherosclerotic plaques

Thrombosis

A thrombus is a solid mass of blood constituents formed within the vasculature (it is NOT a blood clot). Layers of platelets, fibrin and red blood cells will adhere in any area with pro-thrombotic properties. Predisposition to thrombus formation occurs when any of the changes described in Virchow's triad occur, namely:

- Alterations in intima of vessel (eg plaque thrombosis, endothelial damage)
- Altered blood flow (eg turbulence, stasis)
- Altered blood constituents (eg hypercholesterolaemia, smoking)

In arteries thrombosis is usually secondary to atheroma, whereas in veins is usually secondary to venous stasis. Plaque thrombosis occurs following injury to the cap. This is either a deep injury where the plaque fissures, or superficial erosion of the surface of the plaque. Either injury predisposes to thrombus formation, in addition to presence of risk factors and alterations in blood flow caused by the atheromatous plaque itself.

Embolism

An embolus is a mass of material within the vasculature that is able to become trapped within small calibre vessels and block the lumen. Most emboli are derived from thrombus, although can also be from tumour, amniotic fluid and fat embolus or gas. Clinical effects depend upon the region supplied by the blocked vessel, and whether it has a sufficient collateral vascular supply. The commonest venous embolic phenomena arise from the leg veins, causing pulmonary emboli. Systemic arterial emboli may cause stroke, ischaemic bowel, renal infarcts along with ischaemic limbs.

Sources of arterial embolism

- Left ventricle (intraventricular thrombus following AF, recent MI, cardiomyopathy)
- Heart valves (infective endocarditis)
- Aneurysm embolus
- Atherosclerotic plaque embolus
- Tumour embolus
- Paradoxical embolus

Pathological consequences of atherosclerosis

- Vessel occlusion (slow occlusion by disease vs rapid occlusion by thrombus, eg MI)
- Vessel stenosis causing ischaemia (eg angina, limb claudication)
- Plaque thrombosis or haemorrhage (increases size of plaque, therefore see acute-on-chronic changes: stable-to-unstable angina, acute-on-chronic limb ischaemia)
- Embolisation of plaque or thrombotic material

Vasculitides

The vasculitides include all inflammatory disorders of blood vessels. Often these are multi-system disorders with a predilection for highly vascular areas such as the skin, kidney, synovium or eye. They are probably due to a variety of pathological inflammatory processes (such as immune complex deposition or complement activation) that damage blood vessels, leading to thrombosis and resulting in ischaemia and infarction. Of the many disorders involving blood vessels, Buerger's disease, giant cell arteritis and Takayasu's arteritis are most likely to be seen in vascular surgical practice.

Buerger's disease (thrombo-angiitis obliterans)

- Progressive obliteration of distal arteries in young men who smoke heavily
- Commonest in Oriental people and Ashkenazi Jews (associated with HLA B5 and anticollagen antibodies in about 50%)
- Medium sized arteries show transmural inflammation, intimal proliferation and thrombosis with surrounding deposition of collagen
- Affects upper and lower limbs

Management includes smoking cessation, sympathectomy (relieves associated arterial spasm), antibiotics, foot care, and analgesia. Prostaglandin infusions have been used to overcome acute ischaemia and allow collateral channels to open. Serial amputations (including upper limbs) are often required.

Giant cell arteritis

- Granulomatous chronic inflammatory process affecting elastic or muscular arteries
- Classically seen in superficial temporal or cranial arteries
- May present with headache and temporal tenderness (artery and overlying skin thickened and tender with decreased pulsation), jaw claudication, blindness
- Biopsy may not confirm diagnosis in 40% (small sample area, steroid treatment commenced, early stage of disease)
- Management with steroid is usually effective

Takayasu's arteritis (pulseless disease)

- Inflammatory infiltrate affecting branches of the aortic arch
- Young or middle-aged females (commonly oriental or Middle-Eastern origin)
- Associated with pain, malaise and elevated ESR
- Present with hypertension or ischaemic symptoms of the upper limb

3.3 ACUTE LIMB ISCHAEMIA

In a nutshell ...

This is a surgical emergency.

Symptoms
Pain, pallor, paraesthesia, perishingly cold, paralysis pulseless.

Management
Includes symptom relief and restoration of arterial continuity:

- Thrombolysis
- Embolectomy
- Arterial bypass

Re-perfusion
It may be necessary to perform fasciotomies to prevent compartment syndrome.

Causes of acute limb ischaemia

- Arterial embolus
- Acute thrombosis (or acute-on-chronic)
- Trauma
- Aortic dissection
- Thrombosed popliteal aneurysm
- Intra-arterial injection (iatrogenic or drug abuse)

Symptoms of acute limb ischaemia

The mechanism of the pain is unknown but possibly related to anoxia, acidosis, metabolite accumulation and substance P accumulation. Acute limb ischaemia can occur in the upper or lower limb. Symptoms vary with speed of occlusion and extent of collateral circulation. Usual presentation is with loss of pulses (eg radial in upper limb or femoral/popliteal/foot pulses in lower limb. The loss of pulses can be confirmed with a hand-held Doppler if unsure, along with the clinical recognition of these six **P**s which are late signs:

Pain
Pallor
Paraesthesia
Perishing cold
Paralysis
Pulseless

Management of acute limb ischaemia

Acute limb ischaemia is a surgical emergency and must be resolved within 4–6 hours to prevent complications from tissue ischaemia. In acute on chronic ischaemia the limb may remain viable for up to 12 hours depending on collateral supply.

Note: Nerve conduction disappears after 15–30 minutes of acute ischaemia; permanent muscle damage occurs after few hours, with the extensor hallucis longus (EHL) being the last muscle to recover on revascularisation. Skin will tolerate ischaemia for up to 48 hours.

Principles of management of acute limb ischaemia

These are:

- Resuscitation (oxygen and IV fluids)
- Immediate anticoagulation (5000 units heparin IV)
- Analgesia
- Restore arterial continuity
- Identify and correct any underlying source of embolus

If the diagnosis is in doubt, or if arterial reconstruction may be needed, arteriography may be performed. Arterial embolism usually causes a sharp cut off at the upper end of the occlusion with poor collaterals.

Thrombolysis

Thrombolysis may be performed if the limb is not too acutely ischaemic, allowing sufficient time for clot dissolution. It is the preferred choice for acute on chronic ischaemia. tPA, urokinase or streptokinase are introduced through a catheter inserted under fluoroscopic control, directly into the clot. Clot dispersal can be monitored by serial arteriography.

Complications of thrombolysis

- Puncture site haemorrhage/false aneurysm
- Retroperitoneal haemorrhage
- Stroke
- GI bleeding
- Anaphylaxis

Contraindications of thrombolysis

- Extreme old age
- Recent surgery
- Peptic ulceration
- Recent stroke
- Bleeding tendencies

Embolectomy

Op box: Embolectomy (commonly femoral or brachial)

Indications
Identification of embolus as cause of limb ischaemia (usually after urgent angiography or duplex). For acutely ischaemic upper limbs surgical exploration may be undertaken diagnostically. Bear in mind that the embolus may impact at the site of pre-existing occlusive disease in the lower limb.

Pre-op
Analgesia and resuscitation. Anticoagulation (IV heparin). Consent with intra-op hazards and post-op complications in mind. GA or regional anaesthetic for femoral embolectomy. Brachial embolectomy may be performed under LA.

Patient positioning
Supine. Arm extended on arm board for brachial embolectomy.

Incision
Femoral: longitudinal incision in groin below inguinal ligament and over femoral artery
Brachial: transverse incision below the skin crease at the elbow

Procedure
- Femoral or brachial artery is identified and dissected free
- Vascular slings are placed proximally and distally to obtain control

- Patient is heparinised (eg 5000u IV bolus)
- Vascular clamp applied proximally and distally and a transverse arteriotomy is performed
- Fogarty embolectomy balloon catheter (of appropriate balloon size) is passed distally, the balloon inflated and the catheter withdrawn slowly (drawing embolus out of the artery) – this is repeated proximally and distally until flow is restored (bear in mind that, once clear of embolus, control of the artery is vital)
- Arteriotomy is closed with non-absorbable sutures (eg fine proline)

Intra-operative hazards

Over-inflation of the Fogharty catheter inside the artery can cause damage to sections of artery and intimal stripping – this causes a very pro-thrombotic state and the artery is likely to thrombose post-operatively.

Closure

Close the wound in layers with absorbable sutures.

Post-op

Continue formal anticoagulation; regular observations of limb perfusion must be performed (pulses, capillary refill, temperature, colour); re-exploration may be indicated if thrombosis occurs; always look for the source of the underlying embolus for definitive management.

Complications

Haemorrhage, post-op thrombosis, limb loss.

Complications of acute limb ischaemia

Reperfusion injury

Reperfusion injury describes the body's response following restoration of arterial continuity, due to release of high concentrations of products of metabolism (eg potassium, lactate, myoglobin) back into the general circulation. This can cause local and systemic effects.

Following reperfusion, local tissue swelling occurs. This is due to osmotically active fragments produced by tissue necrosis and an increase in membrane permeability brought about by hypoxia. If unrelieved this swelling can cause further ischaemia and ultimately contractures (eg Volkman's ischaemic contracture following upper limb ischaemia). This can be prevented by timely fasciotomy.

Systemically, reperfusion can cause rhabdomyolysis and renal failure. It may also cause pulmonary oedema/ARDS, myocardial dysfunction and clotting disorders.

Compartment syndrome

The anatomy of the muscle compartments in the limbs

The lower leg is divided into three compartments by the tibia and fibula, interosseous membrane and intermuscular septae; the posterior compartment has two components. These divisions become especially important following reperfusion of an ischaemic limb, and knowledge of the actions of the muscles and innervation of nerves within each compartment is essential in diagnosis of compartment syndrome.

Lateral (peroneal) compartment

- Bounded by anterior and posterior intermuscular septae and peroneal surface of fibula
- Contains peroneus longus and brevis and superior peroneal nerve

Extensor compartment

- Bounded by medial tibial surface, interosseous membrane and anterior intermuscular septum
- Contains EHL, EDL, tibialis anterior muscle, peroneus, anterior tibial vessels and deep peroneal nerve

Posterior compartment

- Bounded by posterior intermuscular septum and interosseous membrane
- In **deep compartment:** FHL, FDL, popliteus, tibialis posterior muscle, posterior tibial artery, tibial nerve
- In **superficial compartment:** gastrocnemius, soleus, plantaris, short saphenous vein and sural nerve

Injuries causing compartment syndrome

Fractures, crush injury, revascularisation, bleeding, burns or just severe shock. Prophylactic fasciotomies are indicated after some fracture fixations and revascularisation procedures, or in marked crush or vascular injuries.

Pathology of compartment syndrome

The limbs are encircled with layers of deep fascia which divides the muscle groups into compartments. Tissue swelling within the compartment causes an increase in the intra-compartmental pressure. When this pressure rises above the normal tissue perfusion pressure of the capillary bed (5–10 mmHg) the circulation to the tissues essentially ceases and they become ischaemic. Thus there may still be a palpable pulse on examination.

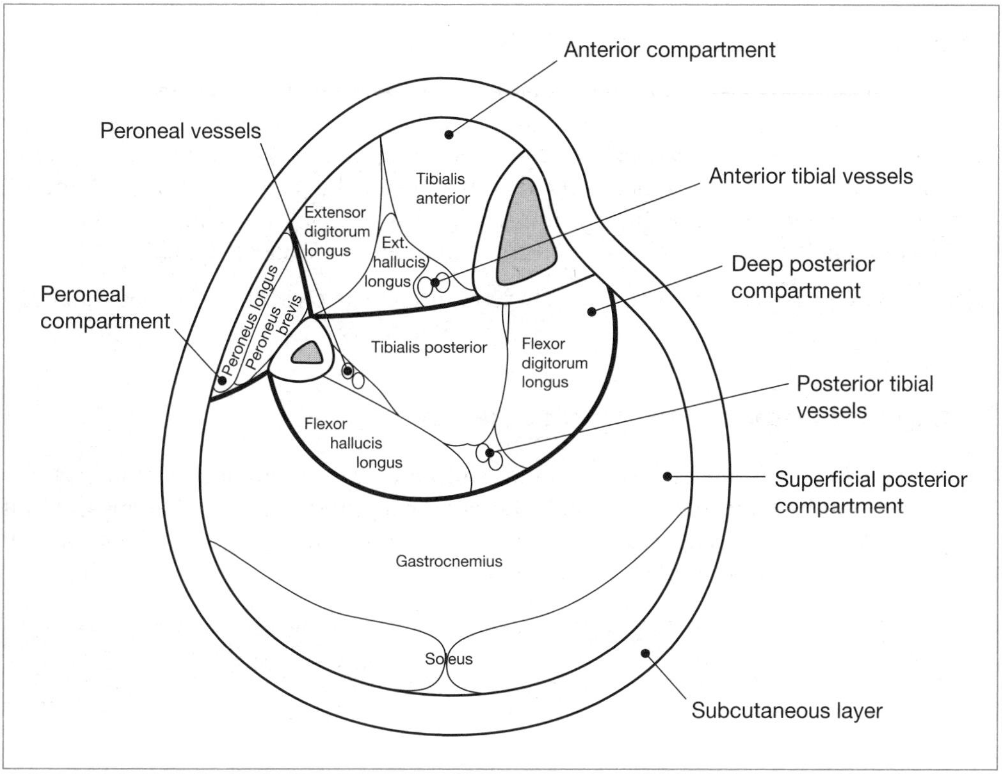

Figure 3.3a *The compartments of the lower limb*

Symptoms and signs of compartment syndrome

Early symptoms and signs

- Pain out of proportion to the condition or injury
- Pain on stretching of the muscle group in the affected compartment
- Weakness and muscle tenderness
- Sensory loss

Very late symptoms and signs

- Absent distal pulse
- Paralysis
- Pale, cold limb

Measurement of compartment pressures

Compartment pressures can be measured using a green needle connected to a pressure transducer. Prepare the skin with antiseptic solution (Betadine™/chlorhexidine). Flush the needle through to ensure a continuous column of fluid to the transducer. Zero the transducer with the needle held at the level of the patient's leg and advance the needle perpendicularly through the skin and superficial fascia into the muscle compartment. Repeat the process for all compartments of the affected limb.

Pressures exceeding 30 mmHg may require surgical intervention in the form of fasciotomy.

Managing compartment syndrome

If compartment syndrome is suspected clinically then plaster immobilisation and any bandaging must be removed immediately. Compartment pressures should be measured if there is doubt about the diagnosis, and, if elevated by > 30 mmHg (or lower if diastolic BP is low), urgent fasciotomy must be performed.

Procedure: Doing a fasciotomy

Once the diagnosis of compartment syndrome has been made there should be as little delay as possible in performing a fasciotomy. The trend is moving away from accident-room fasciotomies as the facilities are better in theatre, but every few minutes could cost the patient viable muscle.

- Confirm elevated compartment pressures if possible pre-operatively, but not if it creates delay
- The usual fasciotomy is a two-incision four-compartment fasciotomy
- The anterior and lateral compartments are decompressed through a lateral incision just anterior to the fibula and the skin is undermined anteriorly and posteriorly to expose these two compartments
- The incision on the medial side of the leg opens the superficial posterior compartment and through this the deeper compartment is released
- The fascia is divided usually via long, medial and lateral incisions, to allow tissue expansion and prevent ischaemia
- All compartments of an affected limb should be fully opened (eg four compartment fasciotomy in the lower limb)
- The visible muscles can be covered with sterile dressings and inspected regularly for perfusion
- Necrotic tissue should be debrided at a later date
- The fasciotomies can be closed later as an elective procedure and skin grafts can be used

The sequelae of compartment syndrome

- Muscle wasting and nerve injury in the affected compartment
- Foot drop if the lateral compartment is affected (superficial peroneal nerve). Compartment syndrome can also occur in the upper limb, especially the volar forearm, and the buttock
- Abdominal compartment syndrome is a different entity caused by swelling of abdominal contents post laparotomy

Long-term management of acute limb ischaemia

Following the restoration of arterial flow to the limb, investigations are performed to identify the underlying cause of embolism.

- Echocardiography to assess LV and heart valves
- US (especially abdominal aorta and popliteal arteries)
- Arteriography to look for other sources of emboli

Long-term anticoagulation is also required, initially with heparin and later with warfarin.

3.4 CHRONIC LOWER LIMB ISCHAEMIA

In a nutshell ...

Chronic lower limb ischaemia is usually caused by atherosclerosis, often secondary to smoking or diabetes. The commonest sites of arterial occlusive disease affecting the lower limb are:

- Aortic bifurcation
- Common iliac artery bifurcation
- Adductor hiatus (SFA)
- Trifurcation disease
- Small vessel disease

Patients present with pain ranging from intermittent claudication through to rest pain, and skin changes ranging from superficial ulceration to gangrene.

Non-limb or life-threatening peripheral arterial disease is best treated conservatively while radiological and surgical interventions are usually reserved for failed medical management.

Sites of arterial occlusive disease

Aorto-iliac occlusive disease

The abdominal aorta may become stenosed or even occluded due to atherosclerotic disease. Occlusion may occur gradually with development of collateral circulation to the lower limbs. Collateral circulation develops from the thoracic aorta via the internal mammary, intercostals, lumbar, SMA and gonadal arteries.

Acute abdominal aortic occlusion presents dramatically with sudden ischaemia of the lower limbs and GI tract. It may also involve the renal arteries if the level of disease is sufficiently high. It may be due to thrombosis during low-flow state in a stenotic aorta, saddle embolus from the heart or aortic dissection.

Infra-inguinal arterial occlusive disease

Infra-inguinal arterial occlusive disease also results from atherosclerosis. Common sites include the level of the adductor hiatus in the superficial femoral artery and at the trifurcation. Over time, collateral circulation may develop (aided by exercise) to supply the lower limb.

Acute-on-chronic ischaemia may occur due to thrombosis on a ruptured plaque or impaction of an embolus at a site of narrowing.

Symptoms of chronic lower limb ischaemia

- **Intermittent claudication (IC)** is the cramping pain experienced on exercise due to muscle ischaemia. It is due to occlusion or stenosis in the relevant proximal arteries. Calf claudication is the most common and usually starts after a consistent walking distance (called the claudication distance), and is relieved by rest. Note that the patient does not have to sit down to relieve the pain (a symptom of spinal stenosis) and once the pain has gone the patient can usually walk the same distance again before the pain recurs
- **Critical ischaemia** implies that without intervention limb loss may be imminent. ABPI is usually less than 0.4
- **Rest pain** is severe, intractable cramping pain, usually experienced at the extremities, due to critical ischaemia. Nocturnal rest pain is classically relieved by hanging the foot over the side of the bed (as dependency of the limb increases blood supply). For this reason these patients often sleep upright in a chair
- **Ulceration** is tissue loss due to critical ischaemia. It typically occurs at the extremities. Arterial ulcers are classically described as being punched out with sloughy, unhealthy bases
- **Gangrene** is tissue necrosis due to critical ischaemia. **Dry gangrene** is due to gradual interruption of the arterial supply to the tissues with black discolouration of the skin

due to staining by free haemoglobin from damaged capillaries. It is insensate, cold and hard, and does not smell. It occurs from distal to proximal. Untreated, gangrenous parts may demarcate (mummify) and auto-amputate. **Wet gangrene** describes ischaemic necrosis associated with infection by putrefactive organisms. It smells and you will see skin blebs. It requires emergency debridement and broad-spectrum antibiotics. **Gas gangrene** is usually due to clostridia infection. There will be crepitus and septicaemia from toxin release

- **Leriche's syndrome** describes buttock, thigh and calf claudication with erectile dysfunction, and proximal muscle wasting due to distal aortic or proximal iliac stenosis or occlusion

Differential diagnosis of chronic leg pain

Arterial
PVD (atherosclerosis)
Popliteal entrapment syndrome
Vasculitis

Venous
Venous claudication
Chronic venous insufficiency
Post phlebitic syndrome

Neurological
Spinal stenosis
Lumbar radiculopathy
Peripheral neuropathy
Reflex sympathetic dystrophy

Rheumatological
Arthritis (OA, RA)
Gout

Orthopaedic
Chronic compartment syndrome
Plantar fasciitis

Examination of the ischaemic leg

What to ask about

- Claudication and rest pain (onset and relieving factors)
- Painful or painless ulceration
- Risk factors for atherosclerotic disease (smoking, hypertension, diabetes, hyperlipidaemia, family history)

What to look for

- **Changes associated with ischaemia:** the ischaemic leg is typically pale but a severely ischaemic leg may be red ('sunset foot') due to acute inflammation and cellulitis secondary to tissue ischaemia, or bluish purple (cyanosis). The leg may be

hairless with shiny skin. Individual toes may show the purple-black hue of a gangrenous digit; this may be hard, well demarcated and painless ('dry gangrene') or infected, soft, and moist with surrounding painful cellulitic tissue ('wet gangrene'). Ulceration may be present (ischaemic/neuropathic)
- **Venous guttering:** in a severely ischaemic foot the veins are collapsed and look like pale blue gutters in the subcutaneous tissue. In a normal circulation the veins never have time to empty fully because the arteries keep refilling them, even if the leg is elevated. Venous guttering on raising the leg 10–15° above the horizontal is a sign of significant ischaemia

What to palpate
Palpate all peripheral pulses starting with the aorta and working downwards. Compare right with left but bear in mind that disease may be bilateral. Test for delayed capillary refill in the feet.

How to carry out Buerger's test
In this bedside test for ischaemia, raise the patient's leg slowly to 90° keeping the leg straight. The foot should remain pink until 90° if there is no vascular compromise. If the foot goes pale at 50° this indicates severe ischaemia, and at 25° it indicates critical ischaemia. This is Buerger's angle. In the second part of Buerger's test, sit the patient up and ask them to swing their legs over the edge of the bed. If the legs become engorged and purple, Buerger's test is positive. The purple colour occurs as sudden additional hypoxia causes a degree of vasodilation and blood flows back more quickly under the influence of gravity.

Conservative management of chronic lower limb ischaemia

Non-limb or life-threatening peripheral arterial disease is best treated 'conservatively' while radiological and surgical interventions are usually reserved for failed medical management.

Conservative management of intermittent claudication

Intermittent claudication is usually managed by correction of risk factors. Walking to the limit of claudication often improves symptoms by improving cardiac performance, and encouraging the development of collateral circulation. Patients with claudication have a high incidence of concurrent cardiovascular and neurovascular disease and a high mortality rate due to MI and CVA.

Patients should:

- Stop smoking
- Exercise
- Improve diet (low fat)
- Lose weight

Management includes:

- Antiplatelet agents (aspirin, clopidogrel, dipyridamole)
- Aggressive BP management in hypertensives
- Aggressive blood sugar control in diabetics
- Management of hypercholesterolaemia/hyperlipidaemia with lipid lowering drugs (statins)

Interventional radiological procedures (eg angioplasty, stenting) or surgery are not usually indicated for intermittent claudication and are reserved for critical ischaemia. However, they are occasionally offered for severe lifestyle-limiting symptoms despite adequate medical management.

Conservative management of chronic critical ischaemia

Chronic critical ischaemia requires active limb re-vascularisation to prevent limb loss. However, concurrent conservative strategies for improving blood flow are also required.

- Stop smoking
- Optimise cardiac output
- Treat infections
- Anticoagulation (heparin)

Investigation is then performed to identify the site/level of the arterial stenosis or occlusion.

Non-surgical interventions for PVD

- **Angioplasty:** a balloon catheter is introduced over a guide wire passed through the stenosis or occlusion under fluoroscopic control. The balloon is then inflated across the stenosis or occlusion to dilate this section of the artery. This technique is good for short occlusions and works better for proximal disease rather than for distal
- **Stenting:** arterial stents are expandable metal prostheses which are placed across stenoses or occlusions to maintain arterial patency. They are usually balloon expandable and introduced under fluoroscopic control, combined with angioplasty. Stenting is indicated for failed angioplasty, and for correction of intimal arterial defects
- **Lumbar sympathectomy:** used if arterial reconstruction is unfeasible. This is usually chemical (phenol, translumbar injection with radiographic control), but it can be surgical. Blockade of the lumbar sympathetic chain improves blood supply to skin, with some relief of rest pain and numbness/tingling associated with chronic ischaemia
- **Drug therapy:** vasodilators can provide some increase in blood supply to the limb, especially in combination with antiplatelet therapy (aspirin). These include (with varying success) nifedipine, Iloprost™ and oxpentifylline among others

Surgery for PVD

These procedures can be divided into two groups.

- **Anatomical procedures** restore vascular continuity through the replacement of the diseased region (eg femoral-popliteal bypass, femoral-distal bypass)
- **Extra-anatomical procedures** restore vascular continuity by diverting blood from other unrelated areas to the diseased region (and are also therefore useful as a salvage procedure if there is infection present) eg axillo-bifemoral and femoro-femoral crossover grafts

Vascular grafts can be fashioned from autologous or artificial materials:

- **Autologous:** the long saphenous vein can be harvested and used in the reverse direction (flow not impeded by vein cusps) or used in situ after destruction of the vein cusps. Composite vein grafts are fashioned by end-to-end anastomosis of sections of arm vein to achieve desired length
- **Prosthetic:** Dacron™ or PTFE grafts are tubes of prosthetic material. They may be woven or plasticised and may be supported by an external wire scaffolding to prevent compression (eg during movement of limbs). They have a much lower patency rate than autologous grafts

ADVANTAGES AND DISADVANTAGES OF VEIN GRAFTS VS PROSTHETIC GRAFTS

	Advantages	Disadvantages
Vein grafts	Better patency rates (75–90% at 5 years)	May not be there (previous surgery including CABG, VV stripping, etc)
	Respond better to angioplasty if required	Insufficient width or length
	More resistant to infection	Points of compression (eg knee joint) may compromise flow in certain positions
	Less neointimal hyperplasia at the anastomosis	
	Easier to suture	
Prosthetic grafts	Limitless supply	Lower patency rates (60% at 5 years)
	External wire scaffolding prevents compression and compromised flow	Higher rates of neointimal neoplasia More expensive

Femoro-popliteal and femoro-distal bypass grafting

Principles of femoro-popliteal and femoro-distal bypass grafting

Indications

Chronic lower limb ischaemia with incapacitating claudication or critical ischaemia; may also be performed for acutely ischaemic limb (acute on chronic thrombosis, occluded popliteal aneurysm, etc).

Pre-op

Elective: angiogram to assess inflow and run off and plan sites for anastomosis; any lesions compromising inflow may be corrected with angioplasty prior to the procedure

Emergency: analgesia and resuscitation; anticoagulation (IV heparin); urgent angiogram to assess cause, underlying disease and plan surgery

GA or regional anaesthetic. Consent with intra-operative hazards and post-op complications in mind

Patient positioning

Supine. Prep and drape with groin and both legs exposed (contralateral long saphenous vein (LSV) harvest or exposure of the arm for arm vein harvest).

Incision

Longitudinal incision in groin below inguinal ligament and over common femoral artery (or alternative site of inflow) for proximal anastomosis

Longitudinal incision at level of above or below knee popliteal artery (or alternative site of outflow such as crural vessels for fem-distal) for distal anastomosis

Short longitudinal incisions over course of LSV for harvesting

Procedure

Femoral and popliteal or crural arteries are identified and dissected free

Vascular slings are placed proximally and distally to obtain control

Vein graft (LSV or segments of arm vein) is harvested and all tributaries ligated

Patient is systemically heparinised and the vessels clamped proximally and distally

A longitudinal arteriotomy is performed and the proximal anastomosis is sutured using non-absorbable suture (fine proline) and then tested for leaks

The graft is tunnelled under the skin and muscle and the distal anastomosis is sutured and tested for leaks

Intra-operative angiography or operative Doppler (op-Dop) testing confirms adequate resting flow rates through the graft

Intra-operative hazards
Excessive undermining of skin flaps during vein harvesting predisposes the patient to flap breakdown and necrosis.

Closure
Close the wound in layers with absorbable sutures.

Post-op
Continue formal anticoagulation; regular observations of limb perfusion must be performed (pulses, capillary refill, temperature, colour) post-operatively; re-exploration may be indicated if thrombosis of the graft occurs; entry into a graft surveillance program for regular duplex is optimal.

Complications
General to all arteriopaths (risk of MI, CVA, renal failure)
Risk of haemorrhage and infection
Risk of graft failure (early; late) and worsening of symptoms
Risk of limb loss

Principles of aorto-bifemoral, axillo-bifemoral and femoro-femoral crossover grafts

Aorto-bifemoral bypass graft
Indication: occlusive or stenotic aorto-iliac disease not amenable to angioplasty or stenting
Procedure: a bifurcated, prosthetic graft is anastomosed proximally to the aorta, and distally to the iliac or femoral vessels. Graft patency rates are excellent. Operative mortality is ~ 5%

Axillo-bifemoral grafting
Indication: aortic or bilateral iliac occlusion or stenoses not amenable to angioplasty or stenting, in the presence of a hostile abdomen, or in a patient not fit for GA
Procedure: a long graft is anastomosed proximally to the axillary artery as it passes under pectoralis major, and distally to the femoral arteries. Patency rates are less good than aorto-bifemoral grafting for this procedure but it is useful in high-risk cases with otherwise untreatable critical ischaemia

Femoro-femoral crossover graft

Indication: unilateral iliac occlusive disease not amenable to angioplasty or stenting

Procedure: a prosthetic vascular graft is anastomosed from one femoral artery, tunnelled subcutaneously and anastomosed to the other to restore flow. Mortality and patency rates are excellent. The procedure does not require GA

Causes of graft failure

- **Early causes** (eg after 1 month) commonly technical failure (low flow state due to poor inflow or insufficient run-off)
- **Mid-term causes** (eg after 1 year) commonly neointimal hyperplasia causing stenosis in the graft
- **Late causes** (eg after 2–5 years) commonly atheromatous disease progression (in inflow or run-off)

Early complications

- Haemorrhage
- Graft thrombosis
- Wound infection
- Swollen leg (reperfusion or DVT)
- Lymphatic fistula

Late complications

- Graft thrombosis
- False aneurysm
- Graft infection

Graft surveillance

- 20–35% of grafts develop haemodynamically significant graft stenosis (which can remain asymptomatic) after 12 months
- Higher risk with longer, artificial grafts with poor distal run off (small or diseased vessels)
- Will progress quickly to critical stenosis and occlude if left untreated
- Most institutions offer graft surveillance for infra-inguinal grafts in form of US scanning at regular intervals, depending on risk to graft
- Management options include angioplasty, atherectomy, vein patching, jump grafting or re-do surgery

3.5 AMPUTATIONS OF ISCHAEMIC LOWER LIMBS

Indications for amputation

The main indications for amputation are indicated by these 3 **D**s:

D ying (eg vascular disease, gangrene)
D angerous (eg tumour, severe infection)
D amned nuisance (eg useless painful limb following trauma, neurological damage)

In the UK the most common reason for amputation is PVD, but worldwide the main indication is trauma.

Indications for amputation in the UK

- Vascular disease and diabetes (80%)
- Trauma (10%)
- Tumour and other reasons (10%)

Levels of amputation

The level for amputation needs to be selected carefully. It needs to be proximal enough for good healing, but more distal amputations have better long-term outcome and rehabilitation. A correctly functioning knee joint should be preserved whenever possible. In below-knee amputations ideally 15 cm of bone below the knee should be conserved. However, a shorter stump is preferable to an above-knee amputation.

Upper limb amputations are much rarer than lower limb amputations and the principles are slightly different. The aims of maintaining length and function by carrying out minimal debridement are paramount. Loss of function is more disabling and less amenable to prosthetics than lower limb loss.

The ideal stump

Heals by primary intention
Is freely mobile
Has good soft tissue cover over bone ends
Has a conical shape
Has a mobile joint above amputation level
Does not transmit pressure through the scar

Levels of lower limb amputation (proximal to distal)

- **Hip disarticulation:** used mainly for soft tissue/bony malignancy in the upper thigh. Very rarely used for vascular disease
- **Above knee:** involves taking a bone section 25–30 cm below the greater trochanter, leaving 12 cm above the knee joint for the knee mechanism. This creates equal anterior and posterior semicircular skin flaps
- **Supracondylar (Gritti Stokes):** involves supracondylar femoral division. The patella is fixed to the end of the femur with wire sutures. It is useful if more length is required than can be obtained from above-knee amputation, such as in bilateral amputees, to aid changing position in bed, etc. It is unpopular because there is a tendency for non-union of the patella to the femur, and it is difficult to fit a prosthesis
- **Through-knee:** quick to perform and is relatively atraumatic. However there is poor healing in ischaemic disease. It is difficult to fit a prosthesis due to the bulbous stump
- **Below-knee:** the most popular level in severe ischaemia (can be done in 80%). Oximetry, thermography and arteriography can be used to help gauge the likelihood of success, but are not standard practice. The best guide to success is clinical judgement and flap bleeding at the time of surgery. The two most widely used methods are the long posterior flap (Burgess), using the posterior calf muscles to cover the bone ends 15 cm below the tibial tuberosity, and the skew flap (Kingsley Robinson). There is little difference in healing rates
- **Syme's:** rarely used in vascular disease. The heel is disarticulated, the malleoli excised and covered with a long posterior skin flap. 30% require revision at a higher level
- **Trans-metatarsal:** useful in diabetic gangrene of the fore-foot. It requires no prosthesis. Individual rays can be amputated, and left to heal by secondary intention
- **Toes:** used in cases of trauma or diabetic infective gangrene in the presence of a good blood supply only

Principles of surgery for amputation

Amputations for PVD and neoplasia tend to be more radical than those for trauma or diabetes in the absence of PVD. In PVD the healing of the distal stumps tends to be compromised by poor blood supply. In neoplastic disease good clearance is a priority.

As a general rule, the total length of flaps will need to be at least 1.5 times the diameter of the leg at the level of the bone section.

During surgery a tourniquet may be applied to provide a bloodless field in trauma or neoplasia, but not in cases where there is PVD.

Post-operative management of amputation

- Analgesia
- Care of the unaffected limb
- Physiotherapy: to prevent flexion contractures and to build up muscle power and co-ordination
- Mobilisation

Patient should be rehabilitated as soon as possible, ideally after 5–7 days.

Complications of amputations

Early complications

Haemorrhage and haematoma formation
Infection (high stumps may have faecal contamination and develop gas gangrene)
Wound dehiscence
Ischaemia and gangrene of flaps
DVT and PE

Late complications

Pain: phantom limb, amputation neuroma, causalgia (intractable burning pain due to sympathetic nerve growth down somatic nerves), scar pain due to adherence to bone, jacitation (sudden jumping of limb)
Chronic infection: osteitis, sinus formation
Ulceration of stump

Prostheses for lower limbs

- Sleeves
- Straps
- Suction devices
- Silicone (suspension) devices
- Foot and ankle devices: depending on the level of activity these can be:
  - Solid-ankle cushioned-heel foot (minimal maintenance)
  - Multi-axial ankle (optimises gait)
  - Energy-storing foot (more active users may benefit)
- Knee mechanisms: free, locking, controlled, intelligent

3.6 THE DIABETIC FOOT

In a nutshell ...

The diabetic foot presents particular surgical problems due to a combination of:
- Atherosclerosis
- Peripheral neuropathy
- Impaired tissue metabolism
- Infection
- AV fistulation

Atherosclerosis

- Accelerated in diabetics (thought to be due to intimal damage by hyperglycaemia)
- Typically trifurcation and distal small vessel disease
- Large vessel disease also occurs earlier and is more severe in diabetics
- May calcify and lead to incompressible vessels (palpable pulses and falsely high ABPI > 1.0)
- Associated with arteriolar constriction and increased ischaemia

Peripheral neuropathy

- Motor nerves: distortion of small muscles (clawing of toes and subluxation of joints) causes abnormal weight bearing and trauma
- Sensory nerves: glove-and-stocking paraesthesiae; unawareness of injury
- Autonomic nerves: disruption of vascular control and sweating (causing dryness of the skin and fissuring)

Impaired tissue metabolism

- Due to hyperglycaemia
- Glycosylation of tissues renders them stiff and less pliable

Infection

- Glucose-rich environment favours infection
- Generalised immunocompromise

AV fistulation

- AV fistulae open shunting blood containing nutrients and oxygen away from the skin and contributing to poor wound healing

Examination of the diabetic foot

Features of diabetes in the leg and foot

- **Ischaemic ulcers:** the heel, malleoli, head of 5th metatarsal, tips of toes, between the toes and the ball of the foot are typical sites for ischaemic ulceration. An ischaemic ulcer typically looks like a poorly healed wound or a punched-out lesion and has no surrounding callus. It may have associated wet or dry gangrene
- **Neuropathic ulcers:** these are commonly seen on the soles of the feet. A neuropathic ulcer typically looks like a punched-out lesion surrounded by a ridge of hard calloused skin. A punched-out or vertical edge to an ulcer follows rapid death and sloughing of a full thickness of skin without successful attempts at self-repair and is therefore seen in both neuropathic and ischaemic ulcers
- **Charcot's joint:** painless disorganised joint due to decreased sensation
- **Loss of foot arches:** due to peripheral neuropathy
- **Shiny hairless leg:** said to be typical but is non-specific
- **Amputated toes:** small vessel disease often leads to loss of digits either by surgery or auto-amputation of a gangrenous digit
- **Necrobiosis lipodica diabeticorum:** erythematous plaques over shins with a waxy appearance and brown pigmentation – can scar, become scaly, or ulcerate
- **Infections:** such as paronychia due to poor circulation

Management of the diabetic foot

All patients require education and good blood glucose control. They should wear accommodative footwear (soft leather or trainers) and skin and nail care should be performed by professionals. They require regular clinical examination and should seek early medical attention for trauma or ulceration.

Superficial ulceration requires good wound care and determination of underlying pathology. Neuropathic ulcers may require debridement and off-loading of pressure. Ischaemic ulcers require revascularisation.

Deep ulceration is often associated with deep tissue infection (and may include osteomyelitis). These ulcers require debridement to a base of healthy tissue, culture-specific antibiotics, and may require partial amputation. Ischaemic limbs will require revascularisation to enable healing.

Section 4
Carotid artery disease

4.1 CAROTID ANATOMY

In a nutshell ...

Common carotid artery
External carotid artery
Internal carotid artery
The circle of Willis (see *Elective Neurosurgery and Spinal Surgery* in Book 2)

Common carotid artery

- Arises from brachiocephalic trunk on right; arch of the aorta on left
- Ascends within the carotid sheath along with the internal jugular veins (laterally), vagus nerves (between and posterior to artery and vein) and ansa cervicalis, from a point postero-lateral to the sternoclavicular joint
- Ends at the upper border of thyroid cartilage (C4)
- Divides (under cover of sternocleidomastoid) into internal and external carotid arteries

External carotid artery (ECA)

- Arises from common carotid artery
- Supplies face, oral and nasal cavities, exterior of head and neck, inner surface of cranial cavity
- Spirals over internal carotid to lie laterally at level of C2
- Crossed by facial vein and hypoglossal nerve
- Gives off superior thyroid and posterior auricular branches before entering parotid gland between superficial and deep lobes (where divides into terminal branches)

Branches of the external carotid artery

3 branches from the front
Superior thyroid
Lingual
Facial

1 deep medial branch
Ascending pharyngeal

2 branches from behind
Occipital
Posterior auricular

2 terminal branches
Superficial temporal
Maxillary

Internal carotid artery (ICA)

- Arises from common carotid artery and continues within the carotid sheath to enter the skull via the carotid canal
- Usually no branches in the neck
- Supplies contents of cranial and orbital cavity (supplemented by vertebrobasilar system)
- Just above the carotid bifurcation there is a slight bulge in the ICA – this is the **carotid sinus**; it contains baroreceptors and is supplied by the glossopharyngeal nerve (stimulation causes bradycardia and hypotension)
- Behind the carotid bifurcation lies the **carotid body**, which contains chemoreceptors for oxygen, CO_2 and pH regulation

Circle of Willis

This is the anatomic arrangement of the intracranial arteries (see *Neurosurgery and Spinal Surgery* in Book 2). It is supplied by both internal carotid arteries and the basilar artery, which forms from the vertebral arteries. It is important because complete occlusion of one ICA in the circle of Willis does not normally cause symptoms due to adequate collateral flow. However the circle of Willis is only complete in about 50% of individuals.

4.2 PHYSIOLOGY OF CEREBRAL CIRCULATION

In a nutshell ...

The brain:

- Has a very high O_2 requirement
- Receives a very high proportion of the cardiac output (13%)
- Has a high blood supply volume per unit weight of tissue (55 mL/min/100 g)
- Is intolerant of ischaemia and protects itself by a phenomenon called autoregulation (preferentially preserving its blood supply at BP of 60–160 mmHg)

Autoregulation occurs via **myogenic** or **metabolic** mechanisms.

Measurement of cerebral blood flow is important during surgery on the carotid artery and can be done using the Fick Principle.

Regulation of cerebral circulation

The brain receives 13% of the cardiac output, that is 750 mL/min of blood. In addition, the brain has a large blood supply per unit weight of tissue, ie 55 mL/min/100 g (100 mL/min/100 g for grey matter) and it is very intolerant of ischaemia.

It has a number of methods by which it regulates constant blood supply despite inconsistent supply to other body parts (autoregulation). This autoregulation is extremely effective for mean BPs of 60–160 mmHg. BP of < 60 mmHg causes syncope, and BP of > 160 mmHg causes brain oedema (as blood–brain barrier permeability increases). The sympathetic nerve supply to cerebral vessels has little effect, allowing local factors to predominate.

Autoregulation is achieved by two mechanisms:

- **Myogenic mechanisms:** these maintain perfusion over wide pressure range; increased pressure causes increased wall tension (Laplace) leading to smooth muscle contraction in vessel walls (constriction)
- **Metabolic mechanisms:** cerebral vessels are very sensitive to changes in $PaCO_2$; increases cause marked vasodilatation locally, and decreases cause vasoconstriction (dizzy sensation when hyperventilating). Changes of as little as 1 mmHg CO_2 can cause a change in cerebral blood flow of up to 5%

Any ischaemia affecting the medulla leads to an increase in systemic BP to improve supply, by alteration in outflow from the medullary centres. The carotid baroreceptors and chemoreceptors ensure that blood supply to the brain is one of the main determinants of systemic BP.

Measurement of cerebral blood flow

The Fick principle

This is used to calculate the blood flow to an organ by applying the law of conservation of mass. If the blood flowing into an organ contains a marker of known concentration and some of this marker diffuses into the organ, then its concentration in the blood leaving the organ will be lower. Remember:

$$\text{Quantity} = \text{concentration} \times \text{volume}$$

Therefore the quantity of marker entering the organ per unit time depends on the concentration of marker and volume per unit time (ie flow). The quantity of marker leaving the organ per unit time depends on the blood concentration and the same blood flow.

Because:

$$\text{Flow in} = \frac{\text{quantity}_{in}}{\text{concentration}_{in}}$$

And:

$$\text{Flow out} = \frac{\text{quantity}_{out}}{\text{concentration}_{out}}$$

Then:

$$\text{Flow to organ} = \frac{(\text{quantity}_{in} - \text{quantity}_{out})}{(\text{concentration}_{in} - \text{concentration}_{out})}$$

NB: $\text{Concentration}_{in}$ – $\text{concentration}_{out}$ is the quantity of marker taken up by the brain per unit time. Nitrous oxide can be used as a marker to calculate cerebral blood flow.

Positron emission tomography (PET)

PET is a nuclear medicine technique whereby radiochemicals (produced in a cyclotron) are injected IV. These substances emit positrons that interact with the body to produce photons. The patient passes through a ring of detectors that receive the photons and create an image. The images reflect physiology rather than anatomic detail and can be used to assess metabolism, for example in tumours.

4.3 CAROTID ARTERY STENOSIS

In a nutshell ...

CVA accounts for 10% of deaths in the UK, often due to thrombosis or emboli
15% of CVAs are caused by carotid artery disease
Current guidelines indicate that patients with symptomatic non-occluded carotid stenosis of 70% or more should be considered for endarterectomy as they have a 20–30% risk of CVA if left untreated
Carotid angioplasty and endovascular stenting is emerging as an alternative

Pathology of carotid artery stenosis

CVA accounts for 10% of deaths in the UK.

Causes of CVA include:

- Thrombosis (53%)
- Emboli (31%)
- Intracerebral haemorrhage (10%)
- Subarachnoid haemorrhage (6%)

Atherosclerosis at the carotid bifurcation is a common and potentially treatable cause of CVA. Carotid atheroma may cause symptoms by causing stenosis, by limiting flow, or by embolisation. The effect of carotid atheroma depends on the degree of stenosis, the presence of collaterals (contralateral carotid and vertebrobasilar via the circle of Willis), and the nature of the plaque. The carotid bifurcation is commonly involved and shearing forces in the blood flow of this region cause the plaque to fracture and expose its thrombogenic core, promoting platelet aggregation.

Presentation of carotid disease

Symptoms of carotid disease

Asymptomatic carotid stenosis (a bruit may be audible on auscultation)
Amaurosis fugax: transient blindness due to temporary retinal artery occlusion
Reversible ischaemic neurological deficit (RIND): reversible defect > 24 hours but < 30 days
Transient ischaemic attack (TIA): focal neurological deficit resolving within 24 hours (may or may not have CT-detectable brain changes)
CVA: focal neurological deficit secondary to a vascular event not resolving within 24 hours

Clinical presentation depends on arterial territory involved:

- Carotid territory: contralateral hemiparesis, dysphasia if dominant hemisphere
- Vertebrobasilar territory: vertigo, diplopia, blurred vision (occipital cortex), loss of consciousness, facial involvement, cerebellar signs

Indications for treatment of carotid stenosis

Approximately 15% of CVAs are caused by carotid disease. In patients with carotid stenosis, the two trials listed below assessed the benefit from surgical intervention compared to best medical management in carotid stenosis.

Rationale for carotid intervention

European Carotid Surgery Trial (ECST)
North American Symptomatic Carotid Endarterectomy Trial (NASCET)

These two large trials randomised patients with ipsilateral symptomatic stenoses (amaurosis fugax, TIA, CVA) within the previous 6 months to surgery or best medical management (control hypertension, antiplatelet therapy, modify risks). Carotid stenosis was assessed by angiography. This suggested that:

- Carotid endarterectomy should be offered to patients with ipsilateral stenoses greater than 70% which have caused symptoms in the previous 6 months; the risk of having a subsequent CVA if there is a > 70% stenosis in the carotid artery is 20–30%
- Urgent surgery can be performed for crescendo TIAs and it may also be performed for stroke-in-evolution to aid reperfusion of the watershed area around the damage

- Intervention for asymptomatic carotid stenosis is controversial; it is suggested that 20 carotid interventions may be needed to prevent a single CVA in these patients (number needed to treat, NNT)
- There is no indication for carotid intervention in patients with occluded carotid arteries at present

Investigating carotid disease

In a nutshell ...

Consider and exclude alternative causes for symptoms of focal cerebral ischaemia:

Embolism: carotid stenosis, atrial fibrillation, endocarditis
Hypercoagulation states: antithrombin III, protein C, protein S, factor V Leiden
Vasculitis: autoantibodies (SLE, antiphospholipid syndrome)
Space-occupying lesion: metastasis from tumours (common in smokers eg lung)

Imaging investigations include:

Doppler US: Duplex of carotid artery, temporal transcranial US
CT scan of brain (areas of infarct) and carotid vessels
Arteriography: IV contrast enhanced, magnetic resonance arteriography

Duplex Doppler ultrasound (US)

This is the gold standard screening test for assessing degree of carotid stenosis. It combines grey-scale US to visualise stenosis with Doppler US which, by measuring velocity in the artery, allows direct measurement of degree of stenosis.

Advantages and disadvantages of Duplex Doppler US

Advantages of Duplex Doppler US	**Disadvantages of Duplex Doppler US**
Non-invasive	Operator dependent
Quick and easy	Poor views in calcified vessels
Gives information on nature of stenosis and plaque morphology	May confuse velocities in ECA and ICA
	Not good for very tight stenoses
	May miss proximal or high lesions

CT scans

Enhanced CT head scanning may be used to exclude other intracranial pathology and may show cerebral infarcts (but it is better at showing haemorrhage).

Reconstructed 3-D CT angiogram images can be used to visualise intracranial and extracranial arteries.

Arteriography

IVDSA

- Less risky but has poor resolution (see section 1)

IADSA

- May use arch flush or selective carotid catheterisation
- Gives accurate anatomic visualisation of arterial lumen
- Good for confirming Duplex findings (especially with tight stenoses and intracranial disease)
- Invasive (may precipitate cerebral infarction by causing embolisation or arterial spasm)
- Needs to be done in two planes
- Risk of TIA (2–3%) and CVA (about 0.1%) during procedure

Transcranial Doppler

This is Doppler US performed through a 'window' of thin temporal bone to visualise middle cerebral artery blood flow. It is good for intra-operative monitoring of cerebral blood flow.

MR angiography (MRA)

This is a non-invasive technique that allows 3-D visualisation of intracranial and extracranial carotid arteries. It is sometimes used as an alternative to IADSA.

Other investigations of carotid disease

These give further information on cerebral blood flow but are not generally used as primary diagnostic tests.

- Near infrared spectroscopy
- Carbon dioxide reactivity studies

Carotid endarterectomy

Op box: Carotid endarterectomy

Indications
Symptomatic ipsilateral carotid stenosis of > 70%.

Pre-op
Carefully document any existing neurological deficits whilst the patient is awake (especially cranial nerves and any deficits due to previous CVA). The procedure may be undertaken under GA or LA.

Positioning
The patient is placed supine on the operating table with 30° head up, and the head tilted to the opposite side.

Incision
A longitudinal incision at the anterior border of the sternomastoid.

Procedure

- Deepen the incision through the platysma
- Identify the internal jugular vein at the anterior border of the sternomastoid; dissect the internal jugular vein free and retract it to expose the common carotid artery
- Continue the dissection proximally and distally to dissect out the common, internal and external carotid arteries
- Once the artery is dissected out, administer 5000 units of heparin IV and allow sufficient circulation time
- Clamp arteries and perform longitudinal arteriotomy; at this stage it may be necessary to place a shunt to maintain cerebral perfusion
- Carefully remove the plaque, ensuring a good end-point is achieved distally
- Close the arteriotomy either directly or with a patch (Dacron or vein)

Intra-operative hazards
Damage to cranial nerves: cutaneous branch of V (upper end of incision, below jaw), and mandibular branch of VII, IX, X, XII (especially due to retractors at the upper end of the wound).

Closure
Place a small drain. Re-oppose other overlying tissues including platysma and skin, usually with a continuous suture.

Post-op

Post-op evaluation of neurological function is performed regularly post-operatively and compared to pre-operative functions.

Complications

Complication and death rates are related to the presenting symptom (CVA > TIA > amaurosis fugax > asymptomatic) and to presence of contralateral carotid disease.

Bleeding: Primary, reactionary or secondary

Haematoma: (may cause respiratory embarrassment)

Cranial nerve injuries: Seen in 15% patients: cranial nerves V (cutaneous branches), VII (mandibular branch), IX, X, XII

TIA: Risk is 3–5% for symptomatic stenoses

CVA: risk 1–2% and may be due to embolisation of debris at surgery or thrombosis of the surgical site (endarterectomy can cause the endothelium to be prothrombotic). Greatest risk is under anaesthetic and within the first 24 hours

Reperfusion syndrome (rare): occurs > 24 hours later and is due to loss of cerebral autoregulation and dramatic increases in cerebral blood flow causing oedema and raised ICP

Death: 1–2% risk (MI is commonest cause of death after carotid endarterectomy)

Options for intra-operative patient monitoring

- Transcranial Doppler
- Near infrared spectroscopy (transcranial pCO_2 monitoring)
- LA carotid endarterectomy with awake monitoring – the patient's neurological function can be continuously monitored during the procedure (conscious level, appropriate responses, speech, contralateral motor function eg by squeezing a squeaky toy on command) and may eliminate the requirement for placement of a shunt (risks of dislodging embolus during placement)
- EEG
- Stump pressure measurements

Carotid angioplasty and stenting

Early results with carotid angioplasty have been satisfactory. This is a less invasive procedure that avoids complications of open surgery, but it is not yet fully evaluated in clinical trials. One potential hazard is dislodging of soft thrombus, causing microemboli. To prevent this, angioplasty catheters with cerebral protection devices have been designed so that any dislodged thrombus can be caught and prevented going downstream to the brain.

Early trials of carotid angioplasty have shown a high re-stenosis rate and in some centres routine stenting is being performed.

4.4 OTHER CAROTID PATHOLOGY

In a nutshell ...

Carotid body tumours
Carotid artery dissection
Carotid artery aneurysms
Fibromuscular dysplasia (FMD)
Vertebrobasilar insufficiency

Carotid body tumours (chemodectoma)

These are composed of paraganglionic cells of neural crest origin. They present equally in males and females, usually affecting people in their 50s.

They present as masses in the neck adjacent to the hyoid bone anterior to sternocleidomastoid. They are relatively smooth, compressible and pulsatile (but not classically expansile) due to their vascular component. Their high vascularity gives them a red-brown appearance, hence the description of 'potato tumours'. They may be mobile horizontally, but not vertically, and they often have a bruit. Size decreases with compression. About 5% are malignant, and this percentage increases with size. They are occasionally bilateral and easily diagnosed on CT scanning. Angiography classically shows splaying of the carotid bifurcation by a vascular mass. The preferred method of excision is dissection of the tumour off the vessel in the subadventitial plane. In elderly patients or in recurrent malignant tumours radiotherapy may be beneficial.

Carotid artery dissection

Dissection of the carotid artery results from fibromuscular dysplasia, trauma, or surgery, and presents with marked neurology. It is initially treated with systemic anticoagulation (unless due to trauma) to prevent thrombus formation and if it fails to settle then it can be surgically repaired using an interpositional vein graft.

Carotid artery aneurysms

Carotid aneurysms are rare and are caused by:

- Degenerative disease (atheroma)
- FMD
- Post-operative false aneurysm
- Mycotic aneurysm

They present with a combination of pulsatile mass, pain, Horner's syndrome, cranial nerve dysfunction (compression) and cerebral ischaemia. They can be treated with interpositional grafting or ligation.

Fibromuscular dysplasia (FMD)

A rare condition affecting long unbranching arteries like the carotid. It occurs bilaterally in 50% cases and is thought to have hormonal, mechanical and genetic aetiology. Looks like a string of beads on angiogram with segmental stenosis and dilatation. Treatment is via progressive angioplasty.

Section 5
Vascular disorders of the upper limb

In a nutshell ...

Vascular disorders of the upper limb encompass a wide variety of pathologies. While atherosclerotic disease of the upper limb arteries is relatively rare, ischaemic symptoms can manifest from pathology such as emboli and aneurysmal disease, or more commonly vasospastic disorders, vasculitides, and connective tissue disease. Assessment of the upper limb is much the same as in the lower limb, with particular attention to comparing sides, and use of duplex scanning and angiography for imaging disease.

5.1 ANATOMY OF UPPER LIMB ARTERIES AND VEINS

In a nutshell ...

Thoracic inlet
Subclavian artery
Axillary artery
Brachial artery
Ulnar artery
Radial artery
Upper limb veins

Thoracic inlet

This is termed the thoracic *inlet* by anatomists but the thoracic *outlet* by surgeons!

- It is the root of the neck, above apex of lungs
- Its borders are:
  - Laterally: the inner border of the first rib
  - Medially: the anterior lip of the upper surface of the 1st vertebral body
  - Anteriorly: the suprasternal notch
- Its plane is obliquely disposed downwards and forwards (low injuries entering the neck can therefore damage structures in this area and then pass intrathoracically)
- It contains the subclavian artery and vein (as they pass over the top of the 1st rib and under the clavicle), the brachial plexus (as it emerges around subclavian artery), and the phrenic nerve (between subclavian artery and vein)

Subclavian artery

This arises on the left directly from the aorta, and on the right from brachiocephalic trunk. It lies on the lateral border of the scalenus anterior.

- Surface marking is a line arching upwards from sternoclavicular joint to 2 cm above middle of the clavicle
- The 1st part has three branches:
  - Vertebral artery
  - Internal thoracic (mammary) artery
  - Thyrocervical trunk (transverse cervical, suprascapular, inferior thyroid)
- The 3rd part gives off costocervical trunk (superior intercostal and deep cervical) and dorsal scapular artery, and this becomes axillary artery at outer border of 1st rib

Axillary artery

This is the continuation of the 3rd part of subclavian artery at outer border of 1st rib. It becomes the brachial artery at lower border of teres major. It is closely related to brachial plexus (cords); both are enclosed in the fascial axillary sheath.

It is divided into three parts by the pectoralis minor muscle; the main branches of each part are:

- 1st part superior thoracic
- 2nd part: thoraco-acromial, lateral thoracic
- 3rd part: subscapular, anterior and posterior circumflex humeral

Brachial artery

This provides the main blood supply to upper limb.

- It is a continuation of axillary artery at lower border of teres major
- It descends in anterior compartment of the arm dividing into the radial and ulnar arteries at the neck of the radius
- Profunda branch supplies the posterior compartment
- Median nerve initially lies laterally but then crosses anteriorly to lie medial to the artery in the antecubital fossa

Ulnar artery

This passes medially and inferiorly in the anterior compartment of the forearm, running deep to flexor carpi ulnaris.

- It lies lateral to the ulnar nerve
- It ends by forming the superficial palmar arch with the superficial branch of the radial artery

Note: Allen's test assesses the relative contributions of the radial and ulnar artery to the blood supply of the hand. Both arteries are occluded at the wrist, the patient makes a fist and the hand goes pale. One artery is released in turn and reperfusion of the hand assessed. It is useful for assessment before AV fistula formation, and gives information about the dominant blood supply to the hand.

The upper part gives off the common interosseous artery, which divides into anterior and posterior branches.

Radial artery

This passes downwards and laterally under brachioradialis, emerging on its medial side near the wrist.

- Distally it lies on the radius, only covered by skin and fascia (its pulsation is felt here)
- Winds laterally before entering the palm between the two heads of the 1st dorsal interosseous muscle
- Supplies neighbouring muscles and ends as the deep palmar arch

Upper limb veins

The veins of the upper limb, like the lower limb, consist of a deep and a superficial system. Knowledge of their course is of surgical importance for two reasons: firstly, for venous harvesting for graft formation; and secondly for the formation of AV fistulae as a means of vascular access (see section 5.7). There are a couple of common variations in the venous anatomy in the elbow region.

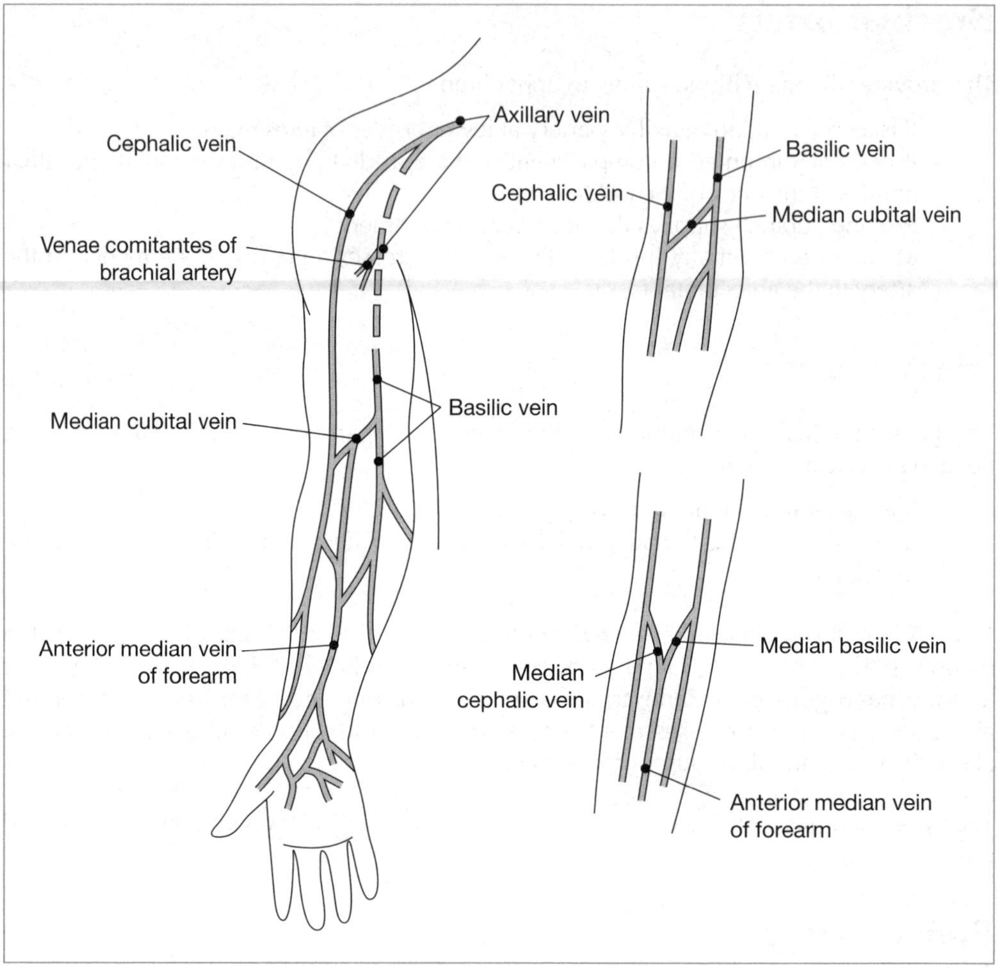

Figure 5.1a *The superficial veins of the upper limb*

Cephalic vein

- On radial side of arm
- Runs in groove between deltoid and pectoralis major muscles
- Pierces clavipectoral fascia and enters axillary vein

Basilic vein

- Ulnar side of arm
- Arises from medial side of dorsal venous arch of hand

Axillary vein

- Formed by union of brachial and basilic veins
- Continues at the 1st rib as the subclavian vein
- Its tributaries correspond to the artery but it also receives the cephalic vein

5.2 ATHEROSCLEROTIC DISEASE OF THE UPPER LIMB

In a nutshell ...

Occlusive (atherosclerotic) disease
Subclavian steal syndrome
Aneurysmal disease
Embolic disease

Occlusive disease

When it occurs, atherosclerotic disease of the upper limb is usually confined to the larger vessels (eg subclavian artery).

Management of occlusive disease

Occlusive disease of the upper limb is managed by:

- Angioplasty
- Stenting
- Bypass grafting (carotid to subclavian, axillary to axillary artery)
- Subclavian transposition (subclavian is divided at origin and re-implanted end-to-side on common carotid artery)

Aneurysmal disease

Upper body aneurysms account for 1% of peripheral aneurysms. They usually require surgical management:

- Either intrathoracic (causing Horner syndrome or venous congestion)
- Or extrathoracic (secondary to atherosclerosis, trauma (eg line placement), fibrous bands, cervical rib)

A complication of radial arterial line insertion is the development of a false radial artery aneurysm at the site of puncture. This may occur more frequently in patients with clotting disorders of any cause.

Subclavian steal syndrome

- Caused by stenosis in the subclavian artery, proximal to the origin of the vertebral artery
- Any increase in demand for blood to the arm (eg cleaning windows!) causes reverse flow of blood from the cerebral circulation, through the vertebral artery, to supply the subclavian artery post-stenosis as the stenosis limits the blood flow obtainable from the aorta
- Loss of blood from the cerebral circulation may cause dizziness, loss of consciousness, ataxia and visual loss

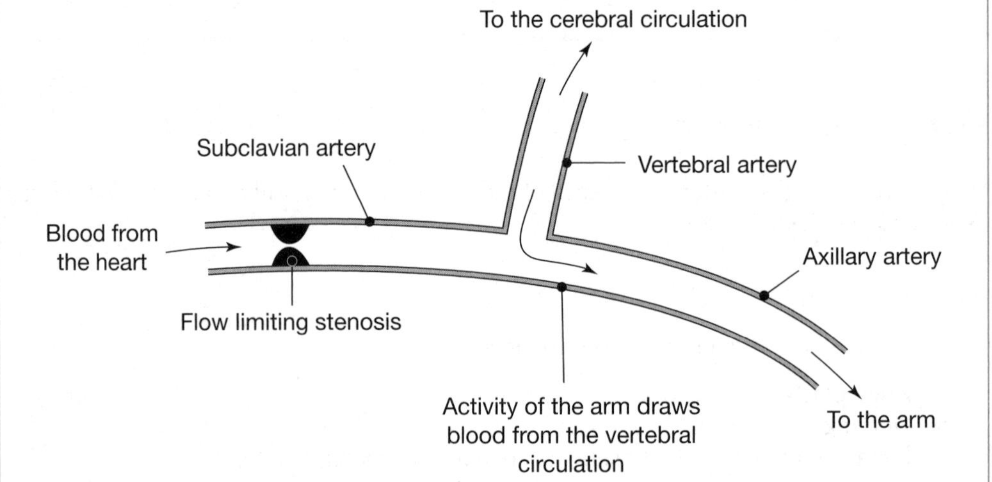

Figure 5.2a *Subclavian steal syndrome*

Embolic disease

Upper limb emboli usually arise from a cardiac source and lodge in the brachial artery. Paradoxical embolus from the venous system can give rise to upper limb emboli (via a cardiac septal defect). Occasionally a shower of smaller emboli may enter the upper limb causing small areas of distal ischaemia (eg digits). Splinter haemorrhages from infective endocarditis represent tiny, infected emboli passing into the upper limb.

Management of upper limb emboli

Upper limb emboli are managed by:

- Analgesia and resuscitation
- Anticoagulation (IV heparin); this sometimes enables conservative management of limb
- Identification of embolus as cause of upper limb ischaemia (angiography/duplex or direct surgical exploration)
- Brachial embolectomy under LA (general if appropriate or necessary) using Fogarty catheter +/– on-table angiograms or radiological intervention if required
- Post-op anticoagulation
- Identification of source of embolus

5.3 RAYNAUD'S SYNDROME

In a nutshell ...

This is characterised by episodic extreme digital vasospasm, often precipitated by cold. It is more common in females.

There are three clinical phases:

- Digital blanching due to arterial spasm (hands go white)
- Cyanosis/pain due to stagnant anoxia (hands go blue)
- Reactive hyperaemia due to accumulation of vasoactive metabolites (hands go red)

This may progress to ulceration, gangrene and digital amputation.

Causes of Raynaud's syndrome

- **Idiopathic:** this is called **Raynaud's disease** (primary cause), and it is commoner in females
- **Connective tissue disorders:** scleroderma, rheumatoid, SLE, PAN
- **Blood disorders:** cold agglutinins, cryoglobulinaemia, polycythaemia
- **Arterial disease:** atherosclerosis, Buerger's disease, subclavian aneurysm, cervical rib, thoracic outlet syndrome
- **Trauma:** vibration injury, frostbite
- **Drugs:** ergot, β-blockers

Investigation of Raynaud's syndrome

This is aimed at ascertaining the underlying cause:

- Bloods: FBC, ESR, rheumatoid and autoantibodies screen
- CXR for cervical rib
- Duplex for arterial component
- CT/MR for thoracic outlet syndrome or subclavian aneurysm

Treatment of idiopathic Raynaud's

This is aimed at symptom control.

- Conservative: gloves, hand-warming devices, smoking cessation
- Drugs: nifedipine, prostacyclin
- Surgery: consider sympathectomy in extreme cases

Other vasospastic disorders

- **Vibration white finger** occurs with prolonged exposure to high-frequency vibrating tools, which causes arterial vasospasm (especially in the cold). Management includes stopping exposure, hand warmers, and nifedipine
- **Hypothenar hammer syndrome** is a rare condition secondary to repeated trauma of the ulnar artery against the hammate in the palm of the hand. It causes digital embolisation
- **Irradiation injury** following radiotherapy to chest wall/axilla (eg breast cancer). This can cause vessel rupture, thrombosis, stenosis, atherosclerosis.

5.4 HYPERHIDROSIS

In a nutshell ...

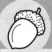

This is excessive sweating that may occur anywhere, but is most common and distressing in the palms, axillae and feet. It is classified with vascular disorders because treatment (sympathectomy) was traditionally performed by vascular surgeons for non-reconstructable critical ischaemia.

Aetiology of hyperhidrosis

Aetiology is either primary (childhood, adolescence, familial) or secondary (hyperthyroid, phaeochromocytoma, hypothalamic tumours).

Treatment of hyperhidrosis

Treatment can be surgical or conservative.

Non-surgical management of hyperhidrosis

- Topical ammonium chloride
- Iontophoresis (electric current to incapacitate sweat glands)
- Botulinum toxin (decreases sympathetic activity)

Surgical management of hyperhidrosis

- Skin excision
- Sympathectomy

Examples of treatments for hyperhidrosis

Palmar hyperhidrosis is treated by thoracoscopic sympathectomy.

Axillary hyperhidrosis is best treated by subcutaneous botulinum toxin injections.

Plantar hyperhidrosis is treated by chemical lumbar sympathectomy.

Thoracoscopic sympathectomy is performed by inserting a laparoscope into the pleural space via the axilla, deflating the lung, then obliterating the 2nd, 3rd and 4th sympathetic ganglia with diathermy or surgery, avoiding the stellate ganglion. Complications of thoracoscopic sympathectomy include:

- Horner syndrome (ptosis, meiosis, anhidrosis due to stellate ganglion damage)
- Haemothorax
- Pneumothorax
- Compensatory hyperhidrosis

5.5 THORACIC OUTLET SYNDROME

In a nutshell ...

This occurs when there is compression of the subclavian vessels or branches of the brachial plexus as they pass from the thorax into the arm. It occurs in 0.4% of the population. 70% are bilateral and 60% are symptomatic.

Causes of thoracic outlet syndrome

- Cervical rib
- Abnormal muscle insertions or muscle hypertrophy
- Fibrous band
- Callus from old clavicular fracture
- Neck trauma
- Malignancy

Symptoms and signs of thoracic outlet syndrome

- Arterial (ischaemic arm/hand); emboli
- Venous (swollen, warm, tender arm)
- Neurologic (pain, paraesthesia, weakness, wasting) (most common)

Differential diagnosis of thoracic outlet syndrome

- Carpal tunnel syndrome
- Cervical spondylosis
- Raynaud syndrome
- Upper limb atherosclerotic disease
- Subclavian aneurysm
- Reflex sympathetic dystrophy
- TIA/CVA
- Trauma (whiplash injury)

Examination and investigation of thoracic outlet syndrome

- Bilateral brachial BP measurement
- Roos' test: abduction and external rotation of the arm may precipitate symptoms
- Reduced or absent pulses
- CXR and thoracic outlet views (note: cervical rib may not be visible on X-ray)
- Cervical spine X-ray

- Nerve conduction studies
- Duplex ultrasound
- MRI/MRA

Treatment of thoracic outlet syndrome

- Physiotherapy
- Surgical decompression: selective nerve root ablation, resection of 1st part of 1st rib, split cervical rib, or divide anterior scalene muscle

5.6 UPPER LIMB VENOUS OCCLUSION

In a nutshell ...

This is less common than lower limb DVT. It may also cause PE.

Presentation of upper limb venous occlusion

- Less common than lower limb DVT
- May also cause PE
- Can occur at any level in the venous drainage of the upper limb (common in the axillary/subclavian veins but may extend)
- Presents as painful, swollen, tender, warm upper limb
- Look for symptoms and signs of underlying cause

Risk factors and causes

- Thoracic outlet syndrome
- Obstructive apical lung lesions
- Hypercoagulable states (congenital, or underlying malignancy)
- Trauma
- Prolonged limb elevation with exercise (eg painting a ceiling)

Treatment of upper limb venous occlusion

Upper limb venous occlusion is treated as for lower limb DVT (see Chapter 6 *Peri-operative Care*)

- Anticoagulate
- Identify and treat underlying cause

5.7 ARTERIO-VENOUS (AV) MALFORMATIONS AND VASCULAR ACCESS SURGERY

In a nutshell ...

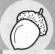

An AV fistula is an abnormal connection between arterial and venous systems. AV malformations consist of a huge spectrum of congenital and acquired vascular abnormalities. They have been placed in the upper limb section for convenience, although they can affect the legs and other parts of the body as well as the upper limbs.

Congenital fistulas
- Cirsoid
- Parkes–Weber
- Klippel–Trenaunay

Acquired fistulas
- Traumatic
- Surgical

Congenital fistulas

These are rare, being seen in approximately 1 per million live births. They are most commonly seen in the head/neck or extremities. Although present from birth they often enlarge during puberty or pregnancy. They may be **localized** or **multiple**.

Localised fistulas (cirsoid aneurysm)

These appear as soft pulsatile swellings that are unsightly and may cause aching pain. The overlying skin/mucosa may ulcerate with brisk haemorrhage. There is often a palpable thrill and machinery murmur present, which may be abolished by compressing the main feeding vessel. Investigation includes CT scanning and selective arteriography. Those that arise during pregnancy should be treated expectantly as many regress after delivery. Treatment may be by embolisation or occlusion of the feeding vessel combined with excision. Direct injections of sclerosants have not been effective.

Multiple fistulas (Parkes–Weber syndrome)

These usually present with an overall enlargement in limb size. They may be dilated superficial veins with ulceration and high-output cardiac failure may develop. The limb is hot with increased width and length associated with bone over-growth. Differential diagnoses include Klippel–Trenaunay syndrome, local gigantism, and lymphoedema. Arteriography characteristically shows rapid blushing through the abnormal communications with early arrival of dye in the veins. Individual fistulas are not visualised unless they are very large. In the absence of heart failure or severe deformity management is usually expectant in early life. Later, ligation of the feeding vessels or injection of microspheres/embolisation may reduce the inflow. Amputation may be required in exceptional circumstances.

Klippel–Trenaunay syndrome (venous abnormality)

These are congenital varicose veins and port-wine stains. There is bone and soft tissue hypertrophy in affected limb, and there are deep venous abnormalities (often).

Acquired fistulas

These may result from accidental trauma (traumatic AV fistula) or be surgically created for renal haemodialysis.

Traumatic AV fistulas

These usually follow simultaneous adjacent arterial and venous injury with a common haematoma. They take days to form, and there is usually a thrill and a bruit. Adjoining veins may become dilated and arterialised, eventually leading to venous hypertension, and possibly ulceration. Limb hypertrophy and lengthening may occur. If blood flow through the distal artery is sufficiently decreased distal ischaemia may occur. A fistula between larger vessels may be sufficient to create a left-to-right shunt, leading to heart failure if severe. Methods for closure include application of Duplex directed pressure, insertion of a covered stent, or surgical closure.

AV fistulas for haemodialysis

These are usually created for long-term dialysis access and once formed can remain patent indefinitely. The connection of the artery to a vein results in a dilated vein, which is suitable for repeated cannulation and can deliver a high flow of blood for dialysis. The ideal site, originally described by Brescia, is the radiocephalic fistula in the forearm, but other sites may be used.

The general rule in fistula formation is that the most distal site on the non-dominant arm is used. The procedure can be carried out under LA by side-to-side anastomosis of the radial artery and cephalic vein, though some surgeons ligate the distal vein or perform an end-to-side anastomosis to prevent the possibility of distal venous hypertension. Post-operatively maintaining a warm limb and adequate hydration are necessary for successful fistula formation. Recently GTN patches have been used on the distal limb to encourage vasodilatation.

Expected patency rates are 60–90% at 1 year and 60–75% at 5 years. Generally, fistulae are not closed following a renal transplant as they may subsequently be required again, though many thrombose spontaneously following transplantation. Indications for fistula closure are cosmetic, large flows leading to heart failure, and occasionally sepsis or distal embolisation.

Section 6

Venous and lymphatic disorders of the lower limb

6.1 VENOUS ANATOMY OF THE LOWER LIMB

In a nutshell ...

The venous system consists of the deep and superficial veins.

Deep veins
Posterior tibial
Anterior tibial
Peroneal
Soleal
Gastrocnemius
Popliteal
Femoral
Iliac

Superficial veins
Long saphenous
Short saphenous

Deep veins

These accompany the arteries.

- Three paired stem veins (no valves): posterior tibial, anterior tibial (smallest, may not see on venogram), and the peroneal veins
- Two muscular veins (with valves): soleal vein, and the gastrocnemius vein

All join and form the popliteal vein in the popliteal fossa, where the short saphenous vein (a superficial vein) also joins the deep venous system.

- Popliteal vein becomes the femoral vein and accompanies the superficial femoral artery
- It is joined by the long saphenous vein (another superficial vein) at the saphenofemoral junction, then becomes the iliac vein

Venous anatomy is very variable, and the deep veins are often multiple. Lower limb occlusive venous pathology is covered in Chapter 6. Upper limb venous occlusion is covered in section 5.6 of this chapter.

Superficial veins

These systems lie in the subcutaneous tissue and are involved in thermoregulation. They become varicose veins. In the lower limb there are two main veins and their tributaries.

Long saphenous vein

This is the longest vein in the body. It runs from anterior to the medial malleolus (site for venous cut-down), along the medial side of the leg, and terminates at the saphenofemoral junction, just medial to the femoral pulse (surface marking 2.5 cm below and lateral to pubic tubercle or 1 fingerbreadth medial to femoral artery in groin crease).

It connects to the deep venous system at the:

- Saphenofemoral junction
- Mid-thigh perforator
- Medial calf perforators (usually three or four)

Short saphenous vein

This commences behind the lateral malleolus and runs along the postero-lateral side of the calf to pierce the deep fascia and join the popliteal vein in the popliteal fossa. It usually communicates with the deep (soleal and gastrocnemius) veins and the long saphenous system.

There are six points of communication between the deep and superficial venous systems:

- Long saphenous (saphenofemoral junction)
- Short saphenous (saphenopopliteal junction)
- Mid-thigh perforating veins
- Medial calf communicating veins (posterior tibial to posterior arch veins)
- Gastrocnemius communicating veins (short saphenous to muscle)
- Lateral calf communicating veins (short saphenous to peroneal)

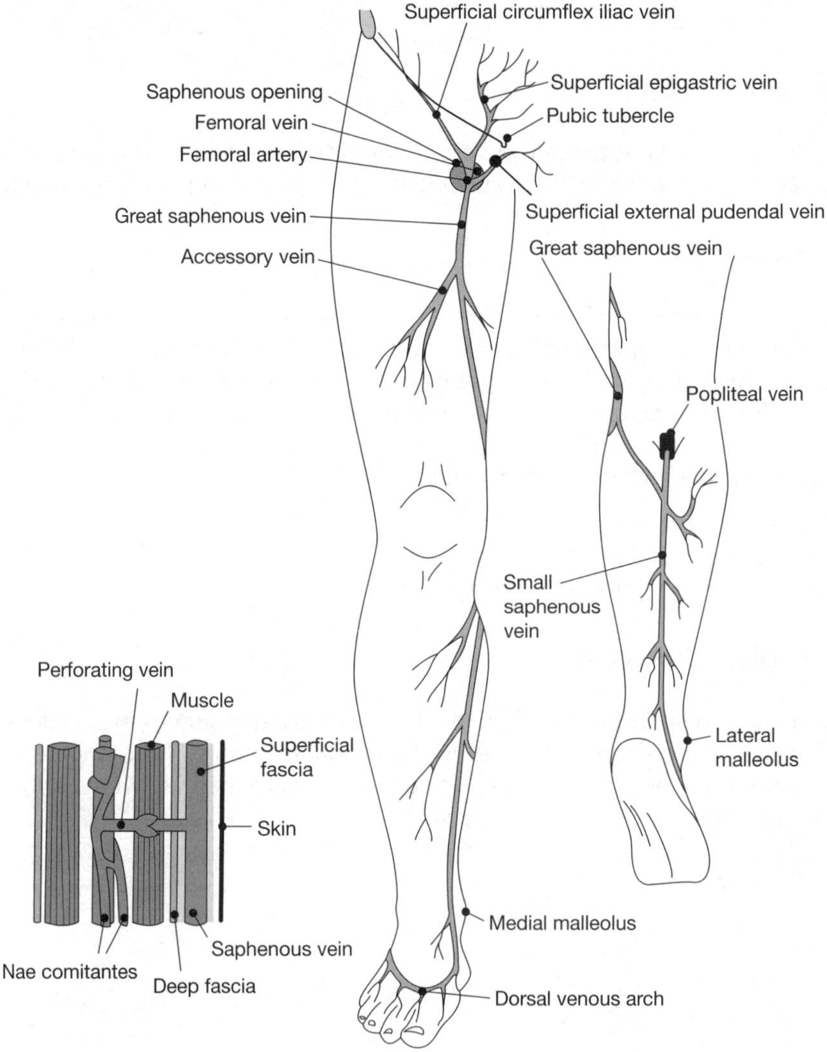

Figure 6.1a *Superficial lower limb venous anatomy*

6.2 PHYSIOLOGY OF LOWER LIMB VEINS

In a nutshell ...

Venous return is maintained by the following:

- Heart (maintains a pressure gradient through the circulation)
- Calf muscle pump
- Venous valves
- Venomotor tone
- Respiratory movements

Venous return is impeded by gravity, which encourages peripheral pooling in dependent limbs.

Venomotor tone

Venomotor tone is maintained by smooth muscle within the vein wall (under control of the sympathetic nervous system). On assuming an upright position, the decreased cardiac output due to dependant pooling leads to increase in sympathetic discharge (which increases venous tone to reduce the capacitance of the system and increase venous return).

Respiratory movements

Changes in intrathoracic pressure with inspiration and expiration influence venous return. When intrathoracic pressure decreases, venous return increases. When intrathoracic pressure increases, venous return decreases (as in the Valsalva manoeuvre) which in turn decreases cardiac output.

Muscular activity and the calf pump

With an upright posture blood should pool in the distal venous system (which can occur with prolonged standing). However, deep veins have valves that prevent reverse flow in the column of blood within the veins. Also, as the calf muscles contract blood is forced upwards resulting in lower pressure in the deep veins during relaxation of muscular activity (this draws blood from superficial to deep veins via the communicating vessels, along the pressure gradient generated). May also have valves to ensure unidirectional flow. The flow is shown in Fig. 6.2a.

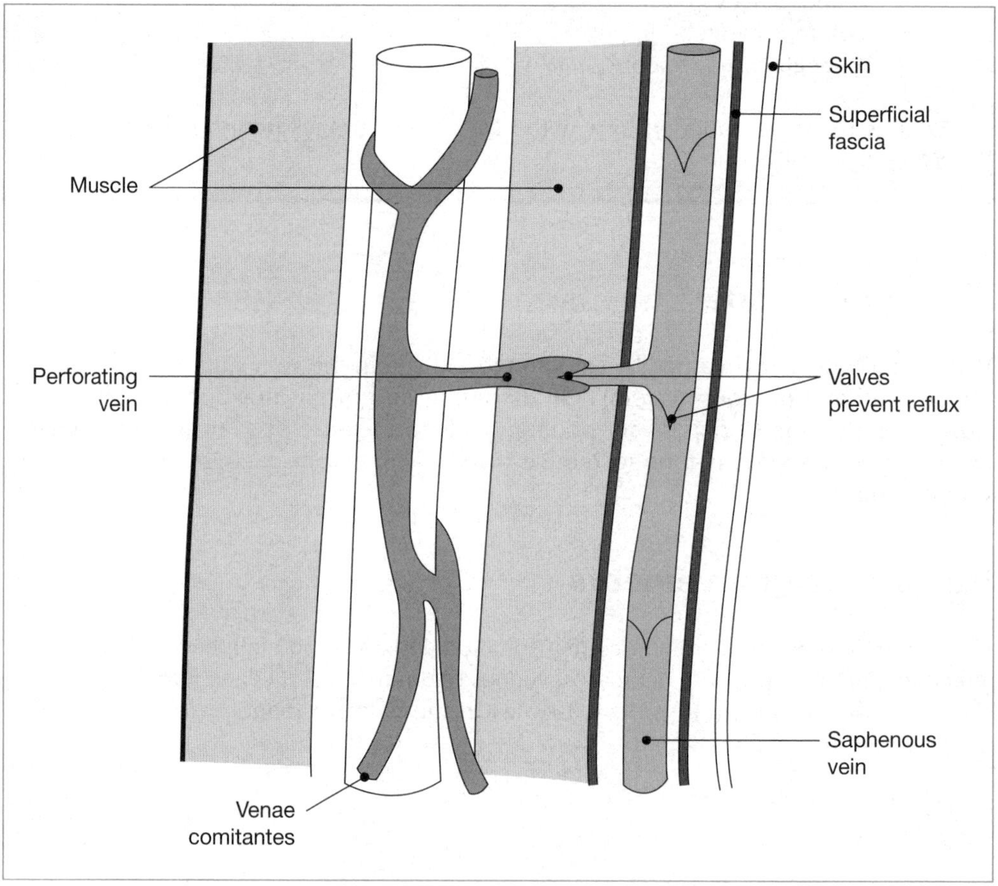

Figure 6.2a *The venous pump*

6.3 VARICOSE VEINS

In a nutshell ...

Varicose veins are dilated, tortuous, elongated superficial veins, which:

- Occur in 2% of the population (increasing incidence with age)
- May be **primary** or **secondary** (due to an obstructed system eg DVT, pelvic malignancy)
- Are commonest in the long saphenous system but may occur in the short saphenous distribution, or may be recurrent (after previous varicose vein surgery)

Primary varicose veins

These form due to gravitational venous pooling and vein-wall laxity causing venous dilatation and valve leakage. In long saphenous varicose veins this usually starts at the saphenofemoral junction, causing more pooling and dilation in the proximal segment of the vein and leakage at the next valve. Eventually all the valves leak and there is a continuous column of blood below the heart, leading to increased venous pressure in the superficial veins of the legs (which may cause leg oedema and tissue damage, leading to complications of varicose veins).

Damage can occur to the valves in the perforating calf veins, such that the calf muscle pump exacerbates the superficial venous pressure. If the superficial venous system is surgically disconnected at the saphenofemoral junction, patients with primary varicose veins generally have a functioning deep venous system which can cope with the venous return of the lower limb.

Secondary varicose veins

If the deep venous system outflow is obstructed (eg DVT, pelvic malignancy) or deep or communicating venous valves are incompetent (eg post-phlebitic) then blood may be forced from the deep to the superficial system resulting in increased superficial venous pressure, and varicose veins. This can also be caused by a congenital absence or abnormality of the venous valves, and rarely by severe tricuspid incompetence causing pulsatile varicosities!

This is significant because secondary varicose veins caused by an absent or poorly functioning deep venous system should not be surgically disconnected as this would leave no alternative effective path of venous return. Secondary varicose veins are associated with symptoms of chronic venous insufficiency, with no alternative effective path of venous return other than the superficial system, secondary varicose veins should never be treated by surgical disconnection of the superficial venous system.

Risk factors for varicose veins

Age (peak 50–60)
Female
Obesity
Pregnancy
Occupations involving long periods of standing
Family history
Pelvic malignancy
Previous DVT
Long bone fracture

Symptoms of varicose veins

- Asymptomatic
- Cosmetic
- Ache
- Itch
- Ankle swelling
- Bleeding
- Thrombophlebitis (painful inflamed thrombosed superficial varicosities)
- Skin discoloration (haemosiderinosis)
- Varicose eczema
- Lipodermatosclerosis (induration/inflammation in skin)
- Ulceration

Examination of varicose veins

In a nutshell ...

Inspect

- Determine whether likely to be primary or secondary (include full exam for potential secondary causes)
- Determine site of incompetence:
  - Tap test
  - Cough test
  - Tourniquet test
  - Perthe's test
  - Hand held Doppler tests

Formal investigation for sites of incompetence using Duplex scanning

This is performed initially with the patient **standing**. Inspect for ankle swelling, haemosiderinosis, varicose eczema, lipodermatosclerosis, and ulceration. Note the distribution and severity of varicosities. Palpate the veins for superficial thrombophlebitis and palpable perforating veins, and examine the popliteal fossa and groin for varices. A saphenovarix is a compressible swelling due to a dilated varix at the saphenofemoral junction (which disappears on lying down).

Sites of incompetence are determined by several tests.

- **Tap test**: palpate the proximal portion of the vein while tapping distally. If you feel an impulse it suggests a column of blood exists between the point of tapping and the vein being palpated
- **Cough test:** the standing patient is asked to cough while you palpate the saphenofemoral junction. A positive cough impulse indicates saphenofemoral junction incompetence. This test is very unreliable
- **Tourniquet test:** the patient is placed in the supine position with the leg elevated and the veins emptied by manual 'sweeping'. A tourniquet is then placed on the mid-thigh and the patient is asked to stand. If veins below the tourniquet do not refill assume that the site of incompetence is above the tourniquet (when the tourniquet is released these veins will then be seen to fill). The test can be repeated with the tourniquet at different levels to ascertain sites of incompetence. This test is more reliable than the cough test but less reliable than handheld Doppler. If done with pressure from hand or tourniquet on the saphenofemoral junction, this is the Trendelenberg test
- **Perthe's test**: once you have controlled the varicose veins by blocking off the superficial venous system with a torniquet, venous drainage of the leg is carried out exclusively by

the deep venous system (as if the patient had surgical disconnection of the saphenofemoral junction). Ask patients to go up and down on their toes increasing arterial blood supply and activating the calf pump. If deep veins are patent this reduces venous engorgement of the limb. If the deep system is not patent or the valves are incompetent the opposite occurs. With the deep system incapable of draining the leg and the superficial system temporarily disconnected, the increased blood supply into the exercising leg has nowhere to drain, and patients experience a bursting pain of venous engorgement. This test shows why it is so important to check the patency of the deep venous system before carrying out varicose vein surgery. If the presenting complaint of venous insufficiency and engorgement of superficial veins secondary to a non-functioning deep venous system (for example, after a DVT) then stripping the superficial system on which the patient is relying will only make it worse

- **Hand-held Doppler**: place the hand-held Doppler probe over the site of incompetence to be assessed (eg saphenofemoral junction) in the standing patient. The vein or leg is then compressed sharply below the probe, and a 'whoosh' is heard as the blood passes the hand-held Doppler. If the site to be assessed is incompetent, a second 'whoosh' is heard as blood passes back through an incompetent section of vein

Finally perform a full examination of the patient, paying special attention to the abdomen and pelvis, looking for secondary causes of varicose veins. Formal investigations of the sites of incompetence may be performed using duplex scanning or venography.

Investigation of varicose veins

- Hand-held Doppler (as described above)
- Duplex Doppler US (see section 1)
- Venography (see section 1)

Management of varicose veins

In a nutshell ...

Management options include:

- Conservative measures
- Compression stockings
- Sclerotherapy
- Laser
- Endoluminal electrocoagulation
- Foam injection
- Surgery

Varicose veins may be treated to relieve symptoms (ache, itch) or to prevent complications (bleeding, ulceration). Management is conservative or surgical. Take care when considering treatment of varicose veins for cosmetic reasons as the benefits of surgery might be outweighed by complications.

- **Conservative measures** are a good option for uncomplicated, asymptomatic varicose veins
- **Compression stockings** press the veins, augment venous return and thus reduce symptoms and complications; they are a good option in the elderly and those not fit enough for surgery, although stockings often not well tolerated by younger patients
- **Sclerotherapy** involves injection of a 'sclerosant' (eg sodium tetradecyl sulphate (fibrovein)) via a fine needle directly into the vein followed by compression bandaging. The sclerosant irritates the venous intima, causing inflammation and ultimately luminal obliteration. It works well for small varicosities (but not large veins or in the presence of significant venous incompetence)
- **Surgery** aims to disconnect the incompetent superficial system from the venous circulation
- **Other treatment modalities** include laser, endoluminal electrocoagulation, and foam injection. These therapies act by damaging the venous endothelium which is then compressed by occlusive bandaging of the treated limb. The damaged endothelium adheres and occludes the lumen of the vessels

Surgery for varicose veins

In a nutshell ...

Surgical options:

- Open surgery with junction ligation and stripping of vein +/– stab avulsions
- Subfascial endoscopic perforator surgery (SEPS)
- Radiofrequency ablation
- Foam ablation

Be aware of common anatomical variations (failure to deal with these leads to recurrence).

Surgical options for varicose veins include open surgery or subfascial endoscopic perforator surgery (SEPS).

SEPS involves the insertion of a rigid endoscope through the skin and superficial fascia to a plane above the muscle. Perforating veins are visible as they exit the muscle. These are dissected free from surrounding tissue and closed by means of metal clips.

Radiofrequency ablation is performed by threading an ablation catheter down the vein (either through an incision at the SFJ and under direct vision or percutaneously). The catheter is heated to 85° C destroying the venous wall.

Pre-operative formal duplex skin marking is used to identify sites of incompetent perforators and the saphenopopliteal junction (SPJ) to aid identification during surgery. Pre-op marking of varicosities with the patient standing is imperative.

Op box: Junction ligation and stripping of varicose veins (long saphenous LSV; short saphenous SSV)

Indications

Symptomatic varicose veins (exclude patients with a non-functioning deep venous system).

Pre-op

ALWAYS carefully mark all varicosities on the skin with the patient standing immediately pre-operatively and ask them to identify any troublesome varicosities (as they will be much less visible when the patient is asleep and supine!). Perforators and the SPJ should be marked on the skin under formal duplex guidance. May be performed under GA, LA or regional anaesthetic. Women taking the OCP should stop and use alternative contraception for 4 weeks prior to the procedure (increased risk of DVT).

Positioning

Supine position with 15° head-down tilt (supine for LSV; prone for SSV).

Incision

LSV: make groin crease incision just medial to the femoral pulse (NB: in obese patients the SFJ will be above the groin crease).

SSV: horizontal incision in the skin crease of the popliteal fossa (at the level of the marked SPJ).

Procedure

LSV

Dissect out and carefully identify the SFJ before any vein is divided. Identify and divide all **5 tributaries** beyond secondary branch points:

- Superficial circumflex iliac
- Superficial inferior epigastric
- Superficial external pudendal

- Postero-medial thigh branch (prevents medial thigh recurrence)
- Deep external pudendal (directly off common femoral vein)

Beware–these tributaries are very variable. Ligate SFJ flush to the common femoral vein – do not narrow the lumen of the common femoral and make sure the ligature does not slip!

Strip long saphenous vein, with an endoluminal stripper, from groin to knee

Avulse below-knee varicosities

SSV

Dissect out and carefully identify the SPJ before any vein is divided

Divide and ligate any small tributaries leading into the SSV/SPJ

Ligate the SPJ

Avulse below-knee varicosities

Intra-operative hazards

LSV: Damage to the saphenous nerve (sensory loss) which runs with the vein below the level of the knee (do not advance endoluminal stripper lower than 1 handbreadth below-knee)

SSV: Damage to the common peroneal nerve (results in foot drop) or sural nerve (sensory loss)

Closure

Close the wound in layers with absorbable sutures

Stab avulsions can be closed with Steri-strips™

Apply compression bandages

Post-operative instructions

Often done as a day case and so standard day-case procedures apply

Compression bandaging remains in place for 24 hours

Replaced with thigh length graduated compression stockings (wear day and night for 1 week; can then be removed at night)

Sit with feet elevated and encourage regular short exercise

Complications

Bruising and leg swelling

Bleeding

Infection

Nerve damage (long saphenous–saphenous nerve, short saphenous–sural nerve)

DVT

Anatomical variation is common and can be identified on duplex scanning. Variants include:

- Double saphenous veins
- Major thigh tributaries including the accessory vein (joins saphenous at mid-thigh)
- Major tributaries joining the superficial external iliac and superficial external pudendal veins

Risk factors and causes of varicose vein recurrence:

- **Re-canalisation**
  - Failure to identify all tributaries at the initial operation (even small vessels can dilate)
  - Leaving segments of the saphenous vein in situ (especially in the thigh)
- **Neovascularisation** around the SFJ or SPJ

6.4 LEG ULCERS

In a nutshell ...

An ulcer is a break in continuity of an epithelial surface
Ulcers are common and an expensive cause of morbidity
Although not all have vascular aetiology, leg ulcers often present to vascular clinics

Causes of leg ulcers

- Venous (varicose veins, post-phlebitic, gravitational)
- Arterial (atherosclerosis)
- Neuropathic (diabetic, CVA, spina bifida, pressure sores)
- Trauma (plaster of Paris, injections, burns)
- Allergic
- Vasculitic and vasospastic (rheumatoid, SLE, PAN, scleroderma, Raynaud's)
- Malignancy (BCC, SCC, malignant melanoma, skin metastases, Marjolin's ulcer – SCC change in previous venous ulcer)
- Infective (TB, HIV)
- Artefactual (patient-induced or iatrogenic)
- Malnutrition (scurvy, UC)
- Lymphatic (infection, trauma)

Associated factors contributing to leg ulcers

- Gravitational stasis
- Immobility
- Obesity
- Malnutrition
- Steroids

In practice, most ulcers are of mixed aetiology.

Pathology of venous ulceration

Raised superficial venous pressure may be due to primary varicose veins, congenital valvular aplasia, or deep venous incompetence. This is marked in the post-thrombotic limb. After significant DVT the thrombus becomes organised and the vessel may partially or totally re-canalise. Thrombus irreversibly damages the valves in the deep venous system leading to incompetence. Chronic venous insufficiency secondary to venous hypertension causes increased hydrostatic pressure from valve dysfunction and blood travelling from the deep to superficial venous systems.

Venous hypertension has several effects:

- Restricts arterial replenishment of capillary blood
- AV shunt formation
- Dilation of venules causes leakage of plasma proteins into the tissues (lipdermatosclerosis is a term given to the combined skin and subcutaneous tissue changes of chronic venous hypertension; a progressive sclerosis of the skin and subcutaneous fat by fibrin deposition, tissue death and scarring – it results in a constricted appearance around the lower leg (oedema above and atrophy below) which resembles an inverted bottle, hence the term 'beer-bottle leg')
- RBCs are forced out into the tissues resulting in pigmentation of the skin called haemosiderin deposition

Together, these changes lead to the clinical picture of raised superficial venous pressure with ankle swelling, haemosiderinosis, varicose eczema, lipodermatosclerosis, and ultimately ulceration.

There are two main theories of ulcer formation:

- Leukocyte trapping theory: raised venous pressure causes increased capillary pressure with fibrin exudation, WBC entrapment, congestion and thrombosis
- Fibrin cuff theory: leaking from capillaries causes fibrin cuffing around the vessel with reduced nutrient and oxygen diffusion

Examination of leg ulcers

First remove all dressings, applications and debris.

- Position – eg gaiter area (venous); sole of foot (arterial or neuropathic)
- Size
- Shape
- Edge – sloping, punched out, undermined, rolled, everted
- Base – slough, granulation tissue, tendon, bone
- Depth
- Discharge – serous, sanguinous, purulent
- Colour
- Temperature
- Tenderness
- Fixity
- Surrounding tissues
  - Arteries/veins (including ABPI)
  - Nerves
  - Bones/joints
- Regional lymph nodes
- General examination

Investigation of leg ulcers

- Duplex Doppler US (arterial and venous)
- Blood tests (FBC, ESR, sugar, autoantibodies)
- Swab (microbiology)
- Biopsy (malignant change, other aetiologies)
- Arteriography/venography (if indicated)

Management of venous leg ulcers

Compression is most usually achieved with stockings or bandaging. Various regimens are described (3-layer, 4-layer, paste). All aim to provide high external pressure at the ankle, graduating down to lower pressure in the upper calf, thus augmenting venous return and allowing ulcer healing. The progress of healing is monitored regularly. Non-healing ulcers require further assessment to exclude other aetiologies (eg Marjolin's change, vasculitis), and antibiotics if infected. If still not healing consider excision and split-skin graft or pinch skin grafts.

Full compression (eg 4-layer bandaging) can be applied for pure venous ulcers (ABPI of > 0.9). When there is an arterial component (ABPI of 0.7–0.9) modified or lighter compression is required. An ABPI of < 0.7 requires correction of the underlying arterial abnormality. 4-layer compression bandaging consists of cotton wool (inner layer), crepe, elastic bandage and a cohesive bandage.

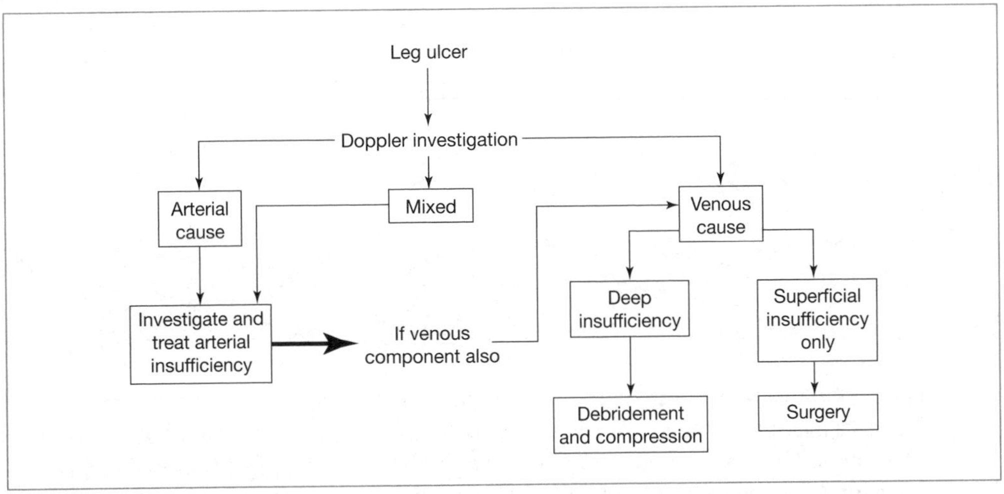

Figure 6.4a *The management of lower limb ulceration*

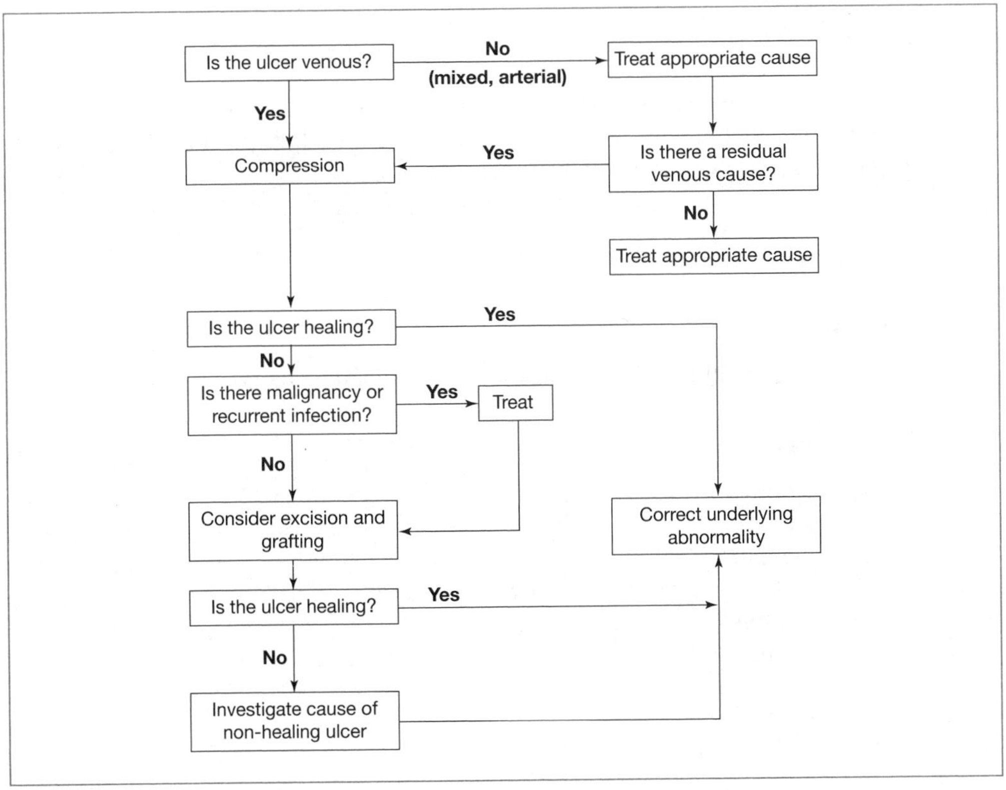

Figure 6.4b *Algorithm for venous ulcer treatment*

Chapter 9

When the ulcer is healed, further management is required to maintain healing. This may be long-term compression stockings, or superficial venous surgery (long saphenous or short saphenous varicose veins) to correct the underlying venous abnormality.

6.5 LYMPHOEDEMA

In a nutshell ...

Lymphoedema is an accumulation of tissue fluid in the extracellular compartment as the result of a failure in the lymphatic system to transport fluid via the lymphatic vessels and lymph nodes. It is commonest in the lower limb (80%) but may occur in the upper limb or scrotum. In contrast, **oedema** is an accumulation of tissue fluid in patients in whom a lymphatic abnormality has not been confirmed (eg cardiac/renal/nutritional).

The lymphatics

The lymphatic system maintains a flow of lymph fluid of approximately 2–2.5 litres per day, maintained by contractility of lymphatic channels and their patency. Lymph nodes absorb water and electrolytes from the lymphatic fluid.

Causes of lymphoedema

Primary causes

- Congenital, idiopathic (Milroy's disease, lymphoedema praecox or tarda)

Secondary causes

- Following groin or axillary surgery
- Post radiotherapy
- Due to malignancy
- Infection (eg filariasis caused by *Wucheria bancrofti*)
- Lymphadenectomy
- Chronic inflammation

Pathology of lymphoedema

Primary lymphoedema occurs due to a developmental lymphatic abnormality. 20% have a family history of swollen legs. This can be lymphatic channel aplasia, hypoplasia or hyperplasia. Secondary lymphoedema follows destruction or obstruction of the lymphatic channels by surgery, radiotherapy, malignancy or filariasis. This results in reduced lymphatic drainage leading to limb swelling. The swelling may be initiated by an infective episode (eg cellulitis) or by minor limb trauma. Initially the oedema is pitting but over time fibrosis occurs leading to classical clinical picture of non-pitting oedema.

Differential diagnosis of lymphoedema

Other causes of leg swelling

- Venous or post-phlebitic oedema
- Cardiac failure
- Hepatic insufficiency (hypoproteinaemia)
- Renal failure
- Gravitational or stasis oedema
- Congenital giant limb (including vascular abnormalities, see section 5)

Investigation of lymphoedema

The clinical diagnosis is usually obvious, but when doubt exists (especially in early primary lymphoedema) it can be confirmed by **lymphoscintography**. A radio active tracer is injected SC into the foot, and its progress is monitored with a gamma camera as it progresses to the proximal lymphatics and beyond. Delayed transit confirms the diagnosis.

More detailed anatomy can be elicited, for example before consideration of lymphatic reconstruction, by **lymphangiography.** A radio-opaque dye is injected directly into lymphatic vessels of the foot using an operating microscope and direct exposure. Conventional X-rays are then used to image the lymphatics.

Management of lymphoedema

This does not include use of diuretics!

- Exclude other causes of oedema
- Elevate affected area
- Antibiotics (treat infections like cellulitis early and aggressively)
- Compression with bandaging or stockings
- Lymphopress (serial pneumatic compression device)
- Surgery

Surgery for lymphoedema

- Reserved for failure of conservative treatment (indicated in < 10% of patients)
- Must be done before distal lymphatics obliterate
- Poor outcome

- **Homan's procedure:** a debulking operation where a wedge of tissue removed from the affected limb, with primary closure
- **Charles operation:** a debulking operation in which subcutaneous tissue is excised. Split skin grafts are applied to the exposed fascia
- **Bridge operation:** a bypass for obstructed iliac lymphatics, from bisected inguinal nodes to an isolated small bowel pedicle

Chapter 10

Paediatric Surgery

Susan Picton and David Crabbe

Section 1
Children as surgical patients

In a nutshell ...

Children are not mini-adults. They differ anatomically, physiologically, and psychologically from adults.

Anatomical differences

- Size and weight
- Respiratory system (eg differences in tracheal length and position)
- Abdominal and pelvic dimensions and the relative size and positions of certain organs
- Skeletal structure and structure of the spine

Physiological differences

- The body's surface area relative to body mass is greater in children than in adults
- Fluids and electrolytes: children have a higher total body water
- Hepatic functions (eg clotting)
- Metabolic rate, thermoregulation and nutritional requirements
- In water loss through the GI tract
- In the urine-concentrating capacity of the kidney
- In respiratory rate and respiratory pattern (eg nose-breathing)
- In heart rate and response to stress
- In neurological functions

Psychological and emotional differences

- Developmental milestones
- Regression with illness

1.1 ANATOMY OF CHILDREN

In a nutshell ...

The important anatomical distinctions between children and adults are:
- Size
- Airway
- Abdomen and pelvis
- Abdominal organs
- Male genitalia (see Chapter 11 *Urology and Transplantation*)
- Spinal cord (see *Elective Neurosurgery and Spinal Surgery* chapter in Book 2)

Size in children

An obvious difference between children and adults is size.

- A child's size varies with age and the most rapid changes occur within the first year
- Fluid and drug dosages are calculated by weight

To estimate a child's weight use:

$$\text{Weight (kg)} = (\text{age} + 4) \times 2$$

The ratio of body surface area to weight decreases with age due to increasing size; neonates and infants are small and therefore lose heat rapidly (see *Thermoregulation* in section 1.2).

Airway in children

Several factors can make endotracheal intubation of an infant difficult:

- The head of an infant is large compared to the rest of the body and the neck is short, thus the resting position of the head is in flexion
- The glottic aperture is more anteriorly inclined and higher than in adults
- The epiglottis is inclined more posteriorly than in adults
- The trachea is significantly shorter (4 cm not 12 cm) and narrower (5 mm not 2 cm) than in adults
- The trachea lies further to the right of the mid-line than in adults
- The tracheal bifurcation lies at T3 not T6 as in adults
- A large tongue and adenoids will obscure the view
- The narrowest part of a child's airway is the cricoid, so uncuffed endotracheal tubes should be used because a cuff can cause pressure necrosis

Until 2 months of age, infants are obligate nasal breathers due to their large tongues. Do not block the nostril of a baby who has an NG tube in the other nostril!

The left brachiocephalic vein runs across the trachea higher in the child than adults – above the suprasternal notch – so it can get in the way if performing a tracheostomy.

Children breathe rapidly because of a high metabolic rate and they have limited oxygen reserves. They become hypoxic rapidly so you have less time to intubate. The normal respiratory rate of a neonate is 30–60 breaths per minute, falling to around 15–20 breaths per minute in a 10-year-old.

Intercostal, subcostal and sternal recession are signs of respiratory distress. Grunting on expiration is a sign of severe respiratory distress in infants.

Abdomen and pelvis in children

The abdomen extends from the costal margin to the pelvic brim. In **adults** the abdomen is longer than it is wide. Therefore in adults the mid-line vertical laparotomy incision gives best access to most intra-abdominal organs. In **neonates** the abdomen is wider than it is long. Therefore in neonates the transverse laparotomy incision gives the best access to most intra-abdominal organs.

Scars will grow with children and get progressively larger, so paediatric surgeons plan their incisions carefully. Scars will migrate – a supra-umbilical scar may end up near the costal margin when the child has grown up.

Abdominal organs in children

There are several differences in the proportions and positions of abdominal organs of children compared to adults:

- Liver and spleen are proportionally larger in children
- Pelvis is shallower in children
- Organs that are housed in the pelvis in adults are above the pelvic brim in children (sitting in the lower abdomen). These are the:
  - Bladder
  - Uterus
  - Ovaries
  - Rectum
- This difference in position of organs means that:
  - Lower abdominal incisions should be made with care
  - Suprapubic catheterisation is quite straightforward in children
- The caecum (and appendix) sit higher in infants, migrating down to the RIF by the age of 3 or 4

Important definitions

Premature infants are those born before 38 weeks' gestation
Neonates are children between birth and 4 weeks' gestation (neonates are also infants)
Infants are children between birth and 52 weeks
Pre-school children are aged between 1 and 4 years old

Abortion is when a child is born dead before 28 weeks' gestation (includes deaths due to natural causes, as well as deliberate termination)
Stillbirth occurs when a child is born dead after 28 weeks' gestation

Perinatal mortality is the number of stillbirths and deaths in the 1st week of life. This accounts for around 1% of deliveries in the UK
Neonatal mortality is the number of deaths in the first 28 days of life regardless of gestational age (about 6 per 1000 live births in the UK)
Infant mortality is the number of deaths in the first year of life (about 10 per 1000 live births in the UK). It includes neonatal mortality

1.2 PHYSIOLOGY OF CHILDREN

In a nutshell ...

The important physiological differences between children and adults include:

- Thermoregulation
- Fluids and electrolytes
- Hepatic immaturity
- Nutrition and energy metabolism
- The gastrointestinal tract
- Renal function
- Respiratory system
- Cardiovascular system
- Nervous system

Thermoregulation

Neonates are more susceptible to hypothermia than adults. They have a larger surface area to weight ratio, less subcutaneous fat and less vasomotor control over skin vessels. Neonates cannot shiver and have no voluntary control over temperature regulation. In addition, premature infants have smaller stores of brown fats.

Precautions should be taken to ensure they do not become hypothermic during surgery:

- Keep the operating theatre temperature high (naked infants need an ambient temperature of 31.5 °C)
- Infants should be well wrapped up
- Respiratory gases should be warmed and humidified
- Use warming blankets
- Infuse warm IV fluids
- During surgery wrap wool around the head and exposed extremities
- Warm the aqueous topical sterilising 'prep'
- Use adhesive waterproof drapes to prevent the infant getting wet
- Limit exposure of the extra-abdominal viscera

Brown fat

Brown fat acts as a heat source – when free fatty acids are oxidised they produce heat via uncoupled ATP production. Neonates can have as much as 200 g of brown fat (less in premature infants). It is situated between the scapulae, between the oesophagus and trachea and predominantly around the kidneys and adrenals (metabolism of brown fat is stimulated by β-adrenergic stimulation). Brown fat has a good blood supply as it needs lots of oxygen and the heat needs to be distributed around the body.

Fluids and electrolytes

- Total body water in a neonate is about 800 mL/kg (80%), falling to about 600 mL/kg (60%) at 1 year
- One third is extracellular fluid, and the remainder is intracellular
- Circulating blood volume is almost 100 mL/kg at birth, falling to 80 mL/kg at 1 year
- Term neonates require transfusion if > 30 mL blood is lost during a surgical procedure (1–2 small swabs)

Signs of dehydration in children

Dehydration in children is traditionally estimated as < 5% (mild), 5–10% (moderate) and > 10% (severe).

SIGNS OF DEHYDRATION IN CHILDREN

	Mild	Moderate	Severe
Thirst	+	+	+
Decreased urine output	+	+	+
Sunken fontanel	–	+	+
Tachycardia	–	+/–	+
Drowsiness	–	+/–	+
Hypotension	–	–	+/–

Fluid requirements are estimated on the following basis:

- Normal insensible losses: respiration, GI losses, sweating
- Maintenance of urine output: excretion of urea, etc
- Replacement of abnormal losses: blood loss, vomitus, pre-existing dehydration, etc

Normal maintenance fluid and electrolyte requirements, based on weight, are shown in the table.

NORMAL MAINTENANCE FLUID AND ELECTROLYTE REQUIREMENTS

Body weight	Fluid requirements	Sodium	Potassium
0-10 kg	100 ml/kg per day (4 ml/kg/hour)	3 mmol/kg/day	2 mmol/kg/day
10-20 kg	50 ml/kg per day (2 ml/kg/hour)	2 mmol/kg/day	1 mmol/kg/day
20+ kg	20 ml/kg/day (1 ml/kg/hour)	1 mmol/kg/day	1 mmol/kg/day

Maintenance fluid and electrolyte requirements incrementally decrease as weight increases so a 25kg child would require (100ml x 10kg) + (50ml x 10kg) + (20ml x 5kg) = 1600ml over 24 hours or 67mls/hour.

- For a newborn infant give 60 mL/kg/day for days 1–2, then 90 mL/kg/day on day 3
- A good choice for maintenance IV fluids for children undergoing surgery is 0.45% saline + 5% dextrose + 10 mmol potassium chloride (per 500 mL of IV fluid)
- Replace NG aspirates with equal volumes of 0.9% saline + 10 mmol potassium chloride per 500 mL

Vitamin K can be given to premature infants if the immature liver is not producing clotting factors, otherwise haemorrhagic disease of the newborn may result. Drug doses in premature infants must be decreased. Glycogen stores are small resulting in hypoglycaemia after short periods of starvation. Poor glucuronyl transferase activity and high haemoglobin load lead to physiological jaundice.

Neonates have a high metabolic requirement compared to adults, mainly because they are so poorly insulated and need to work harder to maintain their core body temperature, and also because they are growing so fast. They therefore need more oxygen (oxygen consumption is 6–8 mL/kg/min compared with 2–4 mL/kg/min in adults). They also need more fuel in the form of calories. They require 100 kilocals/kg/day – more than twice as many as adults.

Enteral fluid requirements are 150 mL/kg/day (more than IV requirements because enterally fed babies use energy to digest the food and lose more fluid in bulky stools). Before birth the principal energy substrate is glucose – after birth it comes from free fatty acids and glycerol.

Gastrointestinal tract

Infants lose more water through their alimentary tract than adults, and this loss can become very important in ill, dehydrated children. The reasons for the increased losses are:

- Small total surface area (villi undeveloped)
- Children lose their absorptive capacity when ill
- Disaccharide intolerance (common)
- Gastroenteritis (common)

Renal function

An adult responds to dehydration by passing a small volume of more concentrated urine, reabsorbing sodium and so retaining water. Neonates are less able to concentrate urine and so dehydrate more easily. They have a lower GFR and lose more sodium in their urine.

Respiratory system

The respiratory rate in neonates is fast due to an increased oxygen demand (see above), usually between 30 and 60 breaths per minute, but it can vary from minute to minute. When increased respiratory effort is required the respiratory rate increases but the tidal volume does not. At birth, 50% of alveoli are not developed and tidal volume is about 20 mL (7 mL/kg). Respiratory distress in infants may lead to hypocalcaemia, which may lead to twitching and seizures.

Surfactant is required for lungs to work properly, and premature neonates do not secrete enough of this.

Cardiovascular system

In utero pulmonary vascular resistance is high. Blood bypasses the lungs (right-to-left shunting) through the foramen ovale at the atrial level and the ductus arteriosus (left pulmonary artery to aorta) – this is the fetal circulation. Before birth the pressure in the right atrium is higher than in the left so the blood moves (shunts) from the right to the left atrium.

At birth, with the first breath, pulmonary vascular resistance falls abruptly. Blood no longer returns to the right atrium from the placenta. These two things reduce the pressure in the right atrium. Simultaneously, blood begins to flow into the left atrium from the lungs. This increases the pressure in the left atrium. Shunting at the atrial level ceases and the ductus starts to close. Any condition which impairs gas exchange in the lungs (eg diaphragmatic hernia) may result in persistence of the fetal circulation (PFC).

Heart rate is high in infants and declines with age:

- Newborn: 120–160 b.p.m.
- 1 year: 110–150 b.p.m.
- 5 years: 80–100 b.p.m.

Stroke volume varies little in infants. Cardiac output increases with increasing heart rate.

Shock is important to recognise and manifests itself differently in children when compared with adults.

- Signs of shock include tachypnoea and tachycardia
- Diminished peripheral perfusion ('shut down') is an early sign
- Assess the capillary refill time: gently squeeze the great toe for 5 seconds to blanch the skin and then release – the colour normally returns within 2 seconds
- Hypotension is a late sign
- Bradycardia is ominous, usually indicative of hypoxia and imminent cardiac arrest

Nervous system

The blood–brain barrier is underdeveloped and myelination is not complete at birth. This means that opiates and fat-soluble drugs have greater efficacy on the brain and can lead to respiratory depression.

1.3 CARING FOR A CHILD IN HOSPITAL

In a nutshell ...

When caring for a child in hospital it is important to:

- Have good communication skills
- Be aware of developmental milestones
- Understand consent issues
- Be able to:
  - Relieve pain
  - Gain vascular access
  - Resuscitate a critically ill child

Communication skills with children and parents

Communication is vital with both accompanying adults and the child. You won't gain their trust if you ignore them and speak only to the adults.

- Say who you are and why you are there
- Find out who they are – don't assume the accompanying adult is a parent
- Sit down – don't tower over the child
- Smile, be friendly, have good eye contact, and avoid jargon
- Do not expect to take a systematic history – be flexible and build a rapport

The priority is to obtain and maintain the trust of the child and parent. You can fill in the gaps of the history at the end of the discussion by quizzing the parents, nurses, social workers etc. Let the child sit on mum's lap while you talk, examine, or take blood. Be honest – don't say 'This won't hurt a bit,' but say something like 'There will be a little sting now and then we'll give you a sticker for being brave.'

Don't push the child for information; they often can't recall timescales ('When did the pain start' is not as good a question as 'Did you feel alright when you were at school today?') and they are poor at localising pain. They may make up an answer if they feel under pressure.

Be reassuring but not unrealistic: wait until you have all the information before you reassure the parents. It's no good saying 'Don't worry, he'll be fine' before you have fully assessed the child. For most parents watching their child be rushed into surgery in the middle of the night is not fine. Find out the facts, then be specific.

Make sure the right people get the right information – do mum and dad know she's in hospital and may be going for surgery, or are aunty and granddad keeping it from them for some reason? You usually need parental or official guardian consent.

Developmental milestones

If you ask a 1-year-old a question and expect a sensible answer, or ask the parents of a 5-year-old girl to put her nappy back on after examining her in clinic, the child's parents will lose confidence in you immediately and assume that all your medical diagnostic skills and advice are worthless. If you have small children in your family these things will be obvious to you; if not, keep them in mind. Don't forget that many children regress by about a year when they are ill – a lucid 4-year-old schoolgirl may cry for mama and go back into nappies; a football-playing 10-year-old may need his favourite blanket, wet the bed, and refuse to speak to anyone he doesn't trust.

The developmental milestones are:

- Social smiles at 6 weeks
- Babbles, puts everything in its mouth, starts teething at 6 months
- Obeys commands at 10–15 months (eg 'Legs up while I change you' or 'Clap')

- Says first word by 12 months (eg 'milk')
- Takes first steps at 12–18 months
- Drinks from a beaker at 18 months
- Puts two words together by age 2 (eg 'want milk' or 'milk please')
- Potty trains between 2 and 3 years
- Knows own name and sex by age 3 (eg 'I'm Ben and I'm a boy!')
- Starts state nursery school at age 3 (may be at private 'nursery' from a few months old)
- Starts 'reception' at age 4
- Starts primary school at age 5
- Starts high school at age 11

Consent and ethics for paediatric patients

Children and consent

At age 16 a young person can be treated as an adult and can be presumed to have capacity to decide. Below the age of 16 children may have the capacity to decide, depending on their ability to understand what is involved.

Where a competent child refuses treatment, a person with parental responsibility or the court may authorise investigation or treatment that is in the child's best interests (except in Scotland). When a child is under 16 and is not competent, a person with parental responsibility may authorise treatments that are in the child's best interest.

Those with parental responsibility may refuse intervention on behalf of an incompetent child aged less than 16, but you are not bound by that refusal and may seek a ruling from the court. In an emergency, you may treat an incompetent child against the wishes of those with parental responsibility if you consider it is in the child's best interests, provided it is limited to that treatment which is reasonably required in that emergency. For example, you can give a life-saving blood transfusion to the incompetent child of Jehovah's Witness parents who refuse to consent, but not to a competent Jehovah's Witness who refuses consent himself, whatever his age. For further discussion see Chapter 8.

Pregnant women and consent

The right to decide applies equally to pregnant women as to other patients, and includes the right to refuse treatment where the treatment is intended to benefit the unborn child.

Analgesia in children

Pain assessment

This can be difficult in small children and they are often under-analgesed.

Look for:

- Advice from the parents: they know the child best and rarely over-estimate the pain
- Signs in the child:
  - Inconsolable crying or being unusually quiet
  - Not moving freely around the bed; reluctant to get up
  - Protecting the painful area
  - Pallor, tachypnoea, tachycardia

Pain charts can be used for older children. You can also try distracting the child with a toy or a story.

ADVANTAGES AND DISADVANTAGES OF ANALGESICS

Pain killer	What is it?	Pros	Cons
Paracetamol	Central cyclo-oxygenase (COX) inhibitor	Widely used Few side effects Oral or PR	Not anti-inflammatory Beware in children with jaundice
Ibuprofen	NSAID	Anti-inflammatory Oral or PR	Beware in asthma, blood disorders, and gastric ulceration
Diclofenac	NSAID	Oral or PR (tastes horrible so give rectally if possible)	
EMLA	Eutectic mixture of local anaesthetic (2.5% lignocaine and 2.5% prilocaine) Topical local anaesthetic	'Magic cream' for taking blood or cannulation Works after 45 mins; lasts for an hour	Not to be used on broken skin
Ametop™	4% amethocaine (tetracaine) Topical local anaesthetic	'Magic cream' as above Works after 35 mins; lasts for 4–6 hours	
Morphine	Opiate	IV or oral in small frequent doses Effective analgesia Nausea not as bad as in adults Sedative	Beware respiratory depression Infants have under-developed blood–brain barrier and so are more susceptible to fat-soluble opiates Excretion by liver and kidney is slower than in adults
Pethidine	Opiate	IV only	

Vascular access in children

The following methods can be used for vascular access.

- **Peripheral line:** cubital fossa, dorsum of hand, scalp, femoral vein, long saphenous vein, foot (remember EMLA)
- **Peripheral long line:** cubital fossa, long saphenous vein
- **Central venous catheterisation** (under expert supervision only): internal jugular, femoral vein
- **Intra-osseous trephine needle into tibia** (1–3 cm below tubercle): This is only for use in children aged less than 6 years. Complications include through-and-through bone penetration, sepsis, osteomyelitis, haematoma, abscess, growth plate injury. Arterial access is via radial artery or femoral artery

Resuscitation of the critically ill child

Read about the basic techniques for resuscitation of children in the *Advanced Paediatric Life Support Handbook* (BMJ Publishing Group 1996).

The basic principles to remember are:

- Summon help
- ABC (Airway, Breathing, Circulation)
- Clear airway. Give 100% oxygen. Ventilate artificially if necessary
- Establish IV access (always difficult in children)
- If child has collapsed insert an intra-osseous needle 2 cm below the tibial tuberosity
- Give initial bolus of 20 mL/kg fluid (0.9% saline, plasma substitutes, 4.5% albumin are all acceptable)
- Repeat boluses according to response. Start maintenance infusions

Section 2

Neonatal surgery

In a nutshell ...

Neonatal surgery demands an understanding of the embryology and neonatal pathologies in the following systems:

- Gastrointestinal tract
- Diaphragm
- Lip and palate
- Spine and neural tube (covered in Chapter 6 *Elective Neurosurgery and Spinal Surgery* in Book 2)

2.1 GASTROINTESTINAL (GI) TRACT

In a nutshell ...

An appreciation of the embryology of the gut is necessary to appreciate neonatal surgical pathology of the gastrointestinal tract.

Anomalies fall into the following categories:

Anatomical anomalies

- Defects of fusion of the anterior abdominal wall (eg gastroschisis, exomphalos)
- Failure of canalisation or 'atresia' (eg oesophageal, duodenal, small bowel atresias)
- Failure of gut rotation

Functional anomalies

- Meconium ileus (failure of electrolyte transport through ion channels)
- Hirshsprung's disease (failure of peristalsis)

Embryology of the GI tract

By the 3rd gestational week the embryo is trilaminar and consists of the notochord, intra-embryonic mesoderm, intra-embryonic coelom, and neural plate. The intra-embryonic coelom is formed by the re-absorption of the intra-embryonic mesoderm. Fig. 2.1a shows the formation of the primitive gut.

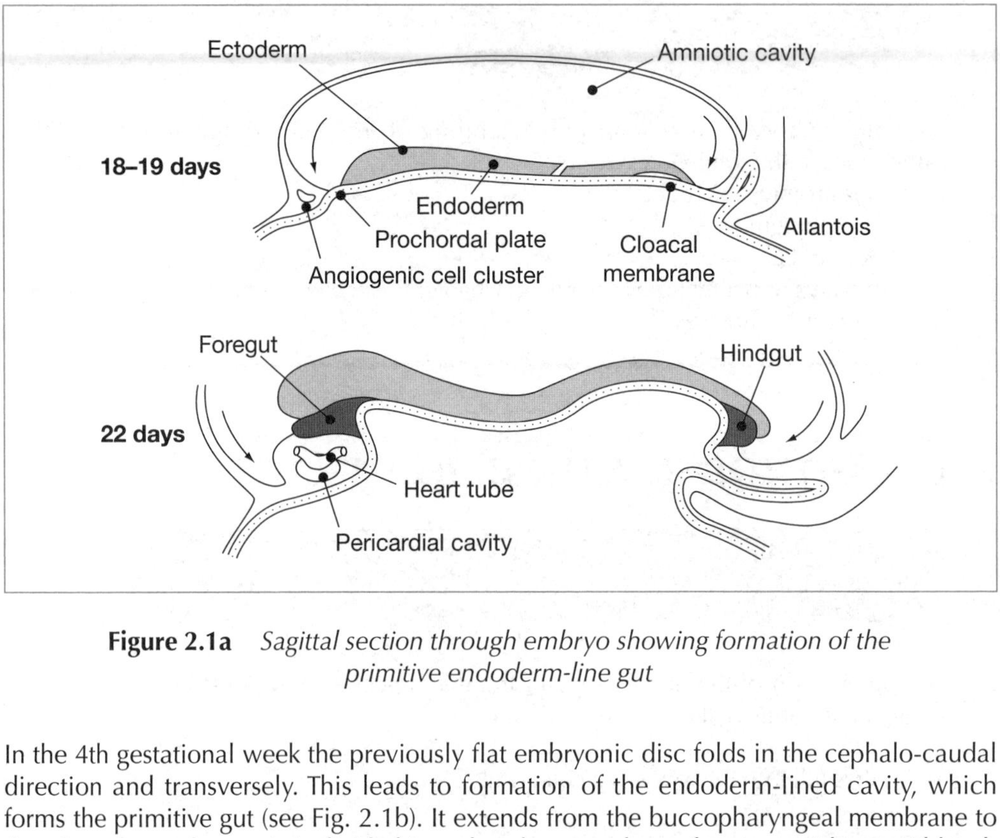

Figure 2.1a *Sagittal section through embryo showing formation of the primitive endoderm-line gut*

In the 4th gestational week the previously flat embryonic disc folds in the cephalo-caudal direction and transversely. This leads to formation of the endoderm-lined cavity, which forms the primitive gut (see Fig. 2.1b). It extends from the buccopharyngeal membrane to the cloacal membrane. It is divided into the pharyngeal gut, fore-gut, mid-gut and hind-gut. The endodermal lining of the primitive gut gives rise to the epithelial lining of the gut whilst mesoderm provides the muscular parts.

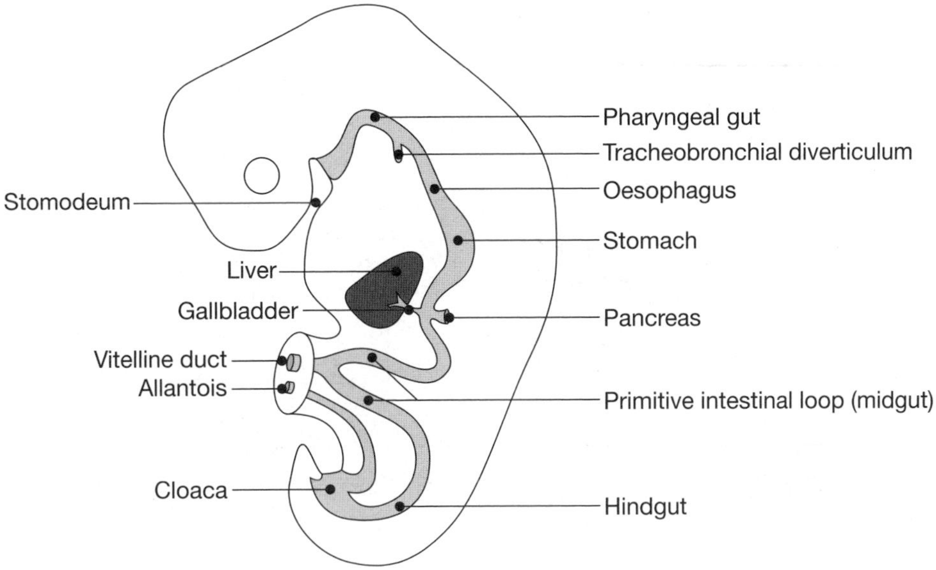

Figure 2.1b *Formation of the GI tract at the 4th week of gestation showing fore-gut, mid-gut and hind-gut*

The pharyngeal gut

This extends from the buccopharyngeal membrane to the tracheobronchial diverticulum.

The fore-gut

This gives rise to the trachea and oesophagus, stomach, duodenum, liver, pancreas and spleen. The **trachea** develops from the tracheobronchial diverticulum, which becomes separated from the fore-gut by the **oesophagotracheal septum**. The lung buds develop from the blind end of the trachea. These lung buds give rise to the segmental bronchi and expand into the pericardioperitoneal cavity. Abnormal closure of the oesophagotracheal septum can lead to tracheo-oesophageal fistula. Fig. 2.1c shows the fore-gut in the 1st week of gestation.

Formation of the **stomach** occurs when the dorsal mesentery lengthens, the gut tube rotates clockwise and the liver bud migrates to the right side of the dorsal body wall. This also gives the **duodenum** its 'C' shape.

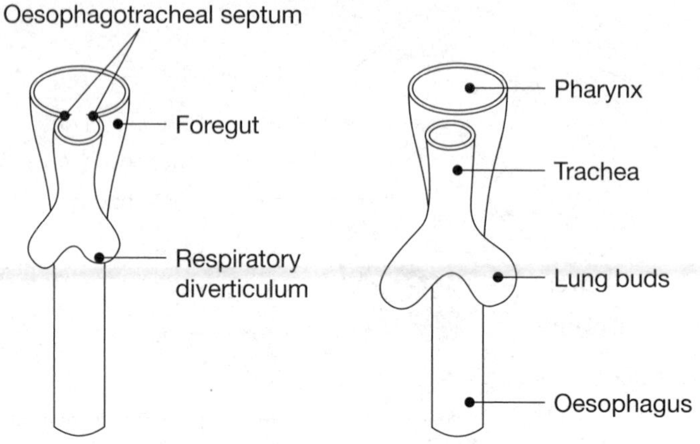

Figure 2.1c *The fore-gut during the 4th week of gestation*

The **liver** develops from the hepatic diverticulum, which is an endodermal outgrowth from the distal end of the fore-gut. The bile duct is formed from the connection between the liver and the fore-gut.

The uncinate process of the **pancreas** is formed from the ventral pancreatic bud which is closely associated with the hepatic diverticulum. The body of the pancreas is formed from the dorsal pancreatic bud. The ventral pancreatic duct rotates clockwise to join the dorsal pancreatic duct.

The **spleen** is a fore-gut derivative of the left face of the dorsal mesentery.

The mid-gut

This extends from the entrance of the bile duct to the junction of the proximal two-thirds and distal one-third of the transverse colon. The mid-gut of a 5-week embryo is shown in Fig. 2.1d. The dorsal mesentery of the mid-gut extends rapidly, producing physiological herniation in the 6th week.

The cephalic limb of the mid-gut grows rapidly to hang down on the right side of the dorsal mesentery. The gut rotates around the axis formed by the superior mesenteric artery (SMA) 270° in an anticlockwise direction. The gut returns to the abdominal cavity in the 10th week.

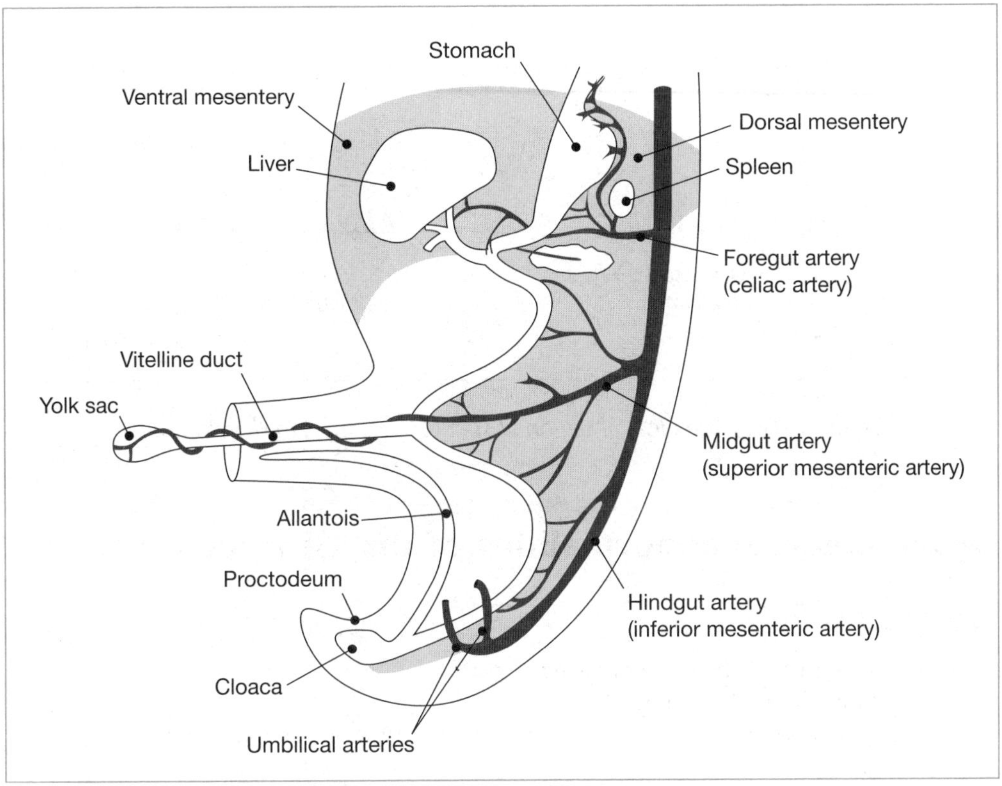

Figure 2.1d *The mid-gut of a 5-week embryo*

The hind-gut

This gives rise to the distal one-third of the transverse colon, descending colon, sigmoid colon, rectum and upper half of the anal canal.

In addition, the endoderm of the hind-gut gives rise to the lining of the bladder and urethra. The **urorectal**, a transverse ridge arising between the allantois and the hind-gut, grows to reach the cloacal membrane, to divide it into the urogenital membrane anteriorly and the anal membrane posteriorly. The **anal pit** forms in the ectoderm over the anal membrane and this ruptures in the 9th week to form a connection between the rectum and outside. Fig. 2.1e shows successive stages of development of the cloacal region.

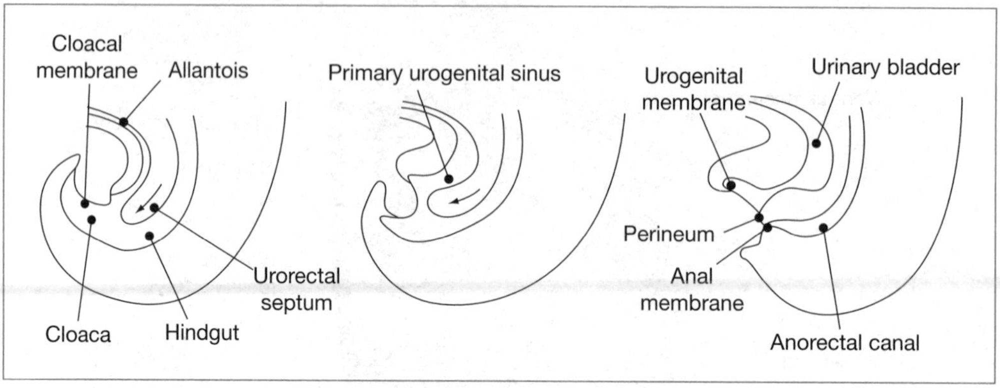

Figure 2.1e *The cloacal region at successive stages in development*

Developmental abnormalities of the GI tract

Gastroschisis

- Incidence 1 in 3000 but increasing
- Most identified on pre-natal US
- Defect in abdominal wall to the right of an otherwise normal umbilicus
- No sac
- The bowel is eviscerated and, as a result of contact with amniotic fluid, thickened and matted
- Associated malformations are uncommon except intestinal atresias (10%)
- Immediate management consists of covering the exposed bowel with Clingfilm™ and closure of the defect as rapidly as possible
- Often has to be staged using a silo
- TPN may be required for many weeks until intestinal function resumes
- Long-term outcome is excellent

Exomphalos (omphalocele)

- Incidence 1 in 3000
- Characterised by a hernia into the base of the umbilical cord – ie covered by a sac (amnion)
- Identifiable on antenatal US
- Classified as exomphalos major if defect > 5 cm diameter and exomphalos minor if < 5 cm
- Associated malformations in 50% – chromosomal defects (trisomies) and cardiac defects
- Treatment consists of closure of the defect in one or more stages
- Prognosis depends on associated malformations

Oesophageal atresia (OA) and tracheo-oesophageal fistula (TOF)

- Incidence 1 in 3500
- Maternal polyhydramnios common, although diagnosis rarely made before birth
- Present at birth as a 'mucousy' baby, choking or turning blue on feeding

Associated malformations present in 50% – the **VACTERL** association:

V **V**ertebral anomalies
A **A**norectal anomalies
C **C**ardiac
TE **T**racheo-o**e**sophageal
R **R**enal
L **L**imb

Diagnosis is confirmed by attempting to pass an NG tube and taking a CXR. Tube coils in upper thorax. Gas in the stomach indicates a fistula between the trachea and the distal oesophagus (TOF). 75% of babies with OA will have a TOF; 10% will have isolated OA, usually associated with a long gap; remainder will have an isolated TOF or upper and lower pouch TOFs.

- Treatment involves disconnection of the TOF and then anastomosis of the upper and lower oesophagus through a right thoracotomy
- Complications include anastomotic leak (particularly if the gap is long), anastomotic stricture, gastro-oesophageal reflux (GOR) and recurrent fistula
- Long gaps may require oesophageal replacement

Duodenal atresia

- Incidence 1 in 5000
- One third have Down syndrome
- Present at birth with bile-stained vomiting
- Diagnosis confirmed by 'double-bubble' sign of gas in stomach and proximal duodenum on AXR
- Treatment consists of side-to-side duodenoduodenostomy
- May be associated with annular pancreas

Small bowel atresia

- Incidence 1 in 3000
- Aetiology is vascular: Barnard (of cardiac transplant fame) and Louw produced experimental atresias in puppies ligating mesenteric blood vessels in utero
- Pathology varies, depending on how deep in the mesentery the vascular accident occurs, from an atresia in continuity with a mucosal membrane to a widely separated atresia with a V-shaped mesenteric defect and loss of gut
- 10% of atresias are multiple

- Babies present shortly after birth with bile-stained vomiting (a cardinal symptom of intestinal obstruction in children) and abdominal distension
- Diagnosis is confirmed by AXR: multiple fluid levels
- Treatment is laparotomy and end-to-end anastomosis

Anorectal malformation (ARM)

- Incidence 1 in 5000
- Associated malformations: VACTERL association (as above)
- Should be identified at birth
- Present with failure to pass meconium, abdominal distension and bile-stained vomiting
- Precise anatomy varies but they can be subdivided into high and low/intermediate anomalies in males and females

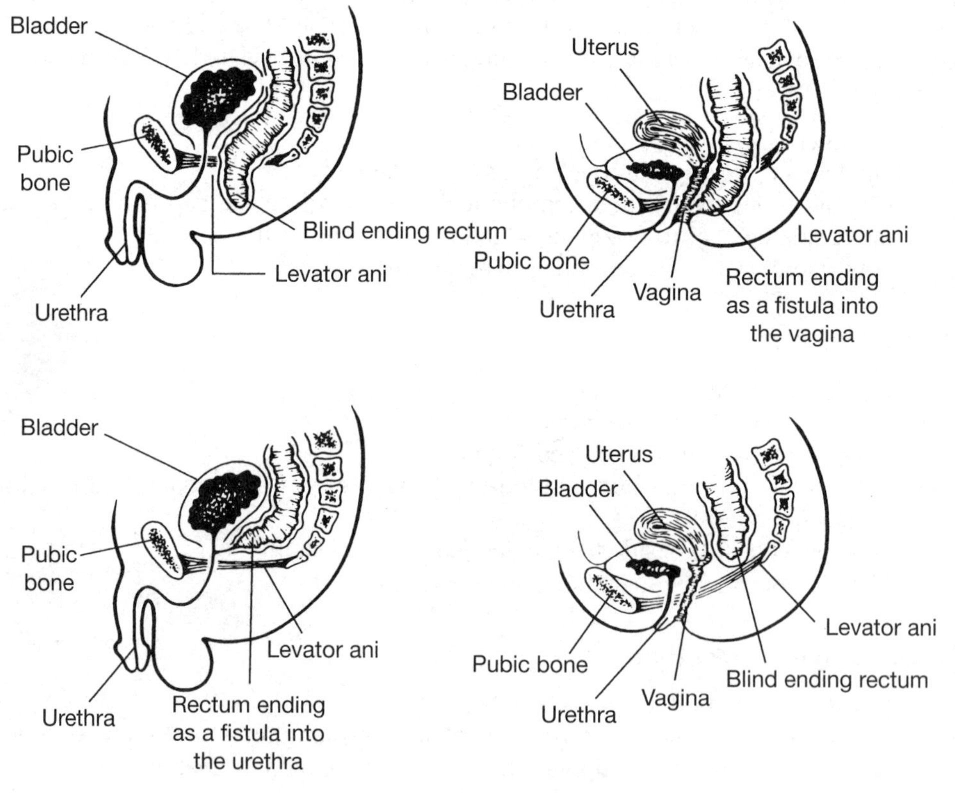

Figure 2.1f *Congenital anorectal anomalies*

Low and intermediate anorectal anomalies

- Rectum present and passes through a normal sphincter complex
- In males there is a tiny fistulous track to the surface of the perineum, often anteriorly onto the scrotum
- If meconium is visible a local 'cut-back' procedure can be performed to open the fistula back to the rectum in anticipation of normal continence

In females the rectum usually opens into the back of the introitus – a rectovestibular fistula. This abnormality is termed intermediate and, though normal continence is ultimately to be expected, reconstruction involves division of a common wall between rectum and vagina. For this reason treatment involves a three-stage procedure with defunctioning colostomy, anorectal reconstruction, and then closure of the stoma.

High anorectal anomalies

- Rare in females, common in males
- Sphincter complex poorly developed and prospects for continence are not good

In males the rectum makes a fistulous connection with the urethra. The three-stage procedure is essential. After the first stage a cystogram and descending contrast study through the colostomy is necessary to define the anatomy of the defect. Reconstruction most commonly involves a posterior sagittal anorectoplasty (PSARP) performed through a mid-line perineal incision.

Mid-gut malrotation and volvulus

As the physiological intrauterine mid-gut hernia reduces, the mesentery normally rotates to bring the caecum to lie in the RIF and D-J flexure to lie to the left of the mid-line. The mid-gut mesentery thus extends diagonally across the back of the abdominal cavity and provides a broad stable pedicle for the SMA to supply the bowel. Malrotation, failure of this normal rotation, leaves caecum high in the right upper quadrant (RUQ) and the D-J flexure mobile in the mid-line. The result is a narrow base for the mid-gut mesentery and a narrow mobile pedicle through which the SMA runs. Malrotation is usually asymptomatic and only detected by contrast meal and follow through.

- Mid-gut malrotation predisposes to mid-gut volvulus – the narrow base to the mesentery twists
- Immediate effect is a high intestinal obstruction at duodenal level, rapidly followed by infarction of the entire mid-gut from the D-J flexure to the splenic flexure
- Symptoms are bile-stained vomiting and later collapse
- AXR is similar to duodenal atresia with a double-bubble and a paucity of gas elsewhere in the abdomen
- Diagnosis confirmed by urgent (middle of the night) upper GI contrast study

Treatment is urgent laparotomy to untwist the bowel. If bowel viability is doubtful perform second-look laparotomy after 24 hours. If the bowel is healthy perform a Ladd's procedure: mobilise the caecum, straighten the duodenal loop. Run the duodenum down to the RIF, return small bowel to the right side of the abdomen and return large bowel to the left side. Caecum then lies in the LUQ so an appendicectomy is performed. Ladd's procedure stabilises the base of the mesentery by reversing normal rotation preventing further volvulus.

Prognosis depends on how much gut is viable.

Meconium ileus

- Incidence about 1 in 2500
- Associated with cystic fibrosis (CF) – 15% of children with CF present with meconium ileus
- Meconium is thick and viscous because of a lack of pancreatic enzymes; this causes an intraluminal intestinal obstruction in the ileum
- Distended obstructed bowel may perforate or undergo volvulus in utero. Although sterile this causes a vigorous inflammatory reaction associated with calcification in the peritoneal cavity, subsequently visible on AXR

Treatment involves relieving the intestinal obstruction. Provided there is no evidence of intrauterine perforation obstruction may be relieved by Gastrograffin enema. Hypertonic contrast draws fluid into the bowel lumen and its detergent effect loosens inspissated meconium. This is frequently not successful, or meconium ileus is complicated by previous perforation, in which case laparotomy is required.

Following correction of the intestinal obstruction careful management of the CF is required; this involves long-term flucloxacillin (to prevent staphylococcal chest infections) and pancreatic enzyme supplements.

Meconium ileus equivalent (MIE) is a complication in later childhood from inadequate levels of enzymes.

Hirschsprung's disease (HD)

- Incidence is 1 in 5000. Sometimes familial and known association with Down syndrome
- HD is caused by a failure of ganglion cells (neural crest origin) to migrate down the hind-gut. Coordinated peristalsis is impossible without ganglion cells and hence there is a functional intestinal obstruction at the junction (transition zone) between normal bowel and the distal aganglionic bowel. In 80% of cases transition zone is in the rectum or sigmoid – short segment disease; in 20% of cases the entire colon is involved – long segment disease

- Presentation: 99% of normal neonates pass meconium within 24 hours of delivery. HD usually presents within the first few days of life with a low intestinal obstruction, failure to pass meconium, abdominal distension and bile-stained vomiting. Occasionally children with short segment disease escape detection in the neonatal period, presenting later with chronic constipation
- Diagnosis: AXR shows a distal intestinal obstruction and the diagnosis is confirmed by rectal biopsy – no ganglion cells in the submucosa. In neonates rectal suction biopsy is performed, in older children open rectal strip biopsy

Treatment is surgical. Traditionally involving a three-stage procedure: defunctioning colostomy with multiple biopsies to confirm the site of the transition zone, a pull-through procedure to bring ganglionic bowel down to the anus, and finally closure of the colostomy. Many surgeons now perform a single stage pull-through in the neonatal period, managing initial intestinal obstruction with rectal washouts. Long-term results of surgical treatment are satisfactory; about 75% of children have normal bowel control, 15–20% partial control, and 5% never gain control.

The main complication of HD is enterocolitis, a dramatic condition characterised by abdominal distention, bloody watery diarrhoea, circulatory collapse and septicaemia often associated with *Clostridium difficile* toxin on the stools. Mortality from enterocolitis is 10%.

The histopathology is illustrated in Fig. 2.1g.

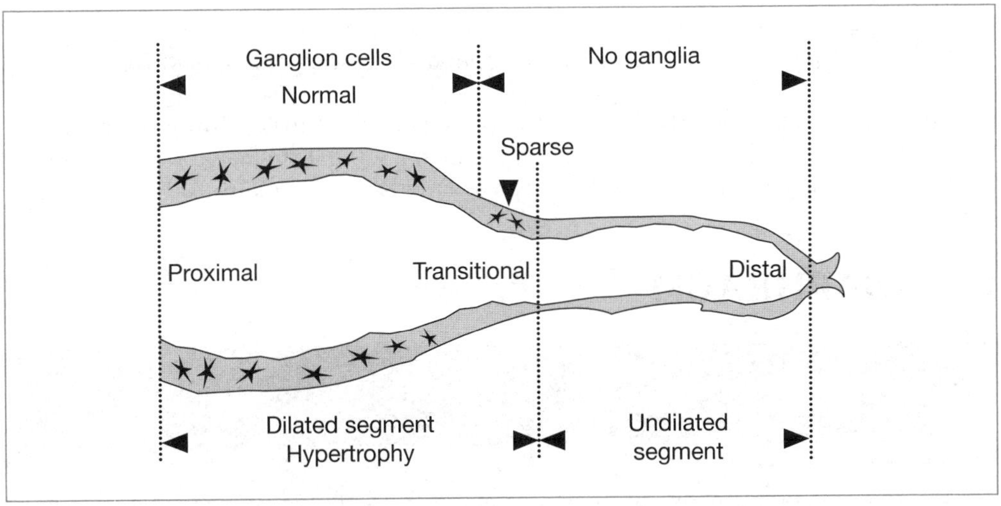

Figure 2.1g *Histopathology of Hirshsprung's disease*

Chapter 10

Necrotising enterocolitis (NEC)

NEC is an acute inflammatory condition of the neonatal bowel which may be associated with areas of bowel necrosis and a systemic inflammatory syndrome. It is more common in premature infants but can also be observed in term babies (incidence 1 in 250 at birth-weight > 1500 g and much higher for babies < 1500 g).

Aetiology is probably multifactorial. Some cases that cluster in epidemics suggest an infectious aetiology; however, a single causative organism has not been identified. Organisms isolated from stool cultures from affected babies are also isolated from healthy babies. The translocation of intestinal flora across an incompetent mucosa may play a role in systemic involvement. Bacteria overwhelm the immature intestine causing local inflammation and a systemic inflammatory response syndrome. Ischaemia and/or reperfusion injury may play a role.

- Symptoms: include feeding intolerance, delayed gastric emptying, abdominal distension and tenderness, ileus, passage of blood per anum (haematochezia). Perforation may occur and cause generalised peritonitis
- Signs: include lethargy, abdominal wall erythema (advanced), gas in the bowel wall and the portal vein, signs of shock (decreased peripheral perfusion, apnoea, cardiovascular collapse)
- Management: supportive: NBM with nutrition delivered parenterally (can cause cholestasis and jaundice); surgical resection is indicated for bowel necrosis and perforation
- Early complications: perforation, sepsis, shock, collapse
- Late complications: strictures, malabsorption syndromes, failure to thrive

Mortality rates range from 10–44% in infants weighing less than 1500 g, compared to 0–20% mortality rate for babies weighing more than 2500 g. Extremely premature infants (1000 g) are particularly vulnerable, with reported mortality rates of 40–100%.

2.2 DIAPHRAGM

In a nutshell ...

The most important neonatal diaphragmatic abnormality is congenital diaphragmatic herniation (CDH) which is associated with pulmonary hypoplasia.

Embryology of the diaphragm

Fig. 2.2a shows the diaphragm in the 4th month of gestation. It develops from the following embryonic structures:

- Transverse septum (the origin of the central tendon)
- Oesophageal (dorsal) mesentery
- Pleuroperitoneal membranes
- 3rd, 4th and 5th cervical somites

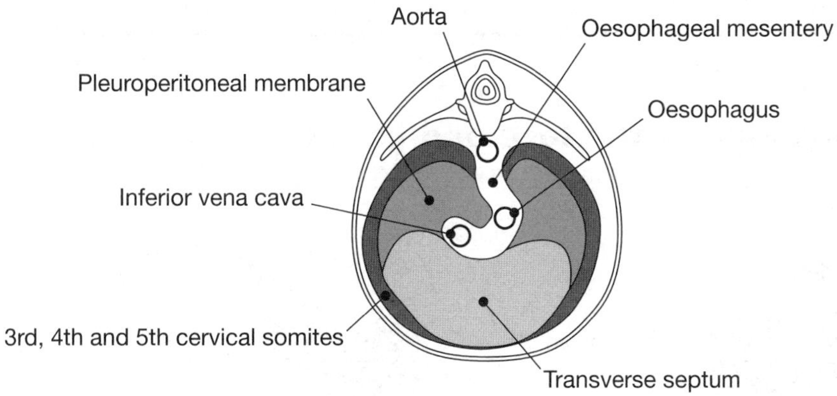

Figure 2.2a *Transverse section of diaphragm at the 4th month of gestation*

Congenital diaphragmatic herniation (CDH)

- Incidence is 1 in 2500
- Main problem is pulmonary hypoplasia and not the diaphragmatic hernia
- Postero-lateral (Bochdalek) defects are most common
- 90% are left-sided
- Anterior (Morgagni) defects are rare
- Most CDHs are now identified on antenatal US
- Initial management consists of endotracheal intubation, paralysis, sedation and mechanical ventilation
- If oxygenation is good (ie pulmonary hypoplasia is not severe) repair of the diaphragmatic defect is undertaken after a few days, either by primary suture or insertion of a prosthetic patch (Gore-Tex™)
- About two-thirds survive and long-term problems are rare

2.3 LIP AND PALATE

In a nutshell ...

Embryological disorders of the lip and palate are common and often need surgical correction. An appreciation of the embryology of the face and palate and an understanding of the main cleft lip and palate abnormalities is probably all you need to know at this stage.

Embryology of the face and palate

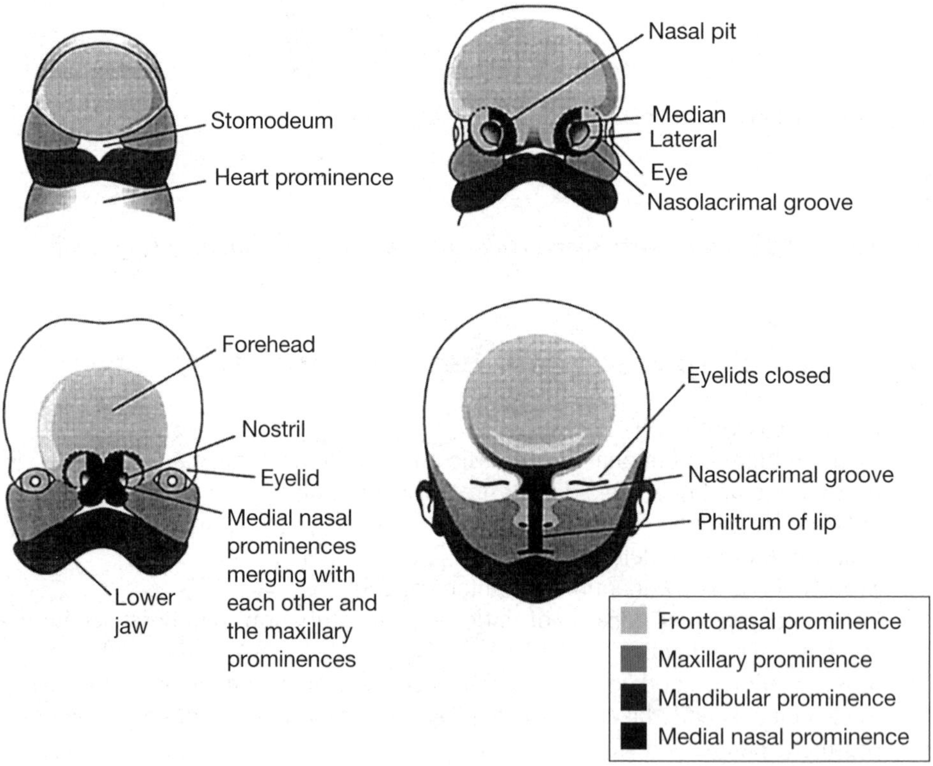

Figure 2.3a *Development of the human face*

Development of the face

The stages of development of the human face are illustrated in Fig. 2.3a. The facial primordia appear in the 4th week around the stomodeum. The five facial primordia are the:

- Frontonasal prominence
- Maxillary prominences (paired)
- Mandibular prominences (paired)

They are active centres of growth and the face develops mainly between the 4th and 8th weeks.

Nasal placodes (the primitive nose and nasal cavities) develop in the frontonasal prominence by the end of the 4th week. The mesenchyme around the placodes proliferates to form elevations, the medial and lateral nasal prominences. The **maxillary prominences** proliferate and grow medially towards each other. This pushes the medial nasal placodes into the mid-line. A groove is formed between the lateral nasal prominence and the maxillary prominence and the two sides of these prominences merge by the end of the 6th week.

As the medial nasal prominences merge they give rise to the **intermaxillary segment**. This develops into the philtrum of the upper lip, septum of the pre-maxilla and the primary palate and nasal septum. The maxillary prominences form the upper cheek and most of the upper lip, whereas the mandibular prominences give rise to the chin, lower lip and lower cheek region.

Development of the palate

The palate develops from the 5th week to the 12th week. It develops from the primary palate and secondary palate. Fig. 2.3b shows the development of the palate. The primary

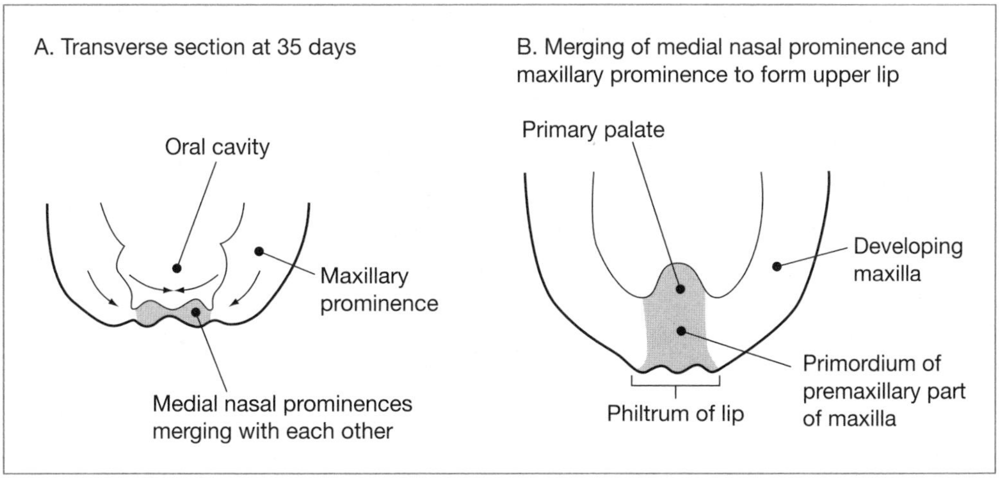

Figure 2.3b *Transverse section through the palate during development*

palate develops from the deep part of the intermaxillary segment of the maxilla, during the merging of the medial nasal prominences. It forms only a small part of an adult's palate. The secondary palate forms the hard and soft palates. It forms from the lateral palatine processes that extend from the internal aspects of the maxillary prominences. They approach each other and fuse in the mid-line, along with the nasal septum and posterior part of the primary palate.

Cleft lip and palate

There are two major groups of cleft lip and palate:

- Clefts involving the upper lip and anterior part of the maxilla, with or without involvement of parts of the remaining hard and soft regions of the palate
- Clefts involving hard and soft regions of the palate

The various types of cleft lip and palate are shown in Fig. 2.3c. Cleft lip and palate is thought to have some genetic basis. Teratogenic factors are largely unknown, but vitamin B complex deficiency in pregnancy may have an aetiological role. The risk of having a second affected child is 4% in comparison to 0.1% in the general population.

- Notochord
- Intra-embryonic mesoderm
- Intra-embryonic coelom
- Neural plate (the ectoderm overlying the notochord)
- Dorsal root ganglia
- Chromaffin tissue in the adrenal medulla
- Melanocytes
- Sheath cells of the peripheral nervous system
- Ganglia of the autonomic nervous system

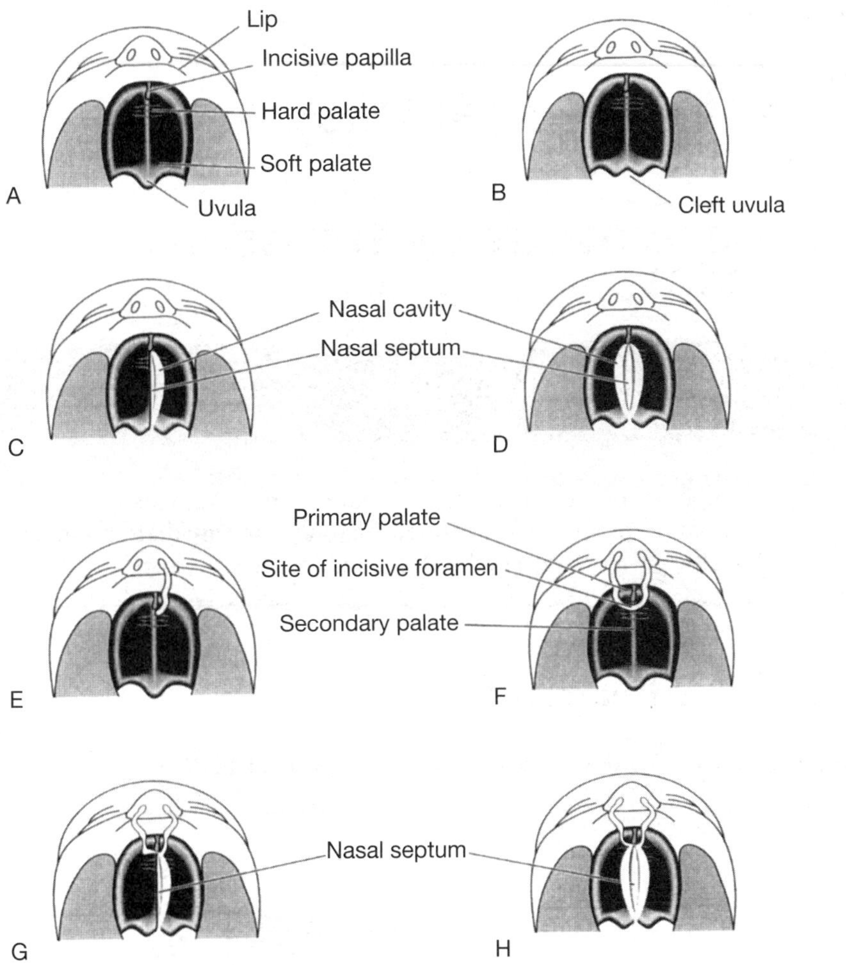

A – Normal lip and palate
B – Cleft uvula
C – Unilateral cleft of the posterior (or secondary) palate
D – Bilateral cleft of the posterior palate
E – Complete unilateral cleft of the lip and alveolar processes of the maxilla with unilateral cleft of the anterior palate
F – As E but bilateral
G – As F plus unilateral cleft of the posterior palate
H – As F plus bilateral cleft of the posterior palate

Figure 2.3c *Types of cleft lip and palate*

Section 3

Paediatric urology

3.1 EMBRYOLOGY OF THE GENITOURINARY TRACT

In a nutshell ...

The development of the urinary and genital system is intimately interwoven. Both develop from a common mesodermal ridge, the **intermediate mesoderm**, which runs along the posterior wall of the abdominal cavity.

Urinary tract embryology

The urinary tract at 5 weeks of development is shown in Fig. 3.1a.

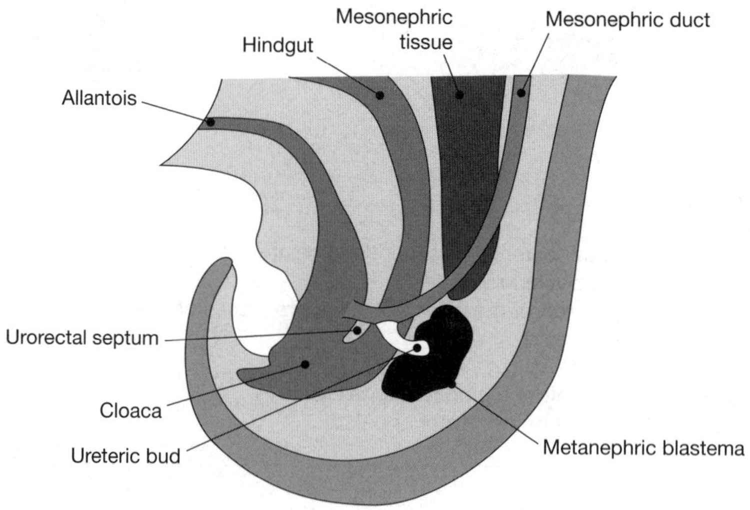

Figure 3.1a *The development of the urinary tract at week 5*

The intermediate mesoderm

The intermediate mesoderm gives rise to three distinct areas, the pronephros, mesonephros and the metanephros. The pronephros and mesonephros represent primitive renal units that disappear ultimately, and the metanephros gives rise to the functioning kidney.

Pronephros

- Extends from the 4th to the 14th somites
- Consists of 6–10 tubular pairs
- Regresses by the end of the 4th week

Mesonephros

- Develops from intermediate mesoderm caudal to the pronephros
- Corresponds to thoracic and upper lumbar segments
- Begins to appear in the 4th week and by 6 weeks forms a large ovoid organ, one on each side of the mid-line
- Lateral to each organ a duct is formed, the **mesonephric duct** (also called the wolffian duct); this drains into the **cloaca**
- By 9 weeks the mesonephric organ has disappeared
- The mesonephric duct plays a role in development of the male genital system but disappears in the female; a bud from it is involved in the formation of the ureter/renal pelvis

Metanephros

- This appears in the 5th week and will give rise to the excretory system of the definitive kidney (see below)

Formation of the definitive kidney

This has two main components:

- The **metanephric organ** gives rise to the excretory system, ie glomeruli and renal tubules all the way to the distal convoluted tubule
- The **ureteric bud** grows out of the mesonephric duct close to its entrance to the cloaca and penetrates the metanephric tissue giving rise to the ureter, the renal pelvis, calyces and the collecting tubules

Nephrons continue to be formed until birth at which time there are about 1 million in each kidney.

The metanephric organ arises in the pelvic region. The kidney comes to lie in the abdomen mainly because of growth of the body in the lumbar and sacral regions. Its blood supply is received sequentially as it ascends directly from the aorta with lower vessels degenerating as new arteries develop above. Abnormalities in ascent are responsible for both **pelvic** kidneys and **horseshoe** kidneys.

Development of the bladder and urethra

The bladder and urethra are derived from the **urogenital sinus**. This is the anterior part of the cloaca, which is separated from the posterior anal canal by the **urorectal septum**.

Three portions of the urogenital sinus can be distinguished:

1. The upper part becomes the urinary bladder; this is initially continuous with the **allantois**. When the allantois is obliterated a thick fibrous cord, the **urachus** remains and connects the apex of the bladder with the umbilicus. In adults it is known as the **median umbilical ligament**
2. The middle narrow part gives rise to the prostatic and membranous parts of the urethra in the male
3. The phallic part develops differently in the two sexes (see below)

Although most of the bladder is derived from the endoderm of the urogenital sinus the **trigone of the bladder is derived from mesoderm**. This is because of absorption of the ureters, which were outgrowths from the mesonephric ducts.

The prostate begins to develop at the end of the 3rd month from outgrowths of endoderm in the prostatic urethra. In the female these outgrowths form the urethral and para-urethral glands.

Genital system embryology

The default situation is female. In the presence of a Y chromosome a testis-determining factor is produced and this leads to male development. The gonads do not acquire male or female morphology until the 7th week.

The development of the urogenital sinus is shown in Fig. 3.1b.

Development of the gonads

These appear initially as a pair of longitudinal ridges medial to the mesonephros. Germ cells migrate here from the yolk sac by amoeboid movement and arrive by the 5th week, invading by the 6th week. At the same time as the germ cells arrive primitive sex cords develop within the gonads.

Testes

- If the germ cells carry an XY sex chromosome complex, **testis-determining factor** is produced and the primitive sex cords proliferate to form the medullary cords. The tunica albuginea forms to separate these from the surface epithelium
- By the 8th week **Leydig cells** in the testis produce testosterone and this influences sexual differentiation of the genital ducts and external genitalia (see below)

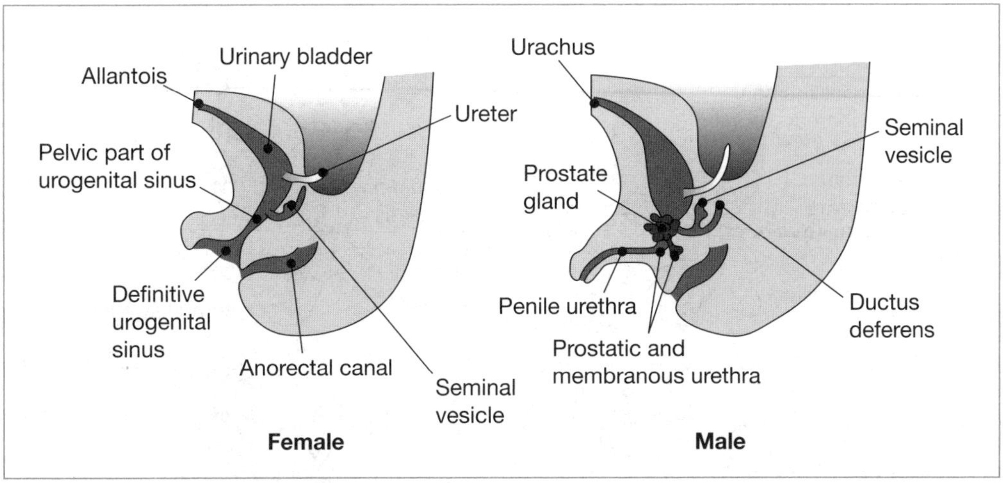

Figure 3.1b *Development of the urogenital sinus*

- The medullary cords remain solid until puberty when they acquire a lumen and form the seminiferous tubules. These join with the excretory tubules of the mesonephric system, which becomes the epididymis, vas deferens, seminal vesicles and ejaculatory ducts

Ovaries

- In the ovary the medullary cords degenerate
- The germ cells become oogonia and these are surrounded by follicular cells

Descent of the gonads

Descent of the testes

The testis is initially an intra-abdominal organ that migrates to the scrotum. The factors that control this are not entirely clear. Abnormalities of descent are important clinically in terms of undescended or ectopic testes. Fig. 3.1c shows the normal descent of the testis.

- The gubernaculum extends from the caudal pole of the testes and extends down to the inguinal region. The testis migrates along this and reaches the inguinal canal by 7 months and the external inguinal ring by 8 months
- During descent the origin of the blood supply to the testis from the lumbar aorta is retained and the testicular vessels lengthen
- An evagination of the abdominal peritoneum, the **processus vaginalis** accompanies the testis as it descends into the scrotum. This evagination forms the **tunica vaginalis**. The processes vaginalis normally closes in the 1st year after birth. If it remains open it can be associated with a congenital inguinal hernia or hydrocele of the testis/cord

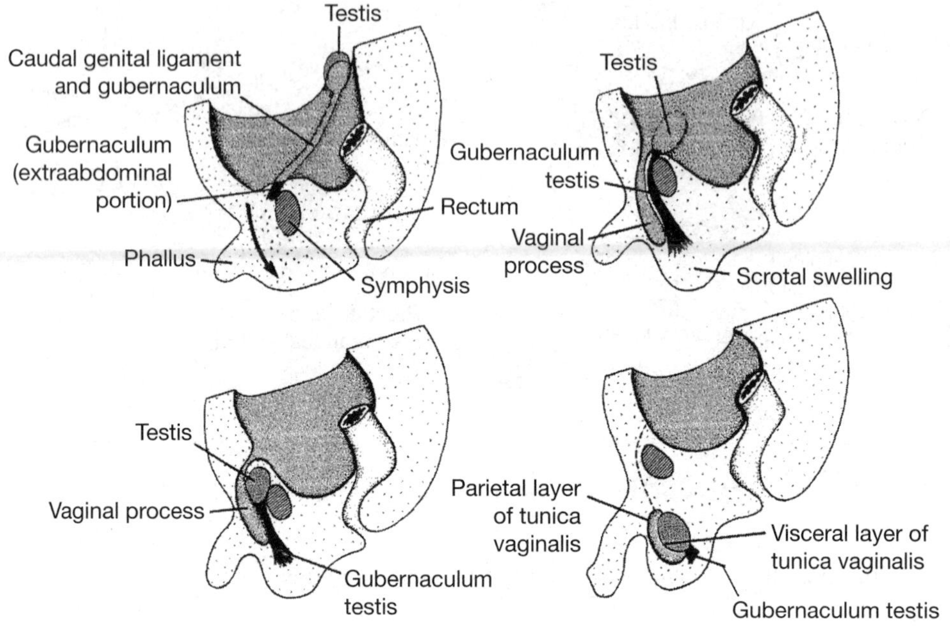

Figure 3.1c *Descent of the testis*

(For discussion of testicular torsion see *Scrotum and penis* in Chapter 11 *Urology and Transplantation*).

Descent of the ovaries

- The ovary becomes attached to the tissues of the genital fold by the gubernaculum and uterovaginal canal, giving rise to the ovarian and round ligaments, respectively
- The mesentery, which descends with the ovary, becomes the broad ligament

The genital duct system

In the indifferent stage of development embryos possess two pairs of genital ducts, mesonephric ducts and **paramesonephric ducts** (also called Müllerian ducts). Essentially the paramesonephric ducts degenerate in the male and the mesonephric ducts degenerate in the female.

Genital ducts in the male

- In the presence of testis-determining factor, **Müllerian inhibiting substance** (MIS) is produced by Sertoli cells in the testis. This causes regression of the

paramesonephric ducts. The only bit that remains is a small portion at their cranial ends, the **appendix testis**
- The mesonephric duct forms the epididymis, the vas deferens, the seminal vesicles and the ejaculatory ducts

Genital ducts in the female

- In the absence of MIS, the paramesonephric ducts remain and develop into the main genital ducts of the female. The upper parts form the uterine tubes (fallopian tubes) and the caudal parts fuse to form the uterine canal
- The upper third of the vagina is also derived from the uterine canal. The lower two-thirds are derived from invagination of the urogenital sinus
- The mesonephric duct system disappears, although occasionally a small caudal portion may remain and later in life this may form a **Gartner's cyst**

Development of the external genitalia

The cloacal folds form around the cloaca and anteriorly these are the **urethral folds** (posteriorly the anal folds). The urethral folds fuse anteriorly to form the **genital tubercle**. **Genital swellings** appear at either side of the urethral folds.

External genitalia in the male

- The genital tubercle becomes the **phallus**
- The urethral folds form the **penile urethra**
- The genital swellings fuse and form the **scrotum**
- Failure of fusion of the urethral folds leads to **hypospadias** – this occurs in 3 in 1000 births

External genitalia in the female

- The genital tubercle elongates only slightly and forms the **clitoris**
- The urethral folds do not fuse as in the male, but develop into the **labia minora**
- The genital swellings enlarge and form the **labia majora**

3.2 CONGENITAL RENAL ABNORMALITIES

In a nutshell ...

Abnormalities of number or size
Renal agenesis and hypoplasia
Supernumerary kidneys

Abnormalities of structure
Aberrant vasculature
Parenchymal anomalies

Abnormalities of ascent
Pelvic kidney
Horseshoe kidney

Bilateral renal agenesis (Potter syndrome)

- Rare – 3.5 in 10 000 births
- Characteristic features are oligohydramnios and secondary characteristic facial appearance
- Pulmonary hypoplasia leads to stillbirth (40%) or death within the first few days

Unilateral renal agenesis

- Incidence 1 in 1100 births
- Often an incidental clinical finding
- Common additional abnormalities include ipsilateral agenesis of vas deferens or ovaries

Aberrant renal vasculature

Aberrant vasculature with multiple arteries or veins is common. This is clearly important to bear in mind during operations on the kidney.

Renal cysts and polycystic kidneys

Cystic disease is the most common space-occupying lesion in the kidney. Cysts may be simple and solitary or part of a polycystic condition. Cystic tumours may also occur (see below).

Simple renal cyst

- May be solitary, multiple or bilateral and are usually benign
- Degenerative cysts can occur in the elderly, lined with cuboidal epithelium
- Asymptomatic unless there is infection or haemorrhage into the cyst
- Complex cysts (calcification, septae) may be associated with malignancy
- Usually untreated unless there is proven tumour or continued symptoms

Infantile polycystic kidneys

This recessive genetic condition causes cystic changes of the renal tubules. Cysts are small and numerous (< 5 mm). Infantile polycystic kidneys cause rapid-onset renal failure and are associated with cystic liver disease with peri-portal fibrosis and portal hypertension.

Adult polycystic kidneys

An autosomal dominant condition causing cystic change in the kidney. Cysts are present at birth and progressively enlarge to compress the renal parenchyma. This occurs at a variable rate and is a common cause of end-stage chronic renal failure (CRF) which often presents in the 4th or 5th decade.

Symptoms

- Abdominal discomfort due to enlarging organs
- Colic and haematuria (spontaneous bleed into cyst)
- Hypertension and CRF

Associations

- Cystic change in other organs (especially liver, spleen and pancreas)
- Berry aneurysms of the circle of Willis
- Mitral valve prolapse

Other cystic conditions

Von Hippel–Lindau syndrome

- Risk of malignant cyst transformation to renal cell carcinoma
- Neurofibromatosis (NF) and cerebral haemangioma

Tuberous sclerosis

- Renal cysts and angiomyolipoma
- Adenoma sebum
- Cerebral hamartoma, retardation and epilepsy

Medullary sponge kidney

- Cystic dilation of the terminal collecting ducts
- Urinary stasis (causes calculi in dilated ducts and infection)
- Often asymptomatic but may have hypercalciuria or renal tubular acidosis

Parenchymal anomalies include lobulation and congenital cysts.

Pelvic kidney

- Arrest of ascent of the kidneys during development causes pelvic kidney
- Incidence 1 in 2500
- More prone to stone disease and infection
- Associated genital abnormalities in 20%

Horseshoe kidney

- Occurs in 1 in 400 individuals
- Fusion occurs before the kidneys have rotated on the long axis and the inferior mesenteric artery (IMA) prevents full ascent
- Blood supply is variable and the horseshoe lies at L3–L5
- Ureter enters bladder ectopically and urinary stasis is common
- May be detected incidentally (33%) or palpated as a mid-line mass
- Complications include UTI, stones and pelvi-ureteric junction (PUJ) obstruction

Crossed renal ectopia

- This is location of a kidney on the opposite side to where its ureter inserts into the bladder.
- It is associated with fusion in 90%
- Most are asymptomatic

3.3 CONGENITAL URETERIC AND URETHRAL ABNORMALITIES

In a nutshell ...

Ureteric congenital abnormalities

- Abnormalities of **number** or **size**
  - Ureteric duplication (unilateral or bilateral)
- Abnormalities of **structure**
  - Ureteric diverticuli

- Ureterocele
- Ectopic and retrocaval ureter
- Abnormalities of **function**
  - Pelvi-ureteric junction obstruction
  - Vesicoureteric reflux (VUR)
  - Urethral congenital abnormalities
- Abnormalities of **structure**
  - Posterior urethral valves
  - Failure of fusion (eg epispadias, hypospadias)

Ureteric duplication

Duplication is common and may predispose to urinary stasis and UTI. It occurs in 1% of the population and is usually unilateral. Most (90%) are incomplete, with fusion of the ureters before the ureteric orifice. In complete duplication, the ureter serving the upper renal moiety will lie distally (Meyer Weigert's law). Renal dysplasia is common in the upper-pole moiety and it is often non-functioning.

Ureterocele

This is cystic dilatation of the intra-mural part of the ureter. It most commonly occurs in association with the upper-pole ureter of a duplex system, but can occur in a single ureter.

Ectopic ureters

Ectopic ureter may drain into the urethra and cause incontinence, commonly presenting in young girls. In boys it may insert into the prostatic urethra and hence continence is preserved. It is diagnosed on IVU and is treated by ureteric re-implantation.

Retrocaval ureter

An abnormality of development of the posterior cardinal veins may lead to the ureter lying behind the IVC and is more common on the right. Compression of the ureter can occur between the IVC and the vertebrae.

Floating kidneys

All kidneys have a small degree of mobility within the abdominal cavity. Occasionally the kidney lies on a fold of peritoneum which acts like a mesentery. This means that the kidney is very mobile and may occasionally cause functional PUJ obstruction.

Pelvi-ureteric junction (PUJ) obstruction

This is a functional obstruction of the ureter at the level of the PUJ that is thought to be congenital in origin. Though it is congenital the problem may not become clinically apparent until later life. 25% of cases are bilateral and boys are more prone to this than girls. It may be due to congenital narrowing, an aperistaltic segment, or kinking of the ureter as it leaves the pelvis. Back pressure causes renal parenchymal damage.

Presentation of PUJ obstruction

- With increasing use of pre-natal US fetal hydronephrosis may be detected, and follow-up of these neonates leads to a diagnosis of PUJ obstruction in 50%
- In children or adults the classic finding is of intermittent abdominal or flank pain. In adults it may occur after ingestion of alcohol for the first time (causes a diuresis and acute renal pelvis distension)
- Other possible presentations are with failure to thrive, recurrent UTIs, or a palpable kidney

Investigation of PUJ obstruction

- **IVU** (intravenous urography) gives classic appearance of a distended pelvicalyceal system with either non-visualisation of the ureter or a ureter of normal calibre. Patients may have a normal IVU in between episodes of pain
- **US** will confirm hydronephrosis but cannot confirm obstruction
- **Diuretic renography** is the gold standard investigation. Isotopes used are DTPA or MAG-3. Frusemide is administered 15 minutes into the investigation to provoke a diuresis. A definitive diagnosis will be obtained in > 90% of patients. The renogram will also provide information on differential renal function

Management of PUJ obstruction

- **Conservative management** may be appropriate in older patients without symptoms. Indications for intervention include:
  - Symptoms
  - Impaired overall renal function
  - Progressive impairment of function on serial scans
  - Development of complications such as stones or infection
- Gold standard treatment is surgical **pyeloplasty** (see Operation Box below)
- **Nephrectomy** may be appropriate if differential function is less than 15%
- Minimally invasive techniques are available and include **endoscopic endopyelotomy** either percutaneously or via the ureteroscope using cautery or laser. An incision is made through the wall of the narrowed segment of the ureter and balloon dilatation is performed. Contrast is injected to confirm that the incision is full thickness. A ureteric stent is then placed between the ureter and renal pelvis across the incision. Healing occurs around the stent which is removed at 6 weeks post-procedure. Minimally invasive measures do not have the same long-term outcome as formal pyeloplasty

Op box: Anderson–Hynes pyeloplasty

Indications
PUJ obstruction.

Pre-op preparation
Prophylactic antibiotic therapy is used for moderate to severe renal pelvic dilatations to reduce the incidence of UTI and damage to the renal parenchyma. Important pre-operative investigations include ultrasonography and renal excretion studies (see above). Consent with intra-operative hazards and post-op complications in mind.

Patient positioning
The procedure is performed under GA. It may be performed open or laparoscopically.

Incision
Flank, dorsal lumbotomy or anterior extraperitoneal approach. Four ports are required for the laparoscopic approach.

Principles of procedure
Essentially the repair consists of transection of the ureter, excision of the narrowed segment, spatulation, and anastomosis to the most dependent portion of the renal pelvis to improve drainage. Anastomosis is performed using fine absorbable sutures and should be watertight and tension free. Placement of a ureteric stent is down to the surgeon's preference (many try to avoid this in children as a further anaesthetic is required to remove the stent).

Intra-operative hazards
Laceration of the vessels to the lower pole (close proximity to the ureter in 40% cases and must be avoided).

Closure
Close in layers with absorbable sutures.

Post-op
Post-operative evaluation is performed by a renal scan or excretory pyelography at 2–3 months. A further evaluation with US is recommended at 12–24 months, but, beyond that, late problems are uncommon in the absence of symptoms. A successful outcome does not always mean an improvement in the differential renal function as measured by renography. In most cases, the pyeloplasty improves the degree of hydronephrosis and washout on the renogram. The symptoms of pain, infection, and haematuria, if present before surgery, resolve along with the improvement of hydronephrosis.

Complications

High success rate (90–95%) with few complications.

Early: anastomotic leak and extravasation of urine

Late: anastomotic stricturing and secondary PUJ obstruction

Vesicoureteric reflux (VUR)

This occurs due to malfunction of a physiological valve at the vesicoureteric junction (VUJ). It may be congenital or acquired secondary to high bladder pressure in neurologic disease or obstruction. It is five times more common in girls, although in the 1st year of life boys predominate.

Renal damage and ureteric dilation occur due to reflux of urine back up the ureter. This is exacerbated if the urine is infected. The condition may disappear spontaneously in many children but ~ 30% develop renal impairment. Although in some cases VUR is diagnosed pre-natally most cases are diagnosed during the investigation of UTI. Management is usually with prophylactic antibiotics; surgery is reserved for patients with breakthrough UTIs or progressive renal damage.

Posterior urethral valves

This is the most common cause of bladder outflow obstruction in boys. Severe forms cause problems in utero with hydronephrosis and oligohydramnios. Less severe obstruction presents later with poor stream, a palpable bladder or non-specific symptoms such as failure to thrive. It is treated with ablation of obstructing valve per urethra.

Epispadias and bladder exstrophy

This results from failed mid-line fusion of mid-line structures below the umbilicus. The bladder mucosa is present as a small plaque on the anterior abdominal wall and the penis is upturned with the meatus opening on to the dorsum. Other features can include split symphysis, low umbilicus, bifid clitoris, apparently externally rotated lower limbs, undescended testes, and poorly developed scrotum. It is more common in boys. **Treatment** is surgical reconstruction of the bladder. However, complications include damage to the upper tracts due to obstruction and reflux and adenocarcinoma of the original bladder mucosa. In adult life, incontinence, renal damage and vaginal stenosis can occur.

Hypospadias

In this condition the external urethral meatus lies on the ventral surface of the penis. Severity varies from a slightly displaced meatus to a perineal meatus (Fig. 3.3a). The incidence is 1 in 125 boys. Associated features include undescended testis, inguinal hernia, bifid scrotum, chordee, and renal and ureteric abnormalities.

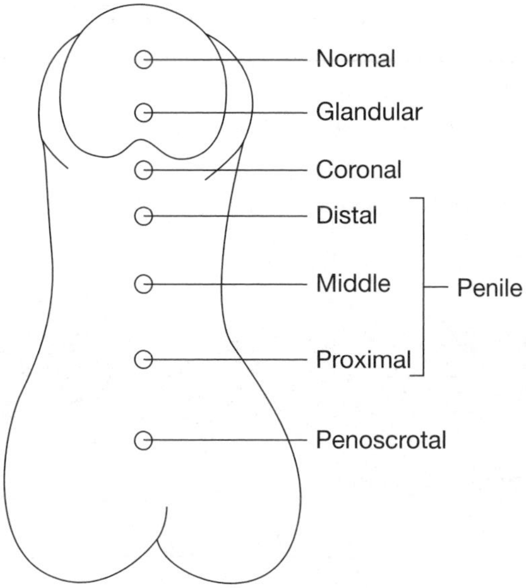

Figure 3.3a *Meatal position in hypospadias*

Classification of hypospadias

These terms describe the position of the meatus after correction of the chordee:

- Glandular
- Coronal
- Anterior penile
- Middle penile
- Posterior penile
- Penoscrotal
- Scrotal
- Perineal

Management of hypospadias

Surgery is performed between the ages of 9 and 18 months and varies according to the classification of the deformity.

- **Meatal advancement and granuloplasty (MAGPI):** this procedure is carried out for glandular abnormalities and consists of creation of a new meatal pit, advancement of the new pit and closure of a sleeve of glandular tissue

- **Mathieu flap:** in coronal hypospadias, a flap is created based on the ectopic meatus; this is folded over and the lateral flaps are closed over the new urethra. Complications of this operation include fistulas and strictures
- **More proximal deformities:** require reconstructive surgery in the form of pedicle grafts, tubes or patches; complications include fistulas, urethral stenosis and meatal regression

3.4 DEVELOPMENTAL ABNORMALITIES OF THE GENITAL TRACT

In a nutshell ...

Disorders of testicular descent
Inter-sex

Undescended testis

Children with a testicle absent from the hemi-scrotum can have:

A **retractile testicle** – sits high in the scrotum or in the inguinal canal but can be milked into the scrotum

An **undescended testicle** – during development the testicle has been arrested somewhere along the course of normal descent

A **maldescended/ectopic** testicle – situated somewhere other than the course of normal descent

A truly **absent testicle** (very rare)

Consider the following.

Is it retractile rather than truly missing?
Parents report seeing it during bath-time. The scrotum is normally developed. The testicle can be felt in the inguinal canal and coaxed into the scrotum on examination. No further intervention is needed – the testicle is likely to descend normally by puberty. Follow-up to check.

Is it undescended in the normal line of descent? (86%)
This carries an increased risk of torsion, malignancy, decreased sperm production and concern to the child. Therefore undescended testes should be re-placed in the scrotum (orchidopexy) in early childhood – ie 2 in the bag by the age of 2.

As surgery is always indicated, investigations such as US (unreliable), MRI and CT (need anaesthetic), and laparoscopy (two-thirds are unnecessary and lead to open surgery) are not indicated. Exploration is via a high inguinal incision allowing first the inguinal canal then the abdominal cavity to be explored.

If a testis is located and is dysplastic it must be removed. If normal, it must be re-placed in the scrotum. Testicular biopsy is not indicated. Cord length is a limitation in orchidopexy, and a two-stage approach may be needed. Alternatively, use the Fowler–Stephen's procedure, which is ligation of the testicular vessels leaving the testicle dependent upon collateral supply to the vas deferens. The orchidopexy is carried out later, but success rates are about 50%.

Is it maldescended or ectopic (not in the normal line of descent? (2%)
See Fig. 3.4a. Management is as for undescended testicles.

Is it truly absent? (6%)
This is usually the result of pre-natal torsion and is the cause of more than half of all truly impalpable testes. It can usually only be confirmed at operation when the testicular vessels and vas end blindly. Any tissue at the distal end of the cord should be excised to avoid a chance of malignancy. Bilateral cryptorchidism should be examined carefully for hormonal or inter-sex abnormalities.

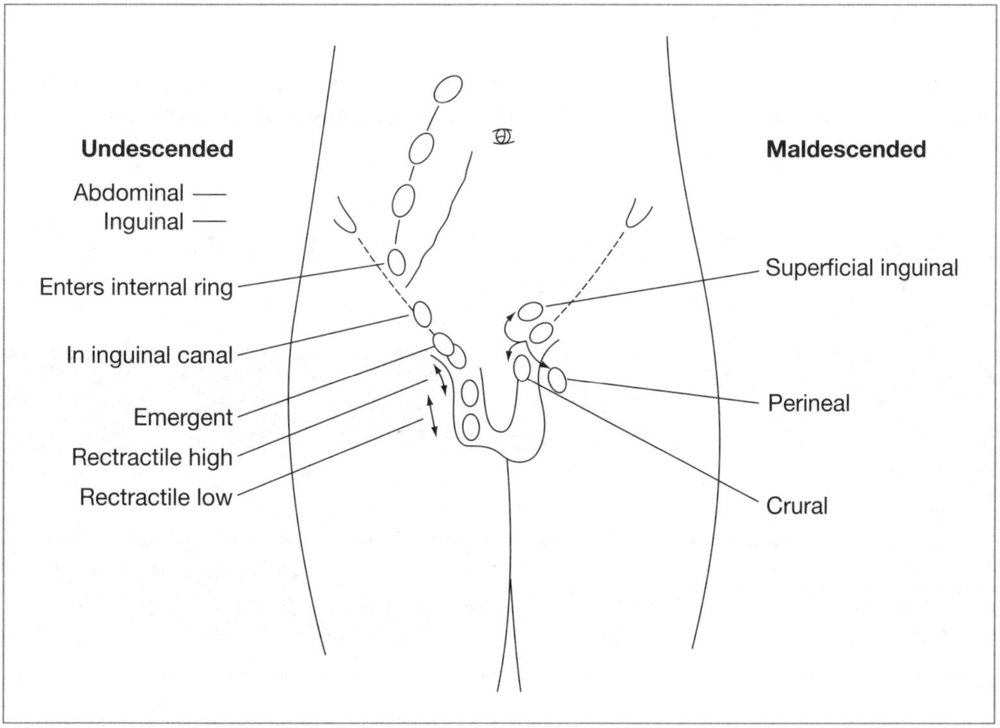

Figure 3.4a *Ectopic positions for an incompletely descended or maldescended testicle*

For discussion of testicular torsion see section 3.8.

Inter-sex

Congenital adrenal hyperplasia (CAH)

This is an autosomal recessive disorder characterised by the absence of certain enzymes in the pathway of cortisol and aldosterone synthesis from cholesterol. It results in excess androgen levels and therefore virilisation in affected females. Affected males may present with adrenal crisis early in life. The most common form is 21-hydroxylase deficiency. Management consists of IV fluids, glucose, and hydrocortisone. Long-term management includes hydrocortisone and surgical correction of virilised external genitalia in females in the 1st year.

Klinefelter syndrome

In this condition males have an extra X chromosome – 47, XXY. The incidence is 1 in 1000 boys. Clinical features include increased height, mild mental retardation, gynaecomastia and infertility. The testes may be small and incompletely descended.

Testicular feminisation

Affected individuals are chromosomally XY but present as females due to complete androgen insensitivity of the genitalia. Patients may present with an inguinal hernia containing a testis or later in life with amenorrhoea.

3.5 GENETIC ABNORMALITIES OF THE UROGENITAL TRACT

In a nutshell ...

The *WT 1* gene is a suppressor gene coding for Wilms tumour (see section 4 *Paediatric oncology*). It is a transcription protein that is expressed primarily in the developing gonads and embryonic kidneys to regulate expression of its target genes. These genes are responsible for differentiation of the renal epithelial cells during development.

Denys–Drash syndrome (DDS)

Denys–Drash is a very rare syndrome caused by point mutations of the *WT 1* gene. It is a triad of:

- Congenital nephropathy (mesangial sclerosis)
- Wilms tumour
- Inter-sex disorders (gonadal dysgenesis with male pseudo-hermaphroditism)

WAGR syndrome

This is due to the complete deletion of the *WT 1* gene and the contiguous loss of neighbouring genes in this region of chromosome 11. WAGR syndrome affects the development of seemingly disparate areas of the body, including the kidney, the genitourinary system, the iris of the eye, and the central nervous system (CNS). It consists of:

- Wilms tumour
- Aniridia
- Genitourinary malformations (structural urinary tract abnormalities without nephropathy)
- Mental retardation

3.6 FORESKIN ABNORMALITIES IN CHILDREN

In a nutshell ...

Phimosis
Balanophosthitis
BXO

Anatomy of the foreskin

The foreskin consists of a single layer of skin which is adherent to the shaft of the penis and is folded over at the end to create the meatus or preputial orifice. The inner layer of the foreskin is called the mucosal layer. In neonates the prepuce is adherent to the glans and does not begin to separate until the age of 1 year. The spontaneous separation of the glans and prepuce may not be complete until age 5 or older, when the dense fibrous adhesions gradually disappear.

Phimosis

The normal infantile adhesion of the prepuce to the glans is referred to as a 'physiological' phimosis. On examination of the normal infant foreskin it has a narrow, blanching bottle-neck appearance and is soft and unscarred. A pathological or 'true' phimosis is due to infection or disease and is characterised by pale hard tissue at the preputial orifice. A 'para-phimosis' occurs when a retracted foreskin has not been correctly replaced, leaving a tight and irreducible band around the penis at the level of the coronal sulcus complicated by preputial and glandular oedema.

Ballooning of the foreskin occurs when urine becomes trapped during micturition. It may then discharge later and can present as wetting. It is otherwise asymptomatic and resolves spontaneously and so is not an indication for circumcision.

Balanoposthitis

This is an acute pyogenic infection of the prepuce. It is commonest in under 5s with non-retractile foreskins. It is treated with antibiotics.

Balanitis xerotica obliterans (BXO)

This affects 0.6% of boys aged up to 15 years. Scarring and collagen deposition occurs on the glans and foreskin. The aetiology is unknown. BXO is the usual cause of 'true phimosis'. It may affect urethra and be associated with strictures. Treatment is circumcision.

Circumcision

Every year many children are circumcised unnecessarily. The normal infant prepuce is not designed to retract from an early age: it is designed to protect the glans from contact with urine in the nappy. A non-retractile prepuce is not an indication for circumcision in young children.

Procedure box: Circumcision

Indications
True phimosis, recurrent balanoposthitis, balanitis xerotica obliterans, recurrent UTIs, religious reasons.

Pre-op preparation and consent
The procedure is usually performed under GA but in very rare cases it may be performed using regional anaesthesia in a penile block. It is commonly performed as a day case.

Patient position
Supine.

Procedure
The penis and foreskin are thoroughly cleaned to remove smegma (cleaning may have to be resumed after the initial incision if the foreskin is very tight). The two layers of the foreskin are cut vertically from the preputial orifice towards the coronal sulcus. The distal skin is then removed circumferentially in layers using scissors, being careful to leave sufficient skin in place for suturing (and in adults, for erection). Bleeding is controlled with bipolar diathermy. The frenular artery may require a suture.

Closure
The edges of the skin are then sutured together using a fine absorbable suture. The suture line is dressed with Gelonet™ and loose coverings.

Intra-operative hazards
Damage to the penile head.

Complications

- Haemorrhage (usually from the frenular artery; often stops with prolonged compression but may require return to theatre)
- Wound infection (uncommon, but may occur)
- Acute retention of urine from pain

Alternatives to circumcision

- Low-dose steroids may speed up separation of preputial adhesions
- Prepucioplasty allows preservation of the foreskin

3.7 URINARY TRACT INFECTIONS (UTIs) IN CHILDREN

In a nutshell ...

UTIs are common in children but may indicate an underlying renal tract abnormality, so need further investigation in the form of urinalysis and ultrasound. Certain groups of children need further investigation. The pathogen is usually *E. coli* and the management is antibiotics and appropriate investigation.

Epidemiology of UTIs in children

Incidence throughout childhood is 5% in girls and 1.5% in boys. UTIs, however, are commoner in boys in the first 12 months of life.

Pathogenesis of UTIs in children

E. coli is the causative organism in 85% of cases. 30–50% of patients investigated for UTI are found to have some underlying urinary tract abnormality but it is doubtful whether all of these are actually responsible for the urinary tract infections. The commonest abnormality found is VUR and this is found in 30% of patients presenting with UTI.

Presentation of UTIs in children

Clinical features often are non-specific particularly in children under the age of 2. Older children have symptoms similar to those found in adults.

Presentation of UTIs in children

Infection
Haematuria
Lethargy
Failure to thrive
Vomiting
Pain
Mass
Abdominal distension

Investigating UTIs in children

It is important to be careful during specimen collection because over-diagnosis of UTI is common due to contamination and leads to unnecessary investigation in many children. Options in very young children include:

- Clean-catch urine in boys
- Collection bags (the routine method)
- Suprapubic aspiration (sometimes required)

All children – regardless of gender – merit investigation after a single proven UTI. Standard tests would include urine analysis and US. US will detect renal dilatation and most urinary calculi and may show renal scarring. US is frequently unreliable in diagnosing both VUR and renal scarring however and further investigation is indicated in:

- All children aged < 2
- Those aged > 2 with febrile infections
- Those with a positive family history of VUR

Further investigations would include:

- **DMSA scintigraphy:** to look for renal scarring
- **Micturating cystography:** this is indicated in all three groups mentioned above and also most children who have scarring on DMSA cystography

There are two main methods for performing a micturating cystogram:

- Contrast cystography which requires urethral catheterisation and is the only method that is accurate in children aged < 4
- Indirect MAG-3 cystography which relies on radioisotope accumulation in the bladder and requires co-operation of the child. It is less invasive than contrast cystography but is relatively insensitive for detecting lesser grades of reflux. It is a standard investigation for follow-up of patients with reflux

Management of UTIs in children

In the acute setting, antibiotic treatment is clearly required and this may be oral or intravenous depending on the severity of the infection. Prophylactic antibiotics are often then prescribed until investigations are completed as there is a risk of continued renal scarring. Further management depends on any other abnormalities found on investigation.

3.8 THE ACUTE SCROTUM IN CHILDHOOD

In a nutshell ...

Acute scrotal pain may also present as lower abdominal pain so always examine the genitalia. Causes of acute scrotal pain in children are:

- **Torsion**
  - Testis
  - Hydatid of Morgagni
- **Infection**
  - Epididymitis
  - Orchitis

- Incarcerated hernia
- Patent processus vaginalis (congenital hydrocele)
- Testicular tumour
- Idiopathic scrotal oedema
- Henoch–Schönlein purpura

Because of the consequences of untreated torsion THE ACUTE TESTICLE IN A CHILD SHOULD ALWAYS BE REFERRED TO A UROLOGIST IMMEDIATELY AND MAY NEED EMERGENCY SURGERY WITHIN THE HOUR.

For in-depth discussion of the pathology, diagnosis and management of these conditions in the adult (see Chapter 11 *Urology and Transplantation*).

Specific differences in children

Torsion

Testicular torsion accounts for 30% of cases of acute scrotum in boys aged < 10 years (and 90% of adult cases of torsion). The hydatid of Morgagni is present in 90% of boys and torsion of this embryological remnant accounts for 60% of the cases of acute scrotum in children. Just prior to puberty the hormonal changes cause an increase in size of the hydatid and it is more prone to torsion. When infarcted it may be seen through the skin as a blue dot on top of a normally lying and non-tender testis. At surgical exploration the hydatid is excised but, unlike torsion of the testis itself, there is no requirement for contralateral scrotal exploration.

Infection

Epididymitis occurs in infancy and the teenage years (due to reflux of infected urine retrogradely through the vas deferens) Torsion of the testis must be excluded by ultrasonography and a UTI demonstrated if possible. Orchitis is very rare before puberty.

Other differences

- Patent processus vaginalis (congenital hydrocele)
- Infantile hydroceles are common
- Caused by failure of the processus vaginalis to obliterate after testicular descent through the inguinal canal

- Clinical signs are identical to adults (see the *Paediatric* section of *Urology and Transplantation*)
- Most resolve by the 2nd year and those that do not should be treated surgically with an inguinal canal ligation
- Scrotal exploration is doomed to failure in children

Testicular tumours have a peak incidence at 2 years and during puberty. Henoch–Schönlein purpura is a vasculitis and presents with a purpuric rash on the legs and buttocks. The rash may also affect the scrotum and cause testicular tenderness. It is usually managed conservatively but sometimes requires steroids.

Section 4
Paediatric oncology

In a nutshell ...

The surgical syllabus requires a basic knowledge of the childhood malignancies you may come across, their clinical features, investigation and principles of management.

4.1 INVESTIGATIONS IN PAEDIATRIC ONCOLOGY

In a nutshell ...

Blood tests
- AFP
- β-HCG
- VMA
- Catecholamines

Imaging
- USS
- X-rays
- Angiography
- CT
- MRI
- MIBG scintigraphy

Alpha-fetoprotein (AFP)

AFP level is used for the diagnosis of:

- Tumours of the ovary or testis
- Liver tumours
- Sacrococcygeal teratomas

And for any other masses which could be teratomas or germ cell tumours (eg mediastinal, retroperitoneal).

AFP levels are also used to monitor the response to chemotherapy or monitor disease after surgical resection of mature teratomas. It is difficult to interpret in the newborn and does not fall to normal adult levels until around 6 months of age.

- Normal ranges for infants have been developed
- Normal adult levels are < 10 kU/L

Beta human chorionic gonadotrophin (β-hCG)

- Normally < 5 mIU/mL
- May be raised in patients with germ cell tumours
- Raised in pregnancy

Vanillylmandelic acid (VMA)

- Raised in patients with neuroblastoma

Catecholamines

Phaeochromocytomas can secrete epinephrine (adrenaline), norepinephrine (noradrenaline), dopamine, metanephrine and normetanephrine.

Most labs will give the dopamine, norepinephrine (noradrenaline) and epinephrine (adrenaline) levels routinely. For phaeochromocytoma it is better to take a timed 24-hour specimen as secretion can be intermittent and a spot urine may therefore be misleadingly normal.

- Increased urinary catecholamine metabolites can be detected in about 90% of patients with neuroblastoma
- Dopamine, HVA (homovanillic acid) or HMMA (4-hydroxy-3-methoxymandelic acid) may also be raised in neuroblastoma. Spot urine tests are adequate for detecting raised levels

Ultrasound scanning (USS) in paediatric oncology

Used initially for flank masses to try and distinguish between Wilms, neuroblastoma and hepatoblastoma. Distinction between Wilms and neuroblastoma is important as the technique of biopsy is different. Wilms tumour should be a needle biopsy (an open biopsy would upstage the tumour) whereas a 1 cm^3 sample is needed for the diagnosis of neuroblastoma because cytogenetics is essential in determining treatment.

- **RUQ masses:** USS of RUQ masses should be able to tell whether the mass is within the liver or not. If a kidney is pushed down by the mass but is intact then neuroblastoma is more likely. Wilms tumour usually replaces the whole of the kidney which is therefore not indentifiable. CT will give further information

- **Wilms tumour:** USS should be used in Wilms tumour to determine whether the renal vessels are patent and if blood flow is normal. Tumour in the renal vein or vena cava is important in the staging of Wilms tumour
- **Abdominal tumours:** Also in liver tumours, tumour in the extra-hepatic vasculature is very important in staging. Therefore, USS with Doppler should be performed for abdominal tumours
- **Masses in the limbs:** USS is the initial investigation for masses in the limbs in order to determine whether the mass is solid or cystic and whether there is blood flow within the mass
- **Pelvic tumours:** USS is useful alongside CT in imaging pelvic tumours such as rhabdomyosarcomas or gonadal tumours

X-rays in paediatric oncology

Plain X-rays are the initial investigation for chest masses particularly to exclude any airway compression. Plain X-rays of the abdomen may identify calcification in an abdominal neuroblastoma – but CT is much more useful now. X-rays of limbs in soft tissue tumours may identify any bony destruction but MRI is much more sensitive.

Angiography in paediatric oncology

Used to aid the surgeon prior to complex resections such as partial hepatectomy.

Computerised tomography (CT) in paediatric oncology

Used for abdominal tumours to distinguish between Wilms tumour and neuroblastoma. Essential for staging as CT will identify whether there is significant local lymphadenopathy. CT is also used for pelvic tumours such as ovarian germ cell tumours and for staging of testicular tumours (looking for lymphadenopathy). Chest CT is used for staging of any tumours likely to metastasise to the chest (eg Wilms tumour, sarcoma, hepatoblastoma, neuroblastoma).

Magnetic resonance imaging (MRI) in paediatric oncology

This has replaced CT for limb tumours such as soft tissue sarcomas. It is also superior to CT for imaging nasopharyngeal tumours such as nasopharyngeal rhabdomyosarcoma and carcinoma (particularly important for identifying the extent eg invasion of the base of skull). MRI is the investigation of choice for para-spinal tumours (such as neuroblastoma, ganglioneuroma, para-spinal rhabdomyosarcoma) and to identify whether there is intra-spinal extension.

Meta-iodobenzylguanidine (MIBG) scintigraphy in paediatric oncology

This is used for staging of neuroblastoma and phaeochromocytoma. It is indicated to evaluate bone and soft tissue sites of disease; it is taken up by catecholaminergic cells (which includes most neuroblastomas) and can therefore be used to assess both the primary site and metastatic sites. 99m-Tc-diphosphonate scintigraphy is used to assess bony metastases and is indicated for all tumours which can metastasise to bone (neuroblastoma, sarcoma).

4.2 CHEMOTHERAPY AND RADIOTHERAPY IN PAEDIATRIC ONCOLOGY

In a nutshell ...

Chemotherapy has a tremendously important role in virtually all malignant tumours in children.

- Most childhood tumours are chemosensitive
- Chemotherapy may be used pre-operatively or post-operatively
- Like adults, children are susceptible to **general** and **organ-specific** complications

Radiotherapy may be indicated for incompletely resected childhood tumours and some metastases.

Principles of chemotherapy in paediatric oncology

Most paediatric tumours are chemosensitive (including Wilms, neuroblastoma, hepatoblastoma, rhabdomyosarcoma, and germ cell tumour) – even for stage 1 completely resected tumours the addition of some chemotherapy will improve survival.

Many tumours are treated with neo-adjuvant chemotherapy (ie tumours are biopsied and then treated with chemotherapy to shrink the tumour prior to surgery).

After resection the child will have further chemotherapy (adjuvant chemo) to ensure that there is no microscopic residual disease.

Main general complications of chemotherapy in paediatric tumours

- Bone marrow suppression
- Sepsis
- Bleeding
- Nausea and vomiting

Organ-specific complications of chemotherapy in paediatric tumours

- Nephrotoxicity
- Ototoxicity
- Hepatotoxicity
- Cardiac toxicity

Radiotherapy in paediatric oncology

Indications for radiotherapy in paediatric oncology

- Radiotherapy is indicated for incompletely resected tumours (Wilms, neuroblastoma, rhabdomyosarcoma)
- Chest radiotherapy is also used for some chest metastases (sarcoma, Wilms tumour)

Principles of radiotherapy in paediatric oncology

- Usually to treat the initially involved area even when initial chemotherapy has resulted in reduction of tumour volume
- Given in fractions on a daily basis
- Young children need a daily GA
- Dose is calculated based on the radiosensitivity and the normal tissue tolerance

Complications of radiotherapy in paediatric oncology

- In the short term skin erythema is common and uncomfortable
- Irradiation of the abdomen involving bowel can cause diarrhoea and mucositis
- Late complications include bowel strictures
- Outside the CNS the main long-term consequences are poor tissue growth resulting in cosmetic problems

Specific paediatric cancers needing surgery

In a nutshell ...

Liver tumours
Rhabdomyosarcoma
Neuroblastoma
Nephroblastoma (Wilms)
Germ cell tumours

Liver tumours (hepatoblastoma and hepatocellular carcinoma)

The median age for hepatoblastoma is 1 year and for hepatocellular carcinoma (HCC) 12 years. They present with an abdominal mass. Hepatoblastoma is a chemosensitive tumour which can occur in association with Beckwith–Wiedemann syndrome.

Staging of liver tumours

- Serum AFP both to aid diagnosis and for monitoring response to treatment, and for follow-up to identify relapse plus CT or MRI scan of the liver and CT of the chest to identify metastases
- Staging of hepatoblastoma is using the PRETEXT system, which considers the number of liver segments involved and whether there is hepatic vein or portal vein involvement

Diagnosis of liver tumours

- By liver needle biopsy, following which patients are treated with chemotherapy. Follow-up imaging prior to tumour resection should be with MRI scan to identify exactly the surgery required to ensure a complete resection

Treatment of liver tumours

- Further chemotherapy is given following resection to treat any microscopic residual tumour
- Successful treatment requires complete surgical excision
- If complete resection is not possible liver transplantation is indicated if disease is localised to the liver
- Overall outlook is very good at over 80%, and even for the most advanced stage survival is about 70%

Rhabdomyosarcoma

Arising from striated muscle, this tumour is the most common soft tissue sarcoma of childhood. It can develop even in sites where striated muscle is not normally found, such as the bladder. It can therefore arise from virtually any site in the body.

Presentation of rhabdomyosarcoma

- Depends on the site, but can vary from a mass in the limbs, a nasopharyngeal tumour presenting with unilateral nasal obstruction and bleeding, to haematuria or urinary obstruction if the tumour is located in the bladder or prostate
- Para-testicular tumours present with a testicular mass

Prognosis of rhabdomyosarcoma

- Depends on the site (eg orbital rhabdomyosarcoma has an excellent outcome), surgical resectability, and histological subtype
- The embryonal subtype has a better prognosis than the alveolar, which has a greater propensity for dissemination
- Head and neck tumours and tumours of the genito-urinary tract are rarely alveolar
- Varies from > 90% for orbital rhabdomyosarcoma to < 10% for widely metastatic alveolar rhabdomyosarcoma

Investigating rhabdomyosarcoma

- Initial investigations include CT or MRI of the primary tumour and identification of local lymphadenopathy
- Bone scan and bone marrow biopsy and CT of the chest for staging
- Various staging systems have been devised and many are based on the degree of surgical removal; the TNM staging system is based on pre-treatment assessment and has also been applied to paediatric sarcomas

Treatment of rhabdomyosarcoma

- Consists of a diagnostic biopsy followed by chemotherapy
- The tumour is resected after shrinkage with chemotherapy
- Complete resection is extremely important for survival and if this is not possible post-op radiotherapy will be needed to ensure adequate local control
- Chemotherapy is also essential to treat metastatic disease. Individual sites of metastatic disease should also be treated with radiotherapy (eg lung metastases and bone metastases)
- Disease which has disseminated to the bone marrow has a poor outlook. Treatment is intensified in this situation using myeloablative chemotherapy

Neuroblastoma

Neuroblastoma is the most common extracranial solid tumour in childhood. It arises from primordial neural crest cells (adrenal medulla and sympathetic ganglia anywhere from the ethmoid to the pelvis). Neuroblastoma displays a diverse clinical behaviour from spontaneous regression and maturation to ganglioglioma in some infants, to widely metastatic malignant behaviour in older children. Patients may present with an abdominal mass, a para-spinal mass, or often symptoms of disseminated disease such as bone marrow failure due to marrow infiltration.

Investigating neuroblastoma

- At presentation this should include: CT scan of the primary tumour to determine whether there is local lymphadenopathy; MRI scan if the tumour is para-spinal to exclude spinal cord compression; MRI of the head if there are deposits obvious such as proptosis; MIBG scan, bone scan, bone marrow aspirate and biopsy and urine catecholamines
- The primary tumour should be biopsied using an open biopsy approach to ensure sufficient tissue is obtained for a fresh sample to be sent to cytogenetics as well as to the histopathologist for diagnosis.

Staging of neuroblastoma

- A specific staging system has been devised – the international neuroblastoma staging system (INSS)
- In infants, stage IVs is a distinct entity with disseminated disease, lack of adverse cytogenetics (ie lack of mycN amplification and other typical poor prognostic cytogenetic abnormalities) and the potential for spontaneous resolution without chemotherapy
- Stage IVs is defined by stage I or II local disease with distant disease in the skin, bone marrow and liver but without bone metastases

Treatment of neuroblastoma

- Localised neuroblastoma stage I or II can be treated with surgical resection alone if the cytogenetics are favourable
- Stage III and IV disease requires intensive chemotherapy followed by surgery after tumour response
- Children with stage IV disease have a poor outlook and are therefore treated aggressively with myeloablative chemotherapy after the delayed surgical resection to try to eliminate microscopic residual disease. This has improved the outcome somewhat

Wilms tumour (nephroblastoma)

This is the most common primary malignant renal tumour of childhood, representing 8% of solid tumours in children. Wilms tumours tend to present at age 3–4 with fever, abdominal swelling and/or haematuria. 5–10% of these tumours are bilateral. They are of embryonic origin and thought to be due to a loss of a tumour suppressor gene on chromosome 11 (the *WT-1* gene).

- May occur as part of a syndrome WAGR (**W**ilms, **a**niridia, **g**enito-urinary **a**bnormalities and mental **r**etardation)
- May also be a part of Denys–Drash syndrome or associated with hemi-hypertrophy

Investigating Wilms tumour

- CT of primary and the chest to identify lung metastases
- Also USS with Dopplers to exclude tumour in the renal vein or vena cava
- Diagnosis is by needle biopsy to exclude other rarer renal tumours
- Open biopsy would upstage the tumour and should be avoided

Treatment of Wilms tumour

- Chemotherapy prior to a delayed surgical resection
- The tumour is often separated from the rest of the kidney by a pseudocapsule although this may be breached by very aggressive tumours
- Radiotherapy to the tumour bed is indicated if the tumour is not completed microscopically excised. Radiotherapy to the lungs is also indicated if there has been lung metastases
- Further chemotherapy after tumour excision, depending on the post-surgical stage
- Partial nephrectomy is only considered if there is bilateral disease, in order to retain some renal tissue

Prognosis of Wilms tumour

- Outlook is very good with survival greater than 90% for stages I and II, > 80% for stage III and about 65% for stage IV (distant metastatic tumour)
- Anaplastic variants of Wilms tumour have a poorer prognosis than classic Wilms tumour

Germ cell tumours

Germ cell tumours can be benign or malignant, within the gonads or extra-gonadal. They arise from pluripotential or primordial germ cells.

Sacrococcygeal teratomas are the most common of the germ cell tumours; 80% of sacrococcygeal teratomas are benign. Presentation is with an obvious mass but some can be entirely pre-sacral without an external mass. These may present with constipation, urinary frequency or lower-extremity weakness. Treatment is surgical resection including the coccyx in the neonatal period. Follow-up should include AFP measurement. Any rise above the normal value for gestational age would indicate relapse of the malignant yolk sac tumour.

Other germ cell tumours include **germinomas**, which most commonly arise in the ovary, anterior mediastinum or in the pineal gland, and can also arise in undescended testes. AFP may be negative in pure germinomas but these are often mixed tumours and therefore other elements of the tumour may produce AFP. **Embyronal carcinomas** are negative for AFP. **Endodermal sinus tumours** (yolk sac tumours) are the most common malignant germ cell tumours in paediatrics. They can arise in the sacrococcygeal area or the ovary in older children and are AFP-positive. **Teratomas** arise from the three germinal layers and can therefore be composed of a wide variety of tissues. They can be mature, immature or with malignant components.

All of these germ cell tumours can present with a mass in the ovary, testis, retroperitoneum or sacrococcygeal region. Those in the chest may be an incidental finding on CXR or present with symptoms of tracheal compression.

Staging of germ cell tumours

- Various staging systems exist but generally are they staged on surgical resectability and the presence or absence of distant metastases
- Spread is to local lymph nodes, lung or liver

Treatment of germ cell tumours

- Benign tumours are treated with surgical resection alone
- Malignant germ cell tumours should be resected totally if possible, followed by chemotherapy, followed by definitive surgery if residual tumour is still present

Prognosis of germ cell tumours

- These are chemosensitive and outlook is generally good (overall > 80% survival)

Section 5
Paediatric general surgery

In a nutshell ...

The field of paediatric general surgery is worthy of an entire textbook in its own right, but for the MRCS exam you should have an appreciation of a few important topics which we have highlighted here. Many of these conditions are covered in more detail in other sections of this book and its companion volume.

General surgical conditions in children
- Pyloric stenosis
- Groin hernia (see also *Abdomen* in Book 2)
- Umbilical conditions
  - Umbilical site problems
  - Umbilical hernia (see also *Abdomen* in Book 2)

Jaundice in neonates
- Biliary atresia
- Choledochal cysts

Conditions causing acute abdominal pain in children (see also *Abdomen* in Book 2)
- Appendicitis
- Gastroenteritis
- Bacterial enterocolitis
- Intussusception
- Malrotation and volvulus
- Bleeding or infected Meckel's diverticulum
- Constipation
- Mesenteric adenitis
- UTI (see *Paediatric Urology* section in this chapter)
- Testicular torsion (see section 8.4 in *Urology and Transplantation*)
- Obstructed/strangulated hernia

For other paediatric conditions see the appropriate chapter (eg for thyroglossal cyst see *Ear, Nose and Throat, Head and Neck* in Book 2).

5.1 PYLORIC STENOSIS

In a nutshell ...

This is a hypertrophy of the circular pyloric muscles that causes gastric outlet obstruction. Its aetiology is unknown. It affects 1 in 300 newborns, is four times commoner in males, and it presents with projectile non-bilious vomiting in the first 2 months of life. Treatment is surgical pyloromyotomy.

Clinical features of pyloric stenosis

- Gradual onset non-bilious vomiting between 3–6 weeks of age – becomes projectile. Symptoms may start earlier but are very rare after 3 months. In between vomiting the baby feeds hungrily
- May be severe dehydration
- Hypochloraemic hypokalaemic metabolic alkalosis: baby vomits repeatedly losing H^+ ions; kidney compensates by exchanging potassium and sodium for hydrogen ions; often associated jaundice (see *Abdomen* in Book 2)

Investigating pyloric stenosis

- Clinical diagnosis: palpate olive-shaped pyloric enlargement (also referred to as a pyloric 'tumour') just above umbilicus during a 'test feed'. May see visible peristalsis
- Confirm diagnosis by US (thickened elongated pylorus) or barium meal

Treatment of pyloric stenosis

- Stop oral feeding
- Give IV infusion of 5% dextrose, 0.45% saline plus 10 mmol potassium chloride per 500 mL until alkalosis corrects (usually 24–48 hours)
- Anaesthesia is not safe until the alkalosis is corrected because of the risk of post-operative apnoea

Principles of Ramstedt's pyloromyotomy

Indications
Pyloric stenosis

Pre-op preparation
NBM and NG tube, correction of alkalosis. The procedure is performed under GA. It may be done as an open procedure or, increasingly, as a laparoscopic technique.

Incision
Right upper transverse incision or a circum-umbilical incision

Principles of procedure
The pylorus is delivered through the incision with care not to put the stomach under too much tension. It can be identified by the pre-pyloric vessel. The pyloromyotomy involves a longitudinal incision from the antrum to the duodenum through the hypertrophied circular muscle layers (note that the muscle fibres change direction at the duodenum). The muscle is further opened by spreading with a pyloric spreader. It is important not to breach the mucosa. Breach of the mucosa can be identified by inflating the stomach with air.

Intra-operative hazards
Perforation of the gastric mucosa.

Closure
Close in layers with absorbable sutures.

Post-op
The NG tube can be removed early if there is no damage to the mucosa but it is left in place if there has been any perforation. Post-op feeding can resume after 6 hours (some vomiting will still occur initially due to gastric atony, but it will settle).

Complications
- Main complication is inadvertent perforation of the duodenal mucosa (repair with absorbable suture and cover with omental patch)
- Incomplete myotomy
- Wound infection

Long-term surgical outcome

Surgery is generally very successful; the pylorus returns to normal. Gastric investigation of these patients when they reach adulthood shows normal capacity and function.

5.2 GROIN HERNIAS

In a nutshell ...

Groin hernias in children are usually indirect inguinal hernias. Emergency management differs from that of adult hernias (reduction by taxis is recommended in children) and surgical treatment is herniotomy, not herniorrhaphy as in adults.

Inguinal hernias

- Almost invariably indirect in children
- More common in males than females; more common on the right side due to later descent of the right testis
- 15% are bilateral
- Bilateral inguinal hernia in a female is a rare presentation of testicular feminisation syndrome; chromosome studies may be necessary
- Treatment is surgical and consists of a herniotomy – the sac is dissected free from vas and vessels then transfixion ligated at the deep ring (see *Abdomen* in Book 2)
- Herniorrhaphy, repair of the posterior wall of the canal, is unnecessary

Incarcerated inguinal hernias in children

Inguinal hernias in infants should be repaired within 2 weeks of diagnosis because the risk of incarceration is high. Risk of incarceration lessens after the age of 1. Incarceration results in an intestinal obstruction and there is 30% risk of testicular infarction due to pressure on the gonadal vessels. Treatment involves resuscitation then reduction by taxis. Most hernias can be reduced safely. If not reduced, proceed to laparotomy. If the hernia has been reduced then herniotomy is performed after 24–48 hours to allow oedema to settle.

Femoral hernias

Very rare in children. Treatment follows the same principles as for adults (see section 1.2 of *Abdomen* in Book 2).

5.3 UMBILICAL DISORDERS

In a nutshell ...

Infection
Herniation

Omphalitis

This is infection of the umbilical site. It is characterised by erythema and discharge of pus. It is common in the developing world and is also associated with immunodeficiency (neutrophil defects cause delay in separation of the cord), peri-natal sepsis, and low birth weight. It can lead to fasciitis and in severe cases may need debridement.

Umbilical hernia

Remember the rule of 3s

3% of live births have umbilical hernias
Only 3 per 1000 need an operation
Operate on after the age of 3 (many surgeons wait until aged 5)
They recur in the 3rd trimester of pregnancy

Epidemiology of umbilical hernia

- 3% of neonates have umbilical hernias; most resolve spontaneously
- 3 in 1000 live births need further surgery
- More common in black children

Anatomy of umbilical hernia

- Peritoneal sac penetrates through linea alba at umbilical cicatrix to lie in subcutaneous tissues beneath skin cicatrix
- There is a narrow, rigid neck at the aponeurosis

Prognosis of umbilical hernia

- All decrease in size as the child grows
- Few persist after puberty
- Some cause disfigurement or incarcerate (but strangulation is virtually unknown)

- Only a minority need an operation
- Must preserve the umbilicus to avoid stigmatising the child
- Similar Mayo 'vest over pants' repair to adult repair (see section 1.2 of *Abdomen* in Book 2)
- Absorbable sutures used

5.4 JAUNDICE IN NEONATES

In a nutshell ...

Physiological causes of neonatal jaundice
Bilirubin is < 200 mmol/l
This can be due to hepatic immaturity or breastfeeding

Medical causes of neonatal jaundice
Rhesus haemolytic disease
ABO incompatibility
Congenital spherocytosis
G-6-PD deficiency
Hypothyroidism
Congenital and acquired infections

Surgical causes of neonatal jaundice
Biliary atresia
Choledochal cysts
Spontaneous perforation of the bile duct
Inspissated bowel syndrome (within the common bile duct)
Tumours of the extrahepatic bile ducts

Gallstones and acute gall bladder distension must not be forgotten when managing children with an unknown cause of jaundice.

Biliary atresia

Unknown aetiology. Extrahepatic bile ducts are destroyed by inflammation. It occurs in 1 in 14 000 live births and is equally common in males and females. Clinical features include jaundice, hepatosplenomegaly, pale stools and dark urine. The inflammation can be confined to the common bile duct or can extend to the right and left hepatic ducts.

Treatment includes biliary–enteric anastomosis, porto-enterostomy or liver transplant if these fail. Long-term sequelae include portal hypertension and cirrhosis.

Choledochal cysts

These occur due to a congenital weakness in the wall of the biliary tree and a functional obstruction at the distal end. They are investigated by US scanning and ERCP. Treatment consists of excision of the cyst.

5.5 CONDITIONS CAUSING ACUTE ABDOMINAL PAIN IN CHILDREN

In a nutshell ...

Conditions causing acute abdominal pain in children

Appendicitis
Gastroenteritis
Intussusception
Malrotation and volvulus
Meckel's diverticulum
Mesenteric adenitis
Constipation
Inflammatory bowel disease in children

Appendicitis

3 children in 1000 per year have their appendix removed. Appendicitis can occur at any age but is more common > 5 years. Children may present with abdominal pain, vomiting and peritonism (McBurney's triad). Infants may show more non-specific features such as anorexia, vomiting, irritability and fever. The mortality of appendicitis is higher in infants than in adults and the diagnosis is often missed and surgery delayed.

Treatment consists of appendicectomy following appropriate IV fluid replacement and antibiotics. See *Abdomen* (Book 2).

Gastroenteritis

This is common in children and toddlers. It presents with diarrhoea and vomiting +/– pyrexia and dehydration (especially in very young children). It is commonly viral but may be bacterial in nature. Common pathogens are:

- Rotavirus
- *Campylobacter*
- *E. coli*
- *Salmonella*

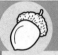

There may be a history of exposure to other infected children (common passage of rotavirus) or potentially infected foodstuffs. Remember parasites as a cause of diarrhoea and vomiting in children who live or have travelled abroad (eg *Giardia*, *Cryptosporidium* and amoebiasis).

Intussusception

Incidence is 1 in 500, with a peak incidence at age 5–9 months. The majority occur in association with viral infections. The enlarged Peyer's patch in the ileum acts as the **lead point**. Intussusception in older children and adults is more likely to have a **pathological lead point** – eg a polyp or Meckel's diverticulum.

The intussusception causes a small bowel obstruction. The intussuscepted segment becomes engorged (with rectal bleeding) and eventually gangrenous – perforation and peritonitis follow this.

The most common site for an intussusception is ileocolic; ileoileal is less common. Small bowel intussusception may occur as post-op complication typically following nephrectomy in infants.

Clinical features of intussusception

- **Typical presentation:** spasms of colic with pallor, screaming and drawing up of legs. The child falls asleep between episodes; later develops bile-stained vomiting and rectal bleeding (redcurrant jelly stools)
- **Clinical signs:** ill, listless, dehydrated child. The child may become desperately ill from shock. Intussusception is palpable as a sausage-shaped mass in about one third. There is blood on rectal examination. Occasionally the tip of the intussusception is palpable PR. Signs of peritonitis indicate perforation

Investigating intussusception

- AXR shows small bowel obstruction. May see a soft tissue mass
- US is characteristic (target sign)
- On barium enema (old-fashioned) intussuscipiens shows up as a 'coiled spring'

Treatment of intussusception

- Resuscitation
- ABC
- Often requires large volumes of plasma to restore perfusion
- IV antibiotics
- Analgesia
- NG tube

If the child can be resuscitated and there is no evidence of peritonitis and an expert paediatric radiologist is available then attempt to reduce the intussusception pneumatically by rectal insufflation of air. Risks are incomplete reduction and perforation. The latter can be particularly dangerous as a tension pneumoperitoneum develops very rapidly. Facilities for immediate laparotomy must be available. Perform laparotomy if pneumatic reduction has failed or is contraindicated. Use a right upper transverse incision. The distal bowel is gently compressed to reduce the intussusception. If the serosa starts to split then reduction should be abandoned and a limited resection performed.

Outcome of treatment

Recurrence rate is about 10% whether treated radiologically or by surgery. Further recurrence raises the question of a pathological lead point.

Malrotation and volvulus

Malrotation of the mid-gut results in a narrow free pedicle with a predisposition to twist around the SMA as a volvulus. Acute volvulus presents during the neonatal period but may occur at any age. It may also be recurrent. Symptoms are bilious vomiting, abdominal distension and tenderness, and may include rectal bleeding. The mid-gut becomes ischaemic and may infarct. AXR shows duodenal obstruction with absent distal bowel gas. Prompt resuscitation and laparotomy for Ladd's procedure and resection of any necrotic areas is indicated.

Meckel's diverticulum

May mimic the presentation of appendicitis or present with bleeding, perforation, intussusception, volvulus or intestinal obstruction. Haemorrhage or perforation may be due to gastric mucosa being present within it. See *Abdomen* (Book 2).

Mesenteric adenitis

Vague central abdominal pain accompanies an URTI, due to inflammation of the mesenteric lymph nodes and subsequent mild peritoneal reaction. Features which distinguish it from appendicitis include cervical lymphadenopathy, headache, mild abdominal pain, shifting tenderness, and pyrexia above 38 °C. It occurs most commonly between the ages of 5 and 10 years. For more details see *Abdomen* (Book 2).

Constipation

Causes of constipation in childhood

- Hypothyroidism
- Hypercalcaemia
- Neuromuscular disorders
- Hirschsprung's disease
- Febrile illness in older children

Chronic constipation may lead to abdominal pain, anorexia, vomiting, failure to thrive, UTIs and faecal soiling.

Soiling occurs due to the accumulation of faeces within the rectum and thus an acquired megacolon. This leads to distension of the external sphincter and eventual failure of the external sphincter.

Anal irritation and tears can occur due to pain on defaecation leading to a cycle of faecal retention.

Management of constipation

- Treat the precipitating cause if applicable
- A short course of oral laxatives is most often successful
- A course of enemas can be considered in more refractory cases
- This should be supplemented with high fluid and roughage intake

Inflammatory bowel disease (IBD) in children

There are about 1000 children with IBD in the UK. The number of children with Crohn's disease is increasing. The presentation, diagnosis and treatment are similar to that in adults – see *Abdomen* in Book 2.

Children tend to present with extra-GI symptoms. Surgery for children who are malnourished because of the severity of their IBD should be performed early to avoid stunting of growth.

Chapter 11

Urology and Transplantation

Sunjay Jain and Kilian Mellon

Section 1

Clinical features and investigation of the urinary tract

1.1 UROLOGICAL SYMPTOMS

In a nutshell ...

Pathology in the urological tract may be asymptomatic, may present as a systemic illness (eg weight loss, fever) or it may present with any of the following urological symptoms:

Pain
Lower urinary tract symptoms
Urinary incontinence
Urinary retention
Haematuria
Pneumaturia

Pain

Pain from the renal tract can be felt anywhere from the renal angle to the genitalia:

- Renal angle pain: kidney
- Flank/loin pain: upper and mid-ureters, non-urological causes (eg abdominal aortic aneurysm)
- Suprapubic pain: bladder (eg retention)
- Perineal/genital pain: lower ureters, epididymis, testes
- Urethral pain: usually infection

Obstructive pain is dull in nature and exacerbated by fluid intake. It is due to distension of the renal pelvis or renal capsule. Chronic progressive obstruction is usually painless.

Colicky pain is due to passage of a calculus or blood clot and is intermittent, severe, and often associated with vomiting. It is due to ureteric spasm and peristalsis. It may classically radiate 'from loin to groin' and into the genitalia (these structures all share a common innervation at T11–T12). Differential diagnosis includes any cause of an acute abdomen but, most importantly, leaking or ruptured AAA must be excluded.

Lower urinary tract symptoms

Lower urinary tract symptoms, or LUTS include storage symptoms and voiding symptoms.

- **Storage symptoms:** these include frequency, nocturia, urgency, dysuria, and/or pyrexia). These are commonly idiopathic but may be due to:
    - Infection
    - Malignancy
    - Reduced functional bladder capacity (inflammation, fibrosis, oedema of the bladder wall)
    - Calculi in the distal ureter (causes trigonal irritation) or in the bladder
- **Voiding symptoms** include hesitancy and/or straining, poor stream, terminal dribbling. These symptoms are commonly due to urethral stricture in young men, and to prostatic hypertrophy or malignancy in older men. As bladder outflow obstruction progresses the detrusor muscle thickens and is less controllable, causing urgency and frequency.

Urinary retention

Urinary retention can be acute, acute on chronic, or chronic.

- **Acute retention** is very painful. It may occur on a background of chronic bladder outflow obstruction or be precipitated by constipation, infection, or around the time of surgery due to location of pain (eg inguinal hernia repair) or use of anaesthetic and analgesic agents
- **Chronic retention** is usually due to bladder outflow obstruction and is usually painless with gradually increasing residual volumes. It may present with overflow incontinence

Urinary incontinence

Urinary incontinence can be subdivided into stress incontinence, urge incontinence and continuous incontinence.

- **Stress incontinence** occurs during raised intra-abdominal pressure and is due to weakness of the external urethral sphincter
- **Urge incontinence** is often neurological in origin and is due to spasmodic loss of control of the detrusor muscle
- **Continuous incontinence** is usually due to an anatomical abnormality

For further details see section 2.3 in *Bladder dysfunction and incontinence.*

Haematuria

This is a common urological symptom and will always need some form of investigation. Although it has a multitude of causes the priority is to exclude neoplasms of the kidney (renal cell carcinoma) or of the transitional epithelium (mostly bladder cancer). Both of these conditions are covered in section 7 *Urological malignancy*.

Clinical presentation of haematuria

Haematuria may be macroscopic (visibly discoloured urine) or microscopic (picked up on dipstick testing). The timing may give an indication as to the site of bleeding.

- Blood early in the stream suggests a urethral/prostatic cause
- Blood at the end of the stream is more indicative of a problem at the bladder neck
- Blood mixed throughout the stream is probably coming from the higher renal tract

The colour of the blood should be noted. Darker blood +/– clots is likely to have come from higher in the renal tract. Urinary discolouration may also occur due to certain drugs (eg rifampicin, allopurinol, laxatives) and ingestion of certain foodstuffs (eg beetroot).

Underlying urological malignancy exists in:

- 20% of patients with macroscopic haematuria
- < 5% of patients with microscopic haematuria

The pick-up rate for malignancy is higher in patients who smoke.

Investigating haematuria

Urgent investigation (within 2 weeks) in the context of a haematuria clinic is suggested for:

- All patients with macroscopic haematuria
- All patients aged > 50 with microscopic haematuria

This is usually a one-stop clinic where patients receive:

- Flexible cystoscopy
- USS of the kidneys or an IVU
- Plain X-ray of the abdomen
- Urinary cytology
- DRE of prostate in men
- Urine culture

Management of haematuria

Patients with negative investigations in whom haematuria resolves can usually be re-assured. If haematuria persists and suspicion for malignancy is high (eg more elderly patients) further investigations should be performed, including:

- IVU (if only US had been performed previously)
- Retrograde studies of ureters
- Rigid cystoscopy and/or biopsy

In younger patients with persistent microscopic haematuria, nephrological referral is warranted.

Pneumaturia

Air in the urine is due to fistulation of any part of the urinary tract with the bowel (commonly the bladder). It is often associated with chronic urinary infection due to passage of enteric bacteria. Common causes include diverticulitis, inflammatory bowel disease, and tumour of the bowel or bladder wall. Full investigation of the bowel is required, and although the fistula is rarely visualised directly at endoscopy, the site of fistulation may be identified by radiological contrast studies, usually barium enema.

1.2 UROLOGICAL INVESTIGATION AND IMAGING

In a nutshell ...

Urological investigation
Urinalysis
Blood tests
Urinary flow rates

Urological imaging
KUB (Kidneys, ureters and bladder)
Contrast studies
Ultrasound (US)
Angiogram
CT and MRI
Radioisotope imaging of the renal tract
Isotope bone scanning
Ureteroscopy

Urological investigations

Urinalysis

Urinalysis is performed on a mid-stream (or clean-catch) urine sample. Tests on urine include:

- **Urine dipstick (eg Multistix™) testing:** initial bedside analysis. Sensitive for blood, protein, leukocytes, ketones, glucose, and nitrites
- **Urine microscopy:** further laboratory analysis looking for RBC, organisms, cellular casts (which imply renal disease), crystals such as oxalate or uric acid (which imply stone disease)
- **Urine culture:** for organism and antibiotic sensitivity. Significant growth is $> 10^5$ organisms per mL
- **Urine cytology:** looking for abnormal transitional epithelial cells. This warrants further investigation for malignancy

Blood tests

- **Urea level:** this is a very insensitive indicator of renal function. Levels are affected by hydration, metabolism and protein intake, as well as glomerular and tubular function
- **Creatinine level:** this is determined by muscle mass and glomerular filtration. It is a more sensitive indicator of renal clearance when used as creatinine clearance measurement
- **Electrolytes:** sodium, potassium and hydrogen (acidosis) and bicarbonate ions give direct evidence of renal concentrating dysfunction

Urinary flow rates

These are used for quantitation of bladder outflow obstruction. Normal flow rates are > 15 mL/second.

Urological imaging

Plain film KUB (kidneys, ureters and bladder)

This X-ray is angled to image the entire length of the urinary tract. Look for the renal outlines (T12–L2) and any visible renal mass. Follow the anatomical path of the ureters into the bladder looking for calcification or opacities that may be calculi.

Contrast studies

- **Intravenous urogram (IVU):** intravenous injection of contrast media is followed by X-ray examination at subsequent time points. This demonstrates the baseline or delayed renal excretion as the contrast is filtered by the kidney the renal outline, including any masses. It shows the renal pelvis and ureters including any filling defects (eg stone or tumour) which can be compared for location with calcification visible on the KUB. And it also demonstrates the bladder-filling and post-voiding films, which give an idea about the degree of bladder emptying
- **Retrograde urogram:** retrograde injection of contrast is used at cystoscopy to visualise ureters
- **Urethrography:** this is useful if traumatic disruption of the urethra is suspected. The meatus only is cannulated and contrast media is introduced. The urethra is visualised by X-ray
- **Micturating cystogram:** this is used for demonstrating fistulation, vesicoureteric reflux, urethral strictures and functional bladder studies

Angiogram

Selective renal arteriography is used to visualise renal arterial anatomy, arterial stenoses, or aneurysms, in staging of renal tumours (for invasion of the renal vein), and for persistent haemorrhage after trauma.

CT and MRI

- **CT** is useful for diagnosis and staging of malignancy, and for abscess and cyst drainage. Non-contrast CT is increasingly the standard investigation for urinary calculi
- **MRI** takes longer than CT but avoids the need for radiation. It is more sensitive than CT for staging of bladder and prostate cancer and detection of lymph node metastases. It is also used for diagnosing vertebral metastases and spinal cord compression

Ultrasound (US)

Ultrasound of the genitourinary system

US is important for visualisation and guided biopsy at many levels of the renal tract.

Kidney US: assesses renal size and cortical thickness, renal masses (cystic/solid), calculi, and hydronephrosis. Also guides nephrostomy insertion, and renal biopsy. The latter carries a small risk of haemorrhage and AV fistulation

Bladder US: residual volume, filling defects (stone, tumour), bladder wall thickness

Testis US: masses, blood flow (eg torsion)

Prostate US: transrectal US (TRUS) is used to guide prostate biopsies

Radioisotope imaging of the renal tract

Nuclear imaging can determine the individual components of glomerular and tubular renal function. Renal excretion or GFR is imaged using a compound filtered by the glomerulus (eg 99m-Tc-DTPA) and split functioning of the individual kidneys (eg before nephrectomy) can be assessed using a compound secreted by the renal tubule (eg 99m-Tc-DMSA).

Isotope bone scanning

Radioisotope uptake in the bone correlates with vascularity. It shows metastatic deposits as areas of increased activity. It is used for staging of malignancy (particularly prostate).

Ureteroscopy

Two forms of ureteroscopy may be performed at cystoscopy:

Rigid/semi-rigid ureteroscopy

- Scopes vary from 4.5 Fr to 9.5 Fr
- In theory they can reach the whole ureter but it's difficult to access the upper one-third
- In males large prostates can make manoeuvring difficult

Flexible ureteroscopy

- Scopes vary from 6.2 Fr to 9.3 Fr
- They are introduced over a wire or through a specially designed access sheath. They give much better access to the upper ureter and can be used within the renal collecting system
- A narrow working channel reduces the range of instrumentation available
- Flexible scopes are expensive and easy to damage

Indications for ureteroscopy

- **Ureteric stones:** rigid ureteroscopy is a good treatment for lower and mid ureteric stones, ESWL is an alternative but may not be successful with these if over bony land-marks. Flexible ureteroscopy is good for upper ureteric stones that are not adequately treated by ESWL
- **Renal stones:** flexible ureteroscopy may be useful for small stones where the drainage does not favour ESWL
- **Haematuria:** ureteroscopy is useful for diagnosing filling defects seen on IVU and biopsies may be obtained

Procedure box: Ureteroscopy

Pre-op

Urinary infection should be excluded with MSU
Appropriate imaging should be available to aid orientation during the procedure
In cases of stone disease antibiotics are given to reduce risk of sepsis (eg IV gentamicin and amoxicillin)
X-ray fluoroscopic imaging is required during the procedure

Operative procedure

Patient in lithotomy position
Initial retrograde ureterogram is usually performed
Dilatation of the ureter can be performed using balloon or graduated dilators
The rigid ureteroscope is usually inserted alongside a guidewire, flexible scope over a wire, or through specially designed access sheath
Methods for stone destruction include Holmium laser and pneumatic lithoclast
A JJ stent may be left in the ureter to ensure adequate drainage, especially after prolonged procedures, or where residual fragments remain

Post-op

Patients with uncomplicated stones (no infection or obstruction) can often go home on the same day
Stent removal is by flexible cystoscopy (under LA)
Plain KUB X-ray will confirm stone clearance in most cases

Complications

Failure to reach stone: leaving a JJ stent in the ureter for a short period often allows easier access subsequently
UTI/Septicaemia: septicaemia is a risk when operating on patients with UTI or infected stones. It's important to monitor these patients closely post-operatively because this situation can be life threatening
Ureteric injury: small perforations are managed by stenting. Major injuries are rare but may require open re-implantation/replacement with ileum

Section 2
Bladder dysfunction and incontinence

2.1 ANATOMY OF THE BLADDER

In a nutshell ...

The bladder is a hollow organ with a capacity of 500 mL in adults. The empty bladder lies within the pelvis and is pyramidal in shape with the apex superiorly, a base inferiorly, a superior surface, and two infero-lateral surfaces.

Anatomic relations of the bladder

Superior

- The apex is joined to the anterior abdominal wall by the **median umbilical ligament** (remains of urachus)
- The superior surface is covered by peritoneum and related to coils of ileum or sigmoid colon. With distension, the bladder rises out of the pelvis and separates the peritoneum from the anterior abdominal wall allowing suprapubic catheterisation to be performed without risk of entry into the peritoneal cavity

Infero-lateral relations

- These surfaces are related anteriorly to a retropubic pad of fat and the pubic bones, and posteriorly to the obturator internus muscle above and the levator ani below

Base of the bladder

- The base of the bladder faces postero-inferiorly and is triangular in shape. The two supero-lateral angles are joined by the ureters and the inferior angle gives rise to the urethra
- In females the base of the bladder lies lower because of the absence of the prostate

- In males the seminal vesicles lie behind the base of the bladder along with the vasa deferentia. Above these is a pouch of peritoneum – the rectovesical pouch
- In females the vagina separates the bladder from the rectum with the uterovesical pouch superior to this
- The pubo-prostatic ligaments in the male and the pubovesical ligaments in the female support the neck of the bladder where it enters the urethra

The trigone relations

- This is the internal surface of the base of the bladder. Like the rest of the bladder it is lined by transitional cell epithelium. Unlike the rest of the bladder the mucosa here is firmly adherent to the underlying muscle and therefore does not form folds
- The ureters enter the trigone at its superior angles. They enter the bladder obliquely with an intramural part that is important in preventing vesico-ureteric reflux

Blood supply of the bladder

Superior and inferior vesical arteries (both are branches of the internal iliac arteries). In addition to these branches the bladder may be supplied by any adjacent artery arising from the internal iliac.

Venous drainage of the bladder

The vesical venous plexus communicates below with the prostatic plexus in males and drains into the internal iliac vein.

Lymphatic drainage of the bladder

This is to the external and internal iliac and obturator nodes.

Nerve supply of the bladder and sphincter mechanism

There are three sources of nerves to the bladder and the sphincter:

- **Parasympathetic autonomic nerves** (S2–S4) are autonomic efferents that arise from the inferior hypogastric plexuses
- **Sympathetic nerves** originate from T10–L2 and run on the pre-sacral fascia into the pelvis. These nerves are at risk during pelvic surgery, especially anterior resection of rectum
- **Somatic nerves** are derived from S2–S4 that are transmitted to the urethra in the pudendal nerves. These originate in a region called **Onuf's nucleus**

2.2 PHYSIOLOGY OF MICTURITION

The normal lower urinary tract should be able to store urine and expel it completely at an appropriate time. This relies on several factors:

Storage of urine depends on the bladder having adequate capacity.
Compliance is the term for the ability of the bladder to increase in volume (to 400–500 mL) with only minimal increases in pressure. It is crucial to normal bladder function and is mediated by relaxation of the detrusor muscle as the bladder fills (due to tonic inhibition of the parasympathetic nerves). At volumes greater than 500 mL the pressure rises sharply and the stretching of the detrusor muscle causes reflex contraction.

Continence and expulsion of urine requires competent sphincters.
There are two urethral sphincters – an internal smooth muscle sphincter in the bladder neck (sympathetically innervated) and an external striated muscular sphincter (in the male membranous urethra and mid urethra of the female) under voluntary motor control via the pudendal nerves. During filling, sacral reflexes increase urethral pressure and maintain continence. The urethral sphincter mechanism should act as a valve for the control of continence and open appropriately during voiding.

Timing of micturition is under the control of the pons.
The centre for co-ordinating bladder and urethral function lies within the pons and is known as the pontine micturition centre. This gives descending input to those centres in the cord that are involved with innervating the muscle of the bladder and sphincter. To commence micturition, the inhibitory input from the higher centres is silenced and this is transmitted via the sympathetic and pudendal nerves allowing the urethra to relax and decrease intra-urethral pressure.

Completeness of micturition depends on parasympathetic nerve supply and detrusor contraction.
The parasympathetic nerves stimulate detrusor muscle contraction. All of the detrusor smooth muscle contracts simultaneously, directing the pressure towards the urethra. Intra-vesicular pressure therefore exceeds intra-urethral pressure and voiding occurs.

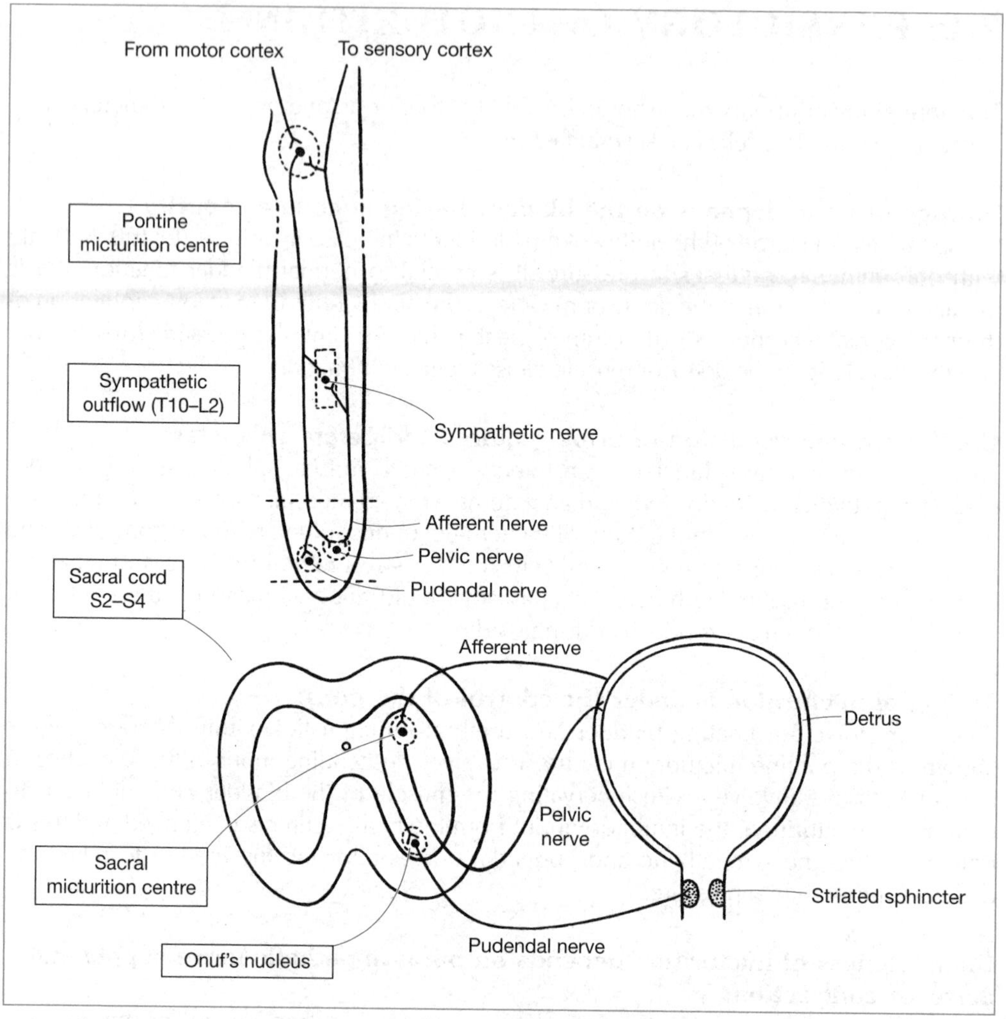

Figure 2.2a *Neural pathways in micturition*

2.3 URINARY INCONTINENCE

In a nutshell ...

Incontinence is defined by the International Continence Society as a condition where involuntary loss of urine is a social or hygienic problem and is objectively demonstrable.

Urine loss can be urethral or extra-urethral

- Extra-urethral loss is secondary to abnormal anatomy (eg ectopic ureter, vesico-vaginal fistula). It presents as constant incontinence
- Urethral loss is usually classified into stress incontinence (sphincter failure) and urge incontinence (bladder dysfunction)

Evaluation of urinary incontinence

- History
- Examination
- Investigations
  - MSU
  - USS
  - Cystoscopy
  - Urodynamic testing

Management of urinary incontinence

Management of stress incontinence

- Conservative
- Mid-urethral tapes
- Colposuspension
- Sphincter reinforcement

Management of urge incontinence

- Bladder training
- Antimuscarinics
- Tricyclic anti-depressants
- Cystoplasty or ileal conduit

Classification of urinary incontinence

Frequently patients will have the picture of mixed incontinence. For example, many women with stress incontinence also have symptoms of urgency.

Stress incontinence

Characteristically this produces symptoms of involuntary loss of urine from the urethra during raised intra-abdominal pressure (eg coughing, sneezing, laughing, or physical exertion). It can be demonstrated by the Valsalva manoeuvre. Stress incontinence is essentially due to failure of the sphincters.

Causes include:

- Pressure denervation of the pelvic floor post-pregnancy and post-childbirth
- External sphincter damage (eg post-TURP)
- Trauma to posterior urethra (eg pelvic fracture)
- Hormonal status (post-menopausal), constipation, and obesity

Urge incontinence

This is the involuntary loss of urine associated with a sudden strong desire to void (urgency). It occurs on a background of normal bladder anatomy and increases with age. It is associated with organic brain damage in the elderly (eg stroke, Parkinson's) and is a common cause of incontinence in this group. Urge incontinence is essentially due to bladder dysfunction.

Causes include:

- Idiopathic detrusor instability (irritable bladder syndrome)
- Infection (bladder wall irritability)
- Loss of cortical control where the bladder fills to capacity and empties spontaneously (eg dementia, paraplegia, MS)

Continuous incontinence

Constant incontinence can result from:

- Overflow incontinence: this occurs in men with chronic urinary retention. There is chronic loss of urine particularly at night
- Bladder fistulas (eg vesicovaginal)
- Anatomical abnormality (eg ectopic ureter, epispadias)

Functional incontinence

In this situation lower UT function is essentially normal but patients are unable to void appropriately because of limitations of mobility or confusion.

Post-void dribbling

This is not true incontinence, but reflects pooling of urine in the bulbar urethra and is common in elderly men.

Evaluation of urinary incontinence

History of urinary incontinence

An accurate idea of the pattern of incontinence is important and a micturition diary may help with this.

Important features in the history are:

- Gynaecological/obstetric history in women
- History of any neurological symptoms
- Drug history
- Details of any previous surgery

A relatively quick onset of urge incontinence symptoms should alert the clinician to the possibility of bladder irritation by infection, stone, or tumour.

Examination for urinary incontinence

Abdominal examination should be performed together with rectal examination in men (to assess the prostate), and pelvic examination in women (which may objectively demonstrate stress incontinence and signs of pelvic floor weakness). Neurological examination should also be performed if indicated from the history.

Investigating urinary incontinence

- **Initial tests** should include MSU, US to assess post-void residual, and possibly cystoscopy
- **Urodynamic testing** is not required in all patients. Essentially it measures the pressure–volume relationships of the bladder during filling (cystometry) and then the pressure–flow relationships during voiding. A catheter in the bladder allows measurement of bladder pressure and also filling. Because bladder pressure consists of both abdominal and detrusor pressure, abdominal pressure is measured separately by an intrarectal pressure sensor and subtracted. Video urodynamics can be performed if the bladder is filled with contrast material. This allows visualisation of the bladder neck to look for hypermobility or sphincter problems. As well as being useful in diagnosing the cause of urinary incontinence, urodynamics has a large role to play in the assessment of bladder outflow obstruction (see section 6.3 *Urinary tract obstruction*)

Management of urinary incontinence

It is important to begin with conservative measures before progressing to pharmacological or surgical treatment. First exclude UTI, diabetes, constipation, diuretic use, and senile vaginitis.

Stress incontinence

Conservative measures

- Weight loss, smoking cessation, and pelvic floor exercises help many women
- Biofeedback mechanisms can improve the results of pelvic floor exercises

Surgical techniques

These aim to either lift the bladder or supplement the sphincter.

- **Burch colposuspension:** this is the traditional operation which involves elevation of the bladder neck and urethra through a lower abdominal incision
- **Needle suspension of the bladder neck (Stamey procedure):** this is a relatively minimally invasive procedure which gives good initial results, but in the long term it is not as good as colposuspension
- **Tension-free vaginal tape (TVT):** this procedure was introduced relatively recently and is very popular. It can be performed under LA. Long-term results are not yet available
- **Peri-urethral bulking agents:** these are not normally a first-line treatment but may give some symptom relief
- **Artificial sphincter implantation:** this is a last-resort measure as there is a high complication rate

Urge incontinence

Re-training is the mainstay of management.

- **Bladder training exercises:** often these improve symptoms
- **Anti-muscarinic agents:** these act on the detrusor muscle (eg oxybutynin, tolterodine)
- **Tricyclic anti-depressants:** these have an anticholinergic effect and also may have central effects
- **Surgery:** this is a last resort in these patients; options include **cystoplasty** which involves augmenting the overactive detrusor with bowel, or in extreme cases urinary diversion with an **ileal conduit**

Overflow incontinence

This is usually due to failure of the detrusor muscle that is irreversible. Men sometimes undergo TURP but the success rate is not high. Intermittent self-catheterisation is an option but if this is not feasible then long-term permanent catheterisation is required.

2.4 NEUROLOGICAL BLADDER DYSFUNCTION

In a nutshell ...

There are several neurological diseases that affect the function of the bladder. Clearly neurological dysfunction may lead either to over-activity or under-activity of the bladder or sphincter and possibly a combination of these.

The balance between the bladder and the sphincter dysfunction will determine the following.

Pressure in the bladder: if this is high it may have implications for renal function because of transmission of this high pressure to the renal pelvis

Effectiveness of bladder emptying: this may manifest as either incontinence or incomplete emptying with recurrent UTIs

Diseases above the brainstem (eg cerebrovascular disease)

Cerebral disease may result in **detrusor hyper-reflexia.** The bladder is hyper-reflexic but retains normal co-ordination of voiding and sensation. Symptoms are frequency, urgency, nocturia and urge incontinence (often due to loss of cortical control). Immediately after a CVA there may be a period where the detrusor becomes atonic (cerebral shock); the reason for this is unclear and it usually recovers.

Spinal cord injury

The spinal cord ends at the level of L2 and becomes the cauda equina. In the initial period after a spinal cord injury there is a period of spinal shock, which is associated with suppression of autonomic and somatic nerve activity and the bladder becomes acontractile and areflexic. This usually results in urinary retention and requires catheterisation. What happens subsequently depends on the level of the spinal cord injury.

Lesions above the sacral spinal cord

- These lead to interruption of fibres passing from the sacral cord to the pontine micturition centre
- Subsequently there is lack of co-ordination between the detrusor and the sphincter, in a condition known as **detrusor sphincter dyssynergia** (DSD)
- The bladder will contract against a closed sphincter and develop high pressure
- These patients are prone to renal damage

Lesions of the sacral cord and cauda equina

- These tend to produce paralysis of the detrusor, so patients have problems with retention because they are unable to empty their bladders

2.5 URINARY FISTULAS

In a nutshell ...

A fistula is an abnormal connection between two epithelial-lined surfaces. Causes of urinary fistulas include:

Obstetric/gynaecological
Birth injury (commonest in developing countries)
Iatrogenic
Malignancy

GI disease
Diverticulitis (50%)
Malignancy (25%)
Crohn's disease (10%)

Trauma
Pelvic fractures

Types of urinary fistulas

- Vesicovaginal
- Vesicocolic
- Vesicocutaneous
- Ureterovaginal or ureterourethral

Symptoms of urinary fistulas

- Recurrent UTI
- Pneumaturia
- Passive incontinence

Investigating urinary fistulas

- MSU
  - Contrast studies
- IVU
  - Barium/gastrograffin enema
  - Cystogram
  - Endoscopy
  - Cystoscopy
  - Speculum examination of vagina
  - Sigmoidoscopy
  - Dye test: if a vesicovaginal fistula is suspected blue dye is instilled into the bladder, and the patient wears a tampon while walking about for 1 hour. The dye will be seen on the tampon if there is a fistula

Treatment of urinary fistulas

- Excision of the fistula and bladder repair or ureteric re-implantation
- Bowel resection and/or temporary colostomy may be needed

Section 3

Urinary tract trauma

3.1 ANATOMY OF THE KIDNEY

In a nutshell ...

The kidneys lie on the posterior abdominal wall in a retroperitoneal position. They are largely under the cover of the costal margin. The right kidney lies slightly lower than the left because of the large size of the right lobe of the liver. The renal hila lie just above and below the trans-pyloric plane, 5 cm from the mid-line.

The average male kidney weighs 150 g and the average female kidney weighs 135 g. The normal size of the kidney is vertically 10–12 cm, transversely 5–7 cm, and AP 3 cm approximately.

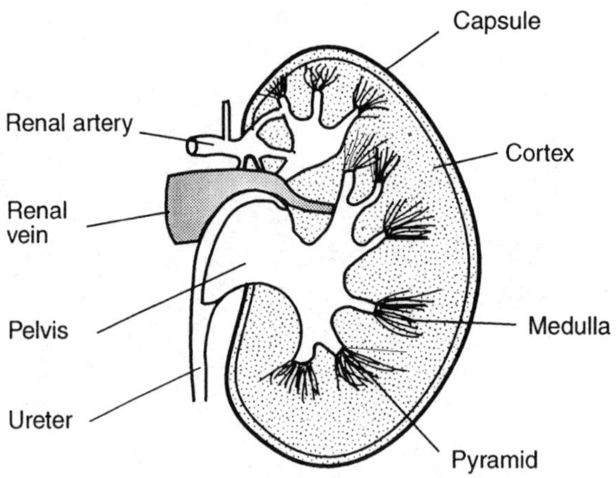

Figure 3.1a *Anatomy of the kidney*

Coverings of the kidneys

The kidneys are covered (from inside to out) by:

- Fibrous capsule
- Peri-renal fat
- Peri-renal or **Gerota's** fascia (dense connective tissue layer surrounding kidneys and adrenal glands and continuous laterally with the fascia transversalis)
- Para-renal fat

Kidney structure

On the medial border of each kidney is the **renal hilum**. This opens into the renal sinus space in the central portion of the kidney occupied by the urinary collecting structures and the renal vessels. The hila lie at the level of the trans-pyloric plane, just lateral to the midline (right hilum lower than the left). The order of the structures at the hilum is (anterior to posterior): renal vein, renal artery, and ureter. Other structures that pass through the hilum are lymph vessels and sympathetic nerve fibres. The kidneys are divided into an outer **cortex** and an inner **medulla**. The medulla is divided into a dozen renal pyramids, each with their base orientated towards the cortex, and a **renal papilla** at the apex. Renal papillae project into the **renal calyces**. Minor calyces fuse to become major calyces of which there are usually two or three. These then coalesce to form the **renal pelvis** (see Fig. 3.1a).

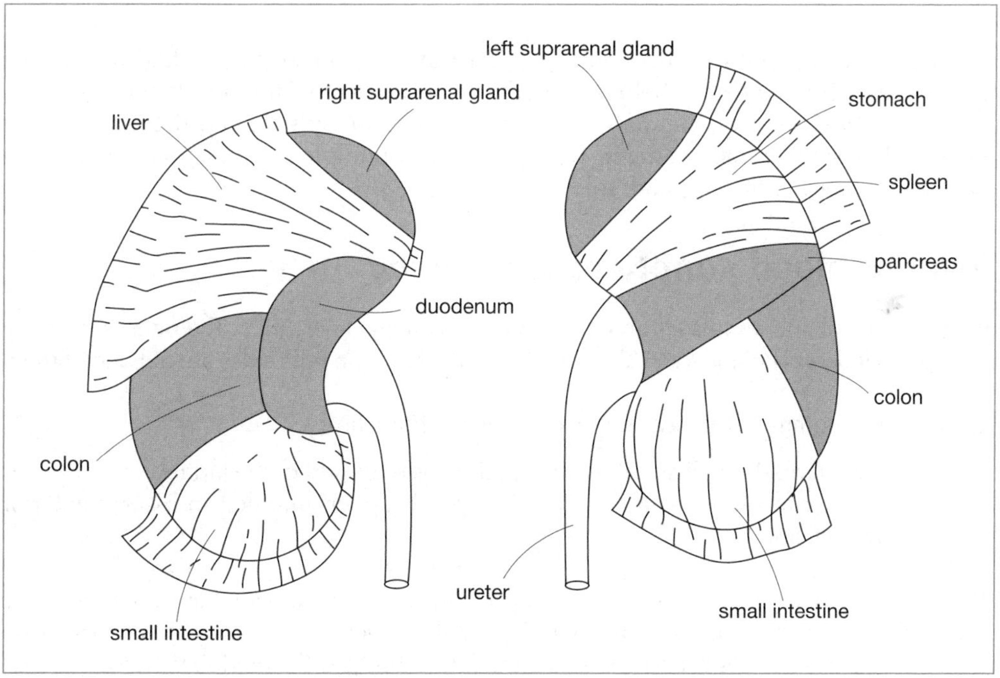

Figure 3.1b *Anterior relations of the kidney*

Anatomic relations of the kidney

ANATOMIC RELATIONS OF THE KIDNEY

	Anterior	Posterior
Left kidney	**Superior** Stomach Spleen (with lieno-renal or spleno-renal ligament) **Medial** Pancreas **Inferior** Left colon	**Superior** Diaphragm covers upper third Costo-diaphragmatic recess **Inferior** Twelfth rib crosses lower pole Ilio-hypogastric nerve Ilio-inguinal nerve **Medial** Psoas muscle **Lateral** Quadratus lumborum and transversus abdominus muscles
Right kidney	**Superior** Adrenal gland Right lobe of liver **Medial** 2nd part of the duodenum **Inferior** Right colon (retroperitoneal) Small bowel	

The peritoneal reflection almost completely separates the upper pole of the right kidney from the liver. This appears to help prevent direct spread of renal tumours to the right lobe. The peritoneum between Gerota's fascia and the inferior splenic capsule is called the **lienorenal** or **splenorenal ligament**. Traction on this during left nephrectomy may cause tears in the spleen and necessitate splenectomy.

Arterial blood supply of the kidney

The paired renal arteries arise from the aorta laterally at the level of L2. The right renal artery is longer as it passes behind the IVC. Multiple renal arteries on both sides are not uncommon.

Renal arteries commonly divide into five segmental branches:

- One posterior branch supplies most of the posterior part of the kidney
- Four anterior branches are called the apical, upper, middle, and lower anterior segmental arteries

All these arteries are end arteries without any collateral circulation (occlusion will produce ischaemia and infarction of the corresponding renal parenchyma). Segmental arteries divide into lobar arteries, to supply a single renal pyramid. Subsequently interlobar arteries give off the arcuate arteries, and these give off several interlobular arteries (eventually become the afferent glomerular arterioles).

Venous drainage of the kidney

Unlike the arteries, renal venous tributaries anastomose freely. Renal veins both drain directly into the IVC.

- The left renal vein is generally three times longer than the right (6–10 cm) and crosses anterior to the aorta. It typically receives the left adrenal vein superiorly, the left gonadal vein inferiorly, and a lumbar vein posteriorly
- The right renal vein is shorter than the left (2–4 cm) and usually has no tributary

Lymphatic drainage of the kidney

This is to the para-aortic nodes around the origin of the renal vessels.

Nerve supply of the kidney

- Sympathetic input is from T8–L1. Para-sympathetic input is from the vagus nerve. The main function of the nerves appears to be vasomotor
- Complete denervation of the kidney as in transplantation appears to have little effect on renal function

Anatomy of the ureters

The ureter represents the tubular extension of the renal collecting system which courses downwards to connect the kidney to the bladder.

- Ureters vary in length from 22 cm to 30 cm
- The ureter is lined by transitional cell epithelium contiguous with that of the bladder

Anatomic relations of the ureters

The position of the ureters is very important as they are at risk of surgical injury in a wide number of abdominal procedures.

Anterior relations

- The right ureter is related to the terminal ileum, caecum, appendix, and ascending colon
- The left is related to the descending colon, the sigmoid, and their mesentery. It lies behind the sigmoid mesocolon as it enters the pelvis
- As they descend both ureters are crossed from medially to laterally by the gonadal vessels anteriorly
- In the female they are crossed anteriorly by the uterine arteries and are closely related to the uterine cervix and therefore are at risk of injury during gynaecology procedures such as hysterectomy
- Within the pelvis in the male the vas deferens crosses anterior to the ureter just before it enters the bladder

Posterior relations

- The ureters on both sides are related to the psoas muscles that separate them from the lumbar transverse processes
- As they enter the pelvis the ureters cross the bifurcation of the common iliac artery

Narrowings in the ureter

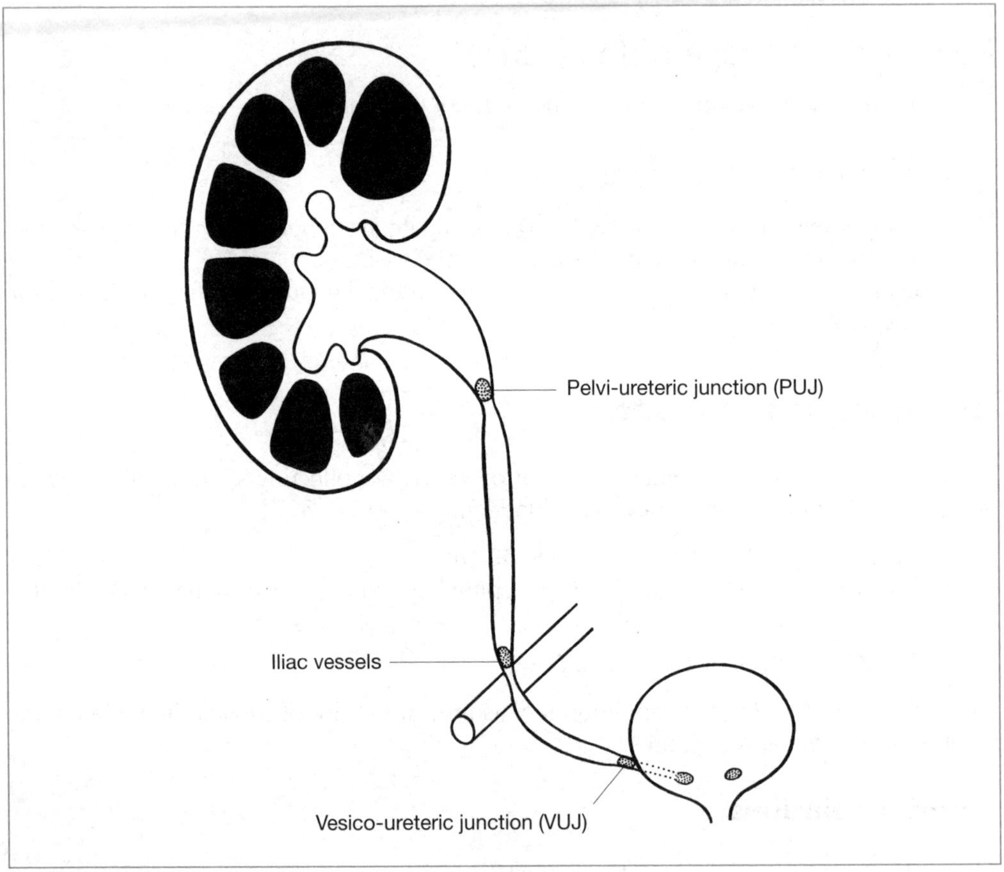

Figure 3.1c *Sites where stones tend to get impacted in the urinary tract*

Classically three points are described at which the ureter is particularly narrow. These are:

- The pelvi-ureteric junction
- At the bifurcation of the iliac vessels where the ureter enters the pelvis
- The vesico-ureteric junction

These are clinically important, as they may be sites of impaction of calculi and may be visible as narrowings on contrast studies.

Blood supply of the ureters

Venous drainage mirrors the arterial supply. This is classically described as corresponding to:

- Upper third: renal artery and vein
- Middle third: gonadal artery and vein
- Lower third: superior vesical artery and vein

Lymphatic drainage of the ureters

- This is to the para-aortic and pelvic lymph nodes

Nerve supply of the ureters

- Autonomic nerves are sympathetic from T10/L2 spinal segments and parasympathetic from S2/S4 segments. Pain fibres leave with the sympathetic nerves and the resulting visceral pain is referred to somatic distributions that correspond to these spinal segments. Pain is therefore produced over the distributions of the subcostal, iliohypogastric, ilioinguinal and/or genitofemoral nerves resulting in flank, groin, or scrotal (or labial) pain.

3.2 RENAL TRAUMA

In a nutshell ...

Injuries to the genitourinary tract account for 10% of all renal trauma.

Most often renal trauma is due to blunt trauma, especially RTAs, and is associated with other abdominal injuries (eg liver or spleen). Penetrating trauma accounts for less than 10% but has a higher association with requirement for intervention.

Injury is more common in children who have relatively larger kidneys and less surrounding fat and muscle bulk than adults and in those with previously abnormal kidneys (eg hydronephrosis or cysts).

Assessment of renal trauma

Clearly these may be multiply injured patients and the ATLS principles of acute trauma should be applied.

- The mechanism of injury is important (eg deceleration in high speed RTA)
- **Gross haematuria means mandatory imaging**. Microhaematuria should be sought either by dipstick or microscopy

Investigating renal trauma

Experience in the USA has shown that not all patients with microscopic haematuria have significant renal injury and therefore imaging is not indicated in all patients. Be suspicious if there is associated systemic shock and loin pain as severe renal pedicle injury may present with only microscopic haematuria. A perinephric haematoma may be palpable. Plain AXR may show loss of psoas shadowing, an enlarged kidney, fractures of overlying ribs or transverse processes of lumbar vertebrae, scoliosis to the affected side due to muscle spasm.

Criteria for renal imaging

- Any penetrating trauma to the flank or abdomen associated with haematuria
- Blunt trauma with gross haematuria
- Blunt trauma with microscopic haematuria and a systolic BP of < 90 mmHg at any stage
- Deceleration injury (classically associated with renal devascularisation and therefore may not present with haematuria)
- Associated major intra-abdominal injury and microscopic haematuria
- Any child with any degree of haematuria

Standard imaging is a CT scan with intravenous contrast (in a *stable* patient). IVU may be used, but CT has advantages in that it more accurately stages renal injuries and also identifies other intra-abdominal injuries and aids in the decision to manage the patient conservatively.

Classification of renal trauma is based on the American Association for the Surgery of Trauma Staging System

Grade 1	Contusion, sub-capsular haematoma but intact renal capsule
Grade 2	Minor laceration of the cortex not involving the medulla or collecting system
Grade 3	Major laceration extending through the cortex and the medulla but not involving the collecting system
Grade 4	A major laceration extending into the collecting system
Grade 5	A completely shattered kidney or renal pedicle avulsion leading to renal devascularisaton

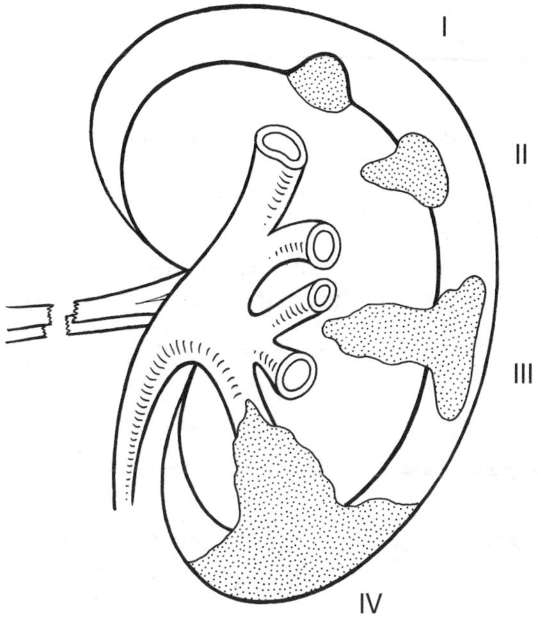

Figure 3.2a *The four stages of renal trauma*

Management of renal trauma

98% of blunt renal injuries are managed non-operatively (hospital admission and bed rest until gross haematuria clears). Serial US may be used to monitor haematoma.

Absolute indications for renal exploration include:

- Persistent hypotension despite resuscitation
- Expanding haematoma
- Disruption of the renal pelvis with leakage of urine

Recent experience suggests not all penetrating trauma requires exploration; 40% of stab wounds and 75% of gunshot wounds were managed non-operatively in a large US series.

Complications of renal trauma

Early complications
Haemorrhage
Urinary extravasation (leading to urinoma and abscess)

Late complications
Penetrating trauma may leave residual AV fistula
Hypertension due to renal ischaemia or renal artery stenosis
Fibrotic change causing obstruction at the renal pelvis and hydronephrosis

3.3 URETERIC TRAUMA

In a nutshell ...

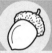

Most ureteric injury is iatrogenic. 50% of iatrogenic injuries to the ureter occur during gynaecological surgery due to the nearby uterine artery.

Management options include stenting or repair, depending on whether the injury is diagnosed immediately or if diagnosis is delayed.

Damage to the ureter after external violence is rare but may be due to penetrating injury.

Most ueretic injuries are due to damage at surgery and include ligation, crush injury due to clamps, complete or partial transection, or devascularisation:

- 50% of iatrogenic ureteric injuries occur during gynaecological surgery, especially during hysterectomy (the ureter lies very close to the uterine artery)
- The remaining 50% occur in colorectal, vascular or urological surgery
- Damage during ureteroscopy occurs in approximately 5% of patients

Presentation of ureteric trauma

- **Early recognition:** often a transected ureter may be obvious at the time of surgery. If ureteric injury is suspected during surgery then the ureter can be directly inspected or a retrograde ureterogram obtained.

- **Late recognition:** post-operative uereteric injury may present with loin pain, and unexplained pyrexia due to abdominal collection of urine or drainage of urine (from a wound drain or per vaginam).

Investigating ureteric trauma

IVU is the first-line investigation. It may show hydronephrosis or delayed excretion of contrast. Urinary extravasation may also be seen.

Management of ureteric trauma

This depends on whether the ureteric injury is recognised at the time of damage, or the diagnosis is delayed.

Immediate recognition of surgical ureteric injury

- **Ligation of the ureter:** treat by removing the ligature and observation. A ureteric stent should be placed across the area of damage to reduce risk of stricture formation
- **Transection recognised immediately:** this may be managed by direct end-to-end repair. The ureter should be spatulated, bearing in mind that the blood supply may be tenuous. If there is likely to be any degree of tension the bladder should be mobilised to allow it to be brought up towards the ureteric injury, with subsequent ureteric re-implantation (methods include the **Boari flap** and the **psoas hitch**). Once again, the ureter is stented to allow for healing without stricturing.

Delayed recognition of surgical ureteric injury

The options are stenting and surgical repair. Occasionally a stent can be passed retrogradely via the bladder. If this is unsuccessful, percutaneous drainage of the kidney (nephrostomy) should be performed, both to relieve obstruction and to prevent urine leak. Subsequent surgical repair should be carried out (about 6 weeks after injury).

Options for repair include:

- **Re-implantation:** if this is feasible
- **Transureteroureterostomy:** anastomosis of the damaged ureter to the normal one on the other side
- **Ureteric substitution** using ileum
- **Autotransplantation** of the kidney to the iliac fossa
- **Nephrectomy:** sometimes this is the simplest solution if there is thought to be associated renal damage and the contralateral kidney has normal function

Ureteroscopic injury

This can usually be treated by insertion of a ureteric stent.

3.4 BLADDER TRAUMA

In a nutshell ...

Blunt trauma can cause injury to the bladder.

- 80% of bladder injuries have an associated pelvic fracture
- 10% of pelvic fractures have an associated bladder injury
- Penetrating injury is rare in the UK

The bladder is also at risk when distended and full from blunt trauma to the abdomen. The tear often occurs at the dome. Iatrogenic injuries may occur during surgery, eg open pelvic surgery such as Caesarean section, or endoscopic surgery such as transurethral resection of bladder tumour (TURBT).

Presentation of bladder trauma

Macroscopic haematuria is present in 95–100% of patients with blunt bladder injury. There may be lower abdominal pain and oliguria or anuria. There may be urinary peritonitis if the diagnosis is made late. Extravasation of urine may also cause a rise in blood urea level due to re-absorption.

Investigating bladder trauma

Retrograde cystography is most accurate method of diagnosing bladder injury. There are two main steps:

- Fill the bladder with contrast via urethral catheter (at least 400 mL)
- Obtain post-drainage views (otherwise small leaks may be missed)

Intraperitoneal and extraperitoneal rupture can be distinguished according to distribution of contrast. Most bladder injuries cause extra-peritoneal rupture.

Management of bladder trauma

Extraperitoneal perforations require catheter drainage for 14 days. Healing should be confirmed with a repeat cystogram. Intraperitoneal bladder perforations all require open surgical repair.

NB: Bladder injuries may co-exist with urethral injuries (see section 3.5) therefore care should be taken with catheterisation if there is blood at the urethral meatus. If a catheter cannot be passed to drain the bladder because of urethral injury one should be inserted **suprapubically** and a cystogram performed by this method.

3.5 URETHRAL AND MALE GENITAL TRAUMA

In a nutshell ...

Urethral injuries can be anterior (associated with fall astride injuries or instrumentation) or posterior (associated with pelvic fractures). They may present with the classic triad of symptoms or with characteristic bruising.

A safe method of investigation is by urethrogram followed by careful urethral catheterisation by an experienced urologist, or suprapubic catheterisation at open cystotomy with inspection of the bladder.

Post-traumatic strictures may need reconstruction.

Classification of urethral trauma

Urethral trauma can be divided into anterior and posterior urethral injuries.

- **Anterior injuries:** these usually affect the penile and bulbar urethra and are often associated with instrumentation of the urinary tract or 'fall astride' injuries
- **Posterior injuries:** these usually affect the membranous urethra and are common sequelae of pelvic fracture (occurring in 4–14%). Some 10–17% of posterior urethral injuries have associated bladder rupture

Presentation of urethral trauma

Urethral trauma may present with the classic triad of:

- Blood at the urethral meatus
- An inability to void
- A palpably full bladder

This triad occurs in a minority of patients, and indeed 50% of patients with significant urethral injury will not have blood at the urethral meatus. Anterior urethral injuries may produce classic **butterfly bruising** of the perineum. Bruising is confined by the Colle's fascia, which fuses posteriorly with the perineal body and extends a little way down each thigh.

Investigating urethral trauma

If there is blood at the urethral meatus there are two schools of thought.

Option 1: try to gently pass a urethral catheter. This should be performed by a urologist and attempts should be abandoned at the slightest resistance. The risk here is the conversion of a partial injury to a complete injury.

Option 2: Perform an **immediate urethrogram**. This is done by inserting a 12 Fr catheter just inside the urethral meatus and slightly inflating the balloon with 1–2 mL of water. Water-soluble contrast is then injected.

Management of urethral trauma

If a catheter cannot be passed, urethral injuries should be treated by **suprapubic catheterisation**. Ideally this should be carried out via an open formal cystotomy at which time the bladder is inspected. Subsequent management will depend on the extent of urethral stricture that develops after conservative management. Injuries may heal with only a small amount of residual structuring. Severe strictures may be treated with urethral reconstruction at a later stage (reduced incidence of long-term stricturing compared to primary repair).

Penile and scrotal trauma

Scrotal haematoma and testicular rupture may occur after a direct blow. Mild haematoma is treated conservatively but a ruptured testis requires surgical reconstruction of the overlying coverings. Penile fracture (ie rupture of the corpus cavernosum) requires surgical intervention to prevent fibrosis and erectile dysfunction.

Section 4
Urological infections

4.1 PATHOGENESIS OF UROLOGICAL INFECTIONS

In a nutshell ...

Most acute infections are due to a single organism (usually *E. coli*).

Chronic infections are often due to multiple organisms and may be related to the presence of a foreign body (eg an in-dwelling catheter) or underlying pathology.

Infection is dependent on bacterial and host factors.

- **Bacteruria:** is the presence of bacteria in the urine. It is subject to the possibility of contamination, and the risk varies according to the technique used for detection. Supra-pubic aspiration is the gold standard
- **Pyuria:** is the presence of white blood cells in the urine
- **Urinary tract infection (UTI):** involves the invasion of urothelium by bacteria. It is usually associated with bacteruria and pyuria
- **Sterile pyuria:** this is pyuria without bacteruria. It warrants evaluation for TB, stones, or cancer
- **Recurrent UTI:** is defined as more than three infections in 1 year. Causes include re-infection (95% of all recurrent infections in women), and bacterial persistence (more common in men). It may also be due to an underlying urological abnormality (eg reflux) or the presence of calculi (eg stag horn). It is common in patients with indwelling catheters
- **Uncomplicated UTI:** this is an infection in a healthy patient with a structurally and functionally normal urinary tract
- **Complicated UTI:** is an infection in a patient with a structural or functional abnormality of the urinary tract or infection associated with immunosuppression or a foreign body

Microbiology of urological infections

Most acute infections are due to a single organism. Chronic infections are often due to multiple organisms and may be related to the presence of a foreign body (eg an in-dwelling catheter) or underlying pathology.

Escherichia coli infection

E. coli causes 90% of community-acquired infections. In hospitals 50% of infections are caused by *E. coli* (usually from a faecal source).

Other pathogens

- **Enterobacter:** such as *Streptococcus faecalis*, *Proteus* spp, *Klebsiella* spp. These are less common causes of acute uncomplicated UTI in both sexes and at all ages
- ***Pseudomonas***: presence of *Pseudomonas* indicates a foreign body, eg a catheter
- ***Proteus***: hydrolyses urea to produce ammonia, which increases urinary pH, and predisposes to stone formation
- ***Staphylococcus saprophyticus***: especially in sexually active women
- ***Staphylococcus aureus***: occurs after surgery on or instrumentation of the urinary tract

Rare causes of chronic infection

- **TB:** this is becoming increasingly common, especially in HIV patients, and may cause a diffuse interstitial picture or localised caseating lesions
- Schistosomiasis
- Hydatid disease

Aetiology of urological infections

Infection is dependent on bacterial and host factors.

Bacterial factors in urological infections

These are thought to be related to the bacteria's adherence to the transitional epithelium. Only a select number of *E. coli* strains possess sufficient fimbriae to allow urinary infection. Different forms of fimbriae allow organisms to colonise different areas of the urinary tract (eg upper UT vs lower UT) and an organism can adapt and change its fimbriae type allowing infection to progress upwards.

Host factors in urological infections

The urinary tract has several defence mechanisms:

- Acidic urine
- High levels of urea
- High osmolality
- Antibacterial secretions, eg:
  - Tamm–Horsfall protein secreted in the loop of Henle
  - Prostatic antibacterial factor
  - Urinary immunoglobulins
- Repeated voiding: prevents urinary stasis

Conditions predisposing to urinary tract infections usually alter or impair defence mechanisms, such as:

- **Female sex** – woman are at greater risk of UTIs than men because:
  - Shorter urethra allows transfer of faecal flora
  - Transfer of vaginal flora occurs during sexual intercourse
  - Hormonal changes cause changes in urine composition during pregnancy and the menopause
- **Diabetes** – this predisposes to UTI because of:
  - Increased glycosuria
  - Immunosuppression
- **Obstruction** – if this occurs in any part of the UT it causes urinary stasis which predisposes to infection
- **Foreign bodies** – eg catheter, calculi predispose to UTI

4.2 LOWER URINARY TRACT INFECTIONS

In a nutshell ...

Lower urinary tract infections include:

- Acute bacterial cystitis (commonly referred to as a UTI)
- Epididymo-orchitis
- Prostatitis

Fournier's gangrene is a serious complication that can result from a lower urinary tract infection, especially in an immunocompromised patient. It needs urgent surgical debridement and is a life-threatening surgical emergency.

UTIs in children are covered in Chapter 10 *Paediatric Surgery*.

Acute bacterial cystitis

50% of women experience at least one attack during their lifetime. Acute bacterial cystitis may also be a cause of confusion and sepsis in the elderly with minimal symptoms.

Remember that procedures performed when the urinary tract is infected can cause severe generalised sepsis, and should be performed under antibiotic cover (eg single-dose gentamicin before catheter insertion).

Clinical features of acute bacterial cystitis

- Frequency and urgency of micturition
- Dysuria +/– haematuria

Investigations of acute bacterial cystitis

Urine culture

It is arguable whether this is needed in all women with symptoms suggestive of acute cystitis and no complicating factors, because treatment is often completed before results are available, and it markedly increases the cost of treatment. A dipstick positive for pyuria, haematuria or bacteruria is usually sufficient. Some dipsticks detect nitrites (produced from nitrate by bacterial degradation) and these are more sensitive for infection.

You should obtain urine culture:

- For all men with suspected cystitis
- For women when symptoms persist or if there are recurrent infections
- For women who are elderly, have diabetes, and are pregnant (because in these situations pathogens may not be typical)

Typical findings from MSU culture in UTI include bacterial growth and pyuria. Causes of a sterile pyuria include:

- Inadequately treated infection
- Atypical organisms (eg TB)
- Inflammation in or near the urinary tract (eg calculi, tumour, chemical or radiation cystitis, interstitial nephritis, prostatitis, appendicitis)
- The degree of symptoms may not be related to the findings of MSU

Further investigations

Further investigations are required in all men and women with severe recurrent UTIs.

- Tests include: renal function, USS (to check kidneys for scarring and assess adequate bladder emptying), plain AXR (to exclude renal calculi)
- IVU may also be used
- Patients with haematuria require a cystoscopy

Treatment of acute bacterial cystitis

- Several studies suggest 3 days of antibiotics are adequate in uncomplicated cystitis in women. Empirical treatment is usually with trimethoprim
- All women should be given general advice about hygiene, adequate fluid intake, and regular bladder emptying (including after intercourse)
- Recurrent UTIs may necessitate prophylactic antibiotics, either taken every night or only after intercourse
- In elderly women HRT may be used to treat atrophic vaginitis, which predisposes to UTI
- Evidence of outflow obstruction requires treatment of its cause

Beware UTIs

In children: see Chapter 10 *Paediatric Surgery*
If planning urological instrumentation: may cause sepsis, so cover with antibiotics
With obstruction: needs urgent decompression
With *Pseudomonas*: look for foreign bodies
With *Proteus*: look for stones
With sterile pyuria: look for TB

Epididymo-orchitis

Clinical features of epididymo-orchitis

- Acute onset of testicular pain with swelling of the scrotum
- Symptoms of UTI may be present
- Occasionally patients are systemically unwell

Pathogenesis of epididymo-orchitis

- Epididymitis is most common (usually bacterial)
- Orchitis is less common (often viral eg mumps, coxsackie virus)
- In older men epididymitis is nearly always related to Gram-negative infection of the urine (usually *E. coli*). This is most often due to bladder outflow obstruction
- In younger men STDs are more common (causative organisms include *Chlamydia* and *Neisseria gonorrhoeae*)

Differential diagnosis of epididymo-orchitis

- In younger men **torsion of the testis** (see section 8). If there is any suspicion of this exploration of the scrotum is mandatory
- About 10% of testicular tumours present with acute symptoms

Investigating epididymo-orchitis

- Urinalysis often reveals abnormalities such as pyuria or bacteruria
- USS is useful to exclude an abscess

Treatment of epididymo-orchitis

- Symptomatic treatment includes bed rest, scrotal support and analgesia
- Antibiotics are also given
  - In elderly men ciprofloxacin is sufficient
  - In younger men doxycycline should be added to cover *Chlamydia*
- In older men, formal assessment for bladder outflow obstruction should be undertaken

Prostatitis

Prostate inflammation is often related to bladder outflow obstruction. In some cases no bacterial cause is found – this chronic pelvic pain syndrome (CPPS) is difficult to treat.

Clinical presentation of prostatitis

- Usually presents with similar symptoms to cystitis
- Acute bacterial prostatitis patients may be systemically unwell, with fever, purulent discharge, tender prostate, pain on ejaculation, and haemospermia

Investigating prostatitis

- Blood culture
- Urine culture
- Trans-rectal ultrasonogrphy (TRUS) (to exclude and treat abscess formation)

Treatment of prostatitis

- Antibiotics appropriate to the organism
- In CPPS there is some evidence for the use of NSAIDs and α-blockers

Fournier's gangrene

Fournier's gangrene is a form of **necrotising fasciitis** of the male genitalia and surrounding areas.

> **If you ever diagnose Fournier's gangrene (eg if you feel crepitus in an infected perineum) you must act quickly. This is a urological emergency and an experienced urologist capable of debriding the perineum should see the patient WITHIN MINUTES of diagnosis. Every minute that the patient is not in theatre means another few centimetres of tissue necrosis. Death can occur within hours. In the few minutes that you are waiting for the urologist you should give fluids, give (not just prescribe) broad-spectrum antibiotics, and book an emergency theatre.**

Clinical presentation of Fournier's gangrene

- Generally occurs in older patients and is particularly common in diabetics
- Cellulitis of the external genitalia with swelling, erythema and necrotic areas
- Crepitus can often be elicited on examination
- Pain is prominent and there is marked systemic upset
- Infection may extend to involve the groin and supra-pubic areas

Investigating Fournier's gangrene

- Cultures often reveal multiple organisms. This is a classical anaerobic/aerobic synergistic infection
- Typical organisms include *Pseudomonas*, β-haemolytic streptococci, *E. coli* and *Clostridium*

Treatment of Fournier's gangrene

- Prompt diagnosis essential
- IV antibiotics and rehydration should be followed by **early surgical debridement**

Mortality is high (10–75%) and reflects the pre-existing morbidity.

4.3 UPPER URINARY TRACT INFECTION

In a nutshell ...

Infection of the renal pelvis and kidneys is referred to as pyelonephritis.

Acute pyelonephritis

Presents with pyrexia, loin pain and rigors on a background of UTI
USS or IVU is useful to exclude infected obstructed system
Treatment is antibiotics

Chronic pyelonephritis

Usually radiologically diagnosed small kidney atrophied by chronic bacterial infections
Investigations aim to assess the damage with ultrasound, IVU and tests of kidney function
Treatment is aimed at the underlying cause (eg VUR) and antibiotic prophylaxis
Nephrectomy may be needed

Acute pyelonephritis

Clinical features of acute pyelonephritis

- Classically presents with pyrexia and loin pain and rigors
- Occasionally present with septic shock
- May be preceding or concurrent symptoms suggestive of UTI
- Alternatively, infection may occur via haematogenous spread from another source

Investigating acute pyelonephritis

- Urine should be tested by dipstick and sent for urine culture
- Blood culture should be taken from all patients with suspicion of septicaemia
- Plain X-ray (KUB) may show stone disease
- USS is used to exclude obstruction
- IVU may show enlargement of the kidney and poor urinary concentration

Treatment of acute pyelonephritis

- Antibiotic therapy is the mainstay of treatment in uncomplicated acute pyelonephritis
- Initial empirical therapy with broad-spectrum antibiotics (eg cefuroxime, gentamicin) can be changed to specific antibiotics when cultures become available
- 14-day course of antibiotics is recommended

Complications of acute pyelonephritis

- **Pyonephrosis (pus in the renal collecting system):** this may result from pyelonephritis associated with distal obstruction. It requires prompt drainage, usually with percutaneous nephrostomy
- **Perinephric abscess (pus around the kidney):** this may rupture and reach adjacent organs. It requires surgical or US-guided percutaneous drainage

Chronic pyelonephritis

Clinical features of chronic pyelonephritis

- Usually radiological diagnosis
- Refers to a small, contracted, atrophic kidney that is the result of chronic bacterial infection
- Though patients may present with recurrent UTIs, the disease may present at an advanced stage when CRF is present
- These patients are susceptible to hypertension, renal impairment and stone formation

Investigating chronic pyelonephritis

- US will confirm a scarred kidney
- IVU will demonstrate loss of renal parenchyma, especially over the renal poles and overlying the calyces
- **Vesicoureteric reflux** (VUR) is often associated with chronic pyelonephritis. This diagnosis can be made by **micturating cystourethrogram**

Treatment of chronic pyelonephritis

- Deal with any predisposing cause
- Antibiotic prophylaxis is often required
- For severely diseased kidneys with minimal function nephrectomy may be appropriate

Chronic inflammation may cause a granulomatous mass that is difficult to distinguish from a renal tumour called chronic xanthogranulomatous pyelonephritis.

4.4 INFLAMMATORY CONDITIONS OF THE BLADDER

Interstitial cystitis

- Causes pain, frequency and urgency
- Characterised by mucosal ulceration and fissures
- Histologically shows chronic inflammatory change
- Exclude carcinoma in situ (CIS)

Radiation cystitis

- Radiation damage to blood supply and bladder wall ischaemia
- May present acutely with severe bleeding
- May cause fistulae and fibrosis in the long term

4.5 BLADDER DIVERTICULI

Congenital diverticuli

- True diverticuli (full thickness wall)
- Tend to occur in urachus and para-ureteric contributing to reflux

Acquired diverticuli

- Usually false diverticuli (mucosal out-pouching only)
- High vesicular pressures associated with obstruction cause trabeculation of bladder wall and formation of diverticuli
- May cause:
  - Stasis with infection
  - Stasis with stone formation
  - Voiding inefficiency

4.6 ANTIBIOTIC PROPHYLAXIS IN UROLOGY

In a nutshell ...

Patients undergoing endoscopic surgery, open surgery, or prostatic biopsies require antibiotic prophylaxis.

Endoscopic surgery

Any patient undergoing endoscopic surgery to the urinary tract is at risk of bacterial infection.

Pre-operative antibiotic prophylaxis required

- Before instrumentation of upper urinary tract
- Where the risk of infection is greater due to the presence of potentially infected urine (eg presence of a catheter, urinary stone disease)
- In patients with increased risk

Patients at increased risk

- Known UTI
- Indwelling catheter
- Congenital cardiac abnormality
- Cardiac valve disease
- Diabetes
- Immunocompromise
- Implanted prosthetic materials (joint, heart valve, pacemaker)

Current antibiotic practice

- A pre-operative dose of gentamicin or a cephalosporin is usually adequate
- Catheter removal following TURP should be covered with a single dose of antibiotic
- At-risk patients covered with a combination of antibiotics (eg amoxycillin and gentamicin) when having catheter removed

Open surgery

Antibiotic prophylaxis for open surgery is as for general surgery with a broad-spectrum cephalosporin plus metronidazole if bowel is used (eg cystectomy).

Prostate biopsy

All patients undergoing trans-rectal prostate biopsies should receive prophylaxis to minimise risk of potentially fatal sepsis. Oral ciprofloxacin is usually given (some units add a dose of IV antibiotic at the time of biopsy).

Section 5

Urinary stone disease

5.1 PATHOLOGY OF URINARY STONES (CALCULI)

In a nutshell ...

Stones in the urinary tract are a common urological problem and the prevalence is estimated at 2–3% in the developed world (1 in 8 white people have stones by the age of 70). Stones tend to affect economically active individuals (ie males under 65) so having a high cost to society. 80% of urinary tract stones are calcium based. Stone formation is encouraged by super-saturation and the presence of a nucleus, and is inhibited by citrate and magnesium.

Certain metabolic abnormalities predispose to stone formation:

- Hypercalciuria
- Hyperoxaluria
- Hyperuricuria
- Cystinuria
- Hypocitraturia
- Infection

Risks factors for urinary tract stones

Higher in carnivores (higher protein intake)
Increased incidence in relatives of sufferers
Warm climate
Metabolic abnormalities (see below)
Dehydration
Previous stones: risk of recurrence is 35–75% at 10 years

The treatment of stones has been revolutionised over the last 20 years with minimally invasive techniques meaning that very few patients now require open surgery for management of their stone disease. The specialty of endourology has developed around these techniques and also encompasses some non-stone disease and also laparoscopy.

Aetiology of urinary tract stones

Composition of the commonest urinary stones is shown in the table. Most (80%) are based on calcium.

COMPOSITION OF URINARY STONES

Calcium oxalate	35%	Hard, brittle, irregular in shape
Calcium phosphate	10%	
Mixed calcium oxalate and phosphate	35%	
Magnesium ammonium phosphate (struvite)	10%	Soft White Fill renal pelvis Associated with infection (eg *Proteus*)
Uric acid	8%	Radiolucent Yellow with fine projections
Cystine	1%	Hard white stones
Others (eg xanthine)	1%	

Stone formation only takes place when urine is super-saturated (solubility product of that particular solute has been exceeded), but in the normal state many stone components in urine are super-saturated (aided by mucoproteins and alanine) and a nucleus is probably needed for further crystal deposition. This may be a small crystal, a protein, a foreign body or sloughed papilla.

Urine contains natural inhibitors of stone formation including citrate and magnesium.

Metabolic abnormalities in stone-formers

Hypercalciuria

30–60% of patients with calcium oxalate-based kidney stones have increased calcium in the urine. The main causes are:

- **Absorptive hypercalciuria**: this is when increased absorption of calcium in the gut takes place in response to vitamin D

- **Renal hypercalciuria**: the kidneys are unable to reabsorb calcium, increasing its concentration in the urine
- **Resorptive hypercalciuria:** this is rare; there is hyper-parathyroidism in most cases, due to increased calcium resorption from bones (associated with hypercalcaemia)

Calcium metabolism is covered in more detail in *Endocrine Surgery* in Book 2.

Hyperoxaluria

- **Primary hyperoxaluria** is a rare genetic disorder
- **Secondary hyperoxaluria** results from any cause of small bowel malabsorption (eg small bowel resection, bowel intrinsic disease, (eg Crohn's disease). The reason is increased colonic permeability to oxalate as a result of exposure of the colonic epithelium to bile salts. Increased intake (eg of tea) is another cause

Hyperuricuria

Most commonly caused by excessive dietary purine intake (eg meat) and contributed to by dehydration. Predisposes to urate stones and calcium oxalate stones. Other causes include ileostomy, chronic diarrhoea, myeloproliferative disease, and gout.

Purine metabolism is covered in more detail in the section on gout in *Orthopaedics* in Book 2.

Cystinuria

This inherited autosomal recessive condition involves a defect in amino acid transport in intestine and kidney.

Hypocitraturia

As stated above, citrate is thought to be an inhibitor of stone formation. A low citrate contributes to formation of urinary stones in up to 60% of patients.

Infection stones

These account for 10% of all urinary stones. They are often large, filling the pelvicalyceal system, giving a characteristic stag-horn appearance. Chemical composition is of magnesium ammonium phosphate (struvite).

They usually arise in response to chronic infection with organisms such as *Proteus*, *Pseudomonas*, and *Klebsiella*. These are urea-splitting organisms that alkalinise urine by production of ammonia and cause deposition of calcium and other ions.

5.2 CLINICAL PRESENTATION OF STONE DISEASE

In a nutshell ...

The usual presentation of stones in the urinary tract is acute ureteric colic. Other modes of presentation include:

Urinary tract infections (UTIs) (see section 4 of this chapter, *Urological Infections*)
Haematuria
As incidental findings during imaging for other symptoms

Ureteric colic

This is the result of a stone impacting in the urinary tract and causing obstruction behind it. The ureter undergoes spasm and hyper-peristalsis.
Stones impact at sites of narrowing in the ureter which can be pathological narrowings (eg stricture) or anatomical narrowings:

- At the pelvi-ureteric junction (PUJ)
- In the pelvis where the ureter crosses the iliac vessels at the sacroiliac joint (SIJ)
- At the vesico-ureteric junction (VUJ)

Clinical features of ureteric colic

- Abrupt onset
- Severe pain from the flank: this radiates laterally from flank, around the abdomen, to the groin and genitals (common innervation of referred pain)
- Patients writhe with pain: they find it impossible to be still. In contrast, patients with peritonitis tend to lie still as movement exacerbates pain
- LUTS: this is caused when the stone nears the bladder and irritates the trigone
- Nausea and vomiting: this is common because the autonomic nervous system transmits visceral pain and the coeliac ganglion serves both kidneys and stomach. Other GI symptoms lead to confusion in the diagnosis
- Tachycardia: this is common
- Pyrexia: obstruction leads to stasis which leads to infection
- Loin tenderness: NB abdominal examination may be normal
- Haematuria: this can be macroscopic or microscopic. It occurs in about 90% of patients

Differential diagnosis of ureteric colic

- Appendicitis
- Diverticulitis
- Ectopic pregnancy
- Salpingitis
- Torsion of ovarian cyst
- Biliary colic
- Ruptured AAA
- Pyelonephritis
- PUJ obstruction

5.3 INVESTIGATING STONE DISEASE

In a nutshell ...

The aims of investigation in urinary stone disease are to:

- Confirm diagnosis
- Elucidate whether infection is present
- Determine location and size of stones
- Determine degree of obstruction
- Determine renal function, both overall and relative for each kidney
- Identify underlying abnormalities that may have caused stone formation (metabolic or anatomic)

Intravenous urogram (IVU)

90% of stones are radio-opaque and visualised on the control KUB film (urate stones are radiolucent). Ideally an IVU will confirm the presence of a stone, its size and location, and also the degree of renal obstruction.

Films can sometimes be difficult to interpret if there is a lot of bowel gas or faeces. Some centres advocate bowel prep before elective IVU.

IVU should be used with caution in patients with poor renal function because it is nephrotoxic – ensure patients are well hydrated pre- and post-procedure) and diabetic patients on metformin (stop 24 hours before the procedure). It is contraindicated in patients with a history of adverse reaction to contrast media.

Ultrasound (US)

This is excellent for determining if there is acute obstruction, it will also detect stones within the kidney. However, it is unreliable for detecting ureteric calculi.

Non-contrast computerised tomography (CT)

This technique has superseded the use of IVU in some centres. It is rapid to perform, requires no contrast media, and identifies both radio-opaque and radiolucent stones. The main disadvantage is the increased radiation dose administered. CT will not allow assessment of the degree of obstruction or of renal function and it is not as easy to interpret anatomical location or detailed pelvicalyceal anatomy.

Metabolic studies

This is not usually relevant in the acute situation, but if any stones are passed then analysis will allow targeted future treatment if applicable. Metabolic screening usually involves serum levels of calcium and urate and a 24-hour urine collection, which in addition to measuring these ions also measures citrate, oxalate, and phosphate.

5.4 MANAGEMENT OF STONE DISEASE

In a nutshell ...

Stones of < 5 mm mostly pass spontaneously over a 6-week period. Stones of > 6 mm rarely pass spontaneously.

Options for treatment depend on:
- Site of the stone
- Size of the stone
- Any associated infection

Modalities include:
- Watch and wait
- Extracorporeal shock wave lithotripsy (ESWL)
- Ureteroscopy and stone extraction
- Percutaneous nephrolithotomy (PCNL)

Acute management of ureteric colic

- **Supportive treatment:** with analgesia (diclofenac is the drug of choice), anti-emetics and rehydration
- **Drainage:** if there are signs of sepsis (pyrexia, rigors, raised WCC), immediate drainage is required as the risk of renal damage is high. The preferred method is percutaneous nephrostomy under LA. An alternative is retrograde placement of a ureteric stent, but this can be difficult, and carries an increased risk of septicaemia
- **Conservative approach:** use this if there is no evidence of sepsis. Patients may experience further pain (ensure adequate analgesia). Sieve urine to identify the stone. Follow-up with regular KUB until the stone is passed (up to 6 weeks)

The likelihood of a stone passing spontaneously depends on its size and position:

- 90% of stones are < 4 mm and in the lower ureter, and are likely to pass
- 5% of stones are > 6 mm and in the upper ureter, and are unlikely to pass

Management of ureteric stones

For patients with large stones, persistent pain, or who fail conservative management, there are two main options: ESWL and ureteroscopic stone destruction.

Extracorporeal shock wave lithotripsy (ESWL)

- This uses an external energy source which is focused accurately on the stone, causing it to shatter. It relies on accurate localisation of the stone by X-ray or US, which may be difficult if the stone lies over a bony landmark such as a transverse process, or over the pelvis
- ESWL is indicated for all stones with diameter < 2 cm
- Complications include colic due to fragments from large stones, haematuria, failure to shatter harder/larger stones, and renal trauma (rarely)
- Contraindications are pregnancy, aortic aneurysm, urosepsis, and uncorrected coagulopathy

Ureteroscopy

With modern ureteroscopy most ureteric stones are accessible. Results are better for lower ureteric stones. Details of ureteroscopy are given in section 1.3.

Management of renal stones

There are several management options for renal stones.

Conservative treatment of renal stones

- Can be used for asymptomatic patients with small renal calculi (< 5 mm)

Extracorporeal shock wave lithotripsy (ESWL)

- Good results can be obtained for stones of < 2 cm
- Ensure that the renal anatomy is appropriate to allow drainage of the fragments
- For larger stones place a ureteric stent to prevent *steinstrasse* or 'stone street' (a column of obstructing stone fragments in the ureter)

Percutaneous nephrolithotomy (PCNL)

- Access is gained to the renal collecting system percutaneously with dilatation of a track to allow insertion of a nephroscope
- Stones are then broken by various methods including electrohydraulic lithotripsy and US
- PCNL is the preferred method for larger stones (eg stag-horn calculi)

Flexible ureterorenoscopy and laser lithotripsy

- This is ideal for small stones in the renal collecting system that are unfavourable for ESWL because of poor anatomical drainage
- It is the method of choice for patients who have both ureteric and renal calculi

Open surgery

- **Open nephrolithotomy:** this is very rarely required because of increasing expertise in endoscopic techniques. It may be combined with pyeloplasty in patients with PUJ obstruction and secondary stones
- **Nephrectomy:** this should be considered in patients with symptomatic renal stones and a kidney contributing < 15% of overall function (assuming overall renal function is normal)

Bladder stones

These are fairly rare except in certain geographical areas.

Causes of bladder stones

- Bladder outflow obstruction and urinary stasis
- Chronic infection
- Foreign body (eg non-absorbable suture)
- Renal calculus

Presentation of bladder stones

- Pain, frequency and haematuria
- Infection
- Chronic irritation of urothelium and increased risks of transitional cell carcinoma

Management of bladder stones

- Usually radio-opaque
- Can be removed by lithoclast fragmentation but require open surgery if > 5 cm

Section 6

Urinary tract obstruction and benign prostatic hyperplasia

6.1 ANATOMY OF THE PROSTATE

In a nutshell ...

The prostate lies inferior to the bladder and surrounds the prostatic urethra. It is roughly conical in shape with the base superiorly.

Weight of the normal prostate is about 20 g

Length of the normal prostate is 3 cm

Anatomic relations of the prostate

- **Superior relations:** the base of the prostate is continuous with the neck of the bladder. Smooth muscle passes continuously from one organ to the other
- **Inferior relations:** the apex of the prostate lies on the **urogenital diaphragm**. The urethra leaves at this point to become the membranous urethra (see below). Anteriorly here the prostate is related to the symphysis pubis and separated from it by extra-peritoneal fat in the retro-pubic space. The **puboprostatic ligaments** connect this surface of the prostate to the pubic bones
- **Posterior relations:** the prostate is separated from the rectum posteriorly by the **fascia of Denonvillier**
- **Lateral relations:** the pubococcygeal portion of levator ani cradles the lateral surfaces of the prostate

Structure of the prostate

The prostate is composed of 70% glandular elements and 30% fibromuscular stroma. It has a discrete zonal anatomy with zones being distinguished by both their location and their differing propensity for pathologic lesions.

- **Transition zone:** this surrounds the urethra proximal to the ejaculatory ducts; this is the area where benign prostatic hyperplasia (BPH) occurs
- **Central zone:** this surrounds the ejaculatory ducts and projects under the bladder base to the seminal vesicles
- **Peripheral zone:** this constitutes the bulk of the apical, posterior and lateral aspects of the prostate; 75% of prostate cancers arise in this zone
- **Anterior fibromuscular stroma:** this is a variable amount of prostatic tissue anteriorly

Clinically the prostate is described as having two lateral lobes separated by a central sulcus that is palpable on rectal examination. A middle lobe is often present in older men and projects into the bladder. These lobes do not correspond to any histologically defined structures.

Blood supply of the prostate

- Branches of the inferior vesical and middle rectal arteries

Venous drainage of the prostate

The veins form the prostatic venous plexus, which receives the deep dorsal vein of the penis and drains with the vesical venous plexus into the internal iliac vein. Drainage also occurs into the vertebral venous plexus and this may be a route of metastasis to the lumber vertebrae for prostate carcinoma cells.

Lymphatic drainage of the prostate

This is to the internal iliac nodes.

Nerve supply of the prostate

Autonomic supply is as with the bladder. Sympathetic nerves with α_1-adrenergic receptors cause contraction of prostatic smooth muscle and are targeted therapeutically in men with BPH.

6.2 ANATOMY OF THE URETHRA, PERINEUM, AND THE FEMALE GENITAL TRACT

Anatomy of the male urethra

The male urethra is about 20 cm long. It extends from the neck of the bladder to the external urethral meatus. It is divided into four parts:

- **Prostatic urethra:** as described above, 3 cm long and is the widest and most dilatable portion of the urethra
- **Membranous urethra:** a 2-cm portion of the urethra that pierces the urogenital diaphragm
- **Bulbar urethra**
- **Penile urethra** (see below)

The female urethra is discussed later in this section.

Anatomy of the pelvic diaphragm

The perineum is separated from the pelvic cavity by a transverse sheet of muscle and covering fasciae called the pelvic diaphragm (formed by the slings of the levator ani and coccygeus muscles). The levator ani has two parts: posteriorly the iliococcygeus, and anteriorly the pubococcygeus. The anterior portion of the sacrospinous ligament also has a muscular component (the coccygeus muscle) which contributes to the pelvic diaphragm.

Iliococcygeus

This joins the muscle of the contralateral side by interdigitating at the ano-coccygeal raphe. It extends from the coccyx to the anorectal junction.

Pubococcygeus

This divides into three parts.

- **Posterior relations:** it interdigitates at the anococcygeal raphe
- **Anterior relations:** it forms the anorectal sling around the anorectal junction; this contributes to formation of the anorectal angle and is important in continence. The fibres also blend with the deep part of the external anal sphincter
- **The puboprostaticus or pubovaginalis:** this is a small portion running in front of the anorectal junction behind the prostate or vagina

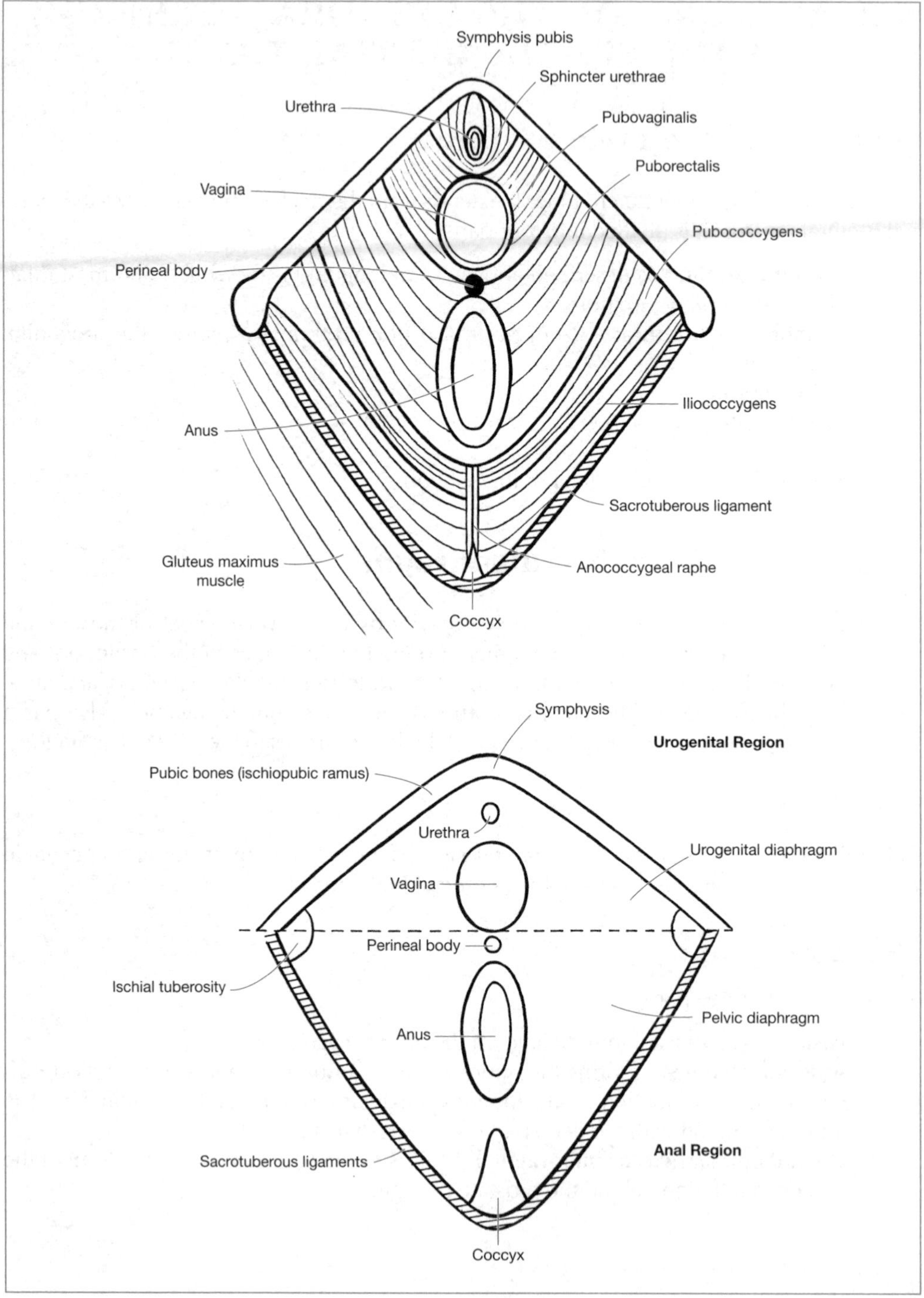

Figure 6.2a *Pelvic diaphragm and diamond-shaped perineum*

Anatomy of the perineum

The perineum has a diamond-shaped outline. This region can be divided into two triangular areas by drawing a line that links the anterior ends of the ischial tuberosities (see Fig. 6.2a).

The anal region

This is delineated by the coccyx posteriorly and the ischial tuberosities laterally. It contains the anal canal as a mid-line structure, and laterally on each side there is a space called the ischioanal fossa which extends superiorly in continuity with the ischiorectal fossae. These are packed with fat and are huge potential spaces for the collection of pus and abscess formation; they can be accessed by an incision in the skin of the buttock.

Borders of the ischioanal and ischiorectal fossae are:

- Medially the anus and rectum
- Superiorly (the roof) the levator ani
- Laterally the medial surface of the obturator internus
- Inferiorly (the floor) the skin of the buttock

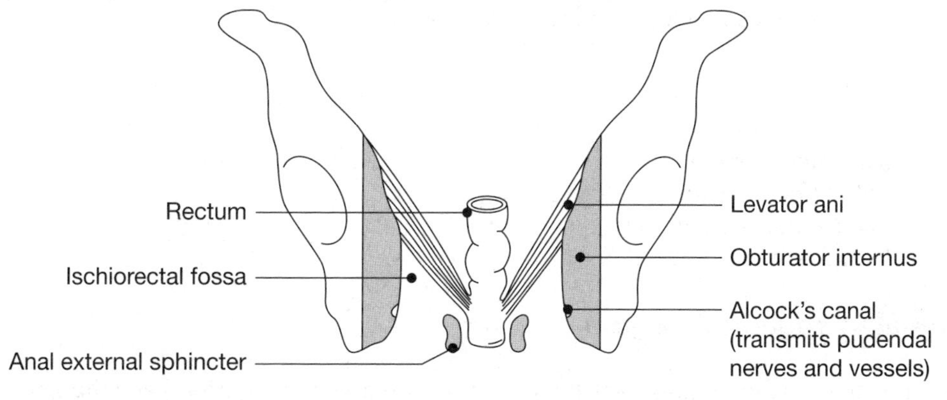

Figure 6.2b *Ischiorectal fossa*

The pudendal nerve and internal pudendal vessels pass along the lateral wall of the fossa in a fascial pudendal canal. The pudendal nerve supplies the external anal sphincter and skin of the perineum. The internal pudendal artery, a branch of the internal iliac, gives rise to the inferior rectal artery and branches to the penis, or labia and clitoris.

See the *Abdomen* chapter of Book 2 for the anatomy of the anal canal and sphincters, and for discussion of perianal sepsis.

The urogenital region

This is an area delineated by the symphysis pubis anteriorly and the ischiopubic rami of the pubic bones laterally. The urethra (and vagina in the female) pass through the incomplete anterior portion of the pelvic diaphragm.

Anterior to the pelvic diaphragm lies the urogenital diaphragm. This has two muscular and fascial layers attached to the margins of the pubic arch laterally and the perineal body posteriorly. Anterior to these layers just under the skin lies the superficial perineal pouch. Between these layers is enclosed the deep perineal pouch.

Male urogenital region

See also the anatomy of the penis (section 8.2). The male urogenital region contains the penis and scrotum.

The superficial perineal pouch contains:

- Root of the penis (the bulb is attached to the urogenital diaphragm and the crura are attached to the pubic bones on either side)
- Muscles covering the root of the penis that also originate in the superficial perineal pouch (bulbospongiosus and ischiocavernosus)

The deep perineal pouch contains:

- Membranous urethra
- Sphincter urethrae
- Bulbo-urethral glands
- Internal pudendal vessels
- Dorsal nerve of the penis

Female urogenital region

See also the female genital tract (below). This contains the external genitalia and the urethral and vaginal orifices.

The superficial perineal pouch contains:

- Structures forming the root of the clitoris (bulbospongiosus and ischiocavernosus)

The deep perineal pouch contains:

- Part of the urethra
- Part of the vagina
- Sphincter urethrae
- Internal pudendal vessels
- Dorsal nerve of the clitoris

Anatomy of the female genital tract

Urethra

The female urethra is much shorter than the male (around 3.5 cm in length) and extends from the bladder into the vestibule. The meatus lies a couple of centimetres below the clitoris.

Vulva

The female external genitalia include the labia majora and minora, the clitoris, the vestibule of the vagina (the area enclosed by the labia minora) and the vestibular glands.

The clitoris has a structure similar to the penis in the male. Its root is made up of three areas of erectile tissue, a bulb attached to the urogenital diaphragm, and two crura. The body and glans of the clitoris have multiple sensory nerve endings supplied by the internal pudendal nerve.

The vestibular glands are located under the labia in the vestibule of the vagina. They are responsible for secreting mucus into a groove leading to the labia minora and hymen during sexual activity.

Vagina

The muscular tube of the vagina is approximately 7–8 cm long with the upper half lying in the pelvis in close proximity to the rectum (separated by a fold of peritoneum which is called the pouch of Douglas) The vagina passes through the pelvic diaphragm where it is supported by the pubovaginalis muscle and the attachment of the posterior wall to the perineal body. The lower half of the vagina lies in the perineum. The cervix of the uterus opens into the vault of the vagina on the anterior surface encircled by the vaginal walls. The vaginal vault can be divided into anterior, posterior, and lateral fornices. Of particular importance is the close passage of the ureters to the lateral fornix of the vagina (these may be injured during hysterectomy).

Anatomic relations of the vagina

Anterior relations

- Uterine cervix
- Base of bladder
- Urethra

Posterior relations

- Pouch of Douglas
- Rectum
- Perineal body
- Anal canal

Lateral relations

- Ureter (superior to lateral fornix)
- Pelvic diaphragm

Arterial supply of the vagina

The uterine, vaginal, middle rectal and internal pudendal arteries form a vascular anastomosis.

Venous drainage of the vagina

A venous plexus drains into the internal iliac veins.

Lymphatic drainage of the vagina

Upper two-thirds drains to the internal and external iliac nodes. Lower third drains to the superficial inguinal nodes.

Uterus

The uterus is a hollow pear-shaped organ which is divided into three anatomically distinct areas: the fundus (above the fallopian tubes), the body, and the neck or cervix. The cervix pierces the anterior wall of the vagina and therefore has two parts, the supravaginal and vaginal parts of the cervix. The cervical canal connects the uterine and vaginal cavities and the ends of the canal are referred to as the internal and external os. The walls of the uterus are thick and muscular and lined with endometrium which is continuous with the lining of the fallopian tube.

Anatomic relations of the uterus

Anterior relations

- Utero-vesicular pouch and bladder
- Anterior fornix of vagina

Posterior relations

- Pouch of Douglas

Lateral relations

- Fallopian tubes
- Broad ligaments
- Uterine artery and vein
- Ureter

Arterial supply of the uterus

This is from the uterine artery (from the internal iliac).

Venous drainage of the uterus

The uterine vein drains into the internal iliac vein.

Lymphatic drainage of the uterus

The fundus drains to the para-aortic nodes. The body and cervix drain to the internal and external iliac lymph nodes.

Ligaments of the uterus

The **round ligament** is the remains of the gubernaculum and thus follows the same pathway through the deep or internal inguinal ring and along the inguinal canal to the labia majora. It maintains the anteverted uterine position but is not essential.

The **broad ligament** is a fold of peritoneum extending from the uterus to the lateral pelvic walls. It forms a mesentery with the fallopian tube running along the superior border. Part of the medial aspect of the broad ligament forms the suspensory ligament of the ovary.

The uterus is supported within the pelvic cavity by the levator ani muscles and three ligaments formed from condensations of pelvic fascia: the transverse cervical ligament, the pubocervical ligament, and the sacrocervical ligament. The round and broad ligaments do not have any supportive function. The uterus usually sits at 90° to the top of the vagina pointing anteriorly (an anteverted position). In some women, however, it may lie flexed and pointing posteriorly into the pouch of Douglas, in a retroverted position.

Fallopian (uterine) tubes

The fallopian or uterine tubes lie in continuity with the cavity of the uterus and extend laterally for approximately 10 cm. They run along the superior border of the broad ligament and have a free opening near to the ovary. This opening is called the ostium and is surrounded by fimbriae. The tubes have a double layer of muscle fibres (inner circular and outer longitudinal) which cause peristalsis. The mucosal lining also has cilia and secretes mucus to aid passage of the fertilised ovum to the uterine body.

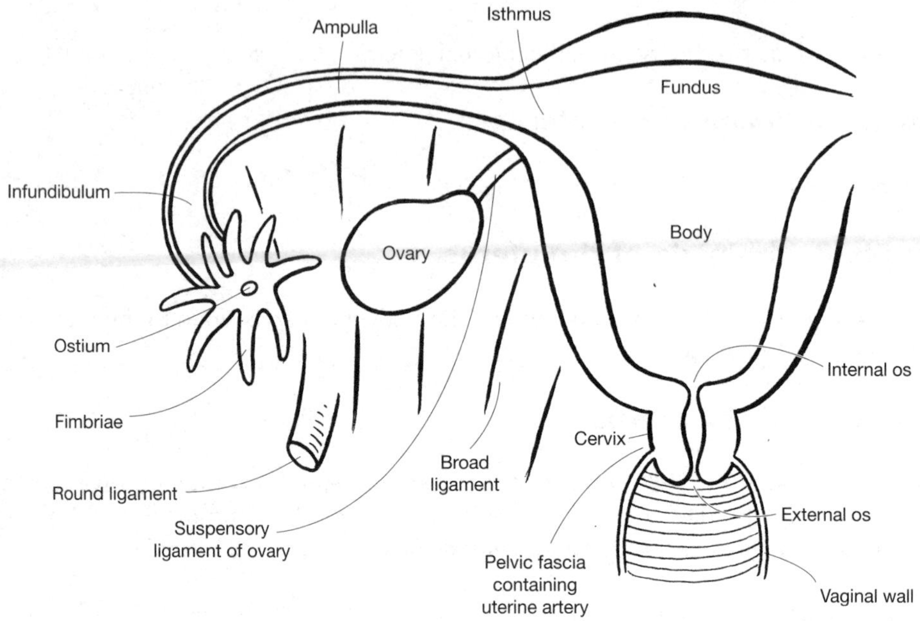

Figure 6.2c *Female reproductive tract*

6.3 URINARY TRACT OBSTRUCTION

In a nutshell ...

The commonest causes of upper urinary tract obstruction are stones, malignancy, and PUJ obstruction.

The commonest causes of lower urinary tract obstruction are benign prostatic hypertrophy and urethral stricture.

Urinary tract obstruction is diagnosed by dilatation of the renal tract (hydronephrosis) although there are other causes of hydronephrosis.

Hydronephrosis

Obstruction of the renal tract usually results in dilatation. Hydronephrosis is defined as a dilatation of the renal pelvis. It is important to remember that there are causes of renal tract dilation other than obstruction (eg vesico-ureteric reflux and congenital mega-ureter).

Urine leaves the kidney by gravity, aided by the peristaltic action of the pelvis and upper ureter. If the collecting system is obstructed the pressure in the renal pelvis quickly rises. A compensatory decrease in muscular tone of the renal pelvis allows a reduction in pressure back towards normal levels and this is followed by a reduction in GFR and impairment of the concentrating ability of the renal tubules.

Obstruction of the renal tract is confirmed by renal excretion studies, usually a DTPA scan.

6.4 BENIGN PROSTATIC HYPERTROPHY (BPH)

In a nutshell ...

This pathological condition is characterised by an increase in both stromal and glandular elements of the prostate gland. It is very common, affecting 50% of men aged > 50, and having almost universal prevalence by age 80.

It occurs in the transition zone of the prostate (the area surrounding the urethra). As the transition zone enlarges, the urethra becomes compressed and the peripheral zone becomes thinner, eventually forming what is known as a 'pseudocapsule'.

The aetiology is not fully understood; local androgen imbalance between testosterone and oestrogen are thought to be important in pathogenesis.

Investigations aim to differentiate BPH from other pathologies and to quantify the degree of obstruction.

Treatment is conservative, pharmacological or surgical (TURP).

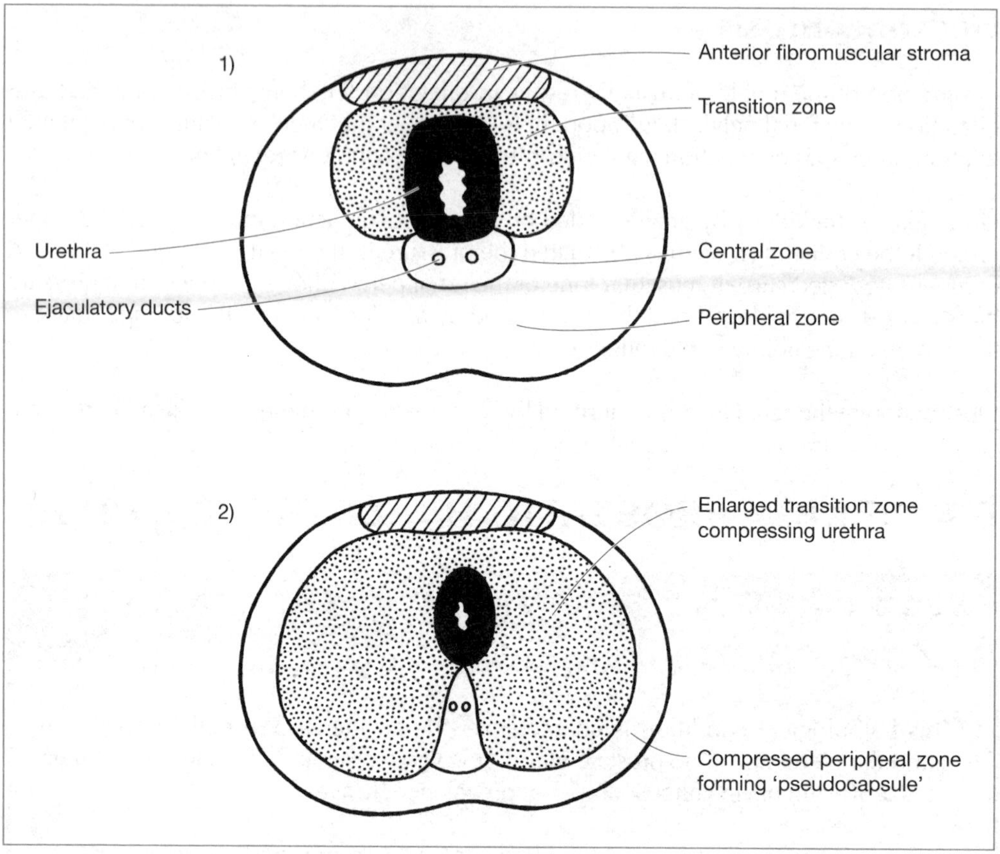

Figure 6.4a *Transverse sections of the prostate: 1) normal 2) benign prostatic hypertrophy*

Presentation of benign prostatic hypertrophy

- Asymptomatic
- Lower urinary tract symptoms (LUTS)
- Acute urinary retention or chronic urinary retention

Evaluation of LUTS

The term 'lower urinary tract symptoms' was coined because of problems associated with previous terms such as 'prostatism'. LUTS are divided into:

- **Voiding symptoms:** eg hesitancy, poor stream, straining, terminal dribbling
- **Storage symptoms:** eg frequency, urgency, nocturia, incontinence

There may also be symptoms associated with complications of BPH, including retention (acute or chronic), infection, bladder diverticulae and stones, and renal impairment due to hydronephrosis.

The major goals of evaluation are:

- To get an overall assessment of the patient including the severity of the symptoms and affect on quality of life
- To perform objective testing to document the cause of the symptoms
- To exclude serious urological pathology

History of benign prostatic hypertrophy

Severity of symptoms can be judged using standardised scoring systems such as the **International Prostate Symptom Score** (IPSS). A voiding diary is useful when discussing lifestyle measures to improve symptoms. Specific symptoms of importance include **haematuria** (mandates investigation for urinary tract cancer) and **dysuria** (suggests infection).

Physical examination in benign prostatic hypertrophy

Abdominal examination will detect a distended palpable bladder if present. Examination of the external genitalia should be done to exclude **meatal stenosis**. Rectal examination will allow identification of any prostatic abnormalities and also a rough estimate of size.

Investigating benign prostatic hypertrophy

Urinalysis

- Should be performed in all patients to exclude UTI
- Detection of haematuria mandates its investigation

Renal biochemistry

- Measurement of serum urea and creatinine are mandatory for all patients with LUTS
- Abnormal results warrant investigation of the upper UT to exclude obstructive uropathy

Prostate-specific antigen (PSA)

- (see section 7.4)
- This is not a specific test for LUTS, but many of these men will be concerned about prostate cancer; therefore it is reasonable to perform this test after appropriate patient counselling

Uroflowmetry

- Simple test of the rate and pattern of urine flow. At least 100 mL needs to be voided to make the test valid
- Obstruction is unlikely in men with a maximum flow (Q_{max}) of > 15 mL/second. Q_{max} of < 10 mL/s is compatible with obstruction

USS for post-void residual volume

- Often performed after uroflowmetry
- A residual of > 300 mL indicates chronic urinary retention

Formal urodynamic studies

- (see section 2.3)
- Performed where there is a strong possibility that symptoms are not due to bladder outflow obstruction (eg equivocal flow rate of 10–15 mL/second, neurological disease such as diabetic neuropathy, men of age < 60, men who have had previous surgery)
- Normograms are available in order to accurately define whether obstruction is present

Management of benign prostatic hypertrophy

It is important to appreciate that not all men require medical treatment. Some may simply be reassured if prostate cancer is excluded. In others, simple lifestyle measures may suffice, such as decreasing fluid at night and reducing caffeine intake. In those in whom this is not sufficient pharmacological or surgical treatment may be appropriate.

Pharmacological treatment of benign prostatic hypertrophy

- **Adrenergic antagonists (eg alfuzosin, tamsulosin):** these act on α_1-receptors within the prostatic and bladder neck smooth muscle. It is thought that about 50% of bladder outflow obstruction caused by prostatic enlargement is due to prostate smooth muscle tone (which is how these drugs have their effect). Their main side effect is postural hypotension
- **5α-reductase inhibitors (eg finasteride, dutasteride):** these block the enzyme 5α-reductase and hence conversion of testosterone to dihydrotestosterone (its active metabolite). They are effective in men with large prostates (> 40 g) and reduce the likelihood of acute urinary retention or surgery. 25% report improved symptoms but the drugs can take 6–9 months to take effect. 5α-reductase inhibitors reduce serum PSA by about 50% and it is important to appreciate this if there are concerns about prostate cancer

Surgical treatment of benign prostatic hypertrophy

Surgery is indicated in patients who do not have adequate symptom relief on pharmacological therapy. Men who have recurrent infections, bladder stones, or present with acute urinary retention also require surgery. Standard surgery is transurethral resection of the prostate (TURP) as described in the operation box.

Op box: Transurethral resection of the prostate (TURP)

Indications

Moderate to severe LUTS
Complications of BPH eg bladder stones, UTI, acute urinary retention, and chronic urinary retention
Failure of medical therapy
Renal impairment due to LUTS

Pre-op

Exclude or treat UTI
Group and save (5% require transfusion)
Broad-spectrum antibiotic prophylaxis
TEDS stockings for DVT prophylaxis, most do not use SC heparin
Spinal or GA

Procedure

Patient in lithotomy position
Initial cystoscopy to exclude urethral stricture or bladder pathology
Urethral dilatation is normally performed before insertion of resectoscope (24–28 French)
Irrigation fluid is glycine 1.5% which allows electrocautery
Resection of prostatic tissue is performed to capsule, from bladder neck proximally to verumontanum distally (to mark level of the external sphincter)
Chips of prostate tissue removed with an Ellik evacuator
Haemostasis is secured and a three-way irrigating catheter placed in the bladder

Post-op

Irrigate for 24–48 hours until urine is clear
In larger resections check Hb and electrolytes post-operatively

Complications

Bleeding: primary, secondary and reactive haemorrhage may occur causing haematuria +/– clot retention
Infection leading to septicaemia
TURP syndrome (see text below)
Failure to void: causes include hypotonic bladder or incomplete resection
Incontinence: sphincter damage or pre-existing detrusor over-activity
Urethral stricture or bladder neck stricture: occurs in 2–5% and requires incision
Impotence: occurs in up to 20%. Warn patients and document existing function
Retrograde ejaculation: occurs in > 80% due to resection of bladder neck

Several minimally invasive therapies (eg laser or microwave ablation of the prostate) have been proposed in order to reduce the morbidity associated with TURP but none has so far replaced it as the gold standard operation. Tissue ablative techniques prevent histological examination of the tissue removed which can be important for excluding malignancy.

In patients with very large prostates (> 90 g) open retropubic prostatectomy may be required.

TURP syndrome

This syndrome develops during or post-TURP surgery due to absorption of large volumes of irrigation fluid through the prostatic venous plexus. It causes electrolyte disturbances (hyponatraemia) and high nitrogen load, hypervolaemia, cerebral oedema and hypothermia. It can cause visual disturbance, nausea, vomiting, mental confusion, seizures, hypertension and bradycardia. It has been observed in 2% of post-TURP patients.

Treatment is with supportive measures (including ICU if necessary), fluid restriction and diuretics.

It is associated with high mortality. The syndrome can be avoided by minimising surgical time (to < 1 hour) and reducing irrigation pressures.

Urethral stricture

Injury to the urethral mucosa will heal as a circumferential scar with subsequent fibrosis. This can cause bladder outflow obstruction.

Causes of urethral stricture

- Traumatic (eg catheterisation, pelvic fracture)
- Neoplastic (eg bladder, penile and prostatic cancer)
- Inflammatory (eg urethritis, *Gonococcus*)

Management of urethral stricture

- Repeated dilatation
- Urethrotomy with stricture excision and/or stenting
- Open reconstruction may be required

6.5 ACUTE URINARY RETENTION

In a nutshell ...

This is an acute painful inability to micturate. It is ten times more common in men than women.

Causes of acute urinary retention

Acute urinary retention is caused by:

- Any cause of bladder outflow obstruction (commonly BPH in elderly men), but also prostate carcinoma and urethral strictures
- Neurological diseases leading to detrusor dysfunction or non-coordination between detrusor contraction and sphincter relaxation (see section 2 *Bladder dysfunction and incontinence*)

Predisposing factors include:

- Constipation
- Urinary infection
- Post-operative factors (pain, immobility, drugs, anaesthetic factors)
- Drugs with an anticholinergic effect (eg antidepressants)
- High fluid intake and bladder over-distension (eg high alcohol intake)

It is likely that in most cases there is a combination of prostatic oedema (eg infection) and detrusor dysfunction (eg due to over-distension or drugs).

Presentation of acute urinary retention

Patients present acutely with an inability to pass urine and severe lower abdominal discomfort. The bladder is usually palpable and tender.

Management of acute urinary retention

- **Urgent catheterisation:** either per urethra or suprapubically, this is initial emergency treatment. The residual volume should be accurately recorded as it may predict likely success of trial without catheter (TWOC). Subsequent management depends on the patient's prior symptoms, residual volume, and fitness for surgery

- **TWOC:** in the past TURP was considered standard treatment for acute urinary retention. But in modern practice many patients will be allowed a TWOC, which has much more chance of success if a recognised predisposing factor had been treated (eg constipation, UTI) and with small residual volumes (< 800 mL)
- **TURP:** patients who have a successful TWOC should be followed up, as a significant number will still come to surgery eventually. However, elective rather than acute surgery has fewer complications
- **Long-term in-dwelling catheterisation:** may be required by some patients

Procedure: Insertion of a urinary catheter

This is probably the commonest urological intervention but is still associated with many problems. The two main forms of catheterisation are urethral or suprapubic.

Urethral catheterisation
Various catheters are available.

- Two-way catheters come in a variety of sizes, the most commonly used being 12–16 Fr
- They can be made of latex rubber for short-term use only (for up to 4 weeks) or of silicone for long-term catheterisation (12 weeks between changes)
- Three-way catheters are available in sizes up to 22 Fr in order to allow bladder washout of blood or debris

When inserting a urethral catheter in a male it is important to remember that the urethra takes a fairly sharp bend anteriorly at the level of the bulbar urethra. If this fact is not appreciated it is easy to create a false passage posteriorly. Once a false passage is created the catheter will naturally head in this direction and it is very difficult to perform subsequent catheterisation.

The commonest causes of difficulty or failure to catheterise are:

- Urethral stricture
- Prostate hypertrophy/bladder neck hypertrophy
- Sphincter spasm

In the case of urethral stricture it is unwise to try and force a catheter and either suprapubic catheterisation or cystoscopy with or without urethrotomy should be performed.

For large prostates or bladder neck hypertrophy a catheter introducer can be used to negotiate the prostatic urethra. This should only be done by somebody with experience.

Sphincter spasm is common and may be eased by lidocaine gel but often it is just patience that allows the catheter to be passed when the spasm temporarily relents.

Suprapubic catheterisation
At the bedside this can only be performed in patients with an easily palpable bladder.

Procedure

The lower half of the abdomen is prepared with antiseptic solution and LA is infiltrated at a point 2 or 3 finger-breadths above the pubic symphysis in the mid-line
As the anaesthetic is infiltrated more deeply the urine can often be aspirated
After a small skin incision the catheter can be inserted percutaneously
Several methods are available for introducing the catheter percutaneously. The commonest involves using a trocar and plastic sheath to introduce a standard 16 French catheter

Contraindications to suprapubic catheterisation

Previous abdominal surgery which may have resulted in small bowel adhesions to the anterior abdominal wall
History of TCC of the bladder because of the risk of seeding into the tract
Any bleeding tendency

6.6 CHRONIC URINARY RETENTION

In a nutshell ...

The strict definition is a residual volume of > 300 mL, however patients often present with residuals much greater than this.

Presentation of chronic urinary retention

- Patients often have no pain
- Low-pressure retention may present with overflow incontinence
- High-pressure retention often presents with renal failure

Management of chronic urinary retention

- **Catheterisation:** this is the standard treatment
- **Monitor diuresis:** patients with renal dysfunction need to be monitored closely as they will have a post-obstructive diuresis. Diuresis is physiological and represents off-loading of salt and water that was retained while the patient was in renal failure. Careful observation and fluid balance is required and IV fluid replacement is usually necessary initially
- **No TWOC:** in contrast to patients with acute urinary retention, patients who have had an episode of high-pressure chronic urinary retention should **not** have a TWOC
- **TURP:** this is the standard treatment after stabilisation of renal function, although success rates in terms of voiding are lower than in patients with acute urinary retention (70% vs 90%)
- **Intermittent self-catheterisation (ISC):** in patients with detrusor failure secondary to chronic obstruction ISC is an option

Section 7
Urological malignancy

7.1 RENAL TUMOURS

In a nutshell ...

The table *Classification of renal tumours* shows many different causes of a tumour in the kidney, but if a mass is identified in the kidney it can rarely be identified until the pathological specimen is obtained.

Thus a mass in the kidney is treated as if it is a renal carcinoma (ie with a radical nephrectomy) unless:

- It can be shown to be benign (eg the diagnostic CT appearance of angiomyolipoma)
- It is < 2 cm and does not enlarge on annual CT

Thus many benign masses are removed with a radical nephrectomy rather than risk missing a cancer.

CLASSIFICATION OF RENAL TUMOURS

	Benign	Malignant
Solid	Angiomyolipoma*	Renal cell carcinoma (adenocarcinoma)
	Oncocytoma**	Wilms tumour (nephroblastoma)
		Metastatic deposits
		Transitional cell carcinoma (renal pelvis)
		Renal sarcoma
Cystic	Simple cyst	Cystadenocarcinoma (cystic renal cell carcinoma)
	Polycystic kidney	Cystic necrosis of renal carcinoma

*Although most are clinically benign, they may occasionally be locally invasive.
**Oncocytoma may metastasise.

Bosniak's classification grades cysts from I to IV according to their CT appearance (calcification, septae, wall thickness, etc). Grade I cysts are almost always benign and grade IV almost always malignant.

Renal cell adenocarcinoma

Also known as renal cell carcinoma or hyper-nephroma renal cell carcinoma is a common malignant solid cancer accounting for 3% of all adult malignancies. The incidence is increasing (mainly due to incidental diagnosis) and there is a sex ratio of 2M to 1F.

Renal cell carcinoma arises from cells of the proximal renal tubule, commonly at the pole of the kidney. It is yellowish (full of fat) and very vascular.

Spread is by:

- Direct extension
  - Peri-nephric fat and fascia
  - Wall and lumen of renal vein/IVC
- Metastasis
  - Cannonball metastases to lung, bone, and brain

Aetiology of renal cell adenocarcinoma

2% of renal cell adenocarcinomas are familial, and these are associated with:

- Von Hippel Lindau disease (70% risk by 60 years)
- Haemangioblastomas of the cerebellum and spine
- Retinal haemangiomas
- Phaeochromocytomas
- Islet cell tumours

Risk factors for non-familial renal cell carcinoma include:

- Acquired renal cystic disease (90% of dialysis patients) has a 17% risk of renal cancer
- Smoking
- Exposure to cadmium, lead, asbestos, polycarbons

Histology of renal cell carcinoma

- Clear cell adenocarcinomas (well over half of all cases)
- Papillary (18% of cases)
- Chromophobe (5% of cases)

Papillary and chromophobe carcinomas carry a slightly better prognosis. Collecting duct type carcinomas have a significantly worse prognosis. Grading of renal tumour is by the Fuhrman system, using a scale of 1 to 4.

Clinical features of renal cell carcinoma

Classic triad of pain, mass and haematuria is now seen in < 10% patients. Commonly an incidental finding (> 50%).

May present with paraneoplastic syndromes due to secretion of renin, erythropoietin or a parahormone. This may result in hypercalcaemia, hypertension, polycythaemia, fever and night sweats, or Stauffer's syndrome (hepatic dysfunction).

- Renal vein involvement in 20%
- IVC involvement in 10%

Investigating renal cell carcinoma

USS is the usual initial diagnostic investigation. CT scan of the chest and abdomen with IV contrast is used for staging and is very sensitive, picking up:

- Renal vein involvement 91%
- IVC extension 97%
- Peri-renal extension 79%
- Lymph node metastases 87%

Staging of renal cell carcinoma

Tumour staging

T_1 Tumour < 7 cm limited to kidney
T_{1a} Tumour < 4 cm
T_{1b} Tumour 4–7 cm
T_2 Tumour > 7 cm limited to kidney
T_3 Tumour extends outside kidney but within Gerota's fascia
T_{3a} Tumour invades adrenals or peri-nephric tissues
T_{3b} Tumour extends into renal vein or IVC below diaphragm
T_{3c} Tumour extends into IVC above diaphragm
T_4 Tumour invades beyond Gerota's fascia

Lymph node staging

N_x Cannot be assessed
N_0 No nodes involved
N_1 Metastasis in a single node
N_2 Metastasis in > 1 node

Metastases staging

M_x Cannot be assessed
M_0 No distant metastases
M_1 Distant metastases present

Chapter 11

Management of renal cell carcinoma

Localised disease

- **Radical nephrectomy:** this is the gold standard (see Op box)
- **Laparoscopic radical nephrectomy:** this is being increasingly performed
- **Partial nephrectomy:** this is performed for selected cases (eg single kidney, poor renal function, multifocal tumours)

IVC involvement does not affect prognosis of the cancer, though it may need cardiac bypass during surgery and this has associated morbidity.

Metastatic disease

30% present with metastases and another 30% develop them.

- **Nephrectomy:** this may be palliative for haematuria. There is a small increase in short-term survival with nephrectomy despite distant metastasis
- **Embolisation:** this can be effective
- **Chemotherapy/radiotherapy:** results with these alone are poor
- **Immunotherapy:** this is effective, and is used in combination with chemotherapy (eg IL-2, IFN-α, 5-FU)

Op box: Nephrectomy

Indications

Radical nephrectomy is indicated for localised renal carcinoma. It involves removal of the kidney with surrounding Gerota's fascia. Simple nephrectomy is indicated in cases of non-functioning kidneys.

Pre-op

Exclude or treat UTI
Cross-match 2–4 units of blood
DVT prophylaxis with TEDS stockings and SC heparin
Ensure adequate imaging to confirm side of operation and anatomy
Some (but not all) surgeons mark the side of surgery

Procedure

Both lateral loin approach (extra-peritoneal) and trans-abdominal approaches are used. In the loin approach, the operating table is 'broken' allowing flexion, with patients lying on their side, to maximise exposure

In the loin approach, the abdominal wall muscles are divided and the incision continues above the level of either the 11th or 12th rib in order to avoid the neurovascular bundle
In both approaches dissection allows exposure of the renal hilum. The renal artery is tied before the vein to prevent renal congestion
On the right, the renal vein is short and care is needed
On the left, undue traction should be avoided to prevent splenic injury. The tail of the pancreas is also at risk

Post-op

IV fluids are required until ileus resolves (longer with the trans-abdominal approach)
Chest physiotherapy and early mobilisation are important

Complications

Bleeding
Chest infection: particularly in smokers and those with pre-existing chest disease
Pain: pain from the incision prevents adequate chest expansion and leads to pulmonary collapse so adequate analgesia and chest physiotherapy are vital
DVT/PE

Prognosis of renal cell carcinoma

This is influenced by tumour grade, degree of local invasion, venous invasion and distant metastasis. 5-year survival is approximately:

- 90% for T_1 disease
- 60% for T_2/T_3 disease
- 0–20% for distant metastasis

Other malignant renal tumours

In a nutshell ...

Apart from renal cell carcinomas, the other important malignant tumours of the kidney are:
Renal nephroblastoma (Wilms tumour). See the oncology section of Chapter 10 *Paediatric Surgery*
TCC of the renal pelvis (see section 7.2 *Bladder cancer and urothelial tumours of the urinary tract*)
Renal sarcoma
Metastasis to the kidney

Renal sarcoma

This accounts for 1–2% of renal neoplasms. This tumour is commonly a leiomyosarcoma. It presents in the 5th decade with flank pain and weight loss. Treatment is with radical nephrectomy.

Metastatic deposits in the kidney

The kidney can be affected by metastasis from the lung (20%), the breast (12%), the stomach (11%) and lymphoma.

Benign renal tumours

Angiomyolipoma

An angiomyolipoma is a benign hamartoma consisting of fat (~ 80%), blood vessels, and smooth muscle. It is rare, accounting for 0.5% of renal tumours.

20–50% of angiomyolipomas are associated with tuberous sclerosis, a syndrome of mental retardation, epilepsy, and adenoma sebaceum, but most commonly angiomyolipoma is asymptomatic. Haemorrhage into the tumour can result in flank pain and hypotension.

Angiomyolipoma may be confidently diagnosed by CT due to diagnostic appearance of a high fat content.

Treatment options include:

- Conservative if < 4 cm
- Consider enucleation or partial nephrectomy for symptomatic lesions or those > 4 cm
- Treatment of acute bleeding requires embolisation or nephrectomy

Oncocytoma

Accounting for 3–7% of solid renal masses, oncocytoma is a solid benign tumour of the kidney. It is a neoplasm of the intercalated cells of the collecting duct, and is usually well circumscribed, encapsulated, and rarely metastasises.

80% are asymptomatic and discovered incidentally.

Unfortunately it cannot be accurately distinguished from renal adenocarcinoma radiologically, so radical nephrectomy (see the Op box) is the standard treatment.

7.2 BLADDER CANCER AND UROTHELIAL TUMOURS OF THE URINARY TRACT

In a nutshell ...

Bladder cancer is most commonly a transitional cell carcinoma, which is a urothelial tumour of the type that affects the entire urinary tract.

95% of urothelial tumours affect the bladder; 5% affect the upper tract. One urothelial tumour in one area of the renal tract increases the risk of another (unstable urothelium).

The grade and stage of the tumour varies widely. Superficial disease, although often recurrent and needing repeated treatment, has a very good prognosis. In aggressive metastatic disease patients are unlikely to survive a year.

Epidemiology and pathology of urothelial cancers and bladder transitional cell carcinoma (TCC)

The renal tract is lined with transitional cell urothelium from the renal pelvis to the urethra. TCC may therefore occur at any point along this tract, including in the kidney.

- Bladder TCC is the second most common urological malignancy
- Incidence is gradually increasing
- Sex ratio is 3M to 1F
- Affects older patients with peak incidence at 65
- There are geographical variations
- Of these cancers > 90% are TCC, 5% are SCC and the rest are adenocarcinomas. Sarcoma is rare. Benign tumours are uncommon

Patterns of bladder TCC include:

- Papillary
- Solid invasive
- CIS (may be ulcerated)

Risk factors for bladder and urothelial cancers

- Smoking: major risk factor in the developed world
- Occupational factors: historically important for workers in the rubber, dye, leather, and textile industries
- Chronic inflammation: eg stone disease, long-term catheters, recurrent infections, bilharzia
- Congenital anomaly: eg remnant of urachus

Presentation of bladder and urothelial cancers

- 80–90% present with painless macroscopic haematuria
- Microscopic haematuria in patients aged > 50 also requires investigation for bladder cancer
- Irritative bladder symptoms may be a presenting feature (a third will have a persistent chronic urine infection)
- 5% present with metastatic disease

Investigating bladder and urothelial cancer

- Diagnosis is usually by flexible cystoscopy
- All patients with haematuria should have an investigation of the upper UT
- Occasionally diagnosis is made on US or IVU when a filling defect in the bladder is demonstrated

Staging of bladder cancer

Tumour staging

T_{IS}	Carcinoma in situ
T_a	Papillary non-I–IV carcinoma
T_1	Tumour invades sub-epithelial connective tissue (through lamina propria)
T_2	Tumour invades muscle
T_{2a}	Tumour invades superficial muscle (inner half)
T_{2b}	Tumour invades deep muscle (outer half)
T_3	Tumour invades peri-vesical tissue
T_{3a}	Microscopically
T_{3b}	Macroscopically (extra-vesical mass)
T_4	Tumour invades adjacent structures
T_{4a}	Invades prostate, uterus, or vagina
T_{4b}	Invades pelvic wall or abdominal wall

Lymph node staging

Nx	Cannot be assessed
N_0	No nodes involved
N_1	Single lymph node metastasis < 2 cm
N_2	Single lymph node 2–5 cm or multiple nodes none > 5 cm
N_3	Lymph node metastasis > 5 cm

Metastases staging

M_X	Cannot be assessed
M_0	No distant metastases
M_1	Distant metastases present

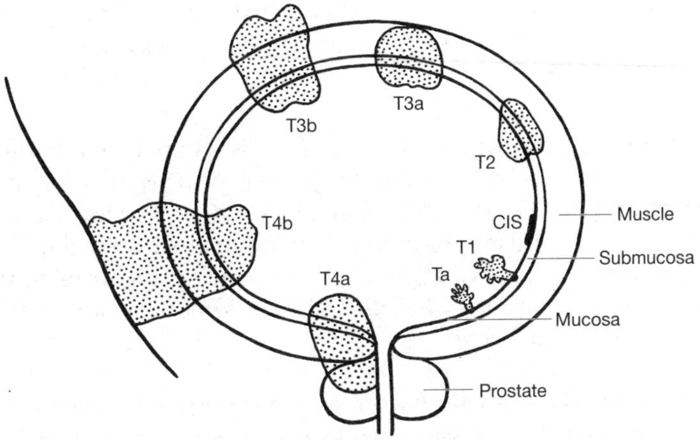

Figure 7.2a *Bladder cancer staging*

The major distinction is between 'superficial' bladder cancer (T_{is}, T_a and T_1) which accounts for 80% of all tumours, and muscle-invasive bladder cancer.

Histological grading of bladder tumours is:

G_1 Well differentiated

G_2 Moderately differentiated

G_3 Poorly differentiated

Management of superficial bladder cancer

'Superficial' bladder cancer is a term that covers stages T_a T_1 and CIS. It covers a wide range of tumours, and these may have quite different clinical behaviours.

Most tumours are managed by **transurethral endoscopic resection (TURBT) with or without intra-vesical therapy**, but there is a risk of progression to muscle-invasive disease so more radical therapy may be required (see below). Risk of progression depends predominantly on the stage and grade.

- G_1 pT_a tumours have a very good prognosis; < 5% will progress
- G_3 pT_1 tumours or CIS are G_3 tumours confined to the urothelium; up to 50% progress

All patients with superficial bladder cancer should undergo regular check cystoscopies (intervals determined by cystoscopic and histological findings). Significant numbers of patients develop a further tumour (even if disease-free for a long time). High-risk patients and those with multiple tumours or frequent recurrences should be considered for intra-vesical therapy. Both chemotherapy and immunotherapy are used.

- **Intravesical chemotherapy:** mitomycin C is the most commonly used drug. A single dose can reduce the recurrence rate after initial transurethral resection. A typical course of mitomycin C is weekly instillations for 6 weeks. There is good evidence that mitomycin C reduces the risk of recurrence, but no evidence that it prevents progression
- **Intravesical immunotherapy:** intravesicular BCG is an immune adjuvant that upregulates the host immune response against the tumour. Also given as a 6-week course and is standard therapy for G_3 pT_1 tumours and CIS. More effective than mitomycin C at preventing recurrence and may have some impact on progression (but this is controversial). Maintenance therapy with further shorter courses improves results. Toxicity is greater than with mitomycin C. Irritative bladder symptoms are common and occasional systemic upset can occur

Patients with high-risk disease who have recurrence despite intra-vesicular therapy are considered for radical therapy (invasive bladder cancer is discussed below).

Management of invasive bladder cancer

This tumour has invaded into the detrusor muscle of the bladder and therefore cannot be completely excised by endoscopic measures. Before trying curative treatment it is important to exclude extra-vesical spread or metastatic disease. Prognosis of invasive bladder cancer is poor with a 5-year survival after surgery and radiotherapy of 30–50%.

- **Thorough investigation** is vital to planning treatment. MRI scan is the best investigation for local staging and would also indicate lymph node involvement in the pelvis. It may be affected by transurethral resection and therefore 4 weeks should be left between TURBT and MRI scan. CXR, serum calcium, serum alkaline phosphatase, and occasionally a bone scan will be required to exclude distant metastases
- **Radical cystectomy** has been the standard treatment for patients with T_2/T_3 non-metastatic bladder cancer. Urinary diversion is needed and is most commonly obtained by formation of an ileal conduit. Patients are increasingly being offered bladder reconstruction using small bowel
- **Radical radiotherapy** is also an option for attempted cure. It has been used particularly for patients who are unfit for cystectomy. An advantage is that the bladder is preserved, however there may be symptoms of radiation cystitis and proctitis. Check cystoscopies are required, and if the tumour recurs, salvage cystectomy may be an option

Treatment of metastatic disease

- Platinum-based chemotherapy for patients with metastatic disease who are fit enough to tolerate its toxicity
- In many patients, palliative care only is appropriate
- Prognosis is poor with survival about 1 year from diagnosis

Op box: Radical cystectomy

Indications

Invasive bladder cancer
Recurrent bladder cancer after radical radiotherapy
High-grade superficial bladder cancer resistant to local treatment

Pre-op

The patient should see a stoma nurse to discuss living with an ileal conduit, and the position should be marked. This should happen even for patients where bladder reconstruction is planned
Bowel prep may be given
DVT prophylaxis with SC heparin and TED stockings is required
Broad-spectrum antibiotic prophylaxis is given
4–6 units of blood should be cross-matched

Procedure

The patient should be supine and catheterised
Lower mid-line incision
A full laparotomy is performed
Initial dissection involves mobilising the urachal remnant (median umbilical ligament) as this should be excised en bloc with the bladder
Bowel mobilisation of the caecum and ascending colon on the right and descending colon on the left allows packing of colon and small bowel into the epigastrium
The ureters are mobilised and divided close to the bladder
A full lymph node dissection is performed to include the obturator lymph nodes, the internal iliac, external iliac and common iliac nodes as far as the aortic bifurcation. As well as providing important staging information, this gives good dissection of the vascular anatomy before cystectomy
The bladder is dissected free. Prostate is also removed in males. Particular care is needed with the dorsal venous complex and while dissecting the prostate and bladder neck from the rectum
In patients with urethral tumours the urethra is dissected through a separate perineal incision and removed en bloc with the bladder and prostate
The standard method of urinary drainage is an ileal conduit, as a loop of small bowel proximal to the terminal ileum is resected and this needs to be long enough to reach the abdominal wall (approximately 25 cm). Once the loop has been isolated small bowel anastomosis is performed to restore continuity of the remaining ileum

Various methods exist to anastomose the ureters to the ileal loop and they can either be anastomosed to the end of the loop or through separate incisions. Stents are placed across the anastomosis
A stoma is formed with a spout to ensure urine does not directly drain onto the skin surface
If continent diversion is planned, various forms of ileal neobladder exist
A tube drain is inserted into the abdomen

Post-op

Patients often need high-dependency care immediately post-operatively
NG drainage should continue until bowel activity returns
Epidural anaesthesia is the optimum method of ensuring that patients are pain free and reducing the risk of chest infections
Chest physiotherapy should be given
Tube drains should be left for at least 48 hours
Ureteric stents can be removed after 10–12 days

Complications

Peri-operative complications
Bleeding
Rectal damage

Early complications
Prolonged ileus
Chest infection
DVT or PE
Urine leak
Pelvic abscess formation (usually follows pelvic haematoma)
Problems related to the bowel anastomosis such as leakage
Wound infection

Late complications
Hernias of the wound or stoma
UTIs or urinary stones
Stenosis of the conduit
Upper tract deterioration is common and electrolytes should be monitored

Other (non urothelial) tumours of the bladder

Squamous cell carcinoma (SCC) of the bladder

This is common in the east and Egypt. It presents late and infiltrates and may be a complication of chronic inflammation with stone disease or bilharzias. It is treated by resection.

Adenocarcinoma of the bladder

This accounts for about 1% of bladder tumours. It may develop in the vault at the site of a urachal remnant and the tumour itself grows outside the bladder. It is managed with surgery and chemotherapy.

Bladder sarcoma

This has a poor prognosis apart from liposarcoma.

Urothelial tumours of the ureter and renal pelvis

These account for 5% of all transitional cell carcinomas. Renal pelvis tumours are three times more common than ureteric tumours and account for 8% of all kidney cancers. Risk factors are similar to those for TCC in the bladder. These tumours are commonly superficial.

Importantly, the risk of a bladder TCC after an upper tract TCC is about 50% (it represents a field change within the urothelium). The risk of upper tract TCC following TCC bladder is low (less than 2%).

Presentation of urothelial tumours of the ureter and renal pelvis

- As in renal cell carcinomas painless haematuria is again the commonest presentation
- US is not good for detecting upper tract TCC, so IVU is recommended for patients with persistent haematuria in whom US and cystoscopy are normal

Treatment of urothelial tumours of the ureter and renal pelvis

- Staging to exclude metastatic disease is as for bladder cancer
- If metastases are excluded curative treatment with **nephro-ureterectomy** is gold standard
- More conservative treatments for patients with solitary kidney or renal impairment (eg ureteroscopic and percutaneous resection)

All patients should have follow-up cystoscopies because of high risk of subsequent bladder cancer.

7.3 PROSTATE CANCER

In a nutshell ...

This is the commonest urological malignancy and the second most common cause of cancer death in males.

Epidemiology of prostate cancer

This is a disease of advancing age, and incidence is increasing with increasing life expectancy.

Autopsy studies show that microscopic foci of prostate cancer are present in up to 80% of men aged 80. This incidence seems to be the same worldwide, and is thought to represent 'latent' cancer, most of which is clinically insignificant. However, the risks of prostate cancer as cause of death is about 3% (men are more likely to die with the disease than because of it).

The incidence of 'significant' prostate cancer is far more common in the developed world. The reasons for this are not clear.

Risk factors for prostate cancer

Environmental factors (eg diet, saturated fats, phyto-oestrogens)
Genetic factors (family history)
Geography/race (more common in people of African origin and less common in people from Asia)

Pathology of prostate cancer

95% of prostate cancers are adenocarcinomas. The rest consist of TCC, SCC, and lymphoma. Most (75%) arise in the peripheral zone of the prostate, unlike BPH which affects the transition zone.

Commonly well differentiated with slow growth in response to androgen, or occasionally poorly differentiated with rapid metastasis. Arises from the epithelium of the prostatic duct acini and preceded by intra-epithelial neoplasia.

Gleason grading system

- Used for histological assessment of prostate cancer
- Correlates with prognosis
- Takes into account heterogeneous nature of the disease by grading the two predominant areas of a tumour
- An individual area may have a Gleason grade of 1 (well differentiated) to 5 (poorly differentiated) leading to a sum score of 2–10 when the scores of the two areas are combined

Presentation of prostate cancer

- **Asymptomatic:** localised prostate cancer often produces no symptoms
- **Incidental finding:** many of these men will also have BPH and present with lower urinary tract symptoms. The prostate cancer is diagnosed on digital rectal examination (hard, craggy prostate, asymmetry, and loss of median sulcus) or by testing for prostate specific antigen (PSA, see below)
- **BOO:** locally advanced disease may present with ureteric obstruction due to local infiltration and renal failure
- **Symptoms of distal disease:** metastatic disease may present with bone pain, pathological fracture or spinal cord compression

Prostate serum antigen (PSA)

This is a proteolytic enzyme produced specifically by the prostate which has a role in the liquefication of the ejaculate. Large amounts are secreted into the semen and small quantities escape into the blood stream.

The PSA level is elevated in prostate cancer but can also be elevated by BPH, urinary tract infection, or urethral instrumentation such as catheterisation or cystoscopy.

The likelihood of diagnosis of prostate cancer rises with the level of PSA (as shown in the table). Because PSA increases with increasing age (probably due to BPH) age-related values have also been defined.

PSA LEVEL AND RISK OF PROSTATE CANCER

PSA level (ng/mL)	Risk of prostate cancer
< 4	Normal
4–10	15–20%
10–20	50–75%
> 20	90%

Chapter 11

Diagnosis and investigation of prostate cancer

Diagnosis of prostate cancer is usually obtained by **prostatic biopsy** performed during **transrectal ultrasonography** (TRUS). Random biopsies are taken (usually 6 to 10) to get a representative sample of prostate gland. Abnormal areas are sometimes seen (classically **hypoechoic** areas on ultrasound) and these should be biopsied although they are not specific for prostate cancer. Because the biopsies are transrectal, infection is a major risk and all patients should have prophylactic antibiotics.

Staging of prostate cancer

This is based on the TNM system.

Tumour staging

T_1 Clinically unapparent tumour not palpable or visible by imaging

T_{1a} Incidental finding at TURP (< 5% of tissue resected involved)

T_{1b} Incidental finding at TURP (> 5% of tissue resected involved)

T_{1c} Identified by needle biopsy (eg because of elevated PSA)

T_2 Tumour confined to prostate (palpable or visible on imaging)

T_{2a} Involving half of one lobe or less

T_{2b} Involving more than half of one lobe, but not both lobes

T_{2c} Involving both lobes

T_3 Tumour extends through prostatic capsule

T_{3a} Extra-capsular extension

T_{3b} Extension into seminal vesicle(s)

T_4 Tumour fixed or invading adjacent structures other than seminal vesicles (eg bladder neck, external sphincter, levator muscles or pelvic side wall)

Lymph node staging

N_x Cannot be assessed

N_0 No nodes involved

N_1 Lymph nodes involved

Metastasis staging

M_X Cannot be assessed

M_0 No distant metastases

M_1 Distant metastases present

Localised and advanced disease

- T_1 or T_2 disease are considered localised and therefore potentially curable
- T_3 disease is locally advanced and therefore unlikely to be cured
- T_4 disease and metastatic disease are advanced disease

In clinically localised disease where curative treatment is proposed, an MRI scan will give information on localised tumour stage and lymph node metastasis in the pelvis.

The most common site of distant spread after the lymph node is the bony skeleton. Bone scan is a sensitive method of detecting skeletal metastases.

Management of localised prostate cancer

It is important to realise that not all prostate cancer requires treatment. Many men with this cancer die of other causes, and do not benefit from treatment (but will be put at risk of any side effects or complications). One of the great challenges in urology at the present time is to identify groups of patients who are likely to have 'aggressive disease' with a high risk of mortality, who therefore require intervention.

There are three main options for men with localised prostate cancer:

- Active monitoring
- Radical prostatectomy
- Radical radiotherapy or brachytherapy

Active monitoring of localised prostate cancer

Ideal for men with well-differentiated tumours and relatively low PSA levels. Morbidity associated with radical treatment is avoided. Monitoring is with regular PSA tests. Usually offered to men with a life expectancy of > 10 years.

Radical prostatectomy of localised prostate cancer

Radical prostatectomy is the removal of the prostate with re-anastomosis of the bladder neck to the urethra. Pelvic lymph node dissection may also be carried out. The traditional approach has been retropubic via laparotomy, but laparoscopic and perineal approaches are also used.

This is a major operation with significant complications (eg bleeding and PE). In the long term 70% have erectile dysfunction and there is a 5% incontinence rate.

Radical radiotherapy of localised prostate cancer

A 6-week course of daily treatments avoids a major operation for localised prostate cancer. Modern conformal therapy is associated with minimal complications, but bladder and bowel toxicity can occur. There are no clinical trials showing a difference in efficacy between radical prostatectomy and radical radiotherapy, but these trials suffer from bias because of differences in patient selection. There is evidence that neo-adjuvant hormone therapy improves the results of radiotherapy.

Monitoring patients with radical radiotherapy can be difficult as PSA levels do not always fall to zero.

Prostate brachytherapy

This method of treating localised disease involves implantation of radioactive seeds into the prostate. Results are comparable with surgery, and complication rates are lower, but there are only a few centres in the country with a long experience of this technique.

Cryotherapy is another method of treatment of localised disease but the long-term results for this are not available.

Management of advanced/metastatic prostate cancer

Locally advanced disease

Radical prostatectomy is not usually indicated in this group of patients. Active monitoring is an option in asymptomatic men. Good 5-year survival figures are obtained with palliative radiotherapy, which is often used in combination with hormonal therapy.

Metastatic disease

Most of these patients require systemic palliative treatment as evidence suggests that in metastatic disease early institution of hormonal treatment may prevent complications such as spinal cord compression and pathological fractures.

Hormonal treatment

The aim of all these treatments is to prevent the action of testosterone on prostate cancer cells. Initial response is normally excellent but eventually prostate cancer cells will become androgen-independent and at that time hormonal therapy is ineffective. Once this occurs median survival is only 6 months.

Luteinising hormone releasing hormone (LHRH) agonists

- These act on the pituitary to prevent the release of **luteinising hormone** (LH). This is because normal stimulation of LH is by pulsed release of LHRH by the hypothalamus and continuous stimulation leads to inhibition
- Lack of LH means that testosterone is not produced by the Leydig cells in the testes. Hence this is a form of medical castration
- Side effects include lack of energy, loss of libido, and hot flushes

Bilateral orchidectomy

- Before the development of LHRH agonists this was the standard treatment for prostate cancer.
- Very effective
- Cheaper than medical therapy
- Avoids repeated injections
- Rarely used in modern practice

Anti-androgens

These drugs compete with testosterone at the androgen receptor and examples include cyproterone acetate, flutamide, and bicalutamide. They are not as effective alone as LHRH agonists but may sometimes be used in combination with LHRH agonists. Anti-androgens do have fewer side effects than LHRH agonists.

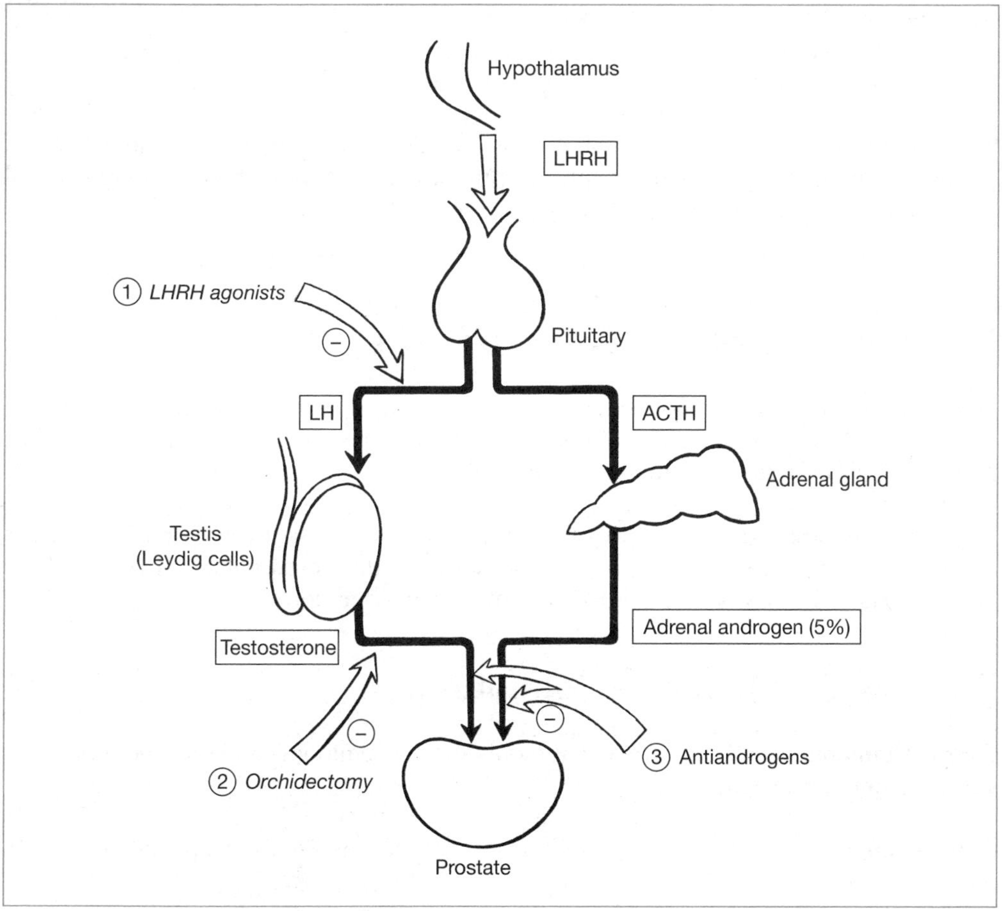

Figure 7.3a *Hormonal control of the prostate and mechanism of action of hormonal therapy*

Management of hormone-escaped prostate cancer

Various chemotherapy regimens have been tried in this situation but prognosis is poor and palliative care alone is usually appropriate. Addition of diethylstilbestrol or prednisolone may provide some benefit. Localised radiotherapy to bone metastases is an excellent form of pain control.

7.4 TESTICULAR CANCER

In a nutshell ...

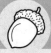

Testicular cancers are the commonest solid tumours in young men. There are two main types:
Seminomas
Non-seminomatous germ cell tumours (NSGCT)

Radical orchidectomy is the treatment of choice in both tumours. Seminomas are usually treated by irradiation with or without chemotherapy. NSGCT may need chemotherapy or (rarely in the UK) retroperitoneal lymph node dissection.

Epidemiology of testicular tumours

Testicular tumour is the commonest tumour in boys and men aged 15–35, and it is increasing in incidence. It is reported to affect 7 men in 100 000, and is four times commoner in white people. 2.5–5% of testicular tumours are bilateral.

A history of undescended testis leads to a 10-fold increased risk, even if orchidopexy has been carried out. The contralateral, normally descended testis is also at risk in these patients, with a 5% risk of CIS, a proven pre-malignant condition.

Pathology of testicular tumours

Germ cell tumours: 95% are germ cell tumours such as seminoma and non-seminomatous germ cell tumours (NSGCTs).

Stromal tumours: these may arise from Leydig or Sertoli cells. They are rare and about 10% are malignant.

Lymphomas occur in older men.

Seminoma

- Accounts for about 50% of germ cell tumours
- Divided into classic (85%), anaplastic and spermatocytic sub-types
- Tend to occur in men in their 30s
- Typically tumours have a homogeneous macroscopic appearance. They consist of sheets of clear cells

Anaplastic seminoma is a more aggressive sub-type and accounts for 30% of all patients dying with seminoma.

Spermatocytic seminoma tends to occur in older men with nearly half occuring in men aged > 50. It appears to have a particularly good prognosis.

Non-seminomatous germ cell tumours (NSGCTs)

There are four main types:

- Embryonal carcinoma
- Yolk sac tumour
- Choriocarcinoma
- Classic teratoma

Most (60%) have a mixed pattern, containing some or all of these histological sub-types.

Presentation of testicular tumours

- Most men present with a painless testicular lump
- 10–20% may have pain, often described as a heaviness or an ache
- Testis may feel firm and bosselated with thickening of the cord (due to infiltration) and a small hydrocele
- Occasionally men present with metastatic disease (eg abdominal mass due to lymph nodes, respiratory symptoms, bone pain)
- Gynaecomastia occurs in about 5% of patients and is related to hCG production

Investigating testicular tumours

- Scrotal US confirms the diagnosis and excludes abnormalities in the other testis
- CXR excludes pulmonary metastases
- Testicular tumour markers (as shown in the table) are used for diagnosis, staging, monitoring response to treatment and predicting prognosis

TESTICULAR TUMOUR MARKERS

α-fetoprotein (AFP)	Normally undetectable after the first year of life Elevated in non-seminomatous tumours only (eg teratoma, yolk sac)
Human chorionic gonadotrophin (β-hCG)	Normally produced by the placenta during pregnancy Produced by all non-seminomatous tumours containing choriocarcinoma elements and 40–60% containing embryonal carcinoma elements 5–10% of patients with pure seminoma have low levels of hCG detectable
Lactate dehydrogenase (LDH)	This is a ubiquitous enzyme and therefore non-specific It is secreted by seminomas and in non-seminomatous disease and seems to be a marker of tumour bulk
Placental alkaline phosphatase (PLAP)	Detected in 65% of seminomas and may be a sensitive marker for metastatic seminomatous disease

Staging of testicular tumours

The UICC (Union Internationale Contre Cancre) 2002 staging system is unique in that addition to the TNM categories there is an 'S category' for serum tumour markers.

Tumour staging (based on pathological information after radical orchidectomy)

T_{is}	Intra-tubular germ cell neoplasia (CIS)
T_1	Tumour limited to testis/epididymis without vascular/lymphatic invasion or tumour may invade tunica albuginea but not tunica vaginalis
T_2	Tumour limited to testis/epididymis with vascular/lymphatic invasion or tumour extends through tunica albuginea with involvement of tunica vaginalis
T_3	Tumour invades spermatic cord with or without vascular/lymphatic invasion
T_4	Tumour invades scrotum with or without vascular/lymphatic invasion

Regional lymph node staging

N_x	Cannot be assessed
N_0	No nodes involved
N_1	Lymph node mass < 2 cm or multiple nodes none > 2 cm
N_2	Lymph node mass 2–5 cm or multiple nodes none > 5 cm or pathological extra-nodal extension
N_3	Lymph node mass > 5 cm

Metastasis staging

M_x	Cannot be assessed
M_0	No distant metastases
M_1	Distant metastases present
M_{1a}	Non-regional lymph node(s) or lung
M_{1b}	Other sites

Serum tumour markers

S_x	Serum markers not available
S_0	Serum markers within normal limits
S_1–S_3	Serum markers outside normal limits (as shown in the table)

SERUM TUMOUR MARKERS LEVELS FOR STAGING

	LDH (mIU/mL)	hCG (mIU/mL)		AFP (ng/mL)	
S1	1.5 × normal level	*and*	< 5000	*And*	< 1000
S2	1.5–10 × normal level	*or*	5000–50 000	*Or*	1000–10 000
S3	> 10 × normal level	*or*	> 50 000	*Or*	> 10 000

Treatment of testicular tumours

Orchidectomy

- Initial definitive treatment is **radical inguinal orchidectomy**. This provides a pathologic diagnosis and will cure about 80% of patients
- Further treatment depends upon histology and staging-CT scans of chest and abdomen to look for metastatic disease

Op box: Radical inguinal orchidectomy

Indication

Testicular tumour

Pre-op

It is important to have measured tumour markers pre-operatively
Testicular prosthesis should be offered

Operative procedure

Patient is placed supine
Inguinal approach similar to that for an inguinal hernia repair is used
External oblique upper aponeurosis is opened from the external to the internal ring
Aspermatic cord is mobilised and clamped at the deep ring
Testis is mobilised in the scrotum and delivered into the inguinal incision
Cord should be transfixed with a heavy suture and then divided at the deep ring
Suture should be left long and haemostasis ensured before allowing the cord to retract
If a prosthesis is to be inserted this can now be sutured to the most dependent part of the scrotal skin

Post-op

Patients can often go home on the same day

Complications

Scrotal haematoma
Wound infection

Post-operative management of seminomas

Seminoma confined to the testis

This may be managed by surveillance alone. 20% of patients relapse. However, surveillance does require repeated CT scans.

Radiotherapy to the para-aortic nodes reduces the recurrence rate to 2%. The main disadvantages of radiotherapy are:

- 80% of patients are over-treated
- Risk of secondary malignancy in the future

Seminoma with lymph node metastases

Treated by radiotherapy. Seminoma with large lymph node metastases (N_3) or metastatic disease is usually treated initially with **combination chemotherapy**.

Post-operative management of non-seminomatous germ cell tumours (NSGCTs)

NSGCTs confined to the testis

Treatment varies in the USA and the UK.

20% of patients have disease in the retro-peritoneal lymph node that is not picked up on imaging, hence in the USA the recommended treatment is **retro-peritoneal lymph node dissection** (RPLND) which has a cure rate > 90%. Because RPLND is over-treatment for many patients the UK approach is for close surveillance.

Patients with high-risk tumours may be given two cycles of chemotherapy.

Metastatic NSGCTs

These are best treated with combination chemotherapy. A standard regimen is bleomycin, etoposide and cisplatin (BEP).

Residual masses in the retro-peritoneum may be resected by RPLND.

Prognosis of testicular tumours

Prognosis depends on the stage but overall 5-year survival is now > 90%. Men with stage 1 testicular cancer of either type should have a 100% 5 year survival rate.

7.5 PENILE CARCINOMA

In a nutshell ...

This is a rare squamous cell cancer, representing 1% of male cancers. It is commoner in the developing world and in the elderly.

Surgical excision and chemotherapy are the main treatment options.

Aetiology of penile carcinoma

Chronic irritation: penile cancer is almost unheard of in men circumcised at a young age. It is associated with an unretractable phimosis and it is thought that chronic irritation with smegma and balanitis are contributory factors.

Human papilloma virus (HPV): incidence is higher in men who have been infected with HPV 16, 18 and 31. It is higher in men whose sexual partners have cancer of the uterine cervix.

Pathology of penile carcinoma

Squamous cell carcinoma is the commonest penile tumour. It is seen as an erythematous indurated area, wart, or ulceration.

Presentation of penile carcinoma

Usually presents with lesion on the glans, prepuce, or foreskin. Most lesions are not painful (may account for the long delay in seeking attention).

Up to 50% of patients delay seeking medical attention for more than 1 year. 50% of patients have palpable inguinal nodes at the time of presentation (these may be inflammatory due to balanitis rather than neoplastic causes).

Diagnosis and staging of penile carcinoma

With small lesions or those involving the foreskin diagnosis is usually combined with treatment. Staging is by the TNM system.

Staging of penile cancer

T_{is}	CIS
T_a	Non-invasive verrucous carcinoma
T_1	Tumour invades sub-epithelial connective tissue
T_2	Tumour invades corpus spongiosum or cavernosum
T_3	Tumour invades urethra or prostate
T_4	Tumour invades other adjacent structures

Regional lymph node staging

N_x	Cannot be assessed
N_0	No nodes involved
N_1	Single superficial inguinal node involved
N_2	Multiple or bilateral superficial inguinal nodes
N_3	Deep inguinal or pelvic node involvement

Metastasis staging

M_x	Cannot be assessed
M_0	No distant metastases
M_1	Distant metastases present

Treatment of penile carcinoma

Local disease

- **Circumcision** or local biopsy may be adequate for T_1 lesions with favourable histology
- **Glans reconstruction** is an option for more extensive lesions
- **Topical chemotherapy** with eg 5-FU
- **Partial or total amputation of the penis** is recommended for poorly differentiated T_1 lesions or for lesions at a more advanced stage. Partial amputation is suitable if a 2-cm margin of palpably normal shaft can be retained (so patients can micturate while standing)

Management of the lymph nodes

The most important predictor of outcome is the status and management of the regional lymph nodes.

50% of patients have palpable adenopathy at presentation, but less than half of these have histological evidence of tumour in the lymph nodes. In the remainder it is thought to be caused by infection or inflammation.

Of patients without palpable nodes 20% have histological evidence of nodal disease, therefore prophylactic lymph node dissection is carried out in high-risk patients with impalpable nodes, ie those that are poorly differentiated T_1 and T_2 (or greater).

In patients with palpable nodes after antibiotic treatment bilateral **radical inguinal lymphadenectomy** with en bloc dissection is recommended (the glans penis drains bilaterally).

Inguinal lymphadenectomy is associated with significant morbidity in terms of lower limb swelling, wound infection, and wound necrosis.

Prognosis in penile carcinoma

5-year survival rates are:

- Localised disease without metastases 60–90%
- Inguinal node involvement 30–50%
- Iliac node involvement 20%

Section 8

Disorders of the scrotum and penis

8.1 ANATOMY OF THE SCROTUM AND TESTIS

In a nutshell ...

The testes are tough, mobile organs lying within the scrotum. The scrotum is an outpouching of the lower part of the anterior abdominal wall. It contains the testes, epididymes, and lower part of the spermatic cords.

Layers of the scrotum

1. Skin.

2. Superficial fascia. This is divided into the superficial and deep layers and contains the dartos muscle. The deep layer of superficial fascia is called Colles' fascia and is continuous with the membranous fascial layer of the anterior abdominal wall (Scarpa's fascia). Posteriorly it is attached to the perineal body and the posterior edge of the perineal membrane.

3. Spermatic fasciae. these are derived from the muscles of the anterior abdominal wall:

- **External spermatic fascia:** derived from the external oblique
- **Cremasteric fascia:** derived from the internal oblique. The cremaster muscle fibres are supplied by the genital branch of the genitofemoral nerve which gives rise to the 'cremasteric reflex' allowing elevation of the testes for warmth and protection
- **Internal spermatic fascia:** derived from the fascia transversalis

4. Tunica vaginalis. Originally an evagination of the peritoneal cavity, this becomes shut off from the processus vaginalis as it closes just before birth. If it remains patent it can be filled with water (infantile hydrocoele) or intraperitoneal contents (indirect hernia).

5. A tough capsule, the **tunica albuginea**, surrounds each testis. Extending inwards from this are a series of fibrous septae that divide the organ into lobules, and within each lobule are coiled **seminiferous tubules**. The tubules open into channels called the rete testis and small efferent ductules connect this to the epididymis

Normal spermatogenesis requires that the testes are maintained at a lower temperature than the abdominal cavity. This lower temperature is achieved by:

- Location outside the abdomen in the scrotum (3° lower than the body temperature)
- Dartos muscle
- Counter-current heat exchange between testicular arteries and the venous pampiniform plexus

Arterial supply of the scrotum and testis

Testicular artery is a branch of the abdominal aorta and follows the embryological descent of the testis down the posterior abdominal wall, into the deep ring, through the inguinal canal, out via the superficial ring, and into the scrotum. There is significant anastomosis between this artery and the epididymal, cremasteric and vasal arteries.

Venous drainage of the scrotum and testis

Testicular veins form several anastomotic channels around the testicular artery, the **pampiniform plexus**. It is thought that this allows counter-current heat exchange and contributes to keeping the testicles cooler than body temperature. The left testicular vein drains into the left renal vein, the right directly into the IVC.

Lymphatic drainage of the scrotum and testis

This is to the para-aortic nodes at the level of L1.

Epididymis

- Lies postero-medial to the testis
- Has an expanded head, a body, and an inferior tail
- Structurally it is a coiled tube of about 6 m long, embedded in connective tissue
- The tail is in continuity with the vas deferens which exits from the medial side

The epididymis has three functions:

- Sperm storage
- Sperm maturation
- Fluid resorption

Vas deferens

- This tube of about 40 cm conveys sperm to the ejaculatory ducts
- It arises in continuity with the tail of the epididymis and passes superior-medially up through the scrotum and through the inguinal canal to the deep inguinal ring to enter the abdominal cavity
- As it enters the abdomen it hooks around the inferior epigastric artery
- It crosses the ureter at the level of the ischial spine and passes inferio-medially on the posterior surface of the bladder towards the seminal vesicle

Seminal vesicles and ejaculatory ducts

- Seminal vesicles are lobulated organs, 5 cm long, lying on the lower posterior aspect of the bladder
- These structurally coiled tubes embedded in connective tissue, which function to produce nourishing secretions that are added to sperm in the ejaculate
- Ducts of the seminal vesicles join the vas deferens medially and become the ejaculatory ducts, which pierce the posterior part of the prostate and enter the urethra close to the prostatic utricle

8.2 ANATOMY OF THE PENIS

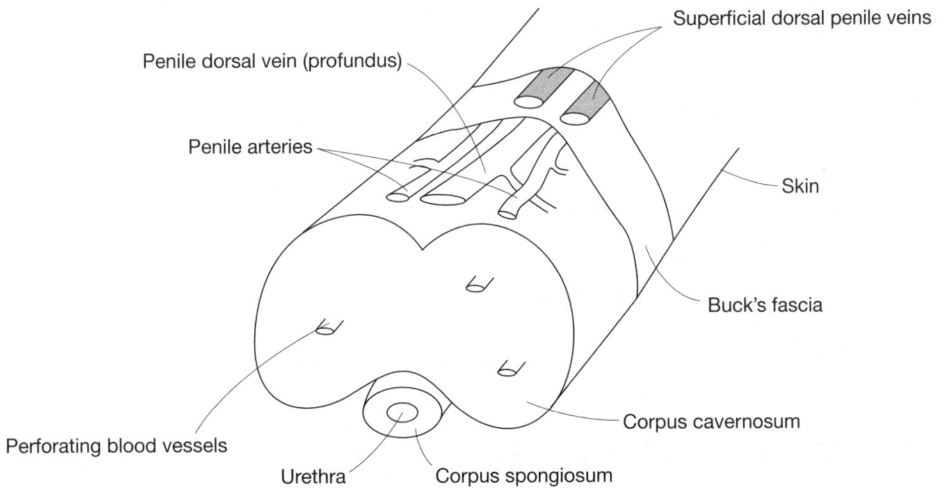

Figure 8.2a *Anatomy of the penis*

The penis has a fixed **root** and a **body** that hangs free.

In a nutshell ...

The right and left **crura** are attached to the inferior pubic rami and perineal membrane. They continue anteriorly as the corpora cavernosa, each surrounded by a tough fascial sheath, the **tunica albuginea.** Each crus is covered on its outer surface by the **ischiocavernosus** muscle.

The **bulb** is attached to the centre of the perineal membrane and surrounded by the **bulbospongiosus** muscle. The forward continuation of the bulb is the corpus spongiosum, which surrounds the penile urethra. Distally the corpus spongiosum expands to form the **glans** penis.

The body of the penis is essentially composed of these three cylinders of erectile tissue enclosed in a tubular sheath of fascia (**Buck's fascia**).

Arterial supply of the penis

The common penile artery is the terminal branch of the internal pudendal artery. It terminates in three branches to supply the erectile bodies.

Venous drainage

The **dorsal vein** of the penis runs in a groove between the corporal bodies and eventually drains into the prostatic venous plexus.

Nerve supply of the penis

This is via the pudendal nerve and pelvic autonomic plexuses.

Lymphatic drainage of the penis

This is to the inguinal and eventually the iliac lymph nodes. The primary route of spread of penile carcinoma is via the lymphatic channels and therefore knowledge of these is important in its management.

8.3 PHYSIOLOGY OF THE MALE REPRODUCTIVE SYSTEM

Testicular function and androgen secretion

The normal hypothalamic–pituitary–gonadal axis has been alluded to in the section on prostate cancer (section 7.3).

The pituitary produces both LH and FSH in response to the pulsatile release of LHRH.

- LH is responsible for stimulating Leydig cells of the testis to produce testosterone
- FSH is important in spermatogenesis and acts on the Sertoli cells in the testis

The Sertoli cells are contained within the seminiferous tubules and surround the developing germ cells (nutritive and supportive role). Tight junctions between the Sertoli cells create an effective blood–testis barrier. Sertoli cells secrete inhibin which acts as negative feedback on FSH secretion via the pituitary.

Spermatozoa are derived from spermatogonia via several stages in which meiosis occurs (see Fig. 8.3a).

Physiology of normal erection

Branches of the **pudendal** nerves containing autonomic fibres from T12–L2 (sympathetic) and S2–S4 (parasympathetic) innervate the cavernosal artery smooth muscle.

Stimulation of parasympathetic nerves leads to the release of neurotransmitters including **nitric oxide** and **prostaglandin**. This causes activation of guanylate and adenylate cyclase increasing local concentrations of **cGMP** and **cAMP.**

These bring about smooth muscle relaxation and dilatation of the cavernosal arteries, leading to blood flow into the cavernosal sinuses. As they fill, the cavernosal sinuses compress the sub-tunical venules resulting in reduced venous outflow, so the corpora become engorged.

Decreased stimulation from neurotransmitters coupled with the metabolism of cGMP and cAMP by **phosphodiesterases** leads to relaxation of the cavernosal arteries and detumescence.

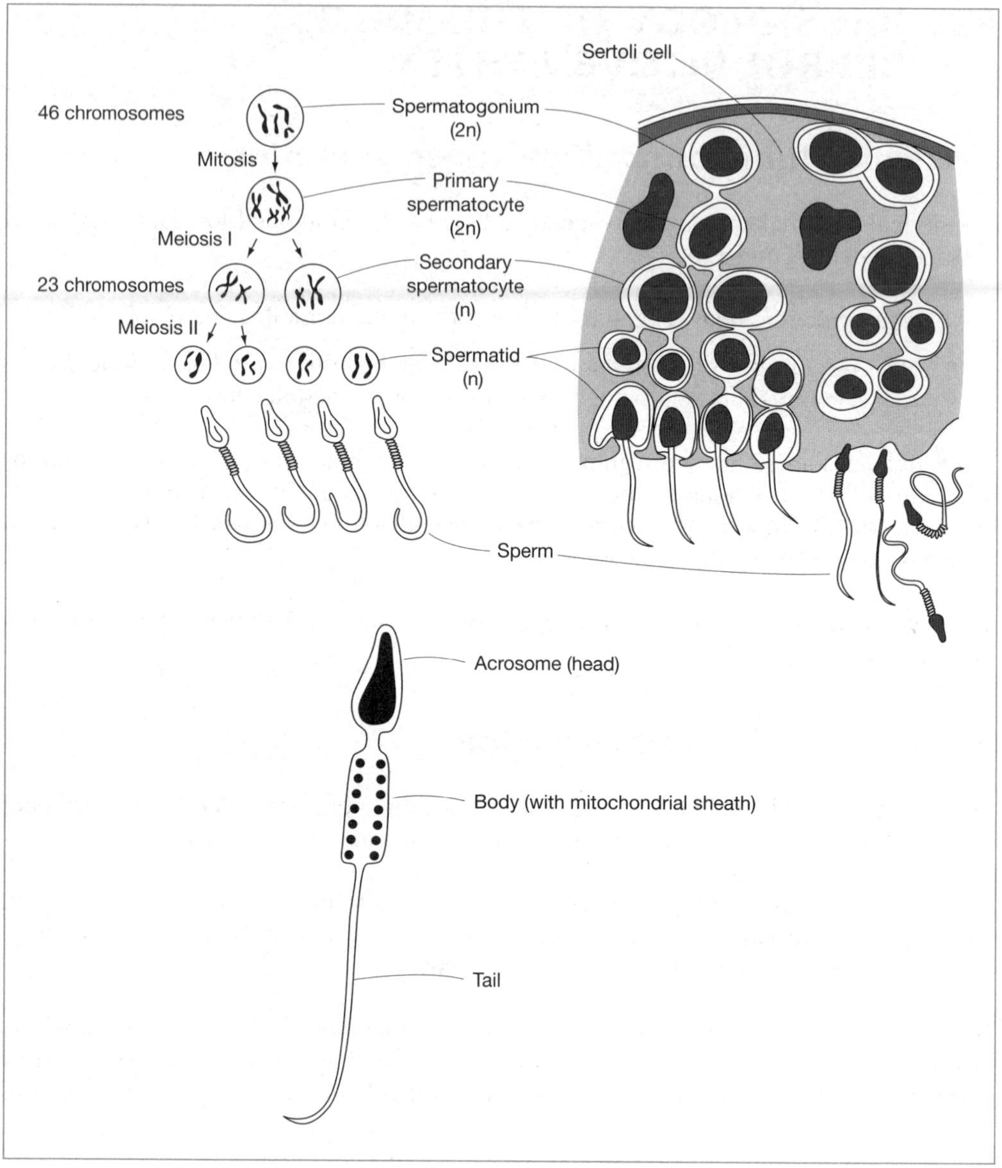

Figure 8.3a *Spermatogenesis*

8.4 DISORDERS OF THE TESTICLE AND SCROTUM

In a nutshell ...

Testicular torsion
Hydrocele
Epididymal cyst
Varicocele
Vasectomy

Testicular torsion

Testicular torsion is a genuine urological emergency. Surgery should be underway within 1 hour of diagnosis so the role of the admitting SHO is crucial – he or she must recognise and confirm a query torsion, ensure the operating surgeon sees it, inform acute theatres and the on-call anaesthetist, arrange consent (including for orchidectomy) and transport of the patient straight to theatre (not to the ward!!) all within minutes of the patient being referred. Irreversible ischaemia occurs within 6 hours of the torsion first occurring.

Epidemiology of testicular torsion

This occurs most commonly in boys aged 10–16, and it is uncommon in men aged > 30. It accounts for 90% of cases of an acute scrotum in males aged 13–21. There is a rare form of torsion that occurs in neonates.

Aetiology of testicular torsion

Essentially the testis twists on its cord structures resulting in venous congestion and eventually infarction. Testicular torsion is classified into two types:

Extra-vaginal testicular torsion

- This is seen in neonates
- Incomplete fixation of the gubernaculum to the scrotal wall allows the entire cord to twist resulting in testicular infarction
- Rarely picked up clinically until the testis is infarcted

Intra-vaginal testicular torsion

- This is the more common form, found in adolescents and adults
- A high investment of the tunica vaginalis on the cord allows the testis to rotate within the tunica on the cord structures

Presentation of testicular torsion

Typically patients present with an acutely painful tender hemi-scrotum. There may be some swelling. Occasionally pain radiates to the groin and even the loin, reflecting the embryological origin of the testis.

- Vomiting can occur
- There may be previous episodes of the pain, suggesting intermittent torsion
- On physical examination the testis is extremely tender
- Classically the testis lies horizontally and slightly higher (bell-clapper testis) although neither of these signs is specific

Differential diagnosis of testicular torsion

- Epididymo-orchitis
- Trauma
- Neoplasia
- Inguinoscrotal hernia
- Torsion of hydatid of Morgagni
- Referred pain from ureteric calculus at VUJ

The main differential is epididymo-orchitis (covered in section 4.2 of *Urological infections*). Presentation is generally less acute and usually there are urinary symptoms, although not always.

Torsion of the **hydatid of Morgagni** can also mimic testicular torsion although there is normally less swelling. This small appendicular attachment to the testis can become twisted and gangrenous in the presence of a completely normal, viable testis. Usually this diagnosis is made at surgery as it is never possible to exclude torsion completely in this situation.

Investigating testicular torsion

If torsion is suspected no investigations are required; indeed time is at a premium so exploration should not be delayed.

Treatment of testicular torsion

Scrotal exploration should be carried out as soon as possible if testicular torsion is suspected (this is the case in almost all young men with an acutely painful testis). Irreversible ischaemic changes can occur within 6 h of torsion so surgery should be performed within 1 hour of presentation. At operation the testis is approached trans-scrotally:

- If torsion is discovered, the testis is untwisted
- If the testis remains dusky after de-torsion it should be wrapped in warm saline-soaked swabs for 15 minutes

If there is still doubt regarding its viability then perform **orchidectomy**. This should be included in the patient consent. If viable the testis should be **fixed** in the scrotum (orchiopexy), as should the contralateral testis.

Hydrocele

This is a common cause of scrotal swelling in all age groups. It represents a collection of fluid around the testis within the tunica vaginalis.

Aetiology of hydrocele

In children they are caused by a **patent processus vaginalis** (see Chapter 10 *Paediatric surgery*) and are a primary hydrocele. In adults they may be primary or rarely secondary hydroceles, due to chronic infection, trauma (and damage to lymphatics) or testicular tumour.

Clinical presentation of hydrocele

This is with painless scrotal swelling. It should be possible to palpate the spermatic cord above the swelling, and if this is not possible it may be a hernia. Classically hydroceles **trans-illuminate** although this is not always the case.

Investigating hydrocele

Carry this out US in young men to exclude testicular tumours. This is not necessary in elderly men.

Treatment of hydrocele

- **None:** do not treat unless they are causing discomfort
- **Aspiration** can be carried out but carries a risk of infection and the hydrocele almost invariably recurs within a few weeks
- **Open repair** is the gold standard treatment. The tunica vaginalis may be plicated as in the Lord's repair or turned 'inside out' as in the Jaboulay repair

Op box: Hydrocele repair

Indication

In adults hydrocele repair is only indicated in large hydroceles that are causing significant symptoms. Pain is not a characteristic feature of hydroceles and patients should be counselled that it will not always resolve after hydrocele repair

Pre-op

In younger patients, pre-operative ultrasound scan should be performed to exclude a testicular tumour as the cause of the hydrocele

Procedure

Either a transverse incision or a median raphe incision can be used. There are two well-described methods for hydrocele repair, the Jaboulay repair and the Lord's repair.

Jaboulay repair

The tunica is dissected free from the dartos and delivered out of the scrotum together with the testicle
The tunica is then divided longitudinally and sutured behind the cord
If the hydrocele is very large some of the tunica may need to be excised

Lord's repair

The incision through skin and dartos is continued through the tunica and the hydrocele is emptied
The tunica is then plicated by using several sutures

Post-op

Wear supportive underwear until recovered
Expect some bruising and swelling initially
Home when patient is comfortable and has passed urine

Complications

Scrotal haematoma
Wound infection
Recurrence

Epididymal cyst

These fluid-filled scrotal masses are thought to arise from congenital diverticula of the epididymal tubules.

Presentation of epidymal cyst

Cysts may be multiple and are usually tense, spherical, and trans-illuminable. The testis can be felt separately (which is how epididymal cyst is differentiated from hydrocele).

Treatment of epidymal cyst

- **None:** if no symptoms, no treatment is required
- **Surgical excision** if there is pain, cysts can be excised. However, the patient should be warned that further cysts might arise and that scarring may affect fertility. Removing the cyst does not always remove the pain and the patient needs to be aware of this

Varicocele

A varicocele is a varicose dilatation of the pampiniform venous plexus that runs within the spermatic cord. Incidence is 15%. It is commoner on the left where the testicular vein drains into the renal vein (the system with the higher pressure).

Presentation of varicocele

Most are asymptomatic. Occasionally there is an aching pain, especially after prolonged standing.

They may be detected during investigation of infertility as they are related to male sub-fertility (due to increased temperature).

Classification of varicocele

Grade 1	Sub-clinical but detectable using Doppler US
Grade 2	Palpable when the patient is standing
Grade 3	Visible as a scrotal swelling and palpable when the patient is lying

Investigating varicocele

Renal US is indicated in older patients because occasionally renal cancer presents with varicocele if the renal vein is involved.

Treatment of varicocele

- **Surgical treatment:** by ligation of the veins in the groin. Clearly the higher the veins are ligated the fewer tributaries there will be
- **Laparoscopic ligation:** of the veins within the pelvis is effective
- **Embolisation:** also an effective treatment that avoids surgery

This may recur or persist (in 20%) due to collateral circulation or incomplete venous ligation.

Vasectomy

Vasectomy is a procedure performed for contraception. Both vas deferens are ligated in the scrotum. It can be performed under LA or GA. Vasectomy is a common cause of medico-legal problems in urology and careful counselling must be performed before the procedure.

Patients must be aware of the following:

- Vasectomy is considered irreversible
- Late re-canalisation of the vas deferens occurs in 1 in 2000 patients and can lead to fertility being re-gained
- The results of vasectomy are not immediate as sperm will continue to appear in the ejaculate for several months. Alternative contraception is essential until consecutive semen analyses show no sperm
- Wound infection or scrotal haematoma may occur
- Chronic scrotal pain is a recognised complication

The procedure should be carried out under GA if the patient is very anxious or has had previous scrotal or groin surgery.

8.5 DISORDERS OF THE PENIS AND FORESKIN

In a nutshell ...

Peyronie's disease
Erectile dysfunction
Priapism
Phimosis
Paraphimosis

Peyronie's disease

This is a fibromatosis of unknown aetiology that affects focal areas of the tunica albuginea of the corpus cavernosum.

Epidemiology of Peyronie's disease

- Incidence is estimated at 1%
- Average age at onset is 53
- Associated with Dupuytren's contracture and plantar fascial contracture

Aetiology of Peyronie's disease

- Uncertain
- Repeated minor trauma in association with vascular insufficiency is postulated to lead to scarring

Presentation of Peyronie's disease

- Symptoms usually start with penile pain on erection
- Gradually deviation of the erection progresses, occasionally reaching a stage where sexual intercourse becomes impossible
- Pain usually resolves within 6–9 months

Treatment of Peyronie's disease

Conservative treatment is appropriate for the 1st year as it takes this long for the disease to stabilise. Various potential drug therapies have been suggested but none have been proven in randomised controlled trials.

ESWL has been used to soften or destroy the penile plaque. This shows promising early results although long-term follow-up is not available.

Surgery: after 1 year, if the deformity has made sexual intercourse impossible, surgery can be offered. There are three main surgical options:

- **Nesbit's operation** (or variation) in which plication with or without excision of the tunica albuginea on the opposite side to the plaque is performed; this procedure is inevitably associated with penile shortening
- **Plaque excision and patching** with a graft such as saphenous vein; this is purported to produce less penile shortening but may lead to problems associated with softer erections
- **Implantation of a penile prosthesis** can be used to straighten the penis in men who have existing erectile dysfunction

Erectile dysfunction

Erectile dysfunction is defined as the persistent inability to obtain and maintain an erection sufficient for sexual intercourse. The prevalence of complete erectile dysfunction varies from 5% at age 40 to 15% at age 70.

Classification of erectile dysfunction

- Broadly this is classified as **psychogenic** or **organic**
- About 50% of men fall into each group, although organic impotence is commoner in older men
- Causes of organic impotence are shown in the table.

CAUSES OF ORGANIC ERECTILE DYSFUNCTION
Vascular disease
Neurogenic eg MS, spinal injury
Trauma eg pelvic surgery, prostatectomy, pelvic fracture
Drugs eg anti-hypertensives, anti-depressants, alcohol
Hypogonadism (pituitary or gonadal)
Peyronie's disease
Chronic illness eg diabetes, renal failure

Evaluation of erectile dysfunction

- **History:** useful for distinguishing psychogenic from organic impotence. Nocturnal erections suggest psychogenic cause. Drug history is important
- **Examination:** should include external genitalia and digital rectal examination
- **Examination of the peripheral pulses:** should be carried out to detect generalised atheromatous disease
- **Urine analysis:** may reveal diabetes
- **Serum testosterone and prolactin:** is indicated if hypogonadism is suggested
- **Further tests:** such as Doppler sonography and cavernosography may be indicated but are not applicable in the vast majority of men

Treatment of erectile dysfunction

General measures

- Patients are advised to stop smoking and to reduce alcohol consumption
- Drugs may be adjusted
- Psychosexual counselling may help in psychogenic erectile dysfunction

Oral drug therapy

- **Phosphodiesterase-5 inhibitors:** eg sildenafil/Viagra™ which maintain high concentrations of cGMP in the cavernosal smooth muscle and facilitate maintenance of an erection. > 70% of erectile dysfunction responds to these drugs. Contraindicated in patients taking nitrates
- **Dopamine agonists:** eg apomorphine. These act on the para-ventricular nucleus in the brain (centre that controls sexual drive)

Local pharmacotherapy to the penis

Prostaglandin E_1 can be administered by intra-corporeal injection or as a urethral pellet. It increases the concentration of cAMP in the cavernosal smooth muscle. An erection is produced in 80% of patients.

- Pain at the injection site can be a problem
- Priapism occurs in 1% of all patients on injection therapy (see below)

Vacuum pump

- Although this is effective it is considered unnatural and is not popular.

Penile prostheses

- These are usually reserved as a last resort
- They can be either solid or inflatable
- Both mechanical failure and infection are problems
- They are expensive

Priapism

This is a prolonged, painful erection that is not associated with sexual desire. It is classified as low flow (veno-occlusive) or high flow (which is rare, and usually due to AV malformation).

Pathophysiology of priapism

The corpora is rigid because of sludging of blood. Ischaemia and hypoxia lead to pain.

- After 3–4 h there is pain
- After 12 h there is interstitial oedema
- After 24–48 h there is smooth muscle necrosis
- After > 1 week there is fibrosis and erectile dysfunction

Causes of priapism

- Therapy for erectile dysfunction: causes 20% of cases, which is common if administered by injection, but rare with oral therapies
- Haematological diseases: such as the hyper-viscosity in sickle cell disease/trait, in other haemoglobinopathies, leukaemia, EPO therapy, or cessation of anti-coagulation
- Malignant infiltration by solid tumours: eg bladder, prostate, renal
- Neurological disease: eg lumbar disc disease, CVA
- Drugs: eg anti-hypertensives, paroxetine, fluoxetine, trazodone

Management of priapism

- Conservative: eg exercise, ice, ejaculation
- Aspiration: (corporal) and irrigation with warm saline
- Oral medication: eg terbutaline 5–10 mg, 36% response
- Intra-cavernosal medication: eg phenylephrine – NB close monitoring of BP is essential
- Surgical intervention, This includes:
  - Glans–cavernosal shunt
  - Cavernosal–spongiosum shunt
  - Cavernosal–saphenous shunt

Prognosis of priapism

Increasing duration results in a higher probability of subsequent impotence:

- < 24 hours leads to impotence in about 43%
- > 24 hours leads to impotence in about 90%

Phimosis

Phimosis is simply non-retraction of the foreskin. It is quite normal at birth because of preputial adhesions (see Chapter 10 *Paediatric Surgery*).

True pathological phimosis occurs secondary to scarring of the foreskin, most commonly due to **balanitis xerotica obliterans** (BXO), which is a fibrosing condition of unknown aetiology. BXO can also affect the urethra, causing problems with voiding.

Pathological phimosis is an indication for circumcision.

Paraphimosis

This is a urological emergency caused by retraction of a tight foreskin. If the foreskin is not replaced it causes constriction of the glans leading to swelling, which makes it more difficult to reduce.

Treatment of paraphimosis

- Aims to reduce swelling using ice-packs and squeezing the oedematous tissue
- Reduction can then be attempted
- LA (penile block or ring block) can be administered
- Occasionally it is necessary to drain the oedematous fluid using a needle
- GA is sometimes required for reduction
- Circumcision (see the Operation box) is recommended in all these patients to prevent the problem recurring

Op box: Circumcision

Indications

Phimosis
Paraphimosis
Recurrent balanitis
Penile tumour

Pre-op

Treat active infection

Procedure

Administer GA or LA with penile nerve block
Mark the incision with the penis on stretch (some use artificial erection) to avoid taking too much or too little skin
Various methods exist to remove the two layers of foreskin. Most surgeons do it in two layers although some take both together and a knife or scissors can be used

Avoid monopolar diathermy as there is a risk of damage to end arteries and subsequent necrosis. Bipolar diathermy or ties are used for haemostasis
Use absorbable sutures for closure

Post-op

This is a day-case procedure
Patient can go home as soon as he is comfortable and has passed urine
Avoid sexual intercourse for 2–3 weeks

Complications

Bleeding (if immediately post-operatively, return to theatre is usually necessary)
Urinary retention
Wound infection

Section 9
Transplantation

9.1 CHRONIC RENAL FAILURE (CRF)

In a nutshell ...

This is a permanent loss in renal function that occurs over several months duration.

Causes of chronic renal failure are:
- Diabetic nephropathy (34%)
- Hypertension (29%)
- Glomerulonephritis (14%)
- Polycystic kidney disease (14%)
- Chronic pyelonephritis (10%)
- Obstructive/reflux nephropathy

Clinical features of chronic renal failure

- **Systemic upset:** this is common and often occurs first (symptoms include fatigue, lack of energy, insomnia, anorexia, nausea and vomiting)
- **Anaemia:** caused by relative lack of erythropoietin
- **Platelet dysfunction** (impaired coagulation): occurs in 60% of patients
- **Pericarditis:** caused by high blood urea levels (indication for immediate dialysis)
- **Neuropathy** (peripheral): caused by loss of myelin from peripheral nerves
- **Encephalopathy:** this is due to high urea levels
- **Renal bone disease 'osteodystrophy':** caused by various factors (eg secondary hyperparathyroidism and vitamin D deficiency)
- **Erectile dysfunction and amenorrhoea:** secondary to hyperprolactinaemia
- **Acquired cystic disease:** particularly common in patients on dialysis (an important predisposing factor for renal carcinoma)

Treatment of chronic renal failure

This is a complex subject. Specialist medical advice should be sought. Several features are relevant to urology:

- Anaemia can be treated with rHu-EPO
- Protein restriction reduces the accumulation of nitrogenous waste products
- Potassium should also be restricted
- Fluid intake should be made to equal daily urine output + 500 mL for insensible losses
- Acidosis should be treated with sodium bicarbonate
- Dialysis and haemofiltration are ways of replacing the excretory functions of the kidney (see below)

Dialysis

Dialysis is used in patients with renal failure to replace the excretory functions of the kidney. It relies on two principles:

- **Diffusion:** this relies on a concentration gradient between blood and dialysis fluid
- **Ultra-filtration:** this relies on a pressure difference between blood and dialysis fluid

Haemodialysis

In this method the blood is pumped from the patient into a dialysis machine where it is separated by a semi-permeable membrane from the dialysis fluid running in a counter-current direction. A pump is used to generate a pressure difference for ultra-filtration.

Large-bore vascular access is required, which can be obtained temporarily through a percutaneous cannula in a central vein, however most patients require formation of an **arterio-venous fistula** (see section on surgical fistula, below).

An adult requires 4–5 hours of haemodialysis three times a week.

Peritoneal dialysis

This is performed by introducing fluid into the peritoneal cavity. Ultra-filtration pressure is generated by increased osmotic pressure within the dialysis fluid. This is usually produced by the addition of dextrose. The two types of peritoneal dialysis are:

- CAPD
- Intermittent PD

Continuous ambulant peritoneal dialysis (CAPD)

CAPD is suitable **for patients who:**

Are mobile and self-caring (to retain independence and continue work)
Have poor arm veins
Have extensive atheroma
Have a needle phobia
Children

CAPD is unsuitable **for patients who:**

Have extensive previous abdominal surgery (intra-abdominal adhesions)
Have with poor dexterity
Have diabetes with poor glycaemic control on CAPD

Advantages of peritoneal dialysis:

- Portable
- Can be carried out by the patient at home
- Does not require anticoagulation
- Patients generally feel better on it

It requires surgical insertion of an in-dwelling peritoneal catheter (Tenchkoff catheter) placed through a lower mid-line abdominal incision and held in place by two cuffs (one in the peritoneum and one just under the skin).

The most important complication is peritonitis (may require laparotomy and abdominal lavage).

Recurrent peritonitis leads to reduced capacity of the peritoneum to act as an exchange membrane for dialysis (recurrent peritonitis leads to scarring and long-term peritoneal dialysis leads to glycosylation of the peritoneal membrane).

Haemofiltration

This is used mainly on ITU for short-term management. Blood is driven through a filter using the patient's BP to allow ultra-filtration. It is simpler than haemodialysis because a pump is not required.

It is very useful for removing large volumes of fluid in fluid-overloaded patients.

Arterio-venous fistula

These are created primarily for ease of vascular access in patients with renal failure who need regular haemodialysis. It avoids the need for a long-term percutaneous central venous catheter which carries risks of infection, venous stenosis, and thrombosis.

Types of arterio-venous fistulas

- **Autogenous:** direct joining of a vein with a neighbouring artery, usually end vein to side artery using the Brescia–Cimino technique
- **Autogenous bridge:** a vein and an artery are joined using a separate vein graft (eg saphenous vein)
- **Synthetic straight bridge grafts:** PTFE or another synthetic graft material is used to bridge between an artery and a vein. Other graft materials include bovine carotid arteries, human umbilical vein or cryopreserved cadaveric vein grafts
- **Loop grafts:** these are usually synthetic. An artery and vein are joined by a loop of graft tunnelled subcutaneously

Sites of arterio-venous fistulas

In order of preference these are: radiocephalic, brachiocephalic, fore-arm loop, upper arm straight. The non-dominant hand and more distal sites are usually considered first.

Pre-operative issues you should consider

- Which is the patient's dominant hand?
- Were there any previous attempts at access and reasons for failure?
- Examine the fore-arm veins, if necessary using a proximal torniquet (40 mmHg)
- Aim for an autogenous but warn the patient of the risks of synthetic bridges in case the veins aren't good enough
- Perform Allen's test (see *Cardiothoracics* in Book 2) to evaluate potential arterial inflow sites. Non-palpable pulses should not be used
- Exclude local or systemic infection

Post-operative complications

- Nerve injury: especially radial and median
- Thrombosis: usually due to poor flow, kinking or compression by haematoma
- Steal phenomenon: claudication symptoms due to inadequate perfusion. Treated by ligating artery just distal to graft except in proximal fistulas which require bypass
- Infection: especially in synthetic grafts
- False aneurysm
- Venous hypertension
- Cardiac failure (high-flow fistulas only)

9.2 PRINCIPLES OF TRANSPLANTATION

In a nutshell ...

In the event of organ failure, transplantation is an option. Most commonly performed in the kidney, liver, heart and lung, other organs are increasingly being transplanted. Donors may be:

Dead (cadaveric)

Brainstem dead
Non-heart beating

Alive

Related
Unrelated

Issues to be addressed when discussing any organ transplantation are consent, compatibility, immunosuppression and rejection.

Organs commonly used for transplantation

Blood (transfusion) – (see Chapter 4 *Haematology*)
Kidney – (see below)
Liver – (see below)
Heart +/– lung – (see *Cardiothoracics* in Book 2)
Pancreas – (see below)
Bone – (see *Orthopaedics* in Book 2)
Small bowel – (see below)
Skin (for treatment of burns) – (see Chapter 1 *Basic Surgical Knowledge and Skills*)

Cadaveric donors

Brainstem-dead donors

Donors who meet the criteria for brainstem death, usually after trauma or intracranial bleed, who continue to be ventilated on ICU are classified as brainstem-dead donors. Organs (usually multiple) are retrieved in the operating theatre where ventilation is ceased. For the definition of brainstem death see *Elective Neurosurgery and Spinal Surgery* in Book 2.

Non-heart-beating donors

Donors who do not meet the criteria for brainstem death and who have arrested, usually in a predictable manner and controlled setting such as ICU are non-heart-beating donors. The time from arrest to organ retrieval is crucial for the recipients in these cases.

Cadaveric surgical organ retrieval

There are three stages of cadaveric organ retrieval.

The warm phase

In the warm phase the heart is still beating and the major vessels are cannulated (thoracic vessels for retrieval of the heart, abdominal aorta and portal system for intra-abdominal organs).

Perfusion of the organs

Perfusion of the organs with ice-cold perfusion solution and cessation of ventilation heralds the start of the cold ischaemic time. Perfusion solutions (eg University of Wisconsin or Marshall's solution) contain:

- Impermeable solutes (minimise cellular swelling)
- Buffers (for pH balance)
- Free radical scavengers and inhibitors
- Membrane stabilisers
- Adenosine (for ATP synthesis)

The cold phase

In the cold phase the organ is removed from the body cavity and packaged in ice for transport. In general kidneys are transplanted within 24 hours and livers within 12 hours.

In non-heart-beating donors the vessels are cannulated after spontaneous cardiac arrest; organs are therefore exposed to a longer warm ischaemia time due to the peri-arrest period of hypotension.

Live donors

There are increasing numbers of live donors who are either related or non-related. Live related donors are usually 1st-degree relatives while unrelated donors include spouses and in some cases, 'good Samaritan' donors.

Kidney donation

There is an increasing frequency of live kidney donation at multiple UK centres, and live renal transplantation now accounts for 20% of transplants). Donor work-up includes recipient cross-match, screening for transmissible disease, IVU, arteriography, and isotope renography (the donor keeps the kidney with a greater functional percentage). Nephrectomy is via loin incision or laparoscope. Donors usually have normal renal function post-transplant but may experience mild hypertension and proteinuria later in life.

Liver donation

Programs for live donation of liver tissue are up and running in the USA and are being incorporated into the UK transplant program, for example:

- Left-lateral segment from adult to child
- Right-hepatectomy specimen from adult to adult

A small number of cases of living donation of lung segments, pancreatic tail and small bowel segments have been reported.

Contraindications for organ and tissue donation

Contraindications for organ donation

- HIV positive
- CJD positive
- Solid organs are rarely retrieved in donors aged over 80

Contraindications for tissue donation

- HIV, Hep B, Hep C, HTLV, syphilis, or risk factors for these infections
- CJD or family history of CJD
- Progressive neurological disease of unknown pathophysiology eg MS, Alzheimer's, Parkinson's, motor neurone disease
- Leukaemia, lymphoma, myeloma
- Previous transplant requiring immunosuppressive treatment
- Systemic malignancy (except for cornea transplant)

Consent issues in organ transplant

The process for organ donation in cadaveric patients is complex and requires a multidisciplinary approach (see Fig. 9.2a). The consent of a live donor involves detailed counselling and it is the clinician's responsibility to ensure that the donor appreciates the short-term and long-term implications of organ donation on his or her own health, as well as the risks of failure of the transplant.

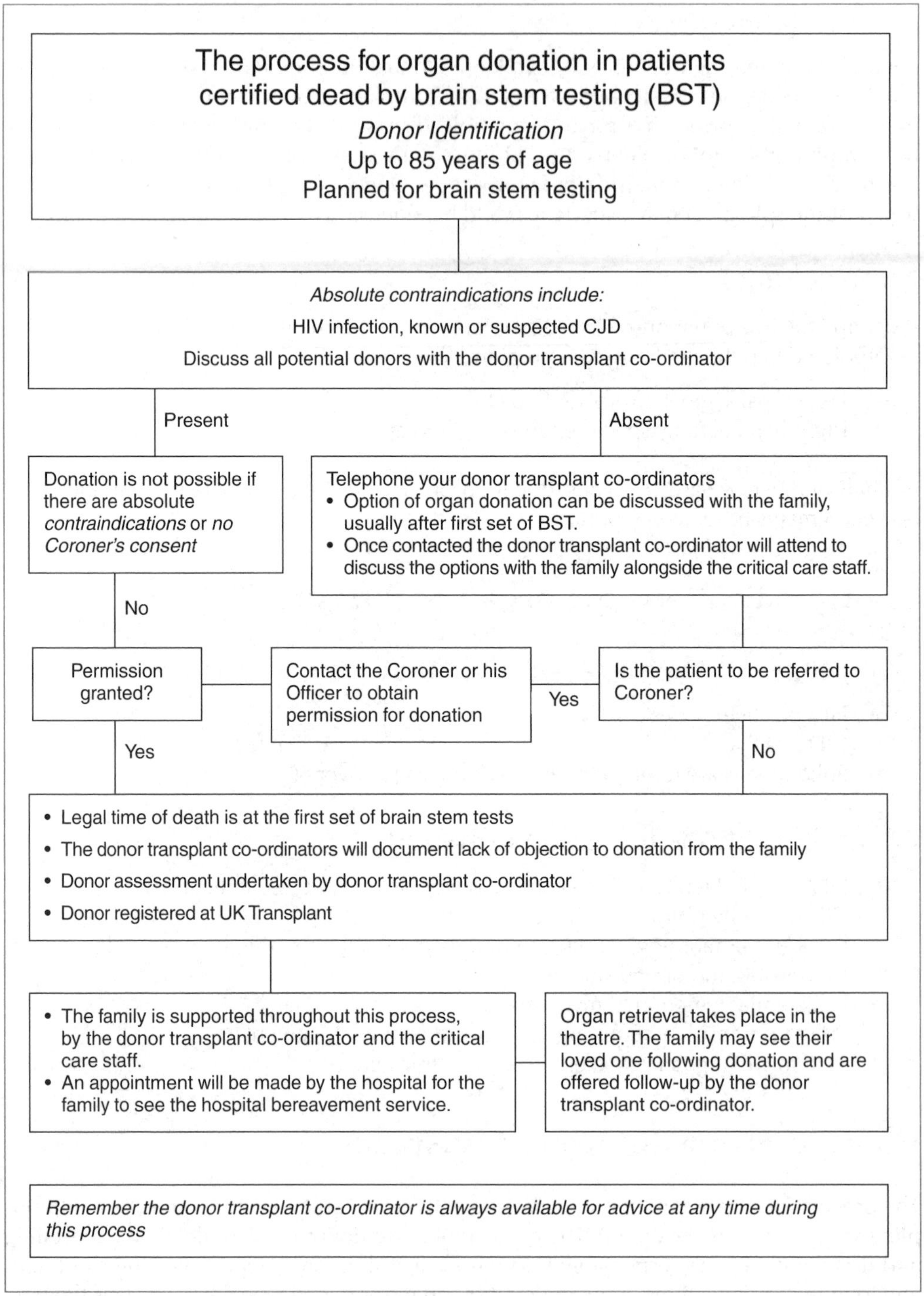

Figure 9.2a *Process for organ donation in patients certified dead by brainstem testing*

Donor–recipient compatibility

Ideally there should be:

- Similarity in donor and recipient age: particularly at extremes of age
- ABO blood group matching
- HLA matching: HLA-A, HLA-B and HLA-DR are the most important with the best matches having all six alleles the same
- Antibody cross matching: recipient serum is tested against donor B and T cells to ensure no cross-reactivity with pre-formed anti-human leucocyte antibodies in the serum. These antibodies arise in response to blood transfusions, pregnancy or previous failed transplants

Immunosuppression

At the time of surgery

Give methylprednisolone 1 g.

Anti-CD25 monoclonal antibody (eg basiliximab): this is starting to be used in several units in the UK. It selectively targets activated T cells. It is given as an intra-operative injection, which is repeated after 4 days. The effects last for several weeks and may reduce the level of ciclosporin or tacrolimus required.

Maintenance therapy

Most units use triple therapy of drugs with synergistic effects, consisting of:

- **A calcineurin inhibitor** (ciclosporin or tacrolimus): this blocks production of IL-2 and thus inhibits recipient T cell activation. A major side effect is nephrotoxicity (can be confused with rejection) and hypertension
- **An anti-proliferative agent** (azathioprine or mycophenolate): this inhibits DNA and RNA synthesis. A major side effect is leukopenia
- **A steroid (prednisolone):** this affects early phases of T cell activation and has non-specific effects on the immune system (including anti-inflammatory cytokine effects and macrophage function). There are many side effects (eg hypertension, poor wound healing)

Complications of immunosuppression

- **Cardiovascular complications (multi-factorial):** diabetes, underlying disease causing hypertension, immunosuppressants causing hypertension, hyperlipidaemia
- **Malignancy:** the risk is about 100 times greater than in the normal population. There is a marked increase in SCC of skin, cervix, lymphoma, and Kaposi sarcoma. There is a marginal increase in malignancy of solid organs (eg breast, colon, lung)

- **Problems associated with long-term steroid use:** hyperglycaemia, hypertension, thin skin, obesity and characteristic fat distribution, confusion, peptic ulcer, poor wound healing
- **Infections:** opportunistic infections occur in the first few months when immunosuppression is at a maximum. CMV infection may occur due to re-activation of endogenous disease or transmission from a donor; this is very common in the general population, and is usually asymptomatic

Rejection of transplanted organs

Patients at higher risk of rejection include those who had previous transplants or multiple blood transfusions, previous rejection reactions, Afro–Caribbean people and children.

There are three mechanisms of transplant rejection.

Hyper-acute rejection

- Due to presence of recipient antibodies against the donor kidney
- Occurs within minutes of revascularisation
- Kidney swells and becomes discoloured
- There is clumping of RBC and platelets, fibrin is deposited, interstitial haemorrhage occurs
- Rarely seen because of antibody cross-reactivity testing (see *Donor–recipient compatibility* above)
- Transplant nephrectomy is required

Acute rejection

- T cell-mediated
- Common in first 2 weeks but can occur up to 6 months after transplant
- Lymphocytic infiltration in interstitium and subsequently in vessel walls
- Treatment with high-dose steroids (often reversible)
- Difficult to distinguish clinically from ATN or drug nephrotoxicity

Chronic rejection

- Occurs months to years after transplant and is probably multi-factorial
- Thickening of the glomerular basement membrane, vascular changes, and renal tubular atrophy
- Less common because of modern immunosuppressive drugs

9.3 RENAL TRANSPLANTATION

In a nutshell ...

In the UK during 2003 and 2004 1838 people received a renal transplant. The commonest indication is end-stage renal failure which has an incidence of 250 per million people. It affects more men than women, and more Afro–Caribbean people than white people.

Before reading this section you may need to refresh your memory by reviewing the following sections:

Normal anatomy of the kidney, ureter and pelvis (sections 3.1 and 6.2 of this chapter)
Renal physiology (Chapter 7 *Critical Care*)
Acute renal failure and chronic renal failure (Chapter 7 *Critical Care* and section 9.1 of this chapter)

Patient selection for renal transplant

Indications for renal transplant

Renal transplant is usually done for chronic renal failure (see section 9.2). The advantages of renal transplant over continued dialysis are:

- Improved quality of life (requirement for dialysis reduced or eliminated)
- Increase in patient survival rate compared to dialysis (Note that selection of fitter patients for surgery may introduce bias)
- Cost-effective in the long term
- It is important that the primary diagnosis is confirmed before considering renal transplantation

Patient assessment for renal transplantation

Risk of recurrent disease in the transplanted kidney

- Will recurrent disease cause graft failure and, if so, how quickly?
- There is a high risk of recurrences in focal glomerular sclerosis, amyloidosis and haemolytic uraemic syndrome
- Renal transplantation may be inappropriate for live related donors with high recurrence risk of primary disease

Technical considerations

- Atheromatous iliac vessels in arteriopaths
- Bladder dysfunction (neurogenic bladder or outflow obstruction)
- Pre-transplant nephrectomy of a native kidney
- APKD: bleeding or infection in cystic spaces
- Large and bulky kidneys with little space for transplant
- Uncontrollable hypertension
- Renal calculi
- Persistent anti-glomerular antibodies

Additional investigations

- ABO and HLA typing
- Virology (hepatitis B, hepatitis C; CMV may require treatment pre-transplant)
- Urinalysis and culture
- Consider effects of common co-morbidities (hypertension, diabetes)
- Cardiovascular assessment
  - High mortality rate from cardiovascular disease in renal transplant patients
  - ECG +/– stress test +/– echocardiography
  - Exclude peripheral vascular disease
- Psychological issues and compliance with life-long immunosuppressive medication

Contraindications for renal transplant

- Active malignancy (cancer free for at least 2 years)
- Active infection: exclude dental sepsis and gallstones (risk of cholecystitis)
- Advanced atheromatous disease (relative contraindication)

Renal transplantation procedure

Anatomy of the transplanted kidney

- The kidney is placed extra-peritoneally in the right or left iliac fossa, usually on the right side (dictated by existing scars or previous transplants)
- Renal vessels are anastomosed (end-to-side) to the recipient's external iliac vessels
- The ureter is taken down into the pelvis where it is anastomosed to the bladder mucosa either directly (extra-vesicular approach) or by threading it through a sub-mucosal tunnel and suturing from inside the bladder through a separate incision in the bladder wall (intra-vesicular approach)
- The ureter is stented (reduces stricture formation) and stent is removed by cystoscopy after 6 weeks

Length of renal vessels

- The right renal vein is anatomically shorter than the left because of the right-sided position of the IVC (may make transplantation of the left kidney more difficult in a large recipient)
- Cadaver kidneys are retrieved with a cuff of tissue taken from the aorta and IVC at the end of the normal renal vessels
- Live donor kidneys do not have this extra tissue and so the renal vessels are shorter

Ureteric blood supply

- Upper 3rd comes from the renal artery
- Middle 3rd comes from the gonadal vessels
- Lower 3rd comes from the common iliacs

It is important not to strip the adventitial tissue from around the ureter as this contributes to its blood supply from the renal artery (other sources of supply ligated at retrieval).

Procedure box: Renal transplantation

Indications

End-stage renal failure

Pre-op

Ensure all cross-matching has been performed and is optimum
Give broad-spectrum prophylactic antibiotics
Start immunosuppression just before surgery in cadaveric organ recipients. In live donor recipients it may be started a week before surgery
The bladder is washed out or filled with approximately 150 mL of antibiotic solution

Procedure

An oblique Gibson incision is made in the iliac fossa. The rectus is preserved
Generally the renal vein is anastomosed at the external iliac vein and the renal artery to the internal iliac artery
During the anastomosis the donor kidney is kept cool on ice or wrapped in a swab soaked with cold saline
The ureter is usually anastomosed to the bladder with an extra-vesical technique. It is tunnelled sub-mucosally in order to prevent reflux. A ureteric stent is placed between the kidney and the bladder (it is removed by cystoscopy at 6 weeks)

Post-op

Careful fluid balance is required (usually urine output + 30 mL/hour)
In situations where the patient remains oliguric or anuric a Doppler scan will assess blood flow and an US will rule out urinary extravasation or hydronephrosis
ATN is associated with increased ischaemia time and may lead to delayed graft function. Renal biopsy may be performed to confirm this and exclude rejection

Complications

Vascular: renal artery or vein thrombosis, renal artery stenosis
Urological: urethral stricture or obstruction
Lymphocele: due to failure of ligation of lymphatics (can be aspirated)

Surgical complications of renal transplant

Early complications of renal transplant

- **Delayed primary function**
  - Kidney may not function for several days and undergoes a degree of ATN
  - Associated with long cold-ischaemic time, warm-ischaemic time and reperfusion injury
  - Requires good patient hydration and supportive management with dialysis (haemodialysis or PD)
  - Usually diagnosed by cortical biopsy
  - Occurs in ~ 25% of transplants
- **Vascular complications**
  - Anastomotic bleed
  - Vessel kinking or vessel thrombosis
- **Urine leak**
- **Lymphocele**
- **Infections:** commonly wound, urinary or respiratory tract

Late complications of renal transplant

- Ureteric stricture
- Reflux nephropathy
- Renal artery stenosis: due to atherosclerosis and hyperlipidaemia

Non-surgical complications of renal transplant

- Complications of immunosuppression (see section 9.2)
- Primary non-function of unknown cause
- Rejection (see section 9.2)

Prognosis after renal transplant

Prognostic factors include:

- Primary diagnosis
- Previous graft failures
- Episodes of rejection
- Kidney total ischaemic time
- Donor factors (eg age)

The 1-year graft survival rate is about 90% in live-related transplants, and 85–90% in cadaveric transplants. The 10-year graft survival rate for first grafts is 60%. In general, live-related recipients fare better than cadaveric recipients.

9.4 LIVER TRANSPLANTATION

In a nutshell ...

In the UK during 2003 and 2004 686 people received a liver transplant. The commonest indication is chronic liver failure although some transplants are performed for acute liver failure.

Before reading this section you may need to refresh your memory by reviewing the following sections:

Normal anatomy of the liver (in the *Liver and spleen* section of *Abdomen* in Book 2)
Pathology of the liver (below)
Portal hypertension (Chapter 4 *Haematology*)

Patient selection for liver transplantation

Chronic liver failure is the most common reason for liver transplantation.

Patients usually have Childs' C level (see *Liver and spleen* in the *Abdomen* chapter of Book 2) disease and life-threatening complications (eg varices); these patients often have significant multiple co-morbidities and require very careful evaluation and work-up.

Early transplantation has improved survival rates in this group over the last 10 years.

Indications for liver transplantation

Chronic liver failure

- Primary biliary cirrhosis
- Primary sclerosing cholangitis (often associated with ulcerative colitis)
- Alcoholic liver disease (abstain from alcohol for at least 6 months)
- Hepatitis B and hepatitis C
- Budd–Chiari syndrome
- Metabolic disease (eg Wilson's disease, α1-anti-trypsin deficiency, haemochromatosis)
- Paediatric conditions: 10–15% of transplants (eg congenital biliary atresia)

Acute liver failure

- Defined as the onset of liver failure within 5 weeks of the development of jaundice. There may be spontaneous recovery. It may be fulminant and rapid. It requires intensive care with cardiorespiratory and renal support. There are strict criteria for supra-urgent listing for transplant as an emergency. Causes of acute liver failure:
  - Drug induced (eg from paracetamol or rifampicin overdose)
  - Metabolic disease (eg Wilson's disease)
  - Viral hepatitis

Liver tumours

- Primary or secondary HCC
- Secondary neuroendocrine tumours
- Cholangiocarcinoma (very rare and only if there is intra-hepatic disease without extra-hepatic disease)

Hepatocellular carcinoma (either primary, or on a background of cirrhosis) is the most common tumour to be treated with transplantation (primary tumours of < 4 cm diameter with no more than two foci of disease).

Contraindications for liver transplantation

- Patient unlikely to survive the procedure
- Extra-hepatic malignancy (individually assessed, but must be cancer-free for 2 years)
- Portal vein thrombosis (relative contraindication)
- Active generalised sepsis
- Psychosocial reasons (eg continued alcohol abuse)

Liver transplant procedures

Types of graft

There are a limited number of donors, so a variety of techniques have been developed to help optimise the number of transplants available.

Whole graft

- **Conventional transplant:** total native hepatectomy plus grafting
- **Accessory transplant 'piggyback':** partial native hepatectomy preserving segments 1–3 with grafting of transplanted liver to the side of the native IVC (a new technique, used as supportive measure for reversible causes of acute liver failure when native liver is expected to recover from the aetiological insult and regenerate). Immunosuppression may be withdrawn after recovery of liver function whereupon graft is rejected, becoming small and fibrosed. Less liver tissue is required, so it can be performed with specimen from split graft

Split graft

- Whole graft can be divided on the basis of its blood supply. Split graft is usually used for two recipients (often an adult and a child)

Live-related graft

- An example is a left lateral segmentectomy specimen from an adult to a child
- Rapid regeneration occurs in the donor
- Transplanted segment grows with the child
- Live-related grafts are becoming part of the transplant program in the UK

Principles of liver transplantation

- **Mercedes or roof-top incision**
- **Hepatectomy**
  - Often this is technically challenging due to intra-abdominal varices and adhesions
  - It may be performed with the patient on veno–veno bypass (femoral vein to internal jugular)
  - The IVC (above and below liver), portal vein and hepatic artery are divided
- **Vascular anastomoses**
  - IVC (above and below liver)
  - Portal vein
  - Hepatic artery
- **Biliary reconstruction**
  - Direct anastomosis of recipient to donor CBD
  - Roux loop for diseased recipient CBD

Surgical complications of liver transplantation

Vascular complications

- **Haemorrhage:** common due to multiple vascular anastomoses, coagulopathy and thrombocytopenia
- **Vessel thrombosis:** due to low flow states or small-diameter vessels (eg accessory arteries)
- **Anastomotic stricture:** late

Biliary tree complications

- Leak
- Anastomotic stricture

Non surgical complications of liver transplantation

Rejection

- **Primary non-function** occurs rarely. There is a climbing prothrombin time and deteriorating clinical condition in first 24–48 hours. This may require re-grafting
- **Early rejection** is fairly common (up to 30%). It is diagnosed by deteriorating LFTs and confirmed on biopsy, and it responds to high-dose steroids

- **Chronic rejection** occurs months after transplant with progressive deterioration of graft function. Re-transplantation is required

Infections

- **General:** eg wound infection, respiratory infection
- **Viral:** eg CMV

Prognosis after liver transplantation

The primary diagnosis, co-morbidity, and stage of disease impact upon outcome measures.

Patients are given individually tailored outcome measures based on risk assessments by an MDT (hepatologist, surgeon, and transplant anaesthetist).

Transplantation for chronic liver failure has the highest survival rates.

9.5 TRANSPLANTATION OF OTHER ORGANS

Pancreas transplantation

Indications

- The main indication for pancreatic transplantation is diabetes mellitus in young patients with brittle disease and end-stage nephropathy. It may be in conjunction with kidney transplant
- Transplant is of either whole organ or isolated islet cell

Complications

- Vascular thrombosis: a common cause of early graft loss
- Rejection which is difficult to diagnose
- Infection (patients are very susceptible)

Small bowel transplantation

Indications

- Intestinal failure with nutritional failure

Graft rejection

- The small bowel is a highly immunological organ requiring high-level immunosuppression. Graft rejection is common and may cause bacterial translocation and sepsis

Multi-visceral transplantation

- May involve transplantation of any combination of kidney, liver, pancreas and small bowel
- Success rates are low but are improving

Other transplant material

Cardiac and lung transplantation is covered in the *Cardiothoracics* chapter of Book 2.

Skin grafting is covered in Chapter 1 *Basic Surgical Knowledge and Skills.*

Bone grafting is covered in the *Orthopaedics* chapter of Book 2.

Blood transfusion is covered in Chapter 4 *Haematology*.

Abbreviations

α-GT	α-glutamyl transpeptidase
2,3-DPG	diphosphoglycerate
5-FU	5-fluorouracil
5-HIAA	5-hydroxyindole acetic acid
5-HT	serotonin
A&E	accident and emergency
AAA	abdominal artery aneurysm
ABGs	arterial blood gases
ACDF	anterior cervical discectomy and fusion
ACL	anterior cruciate ligament
ACT	activated clotting time
ACTH	adrenocorticotrophic hormone
ADH	anti-duiretic hormone (vasopressin)
ADI	atlanto-dens interval
AF	atrial fibrillation
AFB	acid-fast bacillus
AFP	alpha-fetoprotein
AIDS	acquired immunodeficiency syndrome
ALL	acute lymphocytic leukaemia; anterior longitudinal ligament
ALP	alkaline phosphatase
ALS	advanced life support
ALT	alanine aminotransferase
AML	acute myelogenous leukaemia
AMPLE	allergies, medication, past medical history, last meal, events preceding present condition
Ang-1	angiopoietin-1
ANP	atrial natriuretic peptide
AP	antero-posterior
APACHE	acute physiology, age and chronic health evaluation
APBI	ankle brachial pressure index
APC	antigen-presenting cell
APKD	adult onset polycystic kidney disease
APL	abductor pollicis longus
APTT	activated partial thromboplastin time
APUD	amine precursor uptake and decarboxylation
ARDS	adult respiratory distress syndrome
ARF	acute renal failure
ARM	anorectal malformation
ASA	American Society of Anesthesiologists; amino-salicylic acid
ASIS	anterior superior iliac spine
AST	aspartate aminotransferase
ATLS	advanced trauma life support
ATN	acute tubular necrosis
ATP	adenosine triphosphate
AV	arterio-venous
AVM	arterio-venous malformation
AVN	atrioventricular node; avascular necrosis
AVP	arginine vasopressin
AVPU	alert, verbal, painful, unresponsive
AXR	abdominal X-ray
BAL	broncho-alveolar lavage
BBB	bundle-branch block
BEP	bleomycin, etoposide, cisplatin
BIH	benign intercranial hypertension
BiPAP	biphasic positive airways pressure
BIPP	bismuth iodoform paraffin paste
BM	blood glucose monitoring; bone marrow
BMI	body mass index
BMR	basal metabolic rate
BP	blood pressure
BPH	benign prostatic hyperplasia
BUN	blood urea nitrogen
BXO	balanitis xerotica obliterans
Ca	carcinoma
CABG	coronary artery bypass graft
CAD	coronary artery disease
CAGE	cut down, annoyed by criticism, guilty about drinking, eye-opener drinks
CAH	congenital adrenal hypoplasia
CaO_2	arterial content of O_2
CAPD	continuous ambulatory peritoneal dialysis
CAT	computed axial tomography
CAVH	continuous arterio-venous haemofiltration
CBD	common bile duct
CBG	cortisol-binding globulin
CCAD	Central Cardiac Audit Database
CCF	congestive cardiac failure
CCK	cholecystokinin
CCL	carcinoma cell line
CCST	Certificate of Completion of Training

CDH congenital diaphragmatic herniation
CDK cyclin dependant kinase
CEA carcinoembryonic antigen
CEPOD Confidential Enquiry into Peri-operative Deaths
CHOP cyclophosphamide, doxorubicin, vincristine, prednisolone
CIS carcinoma in situ
CJD Creutzfeldt-Jacob disease
CK creatinine kinase
CK-MB creatinine kinase-myocardial bound
CLL chronic lymphocytic leukaemia
CLO *Campylobacter*-like organism
CMF cyclophosphamide, methotrexate, 5-FU
CML chronic myelogenous leukaemia
CMV cytomegalovirus
CNS central nervous system
CO carbon monoxide; cardiac output
COMICE Comparative Effectiveness of MRI in Breast Cancer
COPD chronic obstructive pulmonary disease
COX cyclo-oxygenase
CPAP continuous positive airway pressure
CPP cerebral perfusion pressure
CPPS chronic pelvic pain syndrome
CREST calcinosis, Raynauld's, oesophageal dysfunction, sclerodactyly, telangectasia
CRF chronic renal failure
CRH corticotropin-releasing factor
CRP C-reactive protein
CRPS complex regional pain syndrome
CSF cerebrospinal fluid
CT computerised tomography
CTEV congenital talipes equinovarus
CVA cerebrovascular accident
CvO_2 mixed venous content of O_2
CVP central venous pressure
CVVH continuous veno-venous haemofiltration
CVVHD continuous veno-venous haemodiafiltration
CXR chest X-ray
DAB dorsal abduct
DBP diastolic BP
DCIS ductal carcinoma in situ
DDH developmental dysplasia of the hip
DEXA dual energy X-ray absorptiometry
DHCC dihydroxycholecalciferol
DHS dynamic hip screw
DI diabetes insipidus
DIC disseminated intravascular coagulation
DIP distal inter-pharyngeal
DIT di-iodotyrosine
DLC CO_2 diffusing capacity of lungs for CO_2
DMSA dimercaptosuccinic acid; disodium monomethanearsonate
DO_2 global body oxygen delivery
DoH Department of Health
DPG diphosphoglycerate
DPL diagnostic peritoneal lavage
DSD detrusor sphincter dyssynergia
DTPA diethylenetriaminepentaacetic acid
DU duodenal ulcer
DVT deep vein thrombosis
EBV Epstein–Barr virus
EC enterochromaffin
ECA external carotid artery
$ECCO_2R$ extra-corporeal CO_2 removal
ECF extracellular fluid
ECG electrocardiogram
ECM extracellular matrix
ECMO extra-corporeal membrane oxygenation
ECRB extensor carpi radialis brevi
ECRL extensor carpi radialis longus
ECST European Carotid Surgery Trial
ECU extensor carpi ulnan's
EDC extensor digitorum communis
EDL extensor digitorum longus
EDM extensor digiti minimi
EF ejection fraction
EGF epidermal growth factor
EHL extensor hallucis longus
EI extensor indicis
ELISA enzyme-linked immunosorbent assay
ELN external laryngeal nerve
EMD electro-mechanical dissociation
EMG electromyogram
EMLA eutectic mixture of local anaesthetic
EPB extensor pollicis brevis
EPL extensor pollicis longus
EPO erythropoietin
ER oestrogen receptor
ERC European Resuscitation Council
ERCP endoscopic retrograde cholangiopancreatography
ERV expiratory reserve volume
ESR erythrocyte sedimentation rate
ESWL extracorporeal shock wave lithotripsy
ET endotracheal tube
EtOH ethyl alcohol
EUA examination under anaesthetic
FAP familial adenomatous polyposis

FBC	full blood count
FCU	flexor carpi ulnaris
FDL	flexor digitorum longus
FDP	fibrin degradation product; flexor digitorum profundus
FEC	5-fluorouracil, epirubicin, cyclophosphamide
FEV	forced expiratory volume
FFP	fresh frozen plasma
FGF	fibroblast growth factor
FHH	familial hypocalcuric hypercalcaemia
FHL	flexor hallucis longus
FNAC	fine-needle aspiration cytology
FNH	focal nodular hyperplasia
FOB	faecal occult blood
FRC	functional residual capacity
FSH	follicle-stimulating hormone
FTA	fluorescent *Treponema* antibody
FU	fluorouracil
FUFA	fluorouracil plus folinic acid
FVC	forced vital capacity
G-6-PD	glucose-6-phosphate dehydrogenase
GA	general anaesthesia
GALT	gut-associated lymphoid tissue
GCS	Glasgow Coma Scale
GDC	Guglielmi detachable coils
GFR	glomerular filtration rate
GGT	gamma glutamyl transferase
GH	growth hormone
GHRH	gonadotrophin hormone releasing hormone
GI	gastrointestinal
GIST	gastro-intestinal stromal tumour
GMC	General Medical Council
GORD	gastro-eosophageal reflux disease
GR	glucocorticoid receptor
GRE	glucocorticoid response elements
GRP	gastrin-releasing peptide
GT	glutamyl transpeptidase
GTN	glyceryl trinitrate
GVHD	graft versus host disease
H	histamine
Hb	haemoglobin
HBIG	hepatitis B immunoglobulins
HCC	hepatocellular carcinoma
hCG	human chorionic gonadotrophin
HCl	hydrochloric acid
HD	haemodialysis
HDU	high-dependency unit
Hep-2	human laryngeal tumour cells
HER-2	human epidermal growth factor receptor-2
FGF	fibroblast growth factor
HiB	Haemophilus influenzae type B
HIDA	hepato-imino-diacetic acid; 12-hydroxy-heptadecatrienoic acid
HIPAC	Hospital Infection Control Practices Advisory Committee
HIT	heparin-induced thrombocytopenia
HIV	human immunodeficiency virus
HLA	human leukocyte antigen
HMMA	4-hydroxy-3-methoxymandelic acid
HNPCC	hereditary non-polyposis colon cancer
HOCM	hypertrophic obstructive cardiomyopathy
HPV	human papilloma virus
HR	heart rate
HRT	hormone replacement therapy
HSP	heat shock protein
HSV	herpes simplex virus
HTLV-1	human T cell lymphotrophic virus-1
HUS	haemolytic uraemic syndrome
HVA	homovanillic acid
IADSA	intra-arterial digital subtraction arteriography
IARC	International Agency for Research on Cancer
IBD	inflammatory bowel disease
IBS	irritable bowel syndrome
ICA	internal carotid artery
ICAM	intercellular adhesion molecule
ICNARC	Intensive Care National Audit and Research Council
ICP	intracranial pressure
IDDM	insulin-dependant diabetes mellitus
IFN	interferon
IGF	insulin-like growth factor
IHD	intermittent dialysis; ischaemic heart disease
IJV	internal jugular vein
IL	interleukin
IMA	inferior mesenteric artery
IMV	intermittent mandatory ventilation
INR	international normalised ratio
INSS	international neuroblastoma staging system
IPPV	intermittent positive pressure ventilation
IPSS	International Prostate Symptom Score
IRV	inspiratory reserve volume
ISC	intermittent self-catheterisation
ISS	injury severity score
ITP	idiopathic thrombocytopenic purpura
ITU	intensive therapy unit
IUCD	intra-uterine contraceptive device

IVC inferior vena cava
IVDSA intravenous digital subtraction arteriography
IVU intravenous urography
JVP jugular venous pressure
kCO_2 transfer coefficient
KUB kidneys, ureters, bladder
LA local anaesthetic
LAD left anterior descending artery
LAP left atrial pressure
LCIS lobular carcinoma in situ
LDH lactate dehydrogenase
LFTs liver function tests
LH luteinising hormone
LHRH luteinising hormone releasing hormone
LIF left iliac fossa
LIMA left internal mammary artery
LMP last menstrual period
LMWH low-molecular-weight heparin
LP lumbar puncture
LT leukotriene
LUTS lower urinary tract symptoms
LVEF left ventricular ejection fraction
LVH left ventricular hypertrophy
LVP left ventricular pressure
M&Ms mortality meetings
MAC Mycobacterium avium complex
MAGPI meatal advancement and granuloplasty
MALT mucosa-associated lymphoid tissue
MAOI monoamine oxidase inhibitors
MAP mean arterial pressure
MC&S microscopy, culture, and sensitivity
MCP metacarpophalangeal
MCV mean cell volume
MDT multi-disciplinary team
MEAC minimum effective analgesic concentration
MEN multiple endocrine neoplasia
MESS mangled extremity severity score
MHC major histocompatibility complexes
MI myocardial infarction
MIBG meta-iodobenzylguanidine
MIE meconium ileus equivalent
MIS müllerian-inhibiting substance
MIT mono-iodotyrosine
MMC migrating myoelectric complex
MMP matrix metalloproteinase
MMR measles, mumps, rubella triple vaccine
MND motorneuron disease
MNG multi-nodular goitre
MODS multi-organ dysfunction
MOF multi-organ failure
MOI mechanism of injury
MONA morphine, oxygen, nitrates, aspirin
MPM mortality probability model
MR molecular range
MRCP magnetic resonance choliangopancreatography
MRI magnetic resonance imaging
MRSA methicillin-resistant *Staphylococcus aureus*
MRTB multidrug-resistant TB
MS multiple sclerosis
MST morphine sulfate tablets
MSU mid-stream urine
MTP metatarsophalangeal
MUA manipulation under anaesthesia
MUGA multiple gated acquisition
NAI non-accidental injury
NASCET North American Symptomatic Carotid Endarterectomy Trial
NASH non-alcoholic steatohepatitis
NBM nil by mouth
NCEPOD National Confidential Enquire into Patient Outcome and Deaths
Nd-YAG neodynium-yttrium-aluminium garnet
NF neurofibromatosis
NG nasogastric
NHL non-Hodgkin's lymphoma
NICE National institute for Clinical Excellence
NIDDM non-insulin-dependent diabetes mellitus
NIPPV non-invasive positive pressure ventilation
NJ nasojejunal
NK natural killer cells
NNT number needed to treat
NPI Nottingham Prognostic Indicator
NS nervous system
NSAID non-steroidal anti-inflammatory drug
NSCLC non-small cell lung carcinoma
NSGCT non-seminomatous germ cell tumour
NST no special type
NTD neural tube defect
NYHA New York Heart Association
OA osteoarthritis
OCP oral contraceptive pill
ODP operating department practitioner
OGD oesophago-gastroduodenoscopy
OME otitis media with effusion
ORIF open reduction plus internal fixation
OTC over the counter

p.r.	per rectum
p.r.n.	pain relief negligible!
p.v.	per vaginum
p_A	alveolar pressure
p_a	arterial pressure
PA	pulmonary artery
$PaCO_2$	partial arterial carbon dioxide tension
PAD	palmer adduct
PAF	platelet-activating factor
PAM	physiotherapy, analgesia, mobilisation
PAN	polyarteritis nodosa
PaO_2	partial arterial oxygen tension
PAS	para-aminosalicylic acid
PAWP	pulmonary artery wedge pressure
PBC	primary biliary cirrhosis
PBP	penicillin-binding proteins
PCAS	patient controlled analgesia system
PCI	percutaneous coronary intervention
PCL	posterior cruciate ligament
pCO_2	partial pressure of carbon dioxide
PCP	Pneumocystis carinii pneumonia
PCV	packed cell volume
PDA	patent ductus arteriosus
PDGF	platelet-derived growth factor
PDS	polydioxanone sutures
PE	pulmonary embolism
PEA	pulseless electrical activity
PEEP	positive end expiratory pressure
PEFR	peak expiratory flow rate
PEG	percutaneous endoscopic gastrostomy
PEJ	percutaneous endoscopic jejunostomy
PFC	persistence of fetal circulation
PG	prostaglandin
PGDF	platelet-derived growth factor
PICC	percutaneous indwelling central catheter
PID	pelvic inflammatory disease
PIF	prolactin-inhibiting factor; proteolysis-inducing factor
PIP	proximal inter-pharyngeal
PLAP	placental alkaline phosphatase
PLIF	posterior lumbar interbody fusion
PLL	posterior longitudinal ligament
PMH	past medical history
PMN	polymorphonuclear; polymorphonuclear neutrophil
PND	paroxysmal nocturnal dyspnoea
PNET	primitive neuroectodermal tumour
PNH	paroxysmal nocturnal haemoglobinuria
pO_2	partial pressure of oxygen
PONV	Post-operative nausea and vomiting
POP	plaster of paris
POSSUM	Physiological and Operative Severity Score for enUmeration of Morbidity and Mortality
PP	pancreatic polypeptide; pulse pressure
PPEV	positive pressure filtered ventilation
PPI	proton pump inhibitor
PR	progesterone receptor
PRETEXT	pre-treatment extent of disease
PRF	prolactin-releasing factor
PRV	polycythaemia rubra vera
PSA	prostate-specific antigen
PSC	primary sclerosing cholangitis
PSIS	posterior superior iliac spine
PT	prothrombin time
PTFE	polytetrafluoroethylene
PTH	parathyroid hormone
PTHC	percutaneous trans-hepatic cholangiography
p_v	venous pressure
PV	plasma viscosity
PVD	peripheral vascular disease
PVR	peripheral vascular resistance
PVS	persistent vegetative state
q.d.s.	four times daily
QALY	quality of life data
RA	rheumatoid arthritis
RAA	renin-angiotensin-aldosterone
RBC	red blood cells
RBG	random blood glucose
RCT	randomised controlled trials
RF	rheumatoid factor
rHuEPO	recombinant human erythropoietin
RIF	right iliac fossa
RLN	recurrent laryngeal nerve
RLQ	right lower quadrant
ROSC	return of spontaneous circulation
RPE	retinal pigmented epithelium
RPLND	retroperitoneal lymph node dissection
RQ	respiratory quotient
RSD	reflex sympathetic dystrophy
RTA	road traffic accident
rTPA	recombinant tissue plasminogen activator
RTS	revised trauma score
RUQ	right upper quadrant
RV	residual volume
Rx	prescription
SA	sino-atrial
SAG-M	sodium chloride, adenine, glucose, mannitol

SAH	subarachnoid haemorrhage
SAPS	simplified acute physiology score
SASM	Scottish Audit of Surgical Mortality
SBE	subacute bacterial endocarditis
SBP	systolic blood pressure
SCC	squamous cell carcinoma
SCID	severe combined immunodeficiency disease
SEPS	sub-fascial endoscopic perforator surgery
SFA	superior femoral artery
SG	stoma-gastric
SIADH	syndrome of inappropriate antidiuretic hormone
SIMV	synchronised intermittent mechanical ventilation
SIRS	systemic inflammatory response syndrome
SLE	systemic lupus erythematosus
SMA	superior mesenteric artery
SMR	standardised mortality ratio
SOB(OE)	shortness of breath (on exertion)
SORM	selective oestrogen receptor modulator
SPJ	sapheno-popliteal junction
SSRI	selective serotonin re-uptake inhibitors
STD	sexually transmitted disease
STIR	short tau inversion recovery
SUFE	slipped upper femoral epiphysis
SV	stroke volume
SVC	superior vena cava
SVT	sinoventricular tachycardia
TART	trans-anal resection of tumour
TBG	thyroid-binding globulin
TBPA	thyroid-binding pre-albumin
TBSA	total body surface area
Tc	technetium
TCC	transitional cell carcinoma
TCR	T cell receptor
TEDS	anti-embolism stockings
TFTs	thyroid function tests
TGF	transforming growth factor
THC	trans-hepatic cholangiography
THR	total hip replacements
TIA	transient ischaemic attack
TIPSS	trans-jugular intra-hepatic porto-systemic shunt
TISS	therapeutic intervention scoring system
TKR	total knee replacement
TLC	total lung capacity
Tl–Tc	thallium–technetium
TME	total mesorectal excision
TOE	trans-oesophageal echocardiography
TP	transverse process
tPA	tissue plasminogen activator
TPHA	*Treponema pallidum* haemagglutination assay
TPMT	thiopurine methyl transferase
TPN	total parenteral nutrition
TPO	thyroid peroxidase
TRALI	transfusion-related acute lung injury
TRAM	transverse rectus abdominus myocutaneous
TRH	thyrotropin-releasing hormone
TRISS	ratio of RTS and ISS
TSH	thyroid-stimulating hormone
TT	thrombin time
TTP	thrombotic thrombocytopenic purpura
TURBT	trans-urethral resection of bladder tumour
TURP	trans-urethral resection of the prostate
TV	tidal volume
TVT	tension-free vaginal tape
TWOC	trial without catheter
UC	ulcerative colitis
UGI	upper gastro-intestinal
UICC	Union Internationale Contre Cancre
URTI	upper respiratory tract infection
URTI	upper respiratory tract infections
US(S)	ultrasound (scan)
UTI	urinary tract infection
V/Q	ventilation–perfusion
VA	alveolar volume
VATS	video-assisted thoracoscopic surgery
VC	vital capacity
vCJD	variant CJD
VDRL	Venereal Disease Research Laboratory
VEGF	vascular endothelial growth factor
VF	ventricular fibrillation
VIP	vasoactive intestinal peptide
VLDL	very low density lipoproteins
VMA	vanillylmandelic acid
VO_2	oxygen consumption
VRE	*Vancomycin*-resistant enterococcus
VT	ventricular tachycardia
VUR	vesico-ureteric reflux
vWF	von Willebrand factor
WAGR	Wilms tumour, aniridia, genitourinary abnormalities, mental retardation
WBC	white blood cells
WCC	white cell count
WLE	wide local excision
ZN test	Ziehl-Nielson

Picture Permissions

The following figures in this book have been reproduced with kind permission from www.resus.org.uk.

Critical care

Fig 3.7a Advanced life support – Tachycardia algorithm
Fig 3.7b Advanced life support – Bradycardia algorithm
Fig 3.7c Advanced life support – Adult advanced life support algorithm

The following figures in this book have been reproduced with kind permission from www.ics.ac.uk.

Urology and Transplantation

Fig 9.2a Process for organ donation in patients certified dead by brain stem testing.

The following figures in this book have been reproduced from Snell, Richard S (2000) *Clinical Anatomy for Medical Students* (6th edition) by kind permission of the publisher Lippincott Williams and Wilkins.

Vascular surgery

Fig 3.3a Compartments of the lower limb
Fig 5.1a The superficial veins of the upper limb
Fig 6.1a Superficial lower limb venous anatomy
Fig 6.2a The venous pump

Urology and Transplantation

Fig 3.1b Anterior relations of the kidney

The following figures in this book have been reproduced from Sadler T (1990) *Langman's Medical Embryology* (6th edition) by kind permission of the publisher Lippincott Williams and Wilkins.

Peadiatric surgery

Fig 2.1a Sagittal section through embryo showing formation of the primitive endoderm-line gut
Fig 2.1b Formation of the GI tract at the 4th week of gestation showing fore-gut, mid-gut and hind-gut
Fig 2.1c The fore-gut during 4th week of gestation
Fig 2.1e The cloacal region at successive stages in development
Fig 2.2a Transverse section of diaphragm at 4th month of gestation
Fig 3.1a The development of the urinary tract at week 5
Fig 3.1b Development of the urogenital sinus
Fig 3.1c Descent of the testis

The following figures in this book have been reproduced from K Burnand *et al.* (1992) *The New Aird's Companion in Surgical Studies* (3rd edition) by kind permission of the publisher Churchill Livingstone.

Paediatric surgery
Fig 3.4a Ectopic postions for an incompletely descended or maldescended testicle

The following figures in this book have been reproduced from H Ellis (2002) *Clinical Anatomy* by kind permission of the publisher Blackwell Science.

Urology and Transplantation
Fig 6.2b Ischiorectal fossa

Bibliography

Anderson ID (1999) *Care of the Critically Ill Surgical Patient*. London: Arnold.

Armstrong RF, Salmon JB (1997) *Critical Care Cases*. New York, Oxford University Press.

Bartlesman JF, Hameeteman W, Tytgat GN, *et al.* (1966) 'Principles and practice of screening for disease' *American Journal of Gastroenterology*, 91: 1507–1516.

Berne RM, Levy MN (eds) (1996) *Principles of Physiology* (2nd edition). London: Mosby.

Bersten A, Soni N, Oh TE (2003) *Oh's Intensive Care Manual* (5th edition). London: Butterworth Heinemann.

Blandy J (1998) *Lecture Notes on Urology* (5th edition). Oxford: Blackwells.

Brown N (1997) *Symptoms and Signs of Surgical Disease* (3rd edition). London: Arnold.

Calne R, Pollard SG (1991) *Operative Surgery*. London: Gower Medical.

Cole LJ, Nowell PC (1965) 'Radiation carcinogenesis: the sequence of events' *Science*, 150: 1782–1786.

Cooke RS, Madehavan N, Woolf N (2001) Surgeons in Training Education Programme (*STEP*™). London: Royal College of Surgeons of England.

Corson JD, Williamson RCN (2001) *Surgery*. London: Mosby.

Craft TM, Nolan J, Parr M (1999) *Key Topics in Critical Care*. Oxford: Bios Scientific Publishers.

Doll R (1994) 'Mortality in relation to smoking: 40 years' observation on male British doctors' *British Medical Journal*, 309: 901–911.

Ellis H (1997) *Clinical Anatomy: A Revision and Applied Anatomy for Clinical Students* (9th edition). Oxford: Blackwell Science.

Farr RF, Allisy-Roberts PJ (1988) *Physics for Medical Imaging*. London: WB Saunders.

General Medical Council (1998) *Seeking Patient's Consent: The Ethical Considerations*. London: GMC.

Geohegan JG, Scheele J (1999) 'Treatment of colorectal liver metastases' *British Journal of Surgery*, 86(2): 158–169.

Goldhill DR, Withington PS (1997) *Textbook of Intensive Care*. London: Chapman & Hall.

Goyal A, Newcombe RG, Mansel RE, *et al.* (2004) 'Sentinel lymph node biopsy in patients with multifocal breast cancer' *European Journal of Surgical Oncology* 30: 475–479.

Green DP (ed) (1993) *Fracture of the Metacarpals and Phalanges in Operative Hand Surgery*. London: Churchill Livingstone.

Helfet DL, Howey T, Sanders R, Johansen K (1990) 'Limb salvage versus amputation: Preliminary results of the mangled extremity severity score' *Clinical Orthopaedics*, 256: 80–86.

Hillman K, Bishop G (1996) *Clinical Intensive Care*. Philadelphia: Lippincott-Raven.

Hinds CJ, Watson JD (1996) *Intensive Care: A Concise Textbook*. London: WB Saunders.

Hobbs G, Mahajan R (2000) *Imaging in Anaesthesia and Critical Care*. Edinburgh: Churchill Livingstone.

Irving M, Carlson GL (1998) 'Interocutaneous fistulae' *Surgery*, 16(10): 217–222.

Jenkins TPN (1976) 'The burst abdominal wound: A mechanical approach' *British Journal of Surgery*, 63: 873–876.

Kenealy, J (1999) 'Cutaneous malignant melanoma' *Surgery* 17(3): 68–72.

Kessler RC, Sonnega A, Bromet E, Hughes M, Nelson CB (1995) 'Posttraumatic stress disorder in the National Comorbidity Survey' *Archives of General Psychiatry*, 52(12): 1048–1060.

Khan S, Sutton R (1997) 'Portal hypertension and oesophagogastric varices' *Surgery*, 15(8): 175–181.

Kirk RM, Mansfield AO, Cochrane JPS (1999) *Clinical Surgery in General* (3rd edition). Edinburgh: Churchill Livingstone.

Kleihues P, Cavanee WK (eds) (2000) *WHO Classification of Tumours of the Nervous System*. Lyon: IARC Press.

Knudson AG Jr (1974) 'Heredity and human cancer' *American Journal of Pathology*, 77(1): 77–84.

Mahadevan V (2001) The pathophysiology of bowel strangulation and gangrene in hernia. In: Surgeons in Training Education Programme (*STEP*™). London: The Royal College of Surgeons of England.

Mann CV, Russell RCG, Williams NS (1995) *Bailey and Love's Short Practice of Surgery* (22nd edition). London: Chapman and Hall.

Marino P (1998) *The ICU Book*. Philadelphia: Lippincott Williams & Wilkins.

Martin E (1990) *Concise Medical Dictionary*. New York: Oxford Press.

McArdle CS (1998) 'Colorectal cancer' *Surgery*, 16(12): 265–271.

McConachie I (1999) *Handbook of ICU Therapy*. Cambridge: Greenwich Medical Media.

Medical Research Council (1976) *Memorandum no. 45. Aids to the examination of the peripheral nervous system*. London: HMSO.

Mitchell CL, Fleming JL, Allen R, Glenney C, Sanford GA (1958) Osteotomy-bunionectomy for halux valgus. *Journal of Bone and Joint Surgery*, 40(A): 41–60.

Mokbel K (1999) *Concise Notes on Oncology*. Newbury: Petroc Press.

Nowell PC (1976) 'The clonal evolution of tumor cell populations' *Science*, 194: 23–28.

Oken MM, Creech RH, Yormey DC, *et al.* (1982) 'Toxicity and response criteria of the Eastern Co-operative Oncology Group' *American Journal of Clinical Oncology*, 5: 649–655.

Pallis C, Harley DH (1996) *ABC of Brainstem Death* (2nd edition). London: BMJ Publishing Group.

Parchment Smith C (2002) *Surgical Short Cases for the MRCS Clinical Examination*. Knutsford, PasTest.

Paw GW, Park GR (2000) *Handbook of Drugs in Intensive Care*. Cambridge: Greenwich Medical Media.

Royal College of Surgeons of England (1993) *Clinical Guidelines on the management of groin hernia in adults*. Report from a working party convened by the Royal College of Surgeons. London: RCS.

Sadler TW (1990) *Langman's Medical Embryology* (6th edition). Philadelphia: Williams & Wilkins.

Salter RB, Harris WR (1963) 'Injuries involving epiphyseal plate' *Journal of Bone and Joint Surgery*, 45(A): 587–621.

Scholefield JH, Northover JMA (1998) 'Anal cancer' *Surgery*, 16(12): 281–284.

Sharma V, Williamson R (1998) 'Endocrine tumours of the pancreas' *Surgery*, 16(12): 271–275.

Singh S, Knight MJ (1997) 'Biliary anatomical abnormalities and their surgical importance' *Surgery*, 15(8): 188–191.
Sinnatamby CS (1999) *Last's Anatomy, Regional and Applied* (10th edition). London: Churchill Livingstone.
Smith AB (2004) *Infectious Diseases: An Exploration* (2nd edition). London: Churchill Livingstone.
Thomas WEG (1997) 'Investigation of the biliary tree and the jaundiced patient' *Surgery*, 15(8): 182–182.
Treacy PJ, Johnson AG (1997) 'Complications of peptic ulceration' *Surgery*, 15(12): 269–273.
Treacy PJ, Johnson AG (1997) 'Presentation and management of peptic ulceration' *Surgery*, 15(12): 265–269.
Trunkey DD, Lewis FR (1998) *Current Therapy of Trauma* (4th edition). Philadelphia: BC Decker.
Webb AJ, Shapiro MJ, Singer M, Suter PM (1999) *Oxford Textbook of Critical Care*. Oxford: Oxford University Press.
Whittaker RH, Borley NR (2000) *Instant Anatomy* (2nd edition). Oxford: Blackwell Science.
Wilson JMG, Junger G (1968) *Principles and practice of screening for disease*. Public Health Papers, no. 34. Geneva: World Health Organization.
Woolf N (1998) *Pathology: Basic and Systemic*. London: WB Saunders.
Yentis SM, Hirsch NP, Smith GB (2000) *Anaesthesia and Intensive Care A to Z: An Encyclopaedia of Principles and Practice*. London: Butterworth Heinemann.

Useful web sites

BMJ clinical evidence database: www.clinicalevidence.com
Cochrane Collaboration: www.cochrane.org
EBM or primary care and internal medicine: www.evidence-basedmedicine.com
European System for Cardiac Operative Risk Evaluation: www.euroscore.org
General Medical Council (GMC): www.gmc-uk.org
National Institute for Clinical Excellence: www.nice.org.uk
NHS cancer screening programmes: www.cancerscreening.nhs.uk
Royal College of Surgeons of England: www.rcseng.ac.uk
The Ileostomy and Internal Pouch Support Group: www.the-ia.org.uk
Turning Research Into Practice: www.tripdatabase.com
UK Resuscitation Council: www.resus.org.uk
US National Library of Medicine citations database: www.pubmed.org
World Health Organization: www.who.int

Index